APPLICATIONS
OF
CLINICAL NUTRITION

Frances J. Zeman, Ph.D., R.D.
University of California, Davis

Denise M. Ney, Ph.D., R.D.
University of Wisconsin–Madison

Medical Consultant: Theodore G. Ganiats, M.D.
University of California, San Diego

PRENTICE HALL, ENGLEWOOD CLIFFS, NEW JERSEY 07632

Library of Congress Cataloging-in-Publication Data

Zeman, Frances J.
    Applications of clinical nutrition.

    Includes bibliographies and index.
        1. Diet therapy.   2. Food—Analysis—Tables.
3. Diet therapy—Examinations, questions, etc.
I. Ney, Denise M.   II. Title.   [DNLM:
1. Diet Therapy.   2. Nutrition.   3. Nutrition Disorders.
WB 400 Z529a]
RM216.Z46 1988   615.8′54   87-11371
ISBN   0-13-039538-2

Editorial/production supervision
and interior design: **Marjorie Borden Shustak**
Cover design: **Diane Saxe**
Manufacturing buyer: **Margaret Rizzi**

Printed in the United States of America

10 9 8 7 6 5 4

ISBN 0-13-039538-2   01

Prentice-Hall International (UK) Limited, *London*
Prentice-Hall of Australia Pty. Limited, *Sydney*
Prentice-Hall Canada Inc., *Toronto*
Prentice-Hall Hispanoamericana, S.A., *Mexico*
Prentice-Hall of India Private Limited, *New Delhi*
Prentice-Hall of Japan, Inc., *Tokyo*
Prentice-Hall of Southeast Asia Pte. Ltd., *Singapore*
Editora Prentice-Hall do Brasil, Ltda., *Rio de Janeiro*

CONTENTS

Preface

This volume is designed to help teach the procedures of nutritional care. It is intended to serve as an adjunct to a standard text in diet therapy, not as the sole text. Therefore, the chapters containing the relevant background material in several texts are listed at the end of the Introduction.

Since this volume has potential use for students in dietetics, public health nutrition, nursing, medicine, and the allied health professions, we have chosen to use the generic term "nutritional care specialist" in referring to the individual providing nutritional care. We have organized this volume to provide for maximum flexibility in its use, not only for various groups, but also for courses of variable length. Part I is basic to those that follow. For the remaining chapters, the sequence in which they are studied can be rearranged in order to coordinate with the chosen text.

At intervals within each chapter, exercises entitled "To Test Your Understanding" give the reader an opportunity for review and practice. "Case Studies," included at intervals, provide the student an opportunity for review and integration of material from an entire chapter or several chapters. Alternatively, these questions can be used by the instructor for evaluation of progress. Some questions require modification of diets; for this purpose, it is assumed that the reader will have a diet manual for information on details of individual diets. In Appendix M, some typical menus are provided and may be used for the questions requiring planning of modified diets. If the reader is in a clinical setting, current menus might be used.

We have also included at the end of most chapters a section entitled *Topics for Further Discussion*. This section suggests additional topics for inclusion in the course that are not included in the text due to space limitations. Also at the end of each chapter, sources of information are given in the "References" and "Additional Sources of Information" sections.

We would appreciate suggestions and comments from readers and course instructors using this book.

ACKNOWLEDGMENTS

We gratefully acknowledge the careful review of this manuscript for medical accuracy by Theodore G. Ganiats, M.D., School of Medicine, University of California, San Diego. We also wish to thank Doris Derelian, M.S., R.D., who authored Chapters 3 and 6 of this book.

We wish to express our appreciation to the following for giving us the benefit of their advice: Raymond D. Adelman, M.D., University of California, Davis, CA (Chapter 19); Shawn Bissonnette, M.D., San Diego, CA (Chapters 8, 13); Elizabeth Bowersox, M.S., R.D., Dairy Council of California, Oakland, California (Chapters 3, 6); Lesley Fels Tinker, R.D., formerly of Foundation for Advancement of Diabetes Education (Chapter 18); Louis E. Grivetti, Ph.D., University of California, Davis, CA (Chapter 10); Elizabeth R. Jones, M.S., R.D., San Diego, CA (Chapter 8); Rabbi Bonnie Koppell, Jewish Fellowship of Davis, Davis, CA (Chapter 10); Francene Myers, R.D., formerly of Virginia Mason Hospital, Seattle, WA (Chapters 21, 22); Reed Nishikawa, University of California Medical Center, Sacramento, CA (Chapter 13); Judith Nordquist, R.D., Kaiser-Permanente Hospital, San Diego, CA (Chapter 12).

We also acknowledge the helpful suggestions from graduate students Christina Blais, M.S. and member of the Canadian Dietetic Association, Carol Chase-Deesing, M.S., R.D., Sharon Donovan, Nancy Hess, R.D., Elise Mackenzie, Cheryl Osburn, Jocelyn Reynolds, and Carolyn Shugart. We also appreciate the perspective supplied by the undergraduate students in the diet therapy classes at the University of California at Davis.

Denise M. Ney wishes to thank all those at the University of California at Davis who gave support and suggestions during the preparation of this manuscript.

At Prentice Hall, we would like to thank Susan Willig, executive editor; Shirley Chlopak, her assistant; and Marjorie Borden Shustak, production editor; for all their efforts throughout the production of this book.

Last but not least, we acknowledge the typing and other yeoman services involved in manuscript preparation provided by Jeanne Vadhanasindhu.

Frances J. Zeman
Denise M. Ney

Introduction for the Reader

The purpose of this manual is to give you an understanding of the objectives and procedures of nutritional care. It will introduce the skills required of the professional nutritional care specialist, and provide an opportunity to integrate knowledge of nutritional care with related aspects of clinical care.

When you have completed the assignments in this manual, you will have an understanding of the importance and effect of nutritional therapy in a clinical setting and the contribution it makes to overall patient care. Some of the skills expected of an entry-level professional person providing nutritional care, as well as the medical vocabulary and the means to communicate in the medical record, should become familiar. You also should be able to evaluate laboratory data and other pertinent information, understand the purpose of the main aspects of treatment of the conditions discussed, assess the nutritional status of a patient and the nutritional adequacy of the diets in terms of specific medical conditions, plan the most frequently used diet modifications, recognize the interrelationships between diet and other forms of treatment, and integrate sociological factors into the nutritional care plan. We provide an introduction to some techniques of patient interviewing and patient education. We assume that these skills will be sharpened by further practice and clinical experience.

Within each chapter, exercises labeled "To Test Your Understanding" provide an opportunity to test mastery of the immediately preceding subject matter and to integrate material from previous assignments and from an accompanying text.

The "Case Studies" were designed to develop an appreciation of the contribution of nutrition to the overall care of the patient. They provide a vehicle by which to learn to relate diagnostic procedures, medications, and other forms of treatment to nutritional care. Suggested additional questions and reading resources appear at the end of each chapter.

We assume that you will use this volume in coordination with a textbook which provides background reading on the subject of the assignment. The chapters in several texts providing relevant background for each chapter in this book are indicated at the end of this section. It sometimes will be necessary to seek additional information from standard reference materials; this has been planned in order to introduce you to useful references and develop some skill in their use. In preparing for a professional career in nutrition, acquisition of a professional library is advisable. For the work required in this book, reference to a typical diet manual will be necessary; a manual from any of a number of institutions or regional associations is suitable, and we provide below a list of some that are generally available.

Some questions require you to seek information elsewhere. These sources may vary from pharmacology textbooks in the medical library to the local supermarket. It will be helpful to have a medical dictionary. Suggested choices follow. Food values tables are also necessary, and we also list some available sources of these. In the process of using these resources and completing the work in this volume, you will develop the ability to seek information independently.

SUGGESTED REFERENCES

Textbooks in Diet Therapy

ZEMAN, F.J..*Clinical Nutrition and Dietetics*. New York: Macmillan, 1983.

HUI, Y.H. *Human Nutrition and Diet Therapy*, Parts II and III. Monterey, CA: Wadsworth, 1983.

KRAUSE, M.V. AND L.K. MAHAN. *Food, Nutrition and Diet Therapy*, 7th ed., Part I, Units 2 and 3; Part II. Philadelphia: Saunders, 1984.

WHITNEY, E.N. AND C.B. CATALDO. *Understanding Normal and Clinical Nutrition*, Parts III, IV, V. St. Paul, MN: West, 1983.

Diet Manuals

AMERICAN DIETETIC ASSOCIATION. Handbook of Clinical Dietetics (2nd ed.) New Haven: Yale University Press, 1981.

CHICAGO DIETETIC ASSOCIATION. *Manual of Clinical Dietetics*, 2nd ed. Philadelphia: Saunders, 1981.

Mayo Clinic Diet Manual, 5th ed. Philadelphia: Saunders, 1981.

UNIVERSITY OF CALIFORNIA CENTER FOR HEALTH SCIENCES. *Manual of Clinical Dietetics*. Los Angeles: University of California, 1977.

UTAH DIETETIC ASSOCIATION. *Handbook of Clinical Dietetics*, 2nd ed. Salt Lake City: Utah Dietetic Association, 1986.

Medical Dictionaries

Dorland's Illustrated Medical Dictionary, 26th ed. Philadelphia: Saunders, 1981.

Stedman's Medical Dictionary, 24th ed. Baltimore: Williams and Wilkens, 1982.

MILLER, B.F. AND C.B. KEANE. *Encyclopedia of Medicine, Nursing and Allied Health*, 3rd ed. Philadelphia: Saunders, 1983.

Tables of Food Values

CONSUMER AND FOOD ECONOMICS INSTITUTE. *Composition of Foods*. Agricultural Handbooks No. 8-1 to 8-16. Washington, D.C.: U.S. Dept. of Agriculture, 1976–1987.

LEVEILLE, G.A., M.E. ZABIK, AND K.V. MORGAN. *Nutrients in Foods*. Cambridge, MA: The Nutrition Guild, 1983.

PENNINGTON, V.A.T. AND H.N. CHURCH. *Bowes and Church's Food Values of Portions Commonly Used*, 14th ed. St. Louis, MO: Lippincott, 1984.

SCIENCE AND EDUCATION ADMINISTRATION. *Nutritive Value of Foods*. Home and Garden Bulletin No. 72. Washington, D.C.: U.S. Department of Agriculture, 1986.

Pharmacology References

Compendium of Pharmaceuticals and Specialties, 20th ed. (ed. C.M.E. Krogh). Ottawa: Canadian Pharmaceutical Association, 1985.

Drug Facts and Comparisons, ed. J.R. Boyd. St. Louis, MO: Lippincott, 1985.

Handbook of Nonprescription Drugs, 7th ed. Washington, D.C.: American Pharmaceutical Association, 1982.

Modern Drug Encyclopedia and Therapeutic Index, ed. A.J. Lewis. New York: Yorke Medical Books, 1981.

Physician's Desk Reference, 41st ed. Oradell, NJ: Medical Economics, 1987.

The Physicians' Drug Manual: Prescription and Nonprescription Drugs, eds. R. Bressler, M.D. Bogdonoff and C.J. Subak-Sharpe. Garden City, NY: Doubleday, 1981.

Sources of Laboratory Values and Interpretation

BAKERMAN, S. *ABC's of Interpretive Laboratory Data*, 2nd ed. Greenville, NC: Interpretive Laboratory Data, 1984.

BYRNE, C.V., D.F. SAXTON, P.K. PELIKAN AND P.M. NUGENT. *Laboratory Tests: Implications for Nurses and Allied Health Professionals*. Menlo Park, CA: Addison-Wesley, 1981.

Clinical Guide to Laboratory Tests, ed. N.W. Tietz. Philadelphia: Saunders, 1983.

The Laboratory in Clinical Medicine, 2nd ed. eds. J.A. Halsted and C.H. Halsted. Philadelphia: Saunders, 1981.

RAVEL, R. *Clinical Laboratory Medicine. Clinical Application of Laboratory Data*, 4th ed. Chicago: Year Book Medical, 1984.

TILKIAN, S.M. AND M.H. CONOVER. *Clinical Implications of Laboratory Tests*, 3rd ed. St. Louis, MO: Mosby, 1983.

WIDMANN, F.K. *Clinical Interpretations of Laboratory Tests*, 9th ed. Philadelphia: Davis, 1983.

REFERENCES TO BACKGROUND TEXTS

Zeman & Ney, *Applications of Clinical Nutrition.* Prentice Hall, 1988	Zeman, *Clinical Nutrition and Dietetics.* Macmillan, 1983	Krause & Mahan, *Food, Nutrition Diet Therapy* (7th ed.). Saunders, 1984[a]	Whitney & Cataldo, *Understanding Normal and Clinical Nutrition.* West, 1983[b]	Hui, *Human Nutrition and Diet Therapy.* Wadsworth, 1983[c]
Chapter	Chapter	Chapter	Chapter	Chapter
2	2, 3	19, 21	18, 21	16
4	2, 14	8, 9	18	
5	2	9, 10		
11	2	19	20	23
12	5	35	20	23
13	12	35	20	23
14	4	31		
15	5	22	23	24
16	6	23, 24	23	24
17	6	23	23	24
18	9, 15	25	25	26
19	7	30	27	28
20	8	28	26	27
21	11	24	24	25
22	12, 13	34, 35	22	29

[a]Part 1, Units 2 and 3, and Part 2
[b]Parts 3, 4 and 5
[c]Parts 2 and 3

1

Medical Terminology

The acquisition of vocabulary is an important part of learning a new subject. The nutritional care specialist must acquire an extensive medical vocabulary in order to function effectively. This can seem to be an overwhelming task at first.

This chapter will introduce you to medical terminology and provide some tools to promote easier and faster learning, but learning new vocabulary will continue throughout the use of this manual.

Most medical terms are derived from Greek or Latin; fewer terms are derived from modern languages. As medicine advances, new words must be coined and may be derived from any of these sources. Some terms are composed of elements combined from more than one language.

It is possible to simplify learning, promote understanding of reading material, and increase the ability to communicate by learning to analyze the component parts of words—the root words, prefixes, and suffixes. For example, *tonsillitis* refers to inflammation (*-itis*) of the tonsils. In other cases, the result of such analysis cannot be taken literally but can be used to suggest the meaning. For example, an analysis of the word *anemia* suggests that *an-* (without) *-emia* (blood) means *without blood*. Absence of blood, of course, is incompatible with life, and the term *anemia* is actually used to indicate a deficiency of red blood cells or hemoglobin.

ROOT WORDS

The root word of a medical term indicates the organ or body part that is modified by the prefixes and suffixes. A vowel—a, i, or o—may be inserted in combined forms for easier pronunciation. Some of the root words of particular use to nutritional care specialists include the following:

cardi-	heart	hepat-	liver
enter-	intestine	nephr-	kidney
gastr-	stomach	osteo-	bone

SUFFIXES AND COMPOUNDING WORDS

Suffixes may be prepositions or adverbs added to root words to modify their meaning. Alternatively, adjectives or nouns are used as suffixes to form compound words. Many suffixes indicate a diagnosis, procedure, or symptom. The following are some diagnostic suffixes, with examples of their use:

Suffix	Definition	Examples
-ectasis	dilation of	bronchiectasis
-iasis	presence of	lithiasis
-itis	inflammation of	appendicitis
-megaly	enlargement of	cardiomegaly
-oma	tumor of	hepatoma
-osis	condition	nephrosis
-pathy	disease	cardiopathy

The following are commonly used suffixes indicating procedures:

-ectomy	removal of	appendectomy
-scopy	examination of	gastroscopy
-stomy	opening	ileostomy
-tomy	incision	lithotomy

Symptoms may be indicated by suffixes such as the following:

-algia	pain	myalgia
-genic	originate	cardiogenic
-lysis	breaking down	lipolysis
-oid	resembling	carcinoid
-osis	increase	leukocytosis
-penia	decrease	leukopenia
-spasm	involuntary contraction	cardiospasm

PREFIXES

A prefix may precede a root word to modify its meaning. Some prefixes that are frequently used by nutritional care specialists include the following:

Prefix	Definition	Example
dys-	difficult, painful	dyspnea
endo-	within	endocardium
hemi-, semi-	half	hemiplegic
hyper-	above, excessive	hyperglycemia
hypo-	beneath, below, deficient	hypodermic
para-	beside, around, near, abnormal	parathyroid
peri-	around	perinatal

Some terms have more than one meaning. You can see in the foregoing lists, for example, that the suffix *-osis* can refer to a *condition* or to an *increase*. Also, you can see that both *-osis* and *hyper-* indicate a higher level or amount.

TO TEST YOUR UNDERSTANDING

1. Using the examples in this chapter, define the following terms. The hyphens indicate the separate portions of the words.
   a. Gastr-itis
   b. Hepat-oma
   c. Nephr-ectomy
   d. Osteo-genic
   e. Cardio-megaly

2. Using the examples of root words, suffixes and prefixes in this chapter, compose terms with the following meanings:
   a. Inflammation of the intestine
   b. Enlargement of the liver
   c. Examination of the stomach
   d. Inflammation of the interior lining of the heart
   e. Incision into or opening into the stomach
   f. Removal of the spleen

3. A more extensive listing of terms is contained in Appendix D. Using this list, define the following terms:
   a. Hyperglycemia
   b. Arteriosclerosis
   c. Cholelithiasis
   d. Stomatitis
   e. Nephrolithotomy
   f. Erythropoiesis
   g. Lymphocytosis
   h. Leukocytopenia
   i. Ileostomy
   j. Dysphagia
   k. Hematemesis
   l. Tachycardia

It is also necessary for the nutritional care specialist to be familiar with the abbreviations used in patients' medical records. Many commonly used abbreviations are listed and defined in Appendix D. They will be used in the case studies which are contained in the succeeding chapters. Most of the assignments associated with the case studies require that a chart note be written. You should use appropriate abbreviations in writing these notes in order to become familiar with the medical terminology and the accepted means of communicating in the medical record.

ADDITIONAL SOURCES OF INFORMATION

CHABNER, D.-E. *The Language of Medicine* (3d ed.). Philadelphia: Saunders, 1985.

DUNMORE, C.W. AND R.M. FLEISCHER. Medical Terminology. *Exercises in Etymology* (2d ed.). Philadelphia: Davis, 1985.

FRENAY, A.C. SR. *Understanding Medical Terminology* (5th ed.). St. Louis: Catholic Hospital Association, 1973.

2

The Medical Record

The patient's *medical record,* or *chart,* is an ongoing collection of information which documents a patient's medical care. It is considered a legal document and therefore must be accurate. It includes a complete assessment of a patient's medical condition, including the history, results of the physical examination, summary of the patient's condition at the time of discharge, and results of all diagnostic and laboratory tests. A *patient care plan* followed by *progress notes* monitoring the status of the care plan are also part of the record.

The purpose of the medical record is threefold:

1. to document medical care
2. to facilitate communication between members of the health care team
3. to serve as a basis for the evaluation of health care delivery, including hospital accreditation and peer review (1).

The professional personnel who provide patient care constitute the *health care team,* which consists, at least, of a physician, a nurse, a nutritional care specialist, and a pharmacist. Depending on the patient's needs, others who may be included are physical therapists, occupational therapists, and social workers.

As the member of the health care team most knowledgeable in the field of nutrition, it is essential that you be skilled in documenting relevant nutritional information in the medical record. Your chart entries may include (a) results of the nutritional assessment, (b) plans and suggestions for nutritional care, and (c) the status of patient education efforts (2). Such information is useful in coordinating nutritional care with the care provided by other members of the team.

In this chapter you will learn the appropriate *content* of a medical record entry and the correct *format* in which to record the information. We will focus on the more recent system, known as the *Problem Oriented Medical Record* (POMR). In the completion of case studies in subsequent chapters, you will be asked to use the skills developed in this chapter to summarize your findings and suggestions for nutritional therapy in a chart note.

FINANCIAL IMPLICATIONS OF THE MEDICAL RECORD

Documentation of nutrition services is especially important in the current atmosphere of health care cost reduction. The federal government, through Medicare and Medicaid, is one of the major funders of health care in the United States. In 1983, legislation was approved to establish a Medicare Prospective Payment System which reimburses hospitals for inpatient services as categorized by *diagnosis-related groups* (DRGs). The DRG scheme is intended to control federal spending for health care and requires that hospital dietetics departments define their costs according to the types of patients served. Many health care professionals believe that nutrition services, such as nutritional assessments, consultations, and patient education, will be cut in an effort to reduce hospital costs *unless* the value of these services can be clearly demonstrated. Demonstration of value would include improved health and reduced health care costs as indicated by evidence of decreases in the average length of hospital stay or in the number of hospital admissions or clinic visits and decreased mortality rate.

Documentation of nutrition services is the key to generating data for justification of nutritional services (3). In the words of one chief clinical dietitian, "If a dietitian doesn't chart observations and recommendations for nutritional care, it's as if the patient was never seen." Clinical dietitians working in hospital settings commonly spend 1 to 2 hours of the working day charting.

TYPES OF MEDICAL RECORDS

There are two major styles for organization of the medical record: *source-oriented* and *problem-oriented.* In the *Source-Oriented Medical Record,* the chart is organized according to the category of personnel writing in the record. These charts tend to have numerous sections and may, for example, contain three sets of progress notes—one for physicians, one for nurses, and one for allied health personnel.

The *Problem-Oriented Medical Record* (POMR) is in widespread use, although many institutions have chosen to combine elements of the source- and problem-oriented approaches. The POMR organizes the chart around a patient's problems. A major advantage of the problem-oriented approach is greater use of allied health professionals, including nutritional care specialists, in the health care team, which is headed by the primary care physician. A second advantage of the POMR arises from the fact that the documentation of problem-oriented thought processes is an educational tool for other health professionals and tends to enhance communication among members of the health care team.

COMPONENTS OF THE POMR

The POMR has 4 components: the data base, a problem list, the initial care plan, and progress notes (4).

THE DATA BASE

The data base, which is established at the time care is initiated, is the foundation for the diagnosis and care plan. It includes the history and the results of a physical examination (H&P). The H&P is usually dictated by the admitting physician, and a typed copy is placed in the chart. The history includes the following:

the chief complaint (CC), or the patient's perception of his purpose in seeking medical care,

the history of the present illness (HPI),

the previous medical history (PMH),

the patient profile (PP), which describes the patient's social and family history, and

the review of systems (ROS), which consists of a series of focused screening questions organized by organ system.

The results of laboratory tests and diagnostic procedures and the nutrition history and initial nutritional assessment are also part of the data base. Information included in the data base is found in various parts of the chart.

THE PROBLEM LIST

The problem list is kept at the front of a patient's chart and acts as a table of contents. The master problem list is usually established by the physician, although in many institutions other professionals may add to the problem list. A problem can be defined as anything that requires diagnostic procedures or management. Problems are dated and numbered consecutively, and are dated again when resolved. Problems may be stated in a variety of ways. Here are some examples:

Classification of Problem	Medical Problem	Nutritional Problem
Diagnosis	Hypertension	Anorexia nervosa
Physiological finding	Heart failure	Malnutrition
Symptom	Chest pain	Weight loss
Abnormal lab finding	Elevated fasting blood sugar	Elevated serum cholesterol
Behavior	Refuses medications	Poor compliance with prescribed diet

INITIAL CARE PLAN

For each problem identified, an initial care plan is developed. The plan may include obtaining more information for diagnosis and management, specific intervention measures, and patient education. Physicians, nurses, physical therapists, and nutritional care specialists may each have a care plan to deal with a specific problem with which they are concerned.

In planning for nutritional care, the nutritional care specialist must establish goals and objectives. The objectives should be *patient-centered* and should specify *measurable,* verifiable steps toward achieving the overall goal. Specific activities or interventions must be planned to help the patient achieve the objectives identified. Space limitations in the chart do not usually allow for a detailed discussion of goals and objectives. Instead, patient-centered activities or interventions that are planned or completed are usually charted in the progress notes. In nutritional care, the general types of activity or intervention include the following:

1. prescription of a diet or special supplement,
2. recommendation for the route—either parenteral or enteral—and frequency of nutrient delivery,
3. recommendation for more comprehensive nutritional assessment, including additional laboratory work and measures of food intake,
4. nutrition education, and
5. referrals for public aid, nutrition follow-up, or other social services.

Here are examples of two different types of care plans for two common nutritional problems:

Example #1: Patient refuses to eat hospital food.
Goals:

1. Patient understands the importance of nutrition.
2. Patient's nutritional intake is adequate.

Objectives:

1. Patient will select proper foods from the regular hospital menu, adjusted according to preferences.
2. Patient will demonstrate adequate nutrient intake.

Activities or interventions:

1. Complete a baseline nutritional assessment, including diet history and food preferences.
2. Estimate caloric needs.
3. Modify menus according to patient preferences.
4. Monitor patient-selected menus.
5. Quantify food intake via calorie count or other means.

Example #2: Patient lacks knowledge of low-fat diet for management of cholecystitis. (Note: The physician would include cholecystitis in the problem list, and the item described would be charted under this problem number by the nutritional care specialist.)

Goals:

1. Patient understands the principles of the low-fat diet.
2. Patient is able to apply the principles of the low-fat diet.

Objectives:

1. Patient will verbalize the rationale for a low-fat diet in the management of cholecystitis.
2. Patient will apply the principles of a low-fat diet by selecting proper foods from the hospital menu.
3. Patient will complete a correct sample low-fat menu to be used at home.

Activities or interventions:

1. Instruct patient and significant others in the rationale for the diet and the fat content of the various food groups.
2. Develop a meal plan in accordance with the quantity of fat prescribed.

PROGRESS NOTES

Progress notes are contributed by the various members of the health care team to document the status of the care plan in relation to the initial problem. Notes are of three types: (1) narrative, which are always dated, timed, and headed by the number and name of the problem with which they are associated: (2) flow sheets, or records, of data that are obtained periodically; and (3) the discharge summary, which summarizes the level of resolution of the various problems at the time the patient is discharged.

A standardized format for narrative progress notes is described by the acronym **SOAP*** and contains the following elements:

Subjective: Information that is pertinent to a listed problem and that is obtained from the patient or patient's family or significant others. Information may be recorded as a direct quote—"I can't drink that canned milkshake"—or it may be paraphrased—"Patient refuses supplemental feedings." The key characteristic of the subjective data is that it expresses the *patient's perception* of a problem.

Objective: Factual information relevant to the problem that can be *confirmed by others,* including laboratory and physical findings and observations by health professionals. Factual nutrition information often found in this section of a progress note includes prescribed diet (Diet Rx), height (ht), weight (wt), ideal body weight (IBW), pertinent laboratory values, results of measured food intake, calculation of nutrient needs, and observed difficulties with eating. As a minimum, initial chart notes should state Diet Rx, ht, wt, and IBW under **O.**

Assessment: The health care team member's evaluation or interpretation of subjective and objective data. In this section the nutritional care specialist's judgment about a particular problem, based on patient-provided and factual information, is presented. Examples include the following:

"Patient does not accept value of diet in relation to medical care."

"Present intake is inadequate for nutritional needs. Patient needs to increase caloric intake by 500 kcal/day and protein intake by 15 g/day."

"Pt demonstrates little knowledge of Na content of foods."

Plan: The specific course of action to be taken, based on **S, O,** and **A,** to resolve the patient's problem. The plan may include all or part of the following components:

Dx (diagnosis)—further workup needed, such as a nutrition history, calorie count, lactose tolerance test, or serum albumin or lipid measurement.

Rx (therapy)—suggested diet or diet changes (diet order would have to be written by the physician), supplemental feedings, request for an eating aid.

Pt Ed (patient education)—plans for future individual or group instruction, and notation of teaching just completed, including major instructional materials provided and plans for follow-up.

*Note: A SOAP note is the same as a progress note.

TO TEST YOUR UNDERSTANDING

1. Label the following situation as being either source-oriented (S), problem-oriented (P), or both (B).
   a. a problem list _____
   b. results of laboratory tests _____
   c. SOAP progress notes _____
   d. a history and physical _____
2. Which of the following is appropriately stated for a problem list? How would you improve the statements that are incorrectly worded?

Problem

Marasmus

Sneaking candy from vending machine

Decreased serum albumin

Poorly fitting dentures

3. For each of the following problems, state a goal, a patient-centered measurable objective, and a specific activity or intervention to help reach the goal.

   a. Problem 1: Poorly fitting dentures

   b. Problem 2: Excessive weight gain during pregnancy

4. In the space provided, label the sections of the following two chart notes as **S, O, A,** and **P**—Pt Ed, Dx, or Rx.

Problem 1: CHF (Congestive Heart Failure)

8-6-88 _____ Pt describes previous diet instruction as "Just don't add any salt to your food." Claims to follow no-added-salt diet but admits to using canned pork and beans, luncheon meats, and frozen dinners. Per diet Hx, estimate prior Na, intake at 5–6 g/day.

_____ Diet Rx—2g Na, instruct in diet for DC: Ht—5 ft, 6 in, Wt—150#; 1+ pedal edema; Meds—Lasix, Slow K.

_____ Cooperative pt within IBW who has minimal knowledge of the Na content of foods.

_____ _____ 1. Explain rationale of low-Na diet in relation to CHF; discuss Na content of foods.

2. Pt given copy of 2-g-Na diet with RD name and phone number for future questions.

3. F/U in one month in outpatient nutrition clinic.

Jane Doe, RD

Problem 2: Anorexia

8-14-88 _____ Pt is 25# below IBW of 115#, with continued wt loss; inadequate nutritional intake while hospitalized secondary to general disinterest in food.

_____ Pt says doesn't eat because "has no appetite"; no C/O food.

_____ Diet Rx—Reg; Ht—5 ft, 3 in, Wt—90#, 8# wt loss since admission; present intake is 600–800 kcal/day.

_____ _____ 1. Recommend daily multivitamin and mineral supplement.

2. Offer 4 oz of Ensure t.i.d. between meals.

_____ 1. Recommend examination of factors responsible for patient's anorexia (depression, meds, treatments).

_____ 1. Daily visits to patient, with emphasis on importance of nutritional intake and positive feedback.

Jane Doe, RD

CONTENT OF A NUTRITIONAL CARE PROGRESS NOTE

There is an essential core of nutrition information that belongs in every chart, regardless of format, in which a nutritional care specialist makes entries (5). Throughout this section, the content of a chart note will be linked with the POMR system of SOAP progress notes.

SUBJECTIVE AND OBJECTIVE INFORMATION

Significant History

Any historical data that relates to a patient's nutritional status should appear in a chart note labeled with the number of the problem to which it relates. Historical data may include medical, psychological, social, economic, and environmental factors, such as diet history information (see evaluation of prior or current dietary intake section), a statement reflecting a patient's previous experience with a particular diet regimen, an account of a previous nutritional problem, or details of a patient's life-style.

Many nutritional care specialists make the mistake of failing to restate pertinent data or of restating data that have no bearing on the problem. A good deal of judgment and knowledge is required to glean the *significant* information from patients and from their medical records.

Patient Comments About Prescribed Diet

Noting patients' own observations and opinions about their nutritional problems and dietary management provides valuable information in analyzing and diagnosing problems. It also enhances communication between the patient and the health care team by enabling team members to relate to the patient's problems as the patient perceives them.

Contraindicated Foods

Foods that interact with a patient's prescribed medications or precipitate allergic reactions should be prominently indicated in the chart.

Anthropometric Data

The initial chart notes should state Diet Rx. Measurements of height, weight, skinfold thicknesses, and calculation of ideal body weight (see Chapter 3) should also be recorded under **O.**

Accidents or Unusual Occurrences

An *unusual occurrence* can be defined as any incident, such as an error in patient care, from which medicolegal action may stem. Whenever an unusual incident occurs, the following should be noted: time of the occurrence, time the physician was notified, name of the physician contacted, and confirmation of the filing of an incident report.

For example

O: Pt served brk at 8:15 AM before 9:30 scheduled surgery by food service error. Dr. Smith notified 8:30 AM and incident report filed.

Impaired Ability to Feed Self and Eat

Any physical disabilities that limit a patient's ability to feed himself, masticate, or swallow should be noted in the chart, along with any adaptive equipment used or recommended. Disabilities may include new, poorly fitting, or absent dentures, amputation, use of a prosthesis, paralysis, or perceptual dysfunction. For example

O: Pt requires plate-guard and swivel utensils developed by OT for impaired shoulder motion.

ASSESSMENT OF SUBJECTIVE AND OBJECTIVE INFORMATION

Evaluation of Pertinent Prior Intake

This usually includes a summary of *pertinent* aspects of the diet history, including eating habits and life-style influences and an evaluation of the adequacy of the prior intake and its relationship to the current problem. For example

S: Pt states lives alone and was too sick to go shopping last week so "just didn't eat very much." Summary of 24-hr recall: 800–1,000 kcal/day and less than 20 g pro/day.
O: Diet Rx-Reg; Ht-6 ft, Wt-140#, IBW 175#–185#, estimated calorie needs-2,500 kcal/day

A: Poorly nourished male 35–45# below IBW; intake PTA inadequate in most nutrients.

Note that the 24-hour recall results are part of **S** because they were calculated from what the patient *said* he ate. The *calculation* of nutritional needs is based on fact and thus is part of **O,** and the *evaluation* of the prior intake is part of **A.** (See Chapter 5 for other techniques, such as food records or food frequency lists, that can be used to evaluate prior intake.)

Evaluation of Current Dietary Intake

Current intake usually refers to food consumed within the preceding 72 hours. For a hospitalized patient, then, current intake would be based on the diet received in the hospital. For hospitalized patients, the calorie count allows for a more objective and quantitative estimate of nutrient intake than is provided by food recall methods. An example of quantification and evaluation of the diet of a hospitalized patient follows:

S: "I'm just not hungry."
O: Diet Rx-Reg, Ht-5 ft, 6 in, Wt-100#, IBW-120#–130#. No wt loss since admission 10 days ago. Calorie count: average of 3 days-40 g pro, 1,200 kcal/day. Estimated calorie needs for wt gain: 1,500–1,800 kcal/day.
A: Underweight female undergoing CA therapy consuming inadequate calories secondary to anorexia.

Evaluation of Current Nutritional Status

This involves the evaluation of prior and current diet, and of the anthropometric, laboratory, and physical findings which are summarized in **S** and **O** and interpreted under **A.** For example

A: Wt loss of 10% in past month, low serum albumin, and inadequate calorie and protein intake indicate nutritional depletion.

Interpretation of Significant Laboratory Findings

The dietitian should interpret laboratory values or diagnostic findings (see Chapter 4) only in terms of their relationship to diet and nutritional problems. Laboratory and physical assessment findings should be used to support the diagnosis of a nutritional problem or to monitor an identified nutritional problem. For example:

O: serum albumin = 2.5 mg/dl
A: Visceral protein depletion indicated by low serum albumin level

Evaluation of Patient's Ability to Accept and Understand Diet Instruction

This part of the note documents the nutritional care specialist's assessment of a patient's attitude about and understanding of the prescribed diet. It is important to describe how the patient's attitude was assessed and how understanding of the diet was demonstrated. For example

> **A:** Pt demonstrates adequate knowledge of 2-g-Na diet based on completion of three sample menus for home use and ability to verbalize high-Na "foods to avoid."

ASSESSMENT OR PLAN

Recommendation for Consultation or Evaluation by Others

Institutional policies differ concerning referral to or consultation by non-physician health professionals. The rationale for a referral or consultation would be stated under **A** and the recommendation under **P**lan-Rx. For example

> **A:** Pt unable to purchase special dietary items necessary for 500-mg-Na diet due to financial constraints.
> **P:** Rx—Contact social worker to explore possible financial resources with patient.

Implementing, Monitoring, and Revising the Nutritional Care Plan

The establishment of a nutritional care plan, including goals and patient-centered objectives, is essential to the treatment of a nutritional problem. However, time and space limitations in the medical record usually do not allow for a detailed discussion of goals and objectives. Instead, the patient-centered activities or interventions that are *planned* or *completed* are usually stated, and the goals and objectives are implied. The advantages of stating patient-centered activities are twofold: (1) other health professionals, including other nutritional care specialists, know what has been done and can provide follow-up, and (2) activities are more measurable than goals and can thus be used for audit purposes.

The following is an example of a series of chart notes which state the plans for nutritional care and the progress of the care plan:

9-2-88, 1000 hr.

Problem 1: Excess Body Weight

> **S:** "I want to lose weight while I'm in traction."
> **O:** Diet Rx-House; Ht-5 ft, 2 in, Wt-160# (bed scale), IBW range-110#–120#. Estimated maintenance calorie needs-2,000 kcal/day. Nursing intake records reflect 50% meal consumption. S/P pin placement for compound fracture; 3–6 weeks hospitalization required for traction and IV antibiotic Rx.
> **A:** Obese, immobilized 20 y.o. female w/o major food preferences. Motivated to lose wt but needs education regarding weight reduction diet allowing for 1#/week wt loss during recovery from skeletal fracture.
> **P:** Rx—Contact MD to suggest change to 1,500 kcal wt reduction diet and weekly weight checks. Dx—Obtain diet history.

> Jane Doe RD

9-22-88, 1400 hr.

Problem 1: Excess Body Weight

> **S:** Diet history reflects usual intake of 3,000 kcal/day with high intake of sweetened beverages. No C/O 1,500 kcal diet.
> **O:** Diet Rx—1,500 kcal; weigh weekly on bed scale
> **A:** Prescribed diet is acceptable to pt; will begin pt ed re principles of wt reduction diet.
> **P:** Pt Ed—1. Reviewed concept of exchange lists with elimination of sweetened foods.
> 2. Gave pt exchange booklet with 1,500-kcal meal plan to study.
> 3. Asked pt to categorize a list of foods according to exchange list and to state appropriate portion size.
> 4. F/U next week.
> Rx—1. Maintain flow sheet of pt's weekly weights to be kept in chart.

> Jane Doe RD

9-28-88, 0930 hr.

Problem 1: Excess Body Weight

> **S:** "I finished categorizing that list of foods."
> **O:** Diet Rx-1,500 kcal; Wt-157#
> **A:** Pt correctly used exchange lists to classify foods according to calorie content.
> **P:** Pt Ed—1. Explained 1,500-kcal meal plan in relation to hospital menu.
> 2. Asked pt to complete sample menus for use at home using 1,500-kcal meal plan.
> 3. F/U next week.

> Jane Doe, RD

10-4-88, 0915 hr.

Problem 1: Excess Body Weight

> **S:** "I feel like I lost some weight, and the doctor says my fracture is healing OK."
> **O:** Diet Rx-1,500 kcal; wt-155#. 5# wt loss since 9-2-88.
> **A:** Adequate understanding of diet demonstrated by completion of selective menus and sample menus for home. Pt verbalizes value of diet. No further instruction needed.
> **P:** Pt Ed—1. Pt given RD name and phone number to contact with future questions.

> Jane Doe RD

Disposition Indicated

Nutrition progress notes should come to some logical conclusion. Discharge, referral, or follow-up should be specifically indicated under **P** at the end of a progress note.

Change in Standard Procedure

Variations from standard dietary policy should be documented in the medical record to alert other health professionals that the change has been planned and is not an oversight or error. Examples of such variations or changes in food service procedure include a diabetic patient's being allowed to have a sugar packet on his tray, a patient on a clear liquid diet being allowed to have sherbet, or a patient's being permitted to go to the hospital cafeteria to supplement her dietary intake.

Table 2-1 summarizes the content of a progress note and provides guidelines for placement in the SOAP format. Placement of data in the SOAP format varies somewhat, but the general format, previously outlined in the section on Components of the POMR-Progress Notes, should help to clarify the placement of data.

WRITING STYLE IN PROGRESS NOTES

Dark ink, usually black, should be used for progress notes. Pencil or other colors of ink should not be used. Handwriting should be legible and dark enough to photocopy or put on microfilm. The date, time of entry, and associated problem should precede every note in the chart. All components of the SOAP format need not be used in each entry unless charting is infrequent. The dietitian's signature and credentials should be affixed to the bottom of the chart note.

The objective style, rather than personal pronouns such as *I, my,* or *me,* should be used in the medical record. For example, "Pt's need for protein is increased" is preferable to "I recommend an increase in protein intake." Phrases commonly used in charting are listed in Table 2-2. Accurate spelling and correct medical abbreviations should be used. Medical records

TABLE 2-1. Content of a Progress Note According to Placement in the SOAP Format

Component	Placement
Significant history	**S** or **O**
Patient comments about prescribed diet	**S**
Contraindicated foods	**S** or **O**
Anthropometric data	**O**
Accidents or unusual occurrences	**O**
Impaired motor ability to feed self and eat	**O**
Evaluation of pertinent prior intake	**S, O,** and **A***
Evaluation of current dietary intake	**S, O,** and **A***
Evaluation of current nutritional status	**A**
Evaluation of client's ability to accept and understand diet instruction	**A**
Recommendation for consultation or evaluation by other professionals	**A** and **P**†
Implementation, monitoring, and revision of the nutritional care plan	**P**
Disposition indicated	**P**
Change in standard procedure	**A** and **P**†

*Summary of diet history information should be included under **S,** calculation of nutritional needs and results of measured food intake under **O,** and the evaluation of data under **A.**

†Rationale should be included under **A,** and recommendations under **P-Rx.**

TABLE 2-2. Phrases Commonly Used in Charting

Admits to eating poorly
Admitted for evaluation of
Appetite good, wt stable
Appetite was good
As described previously on (in)
Associated with
Because of the history of
Characterized by
Consistent with
Continuous with
Demonstrated that
Despite these findings
Disregard
Impression at time
Improved with
In consultation with _____ , we suggest the following
Inform
Initially seen at
Instruct
Is not remarkable
It is felt that pt is a candidate for
Markedly increased
Need
Nutritional workup included
Observed
Old records confirm
On this basis
On this regimen she continued to
Oral intake was
Pt continues to have
Pt exhibits difficulty chewing
Pt has no past history of
Pt was initially started on
Pt was noted to be
Pertinent dietary findings
Previously in good health
Recommend
Request
Revealed evidence of
Reviewed previous
Should be followed very carefully
Suggest
To be followed by
Was not felt to be significant

departments usually maintain a list of acceptable medical abbreviations. For our purposes, the abbreviations listed in Appendix D, table 2 will be used.

In general, the traditional rules of grammar are not strictly applied in medical charting. For instance, complete sentences need not be used consistently as long as complete thoughts are expressed. However, subjects and verbs must agree, and verb tenses must be correct. For example, "pt *eats* adequate amounts" is acceptable. "Pt *eat* adequate amounts" is not.

A chart note must be accurate, clear, and concise. The entry should be as brief as it can be without omission of essential elements. Medical personnel do not have time to read rambling chart notes, and you want your notes to be read. In addition, most dietitians record between six and ten short notes a day, so there just isn't time to record information that is not pertinent to the assessment of a nutritional problem. For example, listing certain lab values as objective data, but failing to use these data in the assessment, would be adding nonessential data.

TO TEST YOUR UNDERSTANDING

5. List four items that must be included in initial chart notes under **O.**

6. Fill in the blanks

   _____ ink should be used for all chart entries. Every chart note should be preceded by the _____, _____, and associated _____. At the end of the chart note, the dietitian's _____ and _____ should be provided.

7. A problem and background information are provided for this exercise. For each component listed, extract any appropriate information and fill in the chart. If a factor is not applicable or if the information is not available, state *N/A* (not applicable). This exercise is designed to help you practice selecting key information to include in a SOAP note; it is not critical that you correctly categorize the selected information.

Problem 1-Obesity

Mr. Toone is referred by his physicians to the Nutrition Outpatient Clinic for counseling on a weight-reduction diet. While talking to Mr. Toone, you obtain a quick diet history which you feel is reasonably accurate. You calculate that the diet contains 2,800 kcal per day. Mr. Toone tells you that he is 52 years old, dislikes sweets and fats, is fairly inactive, and eats two large meals a day. You measure Mr. Toone and find that he is 5 feet, 7 inches tall and weighs 195 pounds. You recommend that Mr. Toone eat three meals a day and bring a 3-day dietary record back to the clinic next week for your evaluation.

   Significant history
   Patient comments about prescribed diet
   Contraindicated foods
   Anthropometric data
   Accidents or unusual occurrences
   Impaired motor ability to feed self and eat
   Evaluation of pertinent prior intake
   Evaluation of current dietary intake
   Evaluation of current nutritional status
   Evaluation of client's ability to accept and understand diet instruction
   Recommendation for consultation or evaluation by other professionals
   Implementation, monitoring, and revision of the nutritional care plan
   Disposition indicated
   Change in usual procedure

8. Now write a SOAP progress note for Problem #1 based on the information in question 7. Be sure to use correct and complete format.

9. Write a SOAP progress note for Problem #2.

Problem 2-Tantrums

While working as a consultant at a small nursing home, you are referred by the nursing department to a resident, Ms. Smith, who has started throwing her tray on the floor whenever it is served. You talk with Ms. Smith and she tells you that the hospital food is terrible and that her favorite foods are buttermilk, cheese, and ham. Upon checking the patient's chart, you find that a mild sodium-restricted diet (3 g Na) had been ordered for her at about the time her disruptive behavior began. Some quick calculations indicate that Ms. Smith could have a 6 ounce glass of buttermilk with each meal if she eats salt-free vegetables and meat. You decide to try this and see if it will improve Ms. Smith's appetite. You will return during the evening meal tomorrow to assess whether the patient is accepting her diet.

TOPICS FOR FURTHER DISCUSSION

1. Review the literature for studies that demonstrate a positive relationship between nutritional services and reduced total health care costs. How strong are the data, and how could the methodology be improved?

2. Review the most recent "Guidelines for Dietetic Services" published by the Joint Commission on Accreditation of Hospitals. How does nutritional care documentation fit into these guidelines?

3. Discuss the purpose, organization, and mechanics of a nutritional care audit.

REFERENCES

1. SCHILLER, R. AND V. BEHM. Auditing dietetic services. *Hospitals* 53:(1979)122–127.

2. *American Hospital Association Guidelines: Recording nutritional information in medical records.* Chicago: American Hospital Association, 1976.

3. MASON, M., I. HALLAHAN, E. MONSEN, B. MUTCH, R. PALOMBO, AND H. WHITE. Philosophy, research, documentation: Phase II of the costs and benefits of nutritional care. *J. Am. Diet. Assoc.* 80:(1982)213–214.

4. WEED, L.L. *Medical Records, Medical Education, and Patient Care: The Problem-Oriented Medical Record as a Basic Tool.* Cleveland: Case Western Reserve University Press, 1969, p. 273.

5. ZIMMERMAN, T.P., S.L. SAYERS, M. PRICE, A. LADUCA, J.D. ENGEL, M.E. RISLEY, AND G. GIANNINI. *Medical Dietetics: Medical Recording Skills Manual.* Revised by S. Sayers. Chicago: Center for Educational Development, University of Illinois, 1978.

ADDITIONAL SOURCES OF INFORMATION

THE AMERICAN DIETETIC ASSOCIATION, CODING AND TERMINOLOGY TASK FORCE. *Nutrition Services Payment System.* Chicago: ADA, 1984.

THE AMERICAN DIETETIC ASSOCIATION. *Costs and Benefits of Nutritional Care: Phase 1.* Chicago: ADA, 1979.

THE AMERICAN DIETETIC ASSOCIATION. *Patient Care Audit: A Quality Assurance Procedure Manual for Dietitians.* Chicago: ADA, 1978.

The American Dietetic Association Professional Standards Review Manual. Chicago: ADA, 1976.

Financing Hospital-Based Nutrition Services, ed. J. L. Sharp. Columbus, Ohio: Report of the Fifth Ross Roundtable on Medical Issues, Ross Laboratories, 1984.

Guide to Quality Assurance in Ambulatory Nutrition Care, ed. M. Kaufman. Chicago: ADA, 1983.

JOINT COMMISSION ON ACCREDITATION OF HOSPITALS. *Guidelines on Dietetic Services.* Chicago: JCAH, 1982.

3

Interviewing the Patient

Many of your interactions with patients will consist either of interviewing to gather information or of giving information in the course of teaching or counseling. Since interviewing is the method by which you will gather much of the needed information, it is essential that you master this technique. This chapter will introduce you to interviewing techniques. (Counseling procedures are described in Chapter 6.)

Nutrition practitioners interview and counsel patients in a variety of settings and circumstances. In almost all counselor-client interactions, however, time is limited; thus the counselor must be efficient in order to accomplish the objectives in the time available. The techniques described here emphasize methods that are effective and efficient not only during the interview, but also in the subsequent planning and counseling sessions.

GOALS OF INTERVIEWING

The primary goal of interviewing is the acquisition of information that is useful in planning the patient's nutritional care. The interviewer should seek only information that serves as a foundation for planning and implementing that care; however, enough information should be obtained so that the major problem areas are evident. The problems identified during the interview serve as the basis for the care plan.

BEHAVIORS VERSUS KNOWLEDGE

In order to be able to plan effectively, it is important to learn what the patient *eats*, not what he *knows* about food selection. Nutritional counseling requires the patient to change eating behaviors. Ascertaining, by interview, the patient's current dietary habits thus simplifies and streamlines the entire counseling process. All patients have existing nutrition patterns and experiences. Therefore, you are likely to be most successful if you begin by recognizing the positive behaviors with which the patient enters the treatment process. For example, if you ask a patient, "Do you know what cholesterol is?" she might answer, "Isn't that what is in eggs?" You cannot conclude anything from this answer about the role of cholesterol in this patient's diet. A question about cholesterol consumption provides more valuable information. For example, the interviewer might ask, "How have you changed your diet to decrease cholesterol?" or "How often do you eat eggs, organ meats, and butter?"

Behaviorally worded interview questions pay off in efficiency. Research has shown that learner knowledge—that is, what learners *say* they know—sometimes fools instructors into believing that learners have acquired a behavioral skill when, in fact, no new behaviors have been learned. The patient who knows that salt is made up of sodium and chloride is *not* necessarily able to identify and select a salt substitute made of potassium and chloride. For another example, many people know the names of the four basic food groups, but recent research has shown that almost no one uses this knowledge to plan and select foods on a daily basis.

Behavioral questions also support subsequent problem-oriented charting and help to establish the focus of future counseling efforts. Such questions usually include verbs that describe *doing*, rather than knowing, something. The response to a question like "What do you think about losing weight?" will reflect something different from the answer to a question like "What did you eat the last time you went on a diet to lose weight, and what was the result?" In the second case, the patient must answer by drawing on past experiences and behaviors. The interviewer learns what the patient actually did. Wording questions in such a way as to elicit descriptions of the patient's behaviors is efficient and assists in the preparation of the care plan and the counseling objectives.

TO TEST YOUR UNDERSTANDING

Indicate whether each question below focuses on knowledge or on behavior. If the question is worded for knowledge, rewrite it as a behavioral question.

1. Do you know what a calorie is?
2. Have you heard about the diabetic diet?
3. Do you know what makes a healthy body?
4. What do you eat for a bedtime snack?

OPEN VERSUS CLOSED QUESTIONS

Interview success also depends on the counselor's ability to phrase behavioral questions that demand a narrative response. Questions worded so that they require descriptive responses, instead of a simple yes or no, will garner the most information.

For example, what would the patient be likely to answer to the question, "Do you eat three meals a day?" Possible answers are "yes," "no," or something like "usually," but none of these is especially informative. A better wording for such a question would be "How many times do you eat each day?" The possible answers are infinite and depend upon the patient's actual meal pattern. In addition, patients will often give information that they believe will please the interviewer. A question that has an infinite number of potential responses is more likely to elicit an unbiased answer.

Questions requiring explanatory responses are termed *open;* questions requiring only yes or no answers are termed *closed.* In the following pairs of examples, note the difference in the open versus closed wording formats.

Do you like to eat salty-tasting foods?

compared to

What salty-tasting foods do you like to eat?

Have you ever tried a weight-reduction diet before?

compared to

What weight-reduction diets have you tried?

The closed questions always begin with "Do you . . . ?" or "Have you . . . ?" The open questions used *what, how, when,* and other descriptors. Closed questions are prevalent on diet history forms because yes and no answers are easily quantified and summarized for charting purposes. However, the interview is used to gather more complex information for educational intervention. For this purpose, open-ended questions are much more useful.

In some cases, an open *statement,* rather than a question, works best. For instance, instead of "Do you eat a morning meal?" the counselor might say, "Describe what you usually eat in the morning." The statement obligates the patient to select from his own experience to formulate an answer.

It should be noted that when learners have no previous experience to convey about the subject, they will say so. That is, they will limit their response or give a negative response to the open question or statement. Here is an example:

COUNSELOR: What are your favorite snack foods?
PATIENT: I don't eat any snacks between meals.

This response, although it is in the negative, provides the interviewer with important information about the patient's eating behavior. When counseling begins, the interviewer will not teach information about snacking because it is irrelevant for this patient. Thus, even a negative response serves as a basis for constructing an individualized plan and counseling session.

TO TEST YOUR UNDERSTANDING

Indicate if each question below is open or closed. If a question is closed, rewrite it as an open question.

5. Do you understand the relationship between diet and exercise?
6. What do you eat between meals?
7. Do you eat eggs for breakfast?
8. Have you ever tried to control your diet?

CONTROLLING THE INTERVIEW

Asking open-ended questions may produce tangential conversation, wandering, storytelling, and other deviations from the direction of the interview. These side effects are common in face-to-face discussions between people. Often the interviewer feels a loss of control, and when she finally examines the information obtained during the interview, there is little of practical use. To avoid this inefficient result, the interviewer must develop a strategy for encouraging the patient to provide only pertinent data. Take this example:

COUNSELOR: How often do you eat out in restaurants?

PATIENT: Oh, my husband and I like this little Italian restaurant about three blocks from our house. They serve the best spaghetti and ravioli. My husband's mother used to fix Italian food, but lately she hasn't felt much like cooking. She has arthritis in her hands and can't do the kind of housework she used to do . . .

When the patient responds this way, the interviewer, in the interest of using limited time efficiently, needs to interject a controlling statement to bring the patient back to the question at hand. For example

PATIENT: . . . arthritis in her hands and can't do the kind of housework she used to do . . .

COUNSELOR: I'm sorry to hear that; remember, though, we were discussing the frequency with which you eat out in restaurants.

or

COUNSELOR: The Italian restaurant is one place where you dine out. How *often* do you eat there?

You must practice this skill in order to develop judgment, ability to time interruptions, and ease in realigning the patient's responses in the direction of the interview without offending.

QUESTION FRAMING

Another control-compromising situation may occur in the course of an interview. Sometimes clients will not verbalize, or will provide answers which they believe will please the interviewer, but which do not necessarily reveal their true habits, experiences, and behaviors. This often occurs with overweight or alcoholic patients, children, neurotic or emotionally disturbed patients, and with the counselor's family members or significant others. Here is an example:

COUNSELOR (to an overweight patient): When you eat desserts, approximately how much cake or ice cream or other item might you eat?

PATIENT: I never eat sweets. In fact, I rarely eat dessert.

Let us assume, in this example, that it is the counselor's opinion that the client is not providing an accurate picture of her food intake. Responses such as this can result from both anxiety about the interview and reluctance to share such information with a stranger. To gain control of a situation of this sort, the interviewer may choose to ask one, or a series of, "framed" questions. Framed questions allow the client to hypothesize about an imaginary instance and thereby remove himself from a possibly negative disclosure. For example

PATIENT: I never eat sweets. In fact, I rarely eat dessert.

COUNSELOR: Take another instance. Suppose you went to a friend's home for a party and the only desserts being served were chocolate cake, ice cream parfait, and pecan pie. Which would you choose?

In this example, the "frame" is a hypothetical party, and relatively equal choices of dessert are provided, from which the client must choose an answer. Psychological research demonstrates that the selection of the forced-choice answer will correlate highly with the *actual* choice the client usually makes.

Of course, the interviewer must remain nonjudgmental in accepting the client's answer. The client gradually loses the initial fear of disapproval and begins to open up about actual dietary behaviors.

The interviewer may follow the completely hypothetical question with one more closely related to the client's own life, such as, "Now, if you were planning your own party, what desserts would you include on your menu?" Finally, the interviewer might ask, "Of all these desserts and any others, which ones do you eat?"

If the practitioner senses the client's discomfort and reticence early in the interview, then framing questions allows for safer, nonthreatening interactions and paves the way for the disclosure of truthful information as the interview progresses.

Framed questions could also be useful in an interview with a reluctant school-age child, who could be asked, "If you could buy any foods you wanted in the supermarket, what five foods would you buy?" Or, the quiet child might be asked to choose which foods she would take to the beach or on a camping trip. In either instance, the child fantasizes about foods in hypothetical situations, and his answers are accepted without judgment by the interviewer. This makes possible an increasingly interactive interview session in which the child becomes comfortable talking and answering questions.

For each scenario, create a framed question that will solicit information that the patient is reluctant to provide.

9. A diabetic child is being interviewed about his after-school snacking. He says he eats only carrot and celery sticks, but that response does not fit other evidence.
10. A male renal patient, newly diagnosed, says he doesn't eat much meat. His food record and his wife offer evidence to the contrary.

SUMMARIZING THE PROBLEMS

The interview, then, will reveal the patient's unique problems related to food habits. The practitioner can use this information to identify the behavior changes necessary to fulfill the diet prescription. The most effective way to plan further intervention, stimulate motivation, and ensure long-term adherence is clarified.

Distilling the problems from the interview data requires priority setting. The most critical problem must be defined first, both in the interview itself and in the documented care plan.

For instance, if a diabetic patient states that he already uses the ADA Exchange Lists for meal planning but always gets confused about exactly what the portion sizes should be, the nutrition specialist recognizes that portion identification and control are key problem areas, *not* the definition of the exchange groups. In the course of the interview, the patient supplies the practitioner with a picture of behaviors that are in conflict with prescribed behaviors, allowing definition and identification of problems so that they can be documented in the record.

11. Identify a key problem for the patient being interviewed here:

COUNSELOR: What have been your most successful diet attempts?
PATIENT: I once went to the Weight Watchers meetings and lost about 20 pounds, but then I sort of got tired of eating apricots every day—you know, it says to eat two apricots every day.
COUNSELOR: What other diets have you tried, and what happened when you were on them?
PATIENT: I've tried them all, I get so tired of eating the same thing day after day, especially on those diets where you eat eggs and grapefruit all the time.

INTERVIEWER PERSONALITY AND RAPPORT

The establishment of *rapport* between practitioner and patient is essential to the counseling relationship. It is important to recognize the value of building trust between the nutritional specialist and the patient.

Being nonjudgmental of patient responses may be a good interviewer's most valuable asset. To gain the patient's trust and cooperation, and thus to encourage openness and honest self-disclosure, the interviewer must refrain from appearing to judge behaviors as good or bad. It is better to take the point of view that the patient enters the interview with preexisting experiences which are not open to analysis, but which are simply available data on which planning and counseling will be based.

A word might be added here about personality traits. Sound interviewing techniques, such as open-ended questioning, problem identification, and a non-judgmental manner, correlate better with interview success than do the personality characteristics of the interviewer. Of course, a friendly, interested interviewer who listens makes the entire process more comfortable for both the interviewer and the patient.

INTERVIEWER SUPPORT

Another way in which interviewers can enhance patients' confidence is to begin by recognizing the behaviors that already comply with the dietary prescription. Clients are reassured to discover that many of the decisions they already make about their diets fit the new regimen. For example, if a newly diagnosed diabetic patient related in an interview that she eats a well-balanced night-time snack and has been doing so for many years, the interviewer has an opportunity to reinforce this existing behavior at the time the patient describes it. The counselor might say, "Eating a good night-time snack is exactly the right thing to do on this new diet as well, so keep up the good work."

SUMMARY

The client interview supplies information about the client's behavioral background and identifies dietary problems on which the client's nutritional care plan and later counseling will be based. These two outcomes are the goals of interviewing.

Inquiry must be made using open-ended, behavioral question formats. Control of the interview is maintained by realigning responses to the issues and framing questions when necessary. Nonjudgmental reactions and supportive commentary by the interviewer further the success of the interview.

TO TEST YOUR UNDERSTANDING

For each of the comments presented here, what can be said to reinforce the existing behavior because it complies with the prescribed diet plan?

12. Patient: "Oh, I eat about five or six small meals during the day. I never really eat a huge meal."

13. Patient: "I'm very careful about eating too much butter or margarine or any of those fatty foods. I eat only one or two pats in a whole day."

14. Patient: "When I feel like I might have an insulin reaction, I sometimes eat a special mint that I keep in my purse. I also carry one of those little packages of cheese and crackers, in case I need some protein."

15. Analyze the following scenario, identifying correct and incorrect demonstrations of interviewing skills. If something is incorrect, correct it. Write your comments and corrections on a separate sheet of paper, indicating the lines to which you are referring.

```
1        The interviewer approaches the bedside of a 49-year-old
2    woman, Ms. P., for whom a 1,500-kcal diet for weight reduction has been
3    prescribed. From the chart, the interviewer has obtained the
4    diagnosis (degenerative arthritis), the patient's age, height
5    (Ht = 5 ft, 8 in), weight (Wt = 185 #), and blood pressure, the results of
6    blood and urine analyses, and other medical information.
7        Counselor: "Hello, I'm _____. In order to best
8    assist you with the weight-reduction diet prescribed for you, I
9    need to ask you some questions about what you do at home now with
10   regard to your diet. Let's begin with what you normally eat
11   during a day. Describe your usual day's food intake, beginning
12   with the morning meal."
13       Ms. P.: "Oh, I eat very well, but I know that I have to
14   lose weight. I have juice and coffee for breakfast. Sometimes I
15   have an English muffin. I never eat again before 1:00, when I
16   have a sandwich and coffee. I take my sandwich to work with me."
17       Counselor: "Do you eat meat sandwiches?"
18       Ms. P.: "Yes, I do, and cheese."
19       Counselor: "And for dinner?"
20       Ms. P.: "I live alone, so I usually cook a chicken on Sunday
21   and eat it until Wednesday. You know, I also eat egg salad and
22   tuna salad sandwiches for lunch. I especially like egg salad
23   because the recipe I have came from a famous chef who used to be
24   at the most glamorous restaurant in town. He was once interviewed
25   on TV and he gave his recipes for the delicious potatoes he
26   prepared at this restaurant. I got his egg salad recipe from a
27   magazine . . ."
28       Counselor: "He must have had an excellent recipe. You were
29   saying you often have chicken for dinner. What else do you eat
30   with it?"
31       Ms. P.: "I like vegetables, especially with just a little
32   bit of black pepper. I don't care for butter or sauces because they
33   cover the taste of the vegetables. I always have two or three—
34   raw, cooked, it doesn't matter."
35       Counselor: "Excellent. Your prescribed diet plan suggests
36   exactly that: many vegetables without too much added to them.
37   You will do fine with that. Do you eat desserts?"
38       Ms. P.: "Desserts? Oh, I try not to."
```

39   Counselor: "When you pass a bakery window, which of the
40 items tempts you the most?"
41   Ms. P.: "Oh, the cream-filled pastries. You know I could
42 eat three eclairs without even thinking about it—that is, if I
43 had them around. Fortunately, I don't."
44   Counselor: "What else would you say you include regularly
45 in your diet?"
46   Ms. P.: "I always have lots of juice around. I love
47 nectars and I sometimes buy weird juices, like guava.
48   Counselor: "When you drink juice, how much do you usually
49 have?"
50   Ms. P.: 'About a glass, a large glass, because I always put
51 lots of ice cubes in it to make it very cold."
52   Counselor: "How often do you drink juices during the day?"
53   Ms. P.: "Oh, all day. I have a large glass on my desk at
54 work all the time and all evening while I'm watching TV."
55   Counselor: "I have a list of fruits and vegetables, as
56 well as one for each other type of food—meats, breads, and so
57 on. Please look them over and circle the foods that
58 you eat regularly. I'll be back later to talk with you some more.
59 Thank you for your cooperation. I know we will be able to work
60 together on a successful plan."

16. Write a progress note to identify the dietary problems of the patient in question 15.

4

Evaluating Nutritional Status

Nutritional assessment consists of the gathering of data to (1) identify individuals who require specialized nutritional care, (2) determine the cause and degree of malnutrition, and (3) determine the potential risk for development of malnutrition or related complications. It serves as a basis for planning nutritional therapy and evaluating an individual's response to that therapy. In order to complete a comprehensive nutritional assessment, the nutritional care specialist must be skilled in anthropometric, biochemical, clinical and dietary methods of evaluating nutritional status. This chapter discusses procedures for evaluating nutritional status in adults, including the elderly. Diet evaluation is described in Chapter 5, and nutritional assessment in children is discussed in Chapter 8. You will have an opportunity to practice the skills described in this chapter, which should be studied with the assignments and exercises performed in the order given.

You will find it helpful to review the related material in your text before you begin. In addition, you should have access to the following equipment:

1. Calipers for measuring skinfolds
2. Tape measure (or Inser-Tape from Ross Laboratories, Columbus, Ohio)

EVALUATION OF PROTEIN-ENERGY STATUS

Protein-energy status is evaluated primarily by anthropometric and biochemical methods.

ANTHROPOMETRIC MEASUREMENTS

Anthropometry is the measurement (*-ometry*) of man (*anthropo-*). In clinical situations, anthropometry is used to estimate body energy stores and protein mass. Anthropometric data usually consist of height, weight, skinfold measurements, and measurements of circumferences of various body parts.

Height and Weight

For most patients, height and weight measurements are obtained on admission and are very useful for a rapid preliminary assessment of energy and protein stores.

Measurement. Height and weight, which are measured by the nursing staff when the patient's condition permits, are recorded in the patient's medical record. Weight may be recorded in pounds or in kilograms (1 kg = 2.2#). Height may be recorded in feet and inches or in centimeters (1 in = 2.54 cm). Height is ordinarily based on the patient's stature when standing. Tables of standard values may assume either that the subject is barefoot or that the subject is wearing shoes, in which case the height of the heel is indicated; to use such a table, therefore, the heel height must be added to the height of the barefoot patient. For example, to use a table based on the assumption that the subject is wearing shoes with one-inch heels, a patient who is 5 feet, 5 inches tall without shoes must be considered to be 5 feet, 6 inches tall according to the table. For patients who are unable to stand, *sitting height,* or *crown-rump length,* may be measured, but this is not considered accurate. The total length of a recumbent patient is the *crown-heel length,* or *recumbent length.*

Alternatively, *knee height* can be used to indicate stature in patients who are bedfast, are confined to a wheelchair, or have curvature of the spine. This method is particularly useful with the elderly (1). The patient lies supine (on his back) and bends his left knee to a 90-degree angle. Measurement is made, with an especially large caliper, from under the heel of the foot to the anterior surface of the thigh at the knee. Knee height plus age and sex are used to compute stature using the following equations:

For men

$$\text{Height in cm} = 64.19 - (0.04 \times \text{age in years}) + (2.02 \times \text{knee height in cm}) \quad \textbf{(4-1)}$$

For women

$$\text{Height in cm} = 84.88 - (0.24 \times \text{age in years}) + (1.83 \times \text{knee height in cm}) \quad \textbf{(4-2)}$$

Bed scales may be available to weigh a recumbent patient who is unable to sit or stand on a scale. If measurements of height and weight are not available, the patient may be asked for this information.

TO TEST YOUR UNDERSTANDING

1. List methods of measuring or estimating body height (length).
2. How would you determine or estimate the height of the following patients:
   a. A patient who has a leg in traction and cannot get out of bed?
   b. A patient whose legs have been amputated?
   c. An elderly woman with osteoporosis and spinal curvature?
3. Estimate the height of a 68-year-old male patient who has a knee height of 54 cm. Show your calculations.

Interpretation. There is a great deal of controversy concerning the best standards of weight for height. There is also disagreement on the best terminology. In this manual, we will use the values published by the Metropolitan Life Insurance Company in 1983 (Table F-1).* These values are based on the weights associated with the lowest mortality rate for individuals between the ages of 25 and 59 years. The weights are lower than the average weight for the population group. The subject is assumed to be wearing shoes with one-inch heels and indoor clothing weighing 5 pounds for men or 3 pounds for women. These tables list height and weight ranges for men and women aged 25 to 59 and allow for differences in frame size. In the interest of brevity, we will refer to the weights as *optimal body weights* (OBW).

Body frame size may be estimated in one of two ways:

a. Measurement of elbow breadth (basis for the Metropolitan Life tables)

Procedure: Step 1: The patient extends one arm and bends the forearm up at a 90-degree angle. The palm faces away from the body, and the fingers are straight. Step 2: Measure the distance between the two prominent bones on each side of the elbow with calipers or with the thumb and forefinger. Then measure the space between the thumb and forefinger with a ruler or tape measure. Step 3: Consult Table F-2 for a range of elbow breadth measurements of medium-frame persons of various heights. Measurements lower than these values indicate a small frame; those higher than these values indicate a large frame.

b. Measurement of wrist circumference

Procedure: Step 1: Measure the wrist circumference just distal (toward the hand) to the styloid process at the wrist crease of the right hand (see Fig. 4-1).

*Table F-1 refers to the first table in Appendix F. References to tables in the appendixes will appear this way throughout the book.

Step 2: Calculate the ratio (r) of height (ht) to wrist circumference with this equation:

$$r = \frac{ht \ (cm)}{wrist \ circumference \ (cm)} \quad \textbf{(4-3)}$$

Step 3: Determine frame size by comparing the r value with the following:

	Small	Medium	Large
Men	> 10.4	10.4–9.6	< 9.6
Women	> 10.9	10.9–9.9	< 9.9

If height-weight tables are not available as guidelines, "ideal" body weight (IBW) may be estimated by using the following equations:

For men   IBW = 106# + 6# for each inch > 60 inches   **(4-4)**

For women   IBW = 100# + 5# for each inch > 60 inches   **(4-5)**

Adjustments for frame size are made by subtracting 10 percent for small frames and adding 10 percent for large frames. An additional 10 percent is added for those over 50 years of age. An IBW of 140 pounds, for example, thus becomes 154 pounds. For all values,

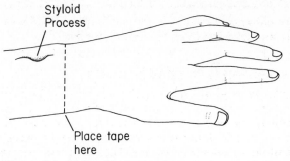

Figure 4-1 Estimating frame size.

normal range is ±10 percent. Weight 20 percent or more above the IBW is often defined as obesity. The IBW values obtained in this manner are not similar to those given in the Metropolitan Life Insurance Company tables.

Two other formulas, which yield values similar to those in the Metropolitan Life tables, have been suggested (2):

For men   OBW = 135# + 3# for each inch > 63   **(4-6)**

For women   OBW = 119# + 3# for each inch > 60   **(4-7)**

These results agree with the values for medium-frame persons, with an error ±1 percent. An adjustment of ±10 percent allows for differences in frame size.

Regardless of the standard used, adjustment must also be made for the patient with an amputated extremity. An estimated weight of the amputated part should be subtracted from IBW or OBW to arrive at the adjusted body weight for the amputee. Following are some estimated weights:

Hand	0.3% of total body weight
Forearm and hand	2.6
Entire arm	6.2
Foot	1.7
Below-knee amputation	7.0
Above-knee amputation	11.0
Entire leg	18.6

For example, a woman 5 feet, 4 inches tall has an estimated body weight of 120 pounds. If she has an above-knee amputation,

$$120 - (120 \times 0.11) = 120 - 13 = 107.$$

adjusted body weight is then 107 pounds ± 11 pounds. The following equations may be used to compare current body weight (CBW) with the chosen standard in adults:

a.   Relative to optimal body weight (OBW)—those given in Metropolitan Life Insurance tables:

$$\%OBW = \frac{CBW}{OBW} \times 100 \qquad \textbf{(4-8)}$$

b.   Relative to the patient's usual body weight (UBW):

$$\%UBW = \frac{CBW}{UBW} \times 100 \qquad \textbf{(4-9)}$$

Similar equations may be used to compare the patient's body weight to IBW, admission weight, weight at previous assessment, or weight prior to a specific course of treatment. One word of caution: If the patient is dehydrated or edematous, the weight data will be misleading.

The significance of the amount of weight change has been variously interpreted. An additional consideration is the rate at which weight loss occurred. One basis for interpretation, including both amount and rate of loss, is given in Table F-3.

An alternative method uses percentiles to show the position of the patient's measurements within the chosen population. A measurement at the fifth percentile, for example, is lower than the same measurement seen in 95 percent of that population. Examples are given in Tables F-4 and F-5. In these tables, measurements below the fifth percentile are considered depleted, while those between the fifth and fifteenth percentiles are considered to be at risk of becoming depleted. This method does not consider the rate at which the weight was lost, however.

The tables just described are primarily based on data for the age range up to 60 years; there are few data for older ages. Some values for the elderly are available, but they are based on a small sample and should be used cautiously (1).

TO TEST YOUR UNDERSTANDING

4. With a tape measure or Inser-Tape, measure the wrist circumference of a classmate and state the frame size indicated. With calipers or a tape measure, measure the elbow breadth of the same classmate and state the frame size indicated. Compare the results of these two methods.

5. A patient's height is 5 feet, 5 inches. What is her height in centimeters?

6. A patient's weight is 132 pounds. How many kilograms does she weigh?

7. What is the frame size of a male patient who is 5 feet, 10 inches tall and has a wrist circumference of 7 inches?

8. A female patient is 5 feet, 6 inches tall and weighs 112 pounds. She has an elbow breadth of 2½ inches and a wrist circumference of 5¾ inches. Giving specific figures, how does this patient's body weight compare with the following:

   a. Optimal body weight associated with the lowest mortality rate?

   b. "Ideal" body weight estimated from a formula?

9. A male patient, age 45, is 5 feet, 9 inches tall with a medium frame. He states that his usual weight is 165 pounds. He recently lost 35 pounds because of illness. How would you evaluate his body weight? Would you consider him at nutritional risk? Why?

10. A male patient, age 70, has a height of 180.9 cm and weighs 80.2 kg. Four weeks ago, he weighed 85 kg. Would you consider this patient to be at risk? Explain your answer.

11. A 57-year-old female patient has an amputation of the right leg above the knee. Knee height obtained from the left leg is 48.75 cm. Calculate
    a. Estimated height
    b. Optimal body weight prior to amputation
    c. Optimal body weight following amputation

Body Fat Stores

Skinfold thicknesses, which include the subcutaneous fat layer, are measured to indicate the body's calorie reserve. The triceps skinfold (TSF), or the area over the triceps muscle on the posterior side of the upper arm, is the most commonly used site. Other sites, often used in combination, are the skinfolds over the biceps muscle and in the subscapular and suprailiac area.

Triceps Skinfold (TSF). Depending on the institution, the accepted procedure may be to use either the nondominant arm or the right arm. When sequential measurements are made, they must be done in exactly the same way. Fat distribution varies with location; therefore, techniques must be precise in order to be reproducible.

Procedure

Step 1—Take the measurement on the bare arm with the patient standing or sitting erect if possible. The arm should be hanging down at the side. Alternatively, a supine patient may be asked to lift the arm so that the elbow is pointed to the ceiling. The arm is bent at a 90-degree angle, and the hand is in a fist with palm facing up.

Step 2—Locate the olecranon process of the ulna and the acromial process of the scapula and mark each point on the skin with a pen or adhesive label (see Fig. 4-2).

Step 3—Place a tape measure between the two points and mark the midpoint in line with the olecranon process. (The Inser-Tape is useful for this purpose.)

Step 4—Pick up, between thumb and forefinger, a *vertical* fold of skin and fat 1 cm above the midpoint, in line with the point of the olecranon process. The fold should be pulled carefully away from the underlying muscle. Ask the patient to contract the underlying muscle to be sure muscle and fascia are not included in the skinfold.

Step 5—Place the caliper jaws perpendicular to the fat fold at the midpoint and release the spring-loaded lever but not the pinch (see Fig. 4-3).

Step 6—Read the measurement in about 2 seconds.

Step 7—Repeat the measurement in Step 5 twice more and average the three results.

Interpretation: Various systems have been suggested as standards for interpretation. The following are the most common:

1. Comparison with a standard value. The values obtained from measurement of the patient may be com-

Figure 4-2 Finding the mid-arm point. (Reproduced with permission from Kabi-Vitrum, Inc., Alameda, Calif 94501.)

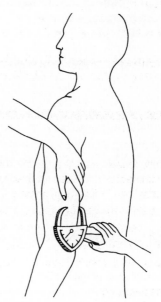

Figure 4-3 Measuring triceps skinfold. (Reproduced with permission from Kabi-Vitrum, Inc., Alameda, Calif 94501.)

pared with standards such as those shown in Table F-6. The patient's values are then calculated as a percentage of this standard using this equation:

$$\% \text{ of standard} = \frac{\text{measurement obtained}}{\text{standard}} \times 100 \quad \textbf{(4-10)}$$

Reduction of triceps skinfold may be interpreted as indicative of a mild, moderate, or severe deficit, as indicated in Table F-7. Values of 190 percent of standard or greater are used to define obesity.

2. Comparison with percentile values. Alternatively, tables classifying TSF values in percentiles are available. These are given in Tables F-8 and F-9. Again, patients below the fifth percentile are considered to be depleted. Those adults between the fifth and fifteenth percentiles are at risk of becoming depleted.

Body Mass Index.   The total body weight in kilograms divided by the square of the stature, or meters squared, is known as body mass index (BMI). This value is also considered a useful simple indicator of the total amount of body fat, and can be used in the elderly or in any situation in which triceps skinfolds are not available.

Procedure: The value is obtained with the following equation:

$$BMI = \frac{\text{Weight}}{\text{Height}^2} \text{ or } \frac{W}{H^2} \quad \textbf{(4-11)}$$

where weight is in kilograms (kg) and height is in meters (M) squared. For example, a woman who weighs 92.5 kg with a height of 162.5 cm, or 1.625 M (2.640 M²), would have a BMI of 35.

Interpretation: The BMI has been shown to be highly correlated with body fatness (3). A BMI greater than 27 is indicative of obesity. BMI of 24 to 27 for females or 24 to 25 for males is considered to indicate excess weight.

Body Density

Procedure

Step 1—Skinfold thicknesses have been used to calculate body density. In one method, skinfolds are measured, as in Steps 5–7 of the procedure for measuring TSF. Measurements are made at the following locations (4):

Biceps	at midpoint over the belly of the muscle
Subscapular	below the tip of the inferior angle of the scapula at an angle 45 degrees from the vertical
Suprailiac	above the iliac crest in the midaxillary line
Triceps	as described for measuring TSF

Step 2—Take the sum of these four measurements (in mm)

Step 3—Obtain the log (S) of this sum.

Step 4—Calculate the density (D) using the following equations:*

Men:	$D = 1.1610 - 0.0632\ S$	**(4-12)**
Women:	$D = 1.5810 - 0.0720\ S$	**(4-13)**
Boys:	$D = 1.1533 - 0.0643\ S$	**(4-14)**
Girls:	$D = 1.1369 - 0.0598\ S$	**(4-15)**

Step 5—Calculate the body fat from the density with this equation:

$$\% \text{ Fat} = \left(\frac{4.95}{D} - 4.5 \right) \times 100 \quad \textbf{(4-16)}$$

Interpretation

The result of this calculation is not often used for routine nutritional assessment, but it may be useful in treatment of obesity. The mean proportion of body fat is 14 percent for men and 27 percent for women.

*These equations disregard age. More detailed equations adjusted for age are available.

TO TEST YOUR UNDERSTANDING

12. Measure the triceps skinfold of a classmate. Repeat the measurement twice more and compare the three results. How reproducible are your results?

13. a. A male patient, age 35, has a triceps skinfold of 8 mm. Calculate the percent of standard.
    b. How would this result be interpreted compared with a standard value?
    c. How would this value be interpreted on a percentile basis?

14. a. A female patient, age 40, is 5 feet, 3 inches tall and weighs 194 pounds. Calculate her BMI.
    b. What do you conclude about this patient's body fat?

Somatic Protein

The somatic protein (skeletal protein mass) is most commonly estimated from a measure of the total midarm circumference (MAC) of the upper arm. Once total arm circumference is known, midarm muscle circumference (MAMC) is then obtained by calculation from the total arm circumference and the triceps skinfold. The rationale for this procedure is based on the fact that muscle protein constitutes the greatest por-

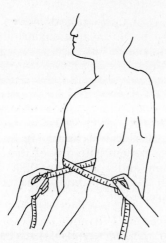

Figure 4-4 Measuring midarm circumference. (Reproduced with permission from Kabi-Vitrum, Inc., Alameda, Calif 94501.)

tion of somatic protein and will reflect changes in the whole.

Procedure

Step 1—Locate the midpoint of the upper arm, as previously described.

Step 2—Measure the midarm circumference of the upper arm with a tape measure or Inser-Tape, aligning the top of the tape with the mark at the midpoint of the arm (see Fig. 4-4).

Step 3—Results are recorded to the nearest 0.1 cm.

Step 4—Calculate midarm muscle circumference (MAMC) from the midarm circumference (MAC) using the equation

$$MAMC = MAC - 3.14\ TSF \qquad (4\text{-}17)$$

where *all* values are in cm.

Interpretation: The results of these procedures are compared with published standards using percent of standard or percentiles as follows:

1. Comparison with a standard value. Calculate the percent of standard using the following equation:

$$\%\ of\ standard = \frac{measurement\ obtained}{standard} \times 100 \qquad (4\text{-}18)$$

This equation may be used with both MAC and MAMC. The results of calculations of arm muscle circumference may be interpreted as normal or as mild, moderate, or severe depletion, as indicated in Table F-7.

2. Based on percentiles. When percentile values are used for interpretation, values in the fifth percentile or less again indicate depletion, and those between the fifth and fifteenth percentiles are considered to indicate a patient "at risk." Percentile values are given in Table F-10 for midarm circumference and arm muscle circumference.

Midarm muscle cross-section *area* (MAMA) is sometimes calculated from the data gathered in the procedures just described. It is useful as an index of the amount of lean tissue in the body and in determining basal metabolic rate (BMR) and drug dosage. It is also useful when applied to children, whose muscle area changes with age. MAMA is calculated using the equation

$$MAMA = \frac{(MAC - 3.14\ TSF)^2}{4 \times 3.14} \qquad (4\text{-}19)$$

where MAMA is in mm² and MAC and TSF are in mm.

Equation 4-19 is based on the equation for the area of a circle found in most elementary geometry texts. Standards of comparison are given in Table F-11.

It has been stated that this equation yields an overestimated value for MAMA. Heymsfield suggests correction factors of −10.0 cm² for men and −6.5 cm² for women to adjust for the presence of bone (5). Average and range of corrected values for normal subjects between ages 20 and 70 are given by Heymsfield as follows

Men	51 cm² (range = 35–68)
Women	28 cm² (range = 17–39).

(It is important to note in these equations whether values must be given in cm or in mm.)

TO TEST YOUR UNDERSTANDING

15. A 42-year-old female patient has a midarm circumference of 27.3 cm and a triceps skinfold of 1.25 cm.

   a. Calculate the midarm muscle circumference.

   b. How would this be interpreted compared with a standard value?

   c. How would this be interpreted based on percentile values?

16. a. Calculate the MAMA of the patient described in the previous question.

   b. Using the values given in Table F-11, how would you interpret your results?

17. a. Using the Heymsfield correction factor, calculate the MAMA for this same patient.

   b. How would you interpret the result?

When MAMA is available, it is also possible to calculate the midarm fat area (MAFA) using the equation

$$\text{MAFA} = \frac{3.14}{4} \times \left(\frac{\text{MAC}}{3.14}\right)^2 - \left[\frac{(\text{MAC} - 3.14\ \text{TSF})^2}{4 \times 3.14}\right]$$

$$(4\text{-}20)$$

where MAFA is in mm² and MAC and TSF are in mm. Note that this equation consists of total cross-section area minus the MAMA obtained in equation 4-19. Percentile values for interpretation are also given in Table F-10. It has been suggested that these values are more useful than are TSF values (6).

BIOCHEMICAL MEASUREMENTS

Biochemical measurements are used in nutritional assessments primarily to evaluate visceral (nonstructural) protein. Criteria are levels of serum proteins and indicators of immune function. Biochemical measurements are occasionally used to supplement anthropometric measurements of somatic protein.

Visceral Proteins

Serum Proteins. Serum proteins have varying half-lives and differing sensitivities to nutritional depletion and repletion.

Serum albumin is usually recorded in the patient's medical record as part of the admission laboratory workup; because of its availability, therefore, this is the value most frequently used. Standards for interpretation are given in Table F-7. The range of normal values is considered to be 3.5–5.5 g/dl. Half-life is about 14 days.

Serum transferrin (TF) may be determined directly; however, it is more common to estimate it from a laboratory determination of total iron-binding capacity (TIBC). Several equations are currently used for this purpose. The equation we will use is

$$\text{TF (mg/dl)} = 0.8\ \text{TIBC (\mu g/dl)} - 43 \qquad (4\text{-}21)$$

This value, however, has been reported to overestimate serum transferrin by 10 to 20 percent. An alternative equation has recently been suggested and is used in some institutions:

$$\text{TF (mg/dl)} = 0.68\ \text{TIBC (\mu g/dl)} + 21 \qquad (4\text{-}22)$$

Half-life is 8 to 10.5 days.

For interpretation, serum albumin, transferrin, and TIBC levels in mild, moderate, and severe depletion are given in Table F-7. Normal TF range is 200 to 355 mg/dl.

Ranges of normal values are given because abnormal increases, as well as decreases, may occur. Fluctuations in serum albumin levels may be the result of factors other than nutritional depletion. Non-nutritional causes of low serum albumin include any factors that result in increased loss, increased degradation, or decreased synthesis, such as may occur in liver disease, kidney disease, some forms of gastrointestinal disease, congenital heart disease, and some endocrine disorders. Increased serum albumin levels may be seen in dehydrated patients. Low transferrin (or TIBC) levels may occur in chronic infection or in liver or kidney disease. In the patient with any of these conditions, serum albumin and transferrin data must be interpreted with caution. Additional diagnostic tests are often necessary.

Immune Function. Currently used estimates of cell-mediated immune function (CMI) are based on total lymphocyte count (TLC) and measures of delayed cutaneous hypersensitivity (DCH).

Total lymphocyte count: To obtain the TLC, note the *total white blood cell* (WBC) count, which is obtained during the admission laboratory workup and is recorded in the patient's chart. In addition, the *differential count* gives the percentage of each of the five types of white blood cells. *Total lymphocyte count* (TLC) is then obtained by applying the following equation:

$$\text{TLC} = \text{Total WBC} \times \%\ \text{lymphocytes}/100 \qquad (4\text{-}23)$$

For example, a patient whose total WBC count is 10,000 and who has 25 percent lymphocytes would have a TLC of $10,000 \times 0.25 = 2500$.

Normal WBC count is usually 5,000 to 10,000 cells/mm³ and lymphocytes are 20 to 35 percent of these. There is some variation in the lymphocyte counts, which is considered normal. Lymphocyte counts of less than 1,200 cells/mm³ may be indicative of depletion. These data must be interpreted with caution since other factors, including injury, radiotherapy, surgery, and immunosuppressive medication, also influence the TLC. In addition, depressed total WBC count, and resulting lower TLC, may be the result of some medications or viral infection even if the patient's nutritional status is normal.

Delayed cutaneous hypersensitivity (DCH): Some institutions test for failure of the cell-mediated immune system (anergy) by testing the response to a battery of skin antigens. The antigens used vary among institutions but are usually chosen from Candida, streptokinase/streptodornase (SK/SD), trychophyton, or mumps.

In this procedure, 0.1 ml of each of the chosen antigens is injected subcutaneously in the inner aspect of the forearm. This is usually done by the nurse. The area of the injection is examined for a reaction in 24 hours, and then again in 48 hours. A reaction consists of a "wheal and flare"—that is, a raised and hardened area of skin (*induration*) surrounded by a reddened area (*erythema*).

A patient who has an induration of 5 mm or more in at least one dimension is considered reactive. If the induration measures 1 to 4 mm, the patient is considered "relatively anergic," a suboptimal response, while lack of response indicates anergy. The area of the erythema is not usually considered relevant.

There is controversy concerning the number and choice of antigens, the necessity to read the results at both 24 and 48 hours, and the number of responses necessary to be considered a positive response.

While anergy may result from malnutrition, other non-nutritional conditions may interfere with the immune response and should be considered in interpretation. These include various infections, renal and hepatic disease, inflammatory bowel disease, sarcoid, neoplastic disease, and primary disorders of the immune system. In addition, treatments affecting the immune response include radiation therapy, anesthesia, and drug therapy with steroids, immunosuppressants, antineoplastic drugs, cimetidine, coumarin, and aspirin. These factors must be taken into account in interpretation of results.

TO TEST YOUR UNDERSTANDING

The medical record of a 65-year-old male patient provides the following information:

Serum albumin	3.0 g/dl
TIBC	165 µg/dl
WBC	4,500 cells/mm³
Differential	
Neutrophils	70%
Lymphocytes	20%
Eosinophils	3%
Basophils	2%
Monocytes	5%
DCH response	
SK/SD	2 mm in 24 hrs
PPD	2 mm in 24 hrs
Mumps	None

18. Using the above information, calculate serum transferrin using Equations 4-21 and 4-22.

19. Calculate the total lymphocyte count (TLC)

20. Fill in the following form:

	Normal	Patient's value
Serum albumin		
Serum transferrin		
White blood cells		
Total lymphocyte count		

21. Evaluate the patient's visceral protein status.

Somatic Protein

The *creatinine-height index* (CHI) is occasionally used as a biochemical method for assessment of somatic protein. Creatinine is released from muscle tissue at a relatively constant rate; therefore, urinary creatinine is proportional to muscle mass.

In this method, a 24-hour urine collection is necessary. The urine sample is analyzed for creatinine, and the creatinine content is compared to the expected creatinine excretion in a man or woman of the same height. The expected excretion is obtained from a table (see Table F-12).

The creatinine-height index is calculated with the following equation:

$$\% \text{ CHI} = \frac{\text{Actual 24-hr creatinine excretion}}{\text{Expected 24-hr creatinine excretion for height}} \times 100$$

(4-24)

Various standards have been established for interpretation. One of these is given in Table F-7. Results are not valid in patients with acute renal dysfunction, amputations, advanced age, or fever, or who eat a high-meat diet or take steroids, methadone hydrochloride, tobramycin sulfate, or Mandol.

The expense and potential inaccuracy of the 24-hour urine collection have reduced the frequency of use of these methods in favor of the measure of arm muscle circumference.

CLINICAL EVALUATION OF PROTEIN-ENERGY MALNUTRITION

Clinical findings indicating protein-energy malnutrition (PEM) generally occur when the deficiency is advanced and already evident by the methods just described. Clinical evaluation of nutritional status is summarized in Table F-13.

Clinical findings in PEM may include the following:

    decreased head circumference
    dry, wiry, brittle, sparse, depigmented, and easily pluckable hair
    hypertrophy of fungiform papillae of tongue
    possible parotid gland enlargement
    bilateral edema in legs and feet
    growth retardation and fat loss

The existence of these conditions may not be diagnostic of nutritional deficiency; other disorders associated with these conditions are also listed in Table F-13.

Conversely, the diet history sometimes provides evidence of nutrient deficiency or excess. When this is the case, certain clinical conditions may occur; these are listed in Table F-14.

OVERALL EVALUATION OF PROTEIN AND ENERGY NUTRITIONAL STATUS

Assessment may determine current status or predict risk factors.

Evaluation of Current Status

Patients may be evaluated to be normally nourished or to be depleted of protein, energy, or both to a mild, moderate, or severe degree. Indications for each type of deficit are as follows:

Evaluation of Risk Factors

Calculations of energy and nitrogen balance may be used to predict risk of malnutrition, to measure the severity of deficits, and to evaluate the adequacy of intake. These calculations are therefore useful for planning therapy.

Energy Balance. Protein nutrition must be considered in concert with an estimate of energy expenditure. Basal energy expenditure (BEE) may be calculated from anthropometric data using the Harris and Benedict equations (7):

$$\text{For men}\quad BEE = 66 + 13.7W + 5H - 6.8A \quad \textbf{(4-25)}$$

$$\text{For women}\quad BEE = 655 + 9.6W + 1.7H - 4.7A \quad \textbf{(4-26)}$$

where W = body weight in kg, H = height in cm, and A = age in years.

In order to more accurately assess total energy expediture and, thus, the maintenance energy needs of patients, factors must be included for activity and injury. Activity factors are as follows:

1.2	for patient confined to bed
1.3	for ambulatory patients
1.5–1.75	for most normally active persons
2.0	for extremely active persons

Injury factors are as follows:

1.2	for patients who have undergone minor surgery
1.35	for patients with skeletal trauma
1.44	for patients who have undergone elective surgery
1.6–1.9	for patients with major sepsis
1.88	for trauma plus steroids
2.1–2.5	for patients with severe thermal burns

The total daily energy expenditure (TDE) for a male would thus be obtained from this adaptation of equation 4-25:

$$TDE = (66 + 13.7W + 5H - 6.8A)(AF)(IF) \quad \textbf{(4-27)}$$

where AF = the activity factor and IF = the injury

			Indicators		
Type of deficit	Body weight	Body fat	Somatic protein	Serum protein	Immune function
Energy (Marasmus)	Decreased	Decreased	Decreased	Moderate or Normal	Decreased
Protein (Kwashiorkor)	Decreased	Normal	Normal	Decreased	Decreased
Protein-energy (Marasmic kwashiorkor)	Decreased	Decreased	Decreased	Decreased	Decreased

factor. For example, a male ambulatory patient's total maintenance energy need following elective surgery would be estimated as follows:

$$TDE = (66 + 13.7W + 5H - 6.8A)\,(1.3)\,(1.44)$$

Similarly, if the patient were female:

$$TDE = (655 + 9.6W + 1.7H - 4.7A)(1.3)(1.44)$$

Estimates of current or future energy needs may be used for several purposes:

1. to evaluate current intake relative to need
2. to plan for future nutritional support
3. to plan weight-reduction diets

This formula might be used, for example, to plan support of a patient currently of normal weight who is to undergo major surgery.

If the patient is already underweight, an additional factor must be used to compensate for that loss.

Nitrogen Balance. Two procedures are useful in estimating nitrogen balance in clinical situations.

Normally, adults are in nitrogen balance—that is, nitrogen balance is approximately zero. Negative nitrogen balance is an abnormal condition, occurring when protein breakdown exceeds formation. Individuals in persistent negative nitrogen balance are at risk of developing protein malnutrition. Positive nitrogen balance occurs during growth in children, during pregnancy, and in wound healing. The goal in nutritional support of the depleted patient is a positive nitrogen balance of 4 to 6 g/day. A preliminary estimate of requirement *for anabolism* is sometimes obtained by using 1.2 to 1.5 g protein/kg actual body weight. This should then be adjusted as will be described next.

Calculations based on nitrogen excretion: Urinary urea nitrogen (UUN) may be used to estimate a patient's nitrogen balance. Like CHI, the use of this method is limited by the need to collect a 24-hour urine sample. The results are sometimes of particular value to the nutritional care specialist, however, so it is important to understand the method.

Step 1: UUN is measured in an aliquot from a 24-hour urine sample.

Step 2: Use the concentration of UUN and the 24-hour urine volume to calculate the total UUN per day using the equation

$$Total\ UUN = \frac{(UUN)\ (urine\ volume)}{100} \quad \textbf{(4-28)}$$

where total UUN is in mg, urinary UUN is in mg/dl, and urine volume is in ml.

Step 3: Estimate the patient's protein intake for the day. (See the next chapter if you did not learn how to do this in your Normal Nutrition course.)

Step 4: Calculate the patient's nitrogen balance (ΔN) using the equation:

$$\Delta N\ (g/day) = \frac{Protein\ intake}{6.25} - (UUN + 4) \quad \textbf{(4-29)}$$

where 6.25 converts protein intake to nitrogen intake (since protein is 16 percent nitrogen); protein intake and UUN are given in grams; and 4 represents grams of nitrogen excretion by routes other than urinary, plus urinary nitrogen other than in urea.

Here is an example: A patient has a protein intake of 62.5 g/day and a urinary excretion of 500 mg/dl UUN in 2,000 ml of urine.

$$UUN = 500 \times 2,000/100 = 10,000\ mg\ or\ 10\ g$$

$$\begin{aligned}\Delta N\ (g/day) &= \frac{62.5}{6.25} - (10.0 + 4) \\ &= 10.0 - 14.0 \\ &= -4.0\end{aligned}$$

Thus, current protein intake is inadequate and should be increased to allow for current needs plus repletion.

Calculations based on estimated energy requirement: Nitrogen balance may also be estimated by comparing a patient's intake with a calculation of estimated need.

Procedure

Step 1: Obtain an estimate of the patient's energy needs as described in equation 4-27.

Step 2: Estimate desired ratio of kcal/g of dietary nitrogen. This varies with the patient's condition and will be discussed in later chapters. For the present, use 150:1 for anabolism and 200:1 for maintenance.

Step 3: Calculate the nitrogen requirement from the following equations:

$$N\ required\ (g) = \frac{kcal}{kcal:N\ ratio} \quad \textbf{(4-30)}$$

For example, assume a patient's estimated energy need is 2,250 kcal/day, and her needed kcal/nitrogen ratio is estimated to be 150:1. Nitrogen need is estimated to be

$$N\ required\ (g) = \frac{2,250}{150} = 15\ g\ nitrogen$$

Step 4: Using this equation, calculate the amount of protein which would contain 15 g nitrogen:

$$Pro\ (g) = Nitrogen\ (g) \times 6.25 \quad \textbf{(4-31)}$$

In our example, the needed 15 g nitrogen would be supplied in 15 × 6.25 = 95.75 g protein.

OTHER INDICATORS OF NUTRITIONAL STATUS

A number of other biochemical tests are used to evaluate the patient's status related to nutrients other than protein and energy when circumstances indicate that

TO TEST YOUR UNDERSTANDING

22. A female patient is 40 years old and is 5 feet, 3 inches tall, with a heavy frame. She has lost 25 pounds in the last 2 months and now weighs 130 pounds. Other assessment values for this patient include the following:

TSF	24.0 mm
MAC	24.5 cm
WBC	4,000 (25% lymphocytes)
DCH	3 mm induration in 48 hours for two antigens of three tested
Serum albumin	3.0 g/dl

How would you evaluate this patient's nutritional status? Explain your reasoning.

23. List procedures for assessing
    a. Somatic protein
    b. Visceral protein
    c. Cell-mediated immunity

24. A male patient, age 62, is 5 feet, 10 inches tall and weighs 150 pounds. He has a protein intake of 70 g/day. The patient is confined to bed with multiple bone fractures.
    Laboratory results include the following:

UUN	600 mg/dl
Urine volume	1,950 ml
Serum sodium	138 mEq/L
BUN	9.9 mg/dl
Blood glucose	100 mg/dl

    a. Calculate the patient's basal energy expenditure (BEE).
    b. Calculate the patient's total daily energy expenditure (TDE).
    c. What is the patient's nitrogen balance?
    d. How would you interpret these results?

25. How might the patient's nitrogen balance and energy expenditure be interrelated?

these values are necessary. Although these tests are less frequently used, they are helpful in certain clinical situations, some of which will be demonstrated in coming chapters.

HEMATOLOGICAL ASSESSMENT

The purposes of hematologic assessment are as follows:

1. to detect the presence of anemia and characterize its type
2. to detect related nutritional deficiency, if any
3. to indicate appropriate nutritional intervention
4. in selected patients, to screen for excess alcohol intake (sometimes indicated by megaloblastic anemia secondary to folate deficiency)

Iron deficiency can result not only from insufficient intake but also from impaired absorption, increased loss, or increased requirements.

The initial screening for anemia usually includes hemoglobin (Hgb) and hematocrit (Hct) or packed cell volume (PCV). *Hematocrit* is the proportion of the total volume of blood that is blood cells. Normal values are given in Table F-15. In addition, the number of red blood cells are counted and reported as the number per mm^3 (see Table E-1). These values will appear in the patient's medical record when a CBC, or complete blood count (see Table E-11), has been ordered. This is a routine procedure upon hospital admission.

The blood cells may be examined under a microscope and classified according to

Size: microcytic (small); normocytic (normal); or macrocytic (large)
Color: hypochromic (pale) or normochromic (normal)
Shape: normocytosis (homogeneous, normal shape) or poikilocytosis (irregular in shape)

Additional calculations, sometimes reported in the medical record, include the following:

Mean corpuscular volume (MCV) indicates the size of the red blood cell.

$$MCV\ (\mu^3) = \frac{Hct \times 10}{Number\ of\ RBC\ (millions\ per\ mm^3)} \quad \textbf{(4-32)}$$

Results are often recorded as femtoliters (FL). MCV is increased in megaloblastic anemia and reduced in microcytic anemia.

Mean corpuscular hemoglobin (MCH) indicates the Hgb content per cell. MCH is obtained with this equation:

$$MCH\ (pg) = \frac{Hgb\ (g/dl) \times 10}{Number\ of\ RBC\ (millions\ per\ mm^3)} \quad \textbf{(4-33)}$$

Results may be given in picograms (pg). A low value would be found if cells were hypochromic. MCH is low in iron deficiency since the RBCs are small. It is high in megaloblastic anemia since the RBCs are larger.

Mean corpuscular hemoglobin concentration (MCHC) indicates the Hgb content per volume of RBC. A low value is obtained when Hgb is decreased more than is Hct. MCHC is obtained with the following equation:

$$MCHC\ (\%) = \frac{Hgb\ (g/dl)}{Hct} \times 100 \quad \textbf{(4-34)}$$

Normal values are given in Table F-15.

In iron-deficiency anemia, MCV, MCH, and MCHC are low. In the macrocytic anemias of vitamin B_{12} or folate deficiency, they may be high or normal. A patient with both a macrocytic and microcytic cause for anemia, such as both a folate deficiency and an iron deficiency, may have normal indices because the effects have averaged out, but the cell morphology will be mixed.

Other values used in evaluation of nutritional anemias are serum iron, folate, and vitamin B_{12} and transferrin saturation. Guidelines for evaluation are given in Table F-15. Since anemia may be caused by other conditions, data for differential diagnosis are given in Table F-16.

TO TEST YOUR UNDERSTANDING

26. Mr. L.'s medical record gives the following data:

Hgb	10.0 g/dl
Hct	35%
RBC	4.6 million/mm³

    a. What is this patient's MCV? (Show your calculations and compare to normal values.)

    b. What is this patient's MCH? (Show your calculations and compare to normal values.)

    c. What is this patient's MCHC? (Show your calculations and compare to normal values.)

    d. A preliminary screening by your assistant reveals that the patient has very limited variety in his diet. You suspect that his diet may be deficient in iron or folate. What nutritional assessment test would help distinguish between these two possibilities and what results would you expect in each case?

    e. You plan to interview Mr. L. in greater depth concerning his previous diet. What foods would you question him about in some detail?

    Iron sources?

    Folate sources?

HYDRATION STATUS

Serum osmolality may be estimated to give an indication of the patient's hydration status.

Procedure

Step 1: Obtain values for serum sodium, blood urea nitrogen (BUN), and blood glucose concentrations from the patient's medical record.

Step 2: Calculate serum osmolality using the equation

$$Serum\ osmolality = (2 \times Serum\ Na) + \frac{BUN}{2.8} + \frac{Blood\ Glucose}{18} \quad \textbf{(4-35)}$$

where serum osmolality is in mOsm/kg, serum Na is in mEq/L, and blood glucose and BUN are in mg/dl.

Interpretation

Normal values = 275–295 mOsm/kg for adults and 270–285 mOsm/kg for children.

Variations from normal are usually the result of changes in serum sodium concentration. Osmolality and the significance of its value in relation to specific diseases will be discussed further in later chapters. At low concentrations, such as in body fluids, osmolarity and osmolality are approximately the same. In high concentrations, they differ. The significance of these differences will be discussed in Chapters 12 and 13.

TO TEST YOUR UNDERSTANDING

27. a. Explain how, in Equation 4-35 for serum osmolality, the values for sodium can be given in mEq and the values for glucose and urea in mg, yet the result is in mOsm.

b. Why are mEq of Na doubled?

28. a. Estimate the serum osmolality in a patient whose laboratory values are as follows:

Na	138 mEq/L
BUN	9.24 mg/dl
Blood glucose	90 mg/dl

b. Interpret your results.

IDENTIFICATION OF RISK FACTORS

Even individuals who are currently well nourished can be at risk of developing malnutrition. Nutritional assessment must include recognition and documentation of nutritional risk. You will need to be able to recognize conditions that interfere with intake, digestion, absorption, or utilization of nutrients, as well as conditions that increase nutrient losses or requirements. In addition to specific diagnoses, the nutritional specialist must consider the effects of medications and other treatments, poverty, age, dental health, and normal developmental stresses, including infancy, adolescence, pregnancy, and lactation. These will be discussed in the chapters which follow. Thus, the material in this chapter will apply throughout the remainder of this book.

TOPICS FOR FURTHER DISCUSSION

1. Differentiate a "screening" from an "in-depth" nutritional assessment. What data would constitute a "screening assessment"?

2. How often should nutritional status be assessed? Which procedures should be used?

3. Discuss the advantages and disadvantages of using each of the following as the standard by which a patient's body weight is evaluated:
a. Standard reference weight of a person of the same height, sex, and age
b. Desirable body weight of a person of the same height, sex, and age
c. The patient's usual weight

4. Compare the relative advantages and disadvantages of using standard values and percentiles as the basis for interpretation of anthropometric data.

5. What are hemosiderin, sideroblasts, and reticulocytes? What is their significance in nutritional assessment?

6. It has been suggested that tests of function can be useful in nutritional assessment. Discuss possible tests and their uses and limitations.

REFERENCES

1. CHUMLEA, W.C., A.F. ROCHE, AND D. MUKHERJEE. *Nutritional Assessment of the Elderly Through Anthropometry.* Columbus: Ross Laboratories, 1984.
2. MILLER, M.A. A calculated method for determination of ideal body weight. *Nutr. Supp. Serv.* 5(3):(1985)31–33.
3. KHOSLA, T. AND C.R. LOWE. Indices of obesity derived from body weight and height. *Brit. J. Prev. Soc. Med.* 21:122–167.
4. DURNIN, J.V.G.A. AND M.M. RAMAHAN. The assessment of the amount of fat in the human body from measurements of skinfold thickness. *Brit. J. Nutr.* 21:(1967)681–689.
5. HEYMSFIELD, S.B., C. McMANUS, J. SMITH, V. STEVENS, AND D. W. NIXON. Anthropometric measurement of muscle mass: Revised equations for calculating bone-free arm muscle area. *Am. J. Clin. Nutr.* 36:(1982)680–690.
6. FRISANCHO, A.R. New norms of upper-limb fat and muscle areas for assessment of nutritional status. *Am. J. Clin. Nutr.* 34:(1981)2540–2545.
7. HARRIS, J.A. AND F.G. BENEDICT. *Biometric Studies of Basal Metabolism in Man.* Washington: Carnegie Institute, 1919.

ADDITIONAL SOURCES OF INFORMATION

GRANT, A. *Nutritional Assessment Guidelines,* 2d ed. Seattle: Ann Grant, 1979.

HEYMSFIELD, S. B., C. B. McMANUS III, S. B. SEITZ, D. W. NIXON, AND J. S. ANDREWS. Anthropometric assessment of adult protein-energy malnutrition. In *Nutritional Assessment,* eds. R. A. Wright and S. Heymsfield. Boston: Blackwell, 1984.

JENSEN, T. G., D. M. ENGLERT, AND S. J. DUDRICK. *Nutritional Assessment: A Manual for Practitioners.* Englewood Cliffs, N.J.: Prentice-Hall, 1983.

KARKECK, J. M. *Assessing the Nutritional Status of the Elderly.* Baltimore: American Society for Parenteral and Enteral Nutrition, 1985.

Nutritional Assessment, eds. R. A. Wright, S. Heymsfield, and C. B. McManus III. Boston: Blackwell, 1984.

5

Evaluating the Patient's Diet

An important part of a comprehensive nutritional status evaluation is the assessment of the patient's nutrient intake and identification of risk factors affecting intake. This chapter will be limited to those methods most frequently used in evaluating the diets of individuals, rather than of groups or populations.

The most commonly used procedure consists of three steps. (1) Information is obtained on the intake of food and fluid and on factors affecting this intake. This step usually requires the use of interviewing techniques you learned in Chapter 3. (2) The nutrient content of the foods specified is determined. (3) These results are then compared with the patient's nutrient requirements. Each of these steps will be described in turn, and you will be given an opportunity to use these methods.

In addition to evaluation of nutritional status and identification of risk factors, the information obtained by these methods is also used in planning for nutritional care and evaluating its effectiveness. These procedures are described in subsequent chapters.

METHODS FOR COLLECTING INTAKE INFORMATION

The methods of collecting information vary in their accuracy and ease of use. Only those that are practical in clinical situations will be described here.

24-HOUR RECALL

The 24-hour recall is one of the easiest methods for collecting information on the patient's intake, but the method is prone to important errors. It consists essentially of obtaining information on food and fluid intake for the previous day or for the previous 24 hours and is based on the assumption that the intake described is typical of daily intake. The information is usually obtained by interviewing the patient or a family member. Interviewing skill (see Chapter 3) can im-

prove the accuracy of the information obtained, but the interviewer should be aware of the following sources of error and seek to avoid them if possible:

1. The patient may not be able to recall the foods eaten. It is often helpful to base questioning on the sequence of activities, beginning with questions such as "What time did you get up in the morning?" "What did you eat first?" and then proceeding methodically in similar fashion through the next 24 hours. Alternatively, you might start with the present and work back through the previous 24 hours. There is a tendency to forget snack foods, fruits, and gravies and sauces in particular, but skillful questioning can jog the patient's memory on these as well as other points.

2. The patient may not be able to estimate the *amounts* of each food eaten. It is helpful to have food models or illustrations of usual portion sizes on hand to provide a basis for comparison.

3. The information given may not be sufficiently specific without skillful questioning. A list of some of the types of information that are needed to provide greater accuracy is given in Table 5-1.

4. The patient may not be telling the truth. The interviewer must be careful not to suggest the answers expected and must not appear judgmental.

5. The intake during the previous 24 hours may not be typical. The patient should be asked about this and, if necessary, questioned about a more typical day's intake.

Many institutions have a form suggesting the line of questioning and providing space for recording information. Form A is an example.

FOOD-FREQUENCY QUESTIONNAIRE

The food-frequency questionnaire is often used in combination with the 24-hour recall. It provides a list of foods or food groups, and the patient answers with information on the frequency with which the food is eaten. Common choices of answers are *never, rarely, occasionally,* or *frequently*. When these terms are used, it

TABLE 5-1.   Checklist for Diet Records

Type of Food	Information Needed
All	Portion size: cups? bottles? cans? length, width, thickness, diameter, shape compared to a model?
Milk and nondairy substitutes	% fat? powder? liquid? evaporated? dairy or nondairy substitutes? type of fat? added sweetening? unsweetened? chocolate?
Eggs and egg substitutes	Fresh? Frozen? Size? How prepared? Added fat? milk? other? Powder? liquid? frozen? Brand?
Meat, fish, poultry	Cut? fat trimmed? bone in or out? cooked weight? How prepared? Added fat, amount, kind? % fat (ground meat)? Source (animal, fish, poultry)? Oil or water pack (fish)? Skin eaten (poultry)?
Vegetables	Cooked or raw? Fresh, frozen, canned? Added sauce or fat? Kind of fat or sauce? Size of serving?
Fruit and juice	Cooked or raw? Fresh, frozen, canned, dried? Sweetened? Heavy, medium, light syrup? Unsweetened? Size of serving (piece or cup)?
Cereals	Ready-to-eat? Cooked? Brand? Additions, such as raisins, sugar, milk? How much? Size of servings?
Baked products	Homemade or commercial? Brand? From scratch or mix? Single or double crust (pie)? Meringue, frosting, topping? Yeast or quick bread (sweet rolls, muffins, and so on)? Dimensions of servings? Weight or number (crackers)?
Fats and oils	Margarine: Major oil? Stick, tub, squeeze, or liquid? Brand? P/S ratio? Diet? Whipped? Oil and shortening: Brand? Major oil? Solid? Salad dressing: Homemade or commercial? Type of oil or brand name? Creamy? Clear? Additions (cheese, bacon)?
Mixed dishes	Homemade: Ingredients and amounts? Cooking methods? Commercial: Brand? Cooking method?
Gravies and sauces	Type of fat? Amount? Liquid, milk or other? Other additions? Amount used?
Soups	Broth or milk base? Type of milk? Principal ingredients?
Beverages	Diet, low-cal, sweetened? Brand? Caffeine or decaf? Added sugar, milk, cream? Cola or noncola? Alcohol content? Type of alcoholic beverage? Amount?
Snacks and candies	Brand? Size? Weight?
Restaurant meals	Name of restaurant? Price range?

is important to define very specifically the terms *occasionally* and *frequently*. In order to avoid this problem, some forms give the choices *never, daily, weekly, monthly,* and *less than monthly.*

The foods on the questionnaire may be listed in a few broad categories or may be categorized in more detail to provide a larger number of groups and more precise definition. For example, a simple grouping might consist of the following four categories: meat and meat substitutes, milk and milk products, fruits and vegetables, breads and cereals. In a more detailed listing, the fruit and vegetable group might be subdivided into deep green and leafy vegetables, dark yellow fruits and vegetables, other vegetables, potatoes, legumes, and others. In any case, the food-frequency questionnaire does not provide information on quantities, but it is useful for checking the accuracy of the 24-hour recall. The form may be general, including all food groups, or it may be specialized for certain categories of patients, providing information on intake of specific nutrients. For example, a special form inquiring about intake of foods containing appreciable amounts of protein, sodium, potassium, and fluid might be used when interviewing patients with certain forms of renal disease. Form B is an example of a general food-frequency questionnaire.

FOOD DIARY

It is sometimes useful to have the patient keep a record of food and drink intake for a specified period. Three days, often two weekdays and one weekend day, are most commonly used. A longer period is necessary if the daily food intake is highly variable because it will take more time to obtain an overview of the patient's usual intake.

OBSERVATION OF FOOD INTAKE

Direct observation of food intake may be practical for hospitalized patients or individuals in residential facilities, and it may be required for those unable to provide the necessary information. Very frequently, information on a patient's total energy intake is required. This "calorie count" is obtained by observing the difference between the amounts served on the patient's tray and the amount not eaten. The protein content of the diet eaten is usually also reported.

NUTRITION HISTORY

The nutrition history is used to collect information on the general pattern of food intake and on other factors influencing the patient's food habits. It is a much more thorough and comprehensive procedure and usually includes a 24-hour recall, a food frequency list, and an extensive interview, as well as a thorough reading of the patient's medical record. A list of factors that may be considered is shown in Table 5-2. It should be obvious from the length of the list that obtaining a nutrition history is time-consuming. In addition, it tends to overestimate food intake. You can see that many of the factors to be considered are included in Forms A and B. This procedure will detect risk factors not evident with more abbreviated methods.

FORM A

University Medical Center
24-Hour Recall Form

Patient's name _____   Date _____
Level of activity _____
Person responsible for shopping? _____
Food preparation? _____
Dentition (circle one)   Normal; Dentures, partial or complete; Edentulous

_____

List of food eaten yesterday
Wake-up time? _____   Is this usual? _____

Time	Where eaten	Food	Description	Amount

Was this day typical?
If not, why not?
How much salt do you add to your food at the table?
Do you take vitamins?
What kind and how much?
Are there foods you do not eat because of religious beliefs?

TO TEST YOUR UNDERSTANDING

1. During your interview with a patient, she lists the following items eaten the previous day. In order to make the 24-hour recall as accurate as possible, list the further information you would seek on each item, *exclusive of* serving size.

Coffee
Cornflakes
Chicken salad sandwich
Milk
Canned peaches
Filet of sole
Toast
Mashed potatoes
Buttered broccoli
Tossed salad

2. If a patient mentioned the following items, suggest some procedures you might use to increase the accuracy of the patient's estimate of portion size. (Use your ingenuity and imagination. You will not find the answers in this volume.)

   Pork chop
   Fruit juice
   Buttered frozen peas
   Cooked breakfast cereal

3. Revise the following questions or statements to improve the interviewing technique and increase the accuracy of the information obtained. Explain your reasons for the changes you make. (Consult Chapter 3 if necessary.)
   a. "What kind of vegetable did you have with your steak dinner?"
   b. "Now that we have information on your breakfast, tell me what you had for lunch."
   c. "Do you drink this much beer every day?"

4. Which methods of collecting information on food intake would you choose for each of the following? Why?
   a. Mr. M., a traveling salesman, was admitted this morning for elective minor surgery. He is alert and cooperative. His surgery is scheduled for tomorrow.
   b. Mrs. B., a homemaker, is seen in the outpatient clinic. She is suspected of having a food allergy, but the allergens have not been identified. The symptoms appear at random intervals, sometimes days apart.
   c. Susan L., age 3, and her mother were involved in an automobile accident. Susan has two fractured legs. Her mother is in a coma with head injuries.

FORM B

University Medical Center
Food-Frequency Checklist

Patient's name _____   Date _____

How often do you consume the following foods?

Food	Servings per day	Servings per week	Seldom	Never	Food	Servings per day	Servings per week	Seldom	Never
Beef, hamburger					Potatoes				
Pork, ham					Dried beans, peas				
Bacon									
Liver					Fruit or juice, citrus				
Lamb									
Veal					Other				
Lunch meat					Tomatoes				
Poultry					Dried fruit				
Fish					Margarine				
Shellfish					Butter				
Cheese (type)					Cooking fat/ oil				
Milk (type)									
Yogurt					Salad dressing				
Ice cream					Salt pork				
Ice milk					Cream (type, % fat)				
Bread (type)									
Cereal (type)					Fried foods				
Pasta (type)					Nuts				
Baked goods (type)					Seeds				
					Sprouts				
Dark green vegetables					Snack crackers				
					Chips				
Dark yellow vegetables					Candy				
					Soft drinks				
Other vegetables					Coffee (decaf?)				
					Tea				
					Alcohol (type)				

Are there other foods not listed that you eat regularly?

_____

_____

TABLE 5-2. Information Obtained from a Nutrition History

1. Economics
   a. income—frequency and steadiness of employment
   b. amount of money for food each week or month and individual's perception of its adequacy for meeting food needs
   c. eligibility for food stamps and cost of stamps
   d. public aid recipient?
2. Physical activity
   a. occupation—type, hours/week, shift, energy expenditure
   b. exercise—type, amount, frequency (seasonal?)
   c. sleep—hours/day (uninterrupted?)
   d. handicaps
3. Ethnic or cultural background
   a. influence on eating habits
   b. religion
   c. education
4. Homelife and meal patterns
   a. number in household (eat together?)
   b. person who does shopping
   c. person who does cooking
   d. food storage and cooking facilities (stove, refrigerator)
   e. type of housing (home, apartment, room, etc.)
   f. ability to shop and prepare food
5. Appetite
   a. good, poor, any changes
   b. factors that affect appetite
   c. taste and smell perception and any changes
6. Allergies, intolerances, or food avoidances
   a. foods avoided and reason
   b. length of time of avoidance
   c. description of problems caused by foods
7. Dental and oral health
   a. problems with eating
   b. foods that cannot be eaten
   c. problems with swallowing, salivation, food sticking
8. Gastrointestinal
   a. problems with heartburn, bloating, gas, diarrhea, vomiting, constipation, distention
   b. frequency of problems
   c. home remedies
   d. antacid, laxative, or other drug use
9. Chronic disease
   a. treatment
   b. length of time of treatment
   c. dietary modification—physician prescription?, date of modification, education, compliance with diet
10. Medication
    a. vitamin and/or mineral supplements—frequency, type, amount
    b. medications—type, amount, frequency, length of time on medication
11. Recent weight change
    a. loss or gain
    b. how many pounds, over what length of time
    c. intentional or nonvolitional
12. Dietary or nutritional problems (as perceived by patient)

Reproduced with permission from Krause, M. V. and L. K. Mahan. *Food, Nutrition, and Diet Therapy* (7th ed.). Philadelphia: 1984.

ESTIMATING NUTRIENT CONTENT OF THE DIET

Once you have information on the patient's food intake, you must translate this information into an estimation of the amount of each nutrient under consideration that those foods contain. The method you choose will depend on the degree of precision you require. If, for example, the patient is the subject of a research program, it may even be necessary to have a chemical analysis of an aliquot of the food. In most clinical situations, however, such precision is impractical and unnecessary. The methods more commonly used are more approximate but faster and thus less expensive in labor cost.

CALCULATION WITH EXCHANGE LISTS

Instead of detailed calculations, diets may be evaluated using an appropriate food-grouping system. Such a system is established by grouping together foods that are similar in nutritive value and, to some extent, their use in the meal. The use of food groups is based on the assumption that eating appropriate amounts of foods in each group will provide proper amounts of protein, calcium, iron, and the vitamins A, ascorbic acid, thiamine, riboflavin, and niacin. It is further assumed that if a wide variety of foods within the groups are consumed, the other nutrients will be obtained in sufficient quantities.

A number of these grouping systems are available, and several are useful in clinical situations. One of those most commonly used in an initial diet assessment is described here. Others, used in planning modified diets, will be described in later chapters.

The most commonly used grouping is based on lists of foods called *exchanges* (1). It is assumed that all foods in an exchange list have approximately the same content of protein, fat, and carbohydrate, and thus can be "exchanged" one for another without making a substantial alteration in the average nutrient intake. The lists of exchanges were originally established for use in diets for diabetic patients, but have since been found useful for other purposes. The protein, fat, and carbohydrate content of each exchange list is given in Table C-1, and foods included in each list are given in Tables C-2 to C-8. Additional values which are sometimes useful when the exchanges are used for diet evaluation for nondiabetics include the following:

1 t (teaspoon) sugar	contains	5.0 g carbohydrate
1 t jam or jelly	contains	5.0 g carbohydrate
1 serving fruit in heavy syrup	contains	50.0 g carbohydrate
1 serving sweetened gelatin dessert (5 servings/pkg)	contains	1.6 g protein, and 15.0 g carbohydrate

In addition, values expressed as exchange lists for combination foods are given in Table C-9. Table C-10 gives lists of food values for alcoholic beverages in terms of these same exchanges.

The protein, fat, and carbohydrate contents of a diet may be calculated using these values. For example, let us assume that a patient's daily intake consists of the following items:

Breakfast	Lunch	Dinner
½ grapefruit	½ c tomato jc.	4 oz roast beef
¾ cup (c) cornflakes	Cheese sandwich:	½ c mashed potatoes
½ c milk, skim	2 slices bread	½ c carrots
1 t sugar	2 oz cheddar cheese	Tossed green salad/
1 poached egg	½ c milk, skim	1 Tablespoon (T) French dressing
1 slice toast	1¼ c fresh whole strawberries	½ c fresh fruit
1 t butter		1 c milk, skim

This menu contains the following exchanges, summarized, with the protein, fat, and carbohydrate content indicated:

		Pro (g)	Fat (g)	CHO (g)
2	Milk exchanges (½ + ½ + 1)	16		24
2	Vegetable exchanges (½ c tomato, ½ c carrots)	4		10
3	Fruit exchanges (½ grapefruit, 1¼ c strawberries, ½ c fresh fruit cup)			45
5	Starch/bread exchanges (¾ c cornflakes, ½ c potatoes, 3 slices bread)	15		75
7	Meat exchanges (1 egg, medium fat; 2 cheese, 4 beef, high fat)	7 / 42	5 / 48	
2	Fat exchanges (1 t buter, 1 T French dressing)		10	
1	Other foods (1 t sugar)			5
1	Negligible food value (Tossed salad)	0	0	0
	TOTAL	68	63	159

The values obtained may be used to evaluate the adequacy of protein and energy intake. The adequacy of vitamin and mineral intake may be estimated by comparing with one of the guides described in the next section or by using the vitamin and mineral exchanges in Table B-1.

If you do not have information on common food sources of nutrients, it is important that you develop a store of this knowledge. In this and succeeding chapters, you will be given an opportunity to do so. The vitamin and mineral contents of major food groups are summarized in Table 5-3.

ANALYSIS FROM TABLES OF FOOD VALUES

Tables of food values may be used to calculate nutrient content of diets when more detailed information is necessary. This method is time-consuming when done manually but can be quite rapid when computer analy-

TABLE 5-3.   Vitamin and Mineral Content in Major Food Groups

Nutrient	Milk Group	Breads & Cereals Group	Fruits & Vegetables Group	Meat Group
Protein	x	x		x
Fat	x			x
Carbohydrate	x	x	x	
Thiamin		x	x	x
Riboflavin	x	x		x
Niacin	x	x		x
Folate	x	x	x	
Vitamin B$_{12}$	x			x
Ascorbic Acid			x	
Vitamin A	x		x	x
Vitamin D	x			
Calcium	x		x	
Iron		x	x	x
Fiber		x	x	x

sis is available. The values in the data base for the computer may be those from the United States Department of Agriculture's (USDA) Handbook 8 (2) or other currently available tables (3–5). Some patients eat large quantities of "fast foods." Detailed information on the nutrient content of fast foods can be obtained from the headquarters of the fast food franchise or from other published sources (3, 6). The more detailed food composition values have some specific uses in clinical situations:

1. for calculation of nutrient content of foods with greater precision than that provided by using exchange lists
2. for calculation of intake of nutrients not included in exchange lists—for example, the vitamins and minerals
3. to provide information on nutrient content of foods not included in exchange lists—for example, the nutritional value of a variety of baked desserts
4. as a source of information on food sources of a specific nutrient—for example, the best food sources of riboflavin.

EVALUATING THE ADEQUACY OF THE DIET

Once the nutrient content of the patient's intake is determined, the nutritionist must evaluate the adequacy of the intake compared to the patient's nutritional requirements.

COMPARISON WITH THE RECOMMENDED DIETARY ALLOWANCES

The Recommended Dietary Allowances (RDA) may be used when it is necessary to evaluate the intake of many nutrients. For your convenience, the RDA from the Food and Nutrition Board of the National Research Council (7) is given in Tables A-1 to A-3. The Canadian standards (8) are given in Table A-4.

When you are using the RDA (7), it is important to

keep in mind several facts that you should remember from your courses in Normal Nutrition:

1. The recommendations are set at a level to provide for the needs of most members of the population group, *not for specific individuals*; they therefore exceed requirements of many individuals (except for the energy requirement).
2. On the other hand, the recommendations are designed to apply to healthy populations and do not cover special needs. Thus, the nutritionist must apply professional judgment when evaluating patients' diets compared to these recommendations. An individual who does not receive the amounts recommended each day is not necessarily malnourished. On the other hand, those with increased needs may be deficient even if recommended amounts are obtained. Conditions in which special needs occur will be described in the chapters which follow.

TO TEST YOUR UNDERSTANDING

5. You are asked to report a patient's protein and kcal intake. After observing her food intake and the uneaten food on her tray, you compile the following list of foods which she ate in one day. Using the exchange lists in Appendix C, calculate the values requested and show your calculations on Form C.

½ c orange juice
¼ c farina
½ c skim milk
coffee
1 t sugar
2-egg omelet
1 t margarine
½ whole-wheat roll
2 t butter

FORM C

University Medical Center
Summary of Daily Nutrient Intake

Food Group	No of Exchanges	PRO g	FAT g	CHO g
Starch/Bread exchanges				
Milk exchanges (Circle non-fat, low-fat, or whole)				
Fruit exchanges				
Vegetable exchanges				
Meat exchanges (Circle low, medium, or high fat)				
Fat exchanges Other				
TOTAL g		_____	_____	_____

Kcal = _____ g protein × 4 = _____
_____ g fat × 9 = _____
_____ g carbohydrate × 4 = _____
_____ TOTAL kcal

tea with lemon
1 c bouillon
6 saltines
5 oz chicken (no bone or skin)
½ c green beans
1 large tomato, sliced
1 T French dressing
½ c ice cream

6. In the menu given in the previous question, what are the major sources of

    calcium?
    iron?
    ascorbic acid?
    thiamine?
    riboflavin?
    niacin?
    vitamin A?

7. A patient tells you that she ate the following foods at a meal:

3 oz lean hamburger, broiled
½ c cooked frozen green beans
1 large tomato, sliced
1 T French dressing
½ c ice cream

    a. Using Form D, calculate the nutrient content of these foods using any extended food-value table (2–5). Calculate only those nutrients listed on the long method part of Form D.

FORM D

Diet Analysis—Long Method

Food	Amount	Kcal	Protein (g)	Ca (mg)	Fe (mg)	Vitamin A (IU)	Thiamin (mg)	Riboflavin (mg)	Niacin (mg)	Ascorbic acid (mg)
Ground beef	3 oz									
Cooked green beans	1/2 c									
Tomato	1 large									
French dressing	1 T									
Ice cream	1/2 c									
	TOTAL									

Exchange Lists (Appendix C)

Food	Amount	Kcal	Vitamins & minerals	Protein (g)	Fat (g)	Carbohydrate (g)
Ground beef	3 oz					
Cooked green beans	1/2 c					
Tomato	1 large					
French dressing	1 T					
Ice cream	1/2 c					
	TOTAL					

b. Calculate the protein, fat, and carbohydrate content and caloric value of these foods using the exchange lists given in Appendix C. List the predominant vitamins and minerals contained in these foods. Use the lower part of Form D.

c. How do the results obtained with the two methods compare?

8. Given the degree of accuracy of the information obtained in a 24-hour recall and the time required for calculation, which method do you think is most likely to be useful and practical in most clinical situations?

9. You interview a 22-year-old male patient who is hospitalized for tooth extraction. He is in good health with body weight 5 percent below normal for his height. Your analysis of the patient's 24-hour recall indicates that he has an intake of ascorbic acid which is 10 percent below the RDA. Give your evaluation of his diet.

10. Six months later, you see the same patient. He has been in a motorcycle accident and has multiple fractures. You know that his injuries result in an increase in his metabolic rate.

a. What effect would the healing process have on his ascorbic acid requirement?

b. Assuming his diet had not changed in the 6 months prior to his injuries, what effect would his injuries have on the adequacy of his diet in kcals? ascorbic acid?

11. Write a SOAP note concerning the adequacy of the patient's diet to meet his present needs.

COMPARISON WITH THE DAILY FOOD GUIDE

It is not usually necessary to evaluate the patient's intake in great detail. Instead, if the patient can eat normal foods and does not have a condition that markedly increases nutrient needs, it is often sufficient to compare the intake with one or more of the "food guides" provided for consumer education. A number of variations of this guide, known as the *Daily Food Guide* (9), are available. Known commonly as the "Basic Four," it was originally designed to help consumers make wise food choices and may be used clinically as the basis for a very rough estimate of diet adequacy.

The Daily Food Guide has been criticized for 3 failings:

1. It does not ensure a nutritionally adequate diet.
2. It does not address the current dietary problems of our population, such as overweight, excess dietary sodium, and excess cholesterol.
3. It is not an effective and efficient communication tool (10).

As a result, various suggestions have been made for alterations. In 1979, the USDA issued a revision of the Basic Four which made changes to focus more attention on micronutrients. The revision also added a fifth group, "Fats, Sweets, Alcohol" (11). The addition of this fifth group recognizes the place of these items in menu planning and their contribution to the energy content of the diet. Others have suggested alterations that provide (1) choices in the milk group to provide an equivalent amount of calcium and (2) choices in the meat group to provide an equivalent amount of protein. A chart indicating one version of current adult recommendations for the United States and the Canadian recommendations is given in Table 5-4. Varia-

tions of these recommendations for pregnant and lactating women and for children are given in Chapters 7 and 8, respectively. Detailed lists of serving sizes are given in Appendix Table I-1.

Depending on specific choices within each group, the Guide provides about 1,200 kcal and about 80 percent of the recommended allowances of other nutrients. It is assumed that the additional energy and other nutrients will be provided by more and larger servings of the items in the meat, milk, fruit-vegetable, and cereal groups, as well as by fats and unlisted foods.

A 24-hour recall can be evaluated by comparing its contents with the items on one of these guides. This system has been criticized as superficial and insen-

TABLE 5-4. Daily Food Guide*

Food Group	Recommended Number of Servings	
	United States	*Canada*
Milk and milk products	2	2
Protein foods†	2	2
Animal protein	(1)	
Legumes and/or nuts	(1)	
Fruit & Vegetable	4	4–5
Ascorbic acid–rich	(1)	(1)
Dark green‡	(1)	(1)
Other	(2)	(2–3)
Whole grain or enriched cereal products	4	3–5

*Additional foods are needed for energy. At least one tablespoon/day of fat or oil is recommended.

†May include animal or vegetable sources of protein.

‡Include a minimum of one serving 3 times per week.

sitive; however, a study of the results of this method compared to results of the use of an abbreviated food-composition table demonstrated that scoring with a food guide was sufficiently sensitive to dietary adequacy (12). For the general population, even if foods from all groups are included, deficits in iron, zinc, magnesium and vitamins B_6, E, and folate may exist. Menus following the *Daily Food Guide* may be high in sodium, cholesterol, and saturated fats and low in fiber. When adequacy of the diet for a patient with abnormal needs is being assessed, this method is less applicable and must be used with caution.

COMPARISON WITH CALCULATED REQUIREMENTS

As discussed in Chapter 4, estimates of an individual patient's nutritional requirements may be calculated. This estimate may then be used as a basis for evaluation of the patient's intake. For example, let us assume that a patient's intake is 1,250 kcal and 70 g protein, but the calculated total daily energy expenditure (TDE) is 1,550 kcal with a 70 g protein requirement. It should be clear that the patient needs supplementation of her energy intake.

TO TEST YOUR UNDERSTANDING

12. Ms. J. C. gives you the following 24-hour recall, which she says is typical of her daily diet.

Breakfast:
½ c orange juice
1 fried egg
1 slice white toast, buttered, enriched
coffee, black

Lunch:
1 tuna fish salad sandwich (enriched bread)
Sliced tomatoes with French dressing
1 fresh peach
1 c milk

Dinner:
1 c beef stew with vegetables
½ c spinach
⅛ head lettuce wedge/Thousand Island dressing
½ c serving of cherry cobbler
1 c milk
Tea with lemon

a. Does this day's intake contain all the food groups recommended by the *Daily Food Guide?* If not, what is lacking?

b. Ms. J. C., age 48, is 5 feet, 8 inches tall and weighs 110 pounds. What would you conclude about the adequacy of her diet?

c. Is your conclusion in question B confirmed if you calculate the energy content of the diet using the exchange lists? (Show your calculations.)

REFERENCES

1. *Exchange Lists for Meal Planning.* Washington, D.C.: American Diabetes Association, and Chicago: American Dietetics Association, 1986.

2. *Composition of Foods.* Agricultural Handbooks No. 8-1 to 8-9. Washington, D.C.: Consumer and Food Economics Institute, USDA, 1976–1982.

3. PENNINGTON, J.A.T. AND H.N. CHURCH. *Bowes and Church's Food Values of Portions Commonly Used,* 13th ed. New York: Harper & Row, 1980.

4. UNITED STATES DEPARTMENT OF AGRICULTURE, SCIENCE AND EDUCATION ADMINISTRATION. *Nutritive Value of Foods.* Home and Garden Bulletin No. 72. Washington, D.C.: USDA, 1981.

5. LEVEILLE, G.A., M.E. ZABICK, AND K.J. MORGAN. *Nutrients in Foods.* Cambridge, Mass.: Nutrition Guild, 1983.

6. YOUNG, E.A., E.H. BRENNAN, AND G.L. IRVING. Update: Nutritional analysis of fast foods. *Dietetic Currents* 8(2):(1981)1–12.

7. FOOD AND NUTRITION BOARD, NATIONAL RESEARCH COUNCIL. *Recommended Dietary Allowances,* 9th rev. ed. Washington, D.C.: National Research Council, 1980.

8. COMMITTEE FOR REVISION OF THE CANADIAN DIETARY STANDARD, BUREAU OF NUTRITIONAL SCIENCES, HEALTH AND

WELFARE, CANADA. *Dietary Standards for Canada,* rev. ed. Ottawa: Information Canada, 1975.

9. FOOD AND NUTRITION SERVICE, AGRICULTURE RESEARCH SERVICE. *A Daily Food Guide.* FNS-13 Rev. July 1975. Washington, D.C.: USDA, 1975.

10. LIGHT, L. AND F.J. CRONIN. Food guidance revisited. *J. Nutr. Educ.* 13:(1982)57–62.

11. UNITED STATES DEPARTMENT OF AGRICULTURE, SCIENCE AND EDUCATION ADMINISTRATION. *Food.* Home and Garden Bulletin No. 228. Washington, D.C.: USDA, 1979.

12. GUTHRIE, H.A. AND J.C. SCHEER. Validity of a dietary score for assessing nutrient adequacy. *J. Am. Dietet. Assoc.* 78:(1981) 240–245.

6

Counseling the Patient

Dietary counseling consists of transferring data and skills from counselor to patient in order to effect dietary change. Just as the interview *gathers* data, counseling *gives* data (information).

For many years, education of the patient meant the teacher's recitation of facts, under the assumption that the learner automatically converted those facts into usable skills. A more effective approach to education utilizes teaching techniques which transfer information in such a way that the learner masters useful skills. This chapter describes these teaching techniques and emphasizes those which work especially well under conditions in which time for counseling is limited.

GOALS OF COUNSELING

Just as the goals of interviewing were explained in Chapter 3, goals of counseling must also be examined. Here, the emphasis is on *the patient* and the actual skills *the patient* is able to achieve.

BEHAVIORAL OBJECTIVES

A revolution took place in education in the 1960s. Teachers began to write down and use statements that specified *exactly* what the learner was expected to do during, and at the end of, instruction. These statements became known as *behavioral objectives*. The reason for their success can be summarized easily: Behavioral objectives finally made clear the *precise* expectations of instruction and learning. When they were written down, both the instructor and the student began working toward the same goals. Additionally, the writer of the objectives divided large behaviors into smaller, teachable tasks. Lessons then contained only information that was necessary to the successful mastery of the individual tasks and, eventually, of the overall behavior. In fact, in the POMR described in Chapter 2, the care plan is almost always stated in terms of measurable, patient-oriented behavioral objectives.

OBJECTIVES AS MENTAL IMAGES

Objectives provide *mental images* for instructor and learner. These images so clearly define an action that it is possible for the learner to visualize and reproduce those actions.

This is perhaps easiest to understand when you consider the teaching of a motor skill. Suppose the objective of a tennis lesson describes the action "holding the racket." In order to achieve this skill—correct holding of the racket—the learner must be able to "see" mentally the expected performance. The statement of objective should be worded in such a way as to tell the learner clearly what that mental picture ought to be. It might read as follows:

> The tennis player will hold the racket in his right hand with the thumb parallel to the shaft and with the remaining fingers beside one another in a firm clasp around the outside of the shaft.

From this statement, even the reader who has never played tennis should be able to approximate the action mentally. It is the clarity of the described behavior which makes behavioral objectives useful to both teacher and learner. In this example, would the learner get the same mental picture if the statement read "The tennis player will hold the racket firmly"? If this truly represented the desired skill, then the tennis instructor would have to accept as perfect *any* way the learner held the racket as long as it was firm.

Similarly, in dietary counseling, objectives function to alert the patient to the expectations of the instruction. Research has verified improved learning and consequent behavior change of learners who knew what skills they would be expected to master.

Consider the objective: The patient will follow a balanced diet. Think about the mental images conjured by this objective. Each patient given this statement could rightfully picture any one of many possible actions. A more useful wording of this objective might be "The patient will plan a well-balanced diet including foods from all essential food groups in portions to meet energy and nutrient needs."

TO TEST YOUR UNDERSTANDING

1. In each pair of objectives below, circle the one which provides the learner with the best mental image of its action.

    a. (1) The learner will inject a sample of saline, in lieu of insulin, by measuring the correct amount into a syringe, preparing the injection site, and injecting the saline subcutaneously at the site.

        (2) The learner will inject saline subcutaneously.

    b. (1) The patient will acknowledge the importance of eating a balanced diet during the course of her pregnancy.

        (2) The patient will describe in her own words the importance of eating a balanced diet during pregnancy.

    c. (1) The client will select from a given assortment of foods those foods that he likes to eat that are allowed in the low-sodium diet.

        (2) The client will understand which foods are low-sodium foods.

    d. (1) The patient will be able to tell her physician about her diet.

        (2) The patient will be able to tell her physician how following her diet will affect her symptoms and general health.

FORMULATING BEHAVIORAL OBJECTIVES

After analyzing a task and writing objectives for a particular set of actions, a counselor begins to discern the basic, or *core*, objectives associated with the desired behavior.

Objectives which sequentially build to diet planning are listed in Table 6-1. Most dietary counselors agree that these skills form the basis for almost all normal and therapeutic dietary instruction. After mastery of these skills, a learner may move to the additional skills listed in Table 6-2. Remember to picture mentally the learner's action described by the statement.

Note that these additional skills all require mastery of the core behaviors before true accomplishment could be expected. Trying to counsel about label reading before the patient has mastered at least skills 2 and 3 from the core list, for example, would be futile. Yet counselors often attempt to race through the core and additional behaviors because they think the patient should immediately absorb the material!

On the other hand, remember that behaviors the patient has already mastered do not have to be repeat-

TABLE 6-1. Examples of Core Objectives

1. The patient will classify an assortment of foods into appropriate groups as defined by the diet prescription.
2. The patient will identify foods allowed and not allowed in each food classification according to the diet prescription.
3. The patient will select appropriate portion sizes for foods within the diet prescription.
4. The patient will plan a diet menu according to his preferred foods within the dietary prescription.

TO TEST YOUR UNDERSTANDING

2. Which of the following behavioral statements is a "core" skill for counseling a client on a low cholesterol diet? Which are "additional" skills that the patient might learn after mastering the core actions? Place a C (core) or A (additional) next to each objective.

_____ a. The patient will identify preferred high-cholesterol foods and preferred low-cholesterol foods.

_____ b. The patient will describe the way in which fat is digested in the stomach and small intestine.

_____ c. The patient will plan one day's food intake, not to exceed a total prescribed cholesterol intake of 60 g.

_____ d. The patient will prepare a low-fat gravy, using only beef drippings and flour.

TABLE 6-2. Examples of Additional Objectives

1. The patient will prepare a shopping list which includes both preferred foods and those foods contained within the dietary modification.
2. The patient will modify several favorite recipes to comply with the restrictions of the prescribed diet.
3. The patient will plan food selections for special or unusual situations within the limitations of the dietary prescription.
4. The patient will read nutrient labels as a basis for selection or rejection of packaged food items.

ed. When the assessment interview revealed that Ms. A., for example, is already able to identify the allowed and not-allowed foods in the prescribed diet, there is no point in reteaching it, even though it is a core skill. Ms. A. now moves on to portion sizing if that is the stage at which she no longer has skill mastery according to the information gained in the interview.

INFORMATION CONTROL

Most of the time, patient instruction contains too much "stuff"—that is, too much explanation, data, facts, material. It is often difficult for beginning nutritionists to sort through the vast amount of data and information learned in the pursuit of their careers. Because assimilation of this material was necessary to make the nutritionist an expert, however, it is extremely difficult to sacrifice any of it in the interest of successful dietary counseling. When too much extraneous material is provided, though, the instruction is ineffective because learners do not have the ability to extract the important facts from the total poured out to them by the well-meaning nutritionist. Nonessential data, no matter how interesting or well presented, does little to ensure skill attainment and often confuses the learner about what is essential.

ESSENTIAL AND NONESSENTIAL INFORMATION

Information supplied to the patient may be classified as "nice-to-know" or as "need-to-know." Any material that does *not* relate to the precise objective (nonessential) is *nice-to-know*. Facts and information that provide the basis for the accomplishment of the specified skill (essential) is *need-to-know*.

To the distress of many nutrition counselors, the history, technology, and, often, the *why* of a subject must be construed as nice-to-know. For example, the *history* of the kidney dialysis machine is often included in instructions to newly diagnosed renal patients. The history of hospital policy regarding treatment of a particular disease is sometimes made part of dietary instruction. Unless the objectives of counseling include knowing the history of the diet or the disease, this information should be eliminated. This nonessential information is confusing and wasteful of valuable counseling time.

The *technology* of an apparatus or concept is also nice-to-know. For instance, an elaborate explanation of the way in which supplemental vitamins are manufactured, or an explanation of the heat-conducting properties of aluminum versus stainless-steel cookware is nice-to-know. While these topics sound as if they might be obviously extraneous, many diet instructions include such discussion.

Perhaps most difficult to understand from a nutritionist's viewpoint is why the rationale behind dietary instructions is often nonessential to learners who are pursuing skills that will help them modify their diet. Long, complex descriptions of why a drug works the way it does or why sugar causes the pancreas to produce insulin or why iron and ascorbic acid interact with one another are usually unnecessary. These topics, while interesting to the nutritionist, occupy time that might be better spent in discussion and activities that lead the *patient* to behavioral competence in making dietary changes.

Cutting out potentially interesting but irrelevant information demands serious contemplation and exacting care. The time limits imposed on regular institutional dietary counseling make every second valuable. If nice-to-know conversation is using that time, then the need-to-know material necessary for mastery of useful skills is lost, with the consequence that the patient is too confused and overwhelmed to adhere.

Separating nice-to-know information from need-to-know often leaves the counselors with the feeling that their expertise is being compromised and that there was much more that could have been explained to the patient. Such a feeling stems partly from being an "expert" in nutrition and dietetics and partly from believing that simply hearing a volume of information on a topic stimulates motivation and learning. The research no longer supports this concept. It is the counselor who must delineate the content of the instruction, limiting the transferred information to that which exactly fits the tasks that the patient must accomplish both in the course of the instruction and later, when independent of the care setting. Reducing discourse to meet the patient's needs will be the most difficult aspect of dietary counseling the newly trained nutritional care specialist will face.

INFORMATION AS A MOTIVATOR

The concept that knowing why or understanding the rationale for a dietary instruction is motivating has not been substantiated by research. In fact, giving a complicated explanation of why at the beginning of a counseling session may have the opposite effect—it may reduce motivation! Since learners are usually not well informed on the topics under discussion in the counseling, they cannot easily assimilate the concepts described in the explanation of rationale, especially when given early in the instruction. Only *after* discussion of the need-to-know topics (those directly related to the objectives) is a summary which includes a statement about why an action is important or appropriate.

As a matter of fact, if left to the end of the instruction, the learner can tell the instructor why, and *that* is motivating. The patient's being able to generate a reason for the importance of a regimen or behavior is highly motivating because the reason originates in the head of the learner.

TO TEST YOUR UNDERSTANDING

3. For each stated objective, identify (underline) the topics that are essential for a learner to have been taught in order to fulfill the objective.

   a. Objective: The patient will identify foods allowed and not allowed on the 2-g-sodium diet.
   Possible Discussion Topics:
   Physiological function of sodium
   Food items allowed and not allowed
   History of the 2-g-sodium diet
   Differences between a 500-mg-sodium diet and a 2-g-sodium diet

   b. Objective: The patient will select appropriate portion sizes for foods within the dietary prescription.
   Possible Discussion Topics:
   Portion size of each food on the list
   Portion size of foods patient eats that are on the list
   The number of grams and ounces in a serving of each food
   Ways to decrease portions when served incorrect amounts
   Explanation of differences between various scales and measuring instruments

4. For each objective, identify (underline) the topics the learner must be taught to complete the objective.

   a. Objective: The patient will describe the relationship between his diet and his disease condition.
   Possible Discussion Topics:
   Physiological and biochemical basis of the disease
   Cellular processing of the nutrients in question
   Patient's symptoms and their relationship to diet control
   History of the disease in the United States
   Other similar disease conditions

   b. Objective: The patient will plan a selection of foods for dinner from a restaurant menu.
   Possible Discussion Topics:
   The restaurant menu itself
   Explanation of every food on the menu
   Comparison of this restaurant with others
   Explanation of foods the patient might select from the menu
   How to ask a restaurant to modify a menu item to fit the diet prescription

LEARNER PERFORMANCE

Now that the instructional session has been drastically altered by eliminating much of the superfluous input, what will occupy the time during which the counselor and patient are together? The time *should* be spent in *organized* interaction between patient and counselor in which the patient practices the skills suggested by the objectives. If a patient is expected to select foods from a restaurant menu, then that is exactly what the patient must practice in the counseling session. In fact, it is learner performance which education researchers believe bridges the mental gap between *receiving the information* and *applying the skill.*

Think about it. How many times do people repeat behaviors about which they are uncertain? Perhaps a daredevil might try skydiving without first practicing the process safely by jumping off a two-foot ledge, then a ladder, then a small ledge over sand, then finally something simulating the real event. All those practices enable the skydiver to demonstrate mastery of each small task leading to the overall action called skydiving. What has education investigators so interested in this concept is that it works for mental skills like planning as well as for motor skills like skydiving. If a counselor expects a patient to plan a day's food intake, then the only true practice of that skill is planning that menu right there in the counseling session or as an assignment that can be completed away from the session and returned.

HOW PERFORMANCE CONTRIBUTES TO LEARNING

When learners practice skills during the counseling session, the counselor can provide full support and feedback about the success of the attempts, and learners gain *competence* in their independent performance of the same or similar tasks will be correct. Competent learners repeat behaviors. Learners who are skeptical about their ability to perform a skill successfully do *not* repeat and are therefore not adherent with prescribed treatment.

What does it take to include practice activities in a counseling lesson? First, it is necessary to have a precise objective or objectives in mind, as they clarify for the instructor and learner the behavior to be practiced. Simulation, role play, dramatization, or any other constructed opportunity must then be presented to learners for their response. For example, suppose the objective for a group of second-grade children is "Each child will make a sack lunch which contains at least one food that he or she likes from each of the basic food groups." There are many activities that would enable the youngsters to practice putting together a lunch. For example, each child might be given a small brown bag and three or four food pictures. The children could move around the room trading pictures with one another until each child had four items, each a food they liked and each representing one of the basic food groups. Another age-appropriate activity would be to have the children bring bag lunches from home which contained three out of four food groups; they could then trade food items until each child had the full representation of groups. However, an activity in which the children simply colored food pictures would not help them practice the behavior called for in the objective.

For another example, suppose your adult patient's objective is to be able to select a low-sodium meal from a restaurant menu. You might give the patient a sample menu from a popular restaurant and ask for selections that represent foods she would actually eat that are low in sodium. Or, you might first ask the patient to identify what she usually selects when she goes out to dinner, and then ask her to analyze the meal for high- and low-sodium foods. In either case, the learner would be performing meaningful interactive behaviors to and observable demonstrations of dietary activities.

TO TEST YOUR UNDERSTANDING

5. Check the most appropriate practice activity for each of the following objectives:

a. Objective: The patient will prepare a shopping list using foods within the dietary modification.

_____ Possible Practice 1: Patient reads a label aloud.

_____ Possible Practice 2: Patient describes her favorite supermarket.

_____ Possible Practice 3: Patient writes down foods to be purchased that are not now available to her at home.

_____ Possible Practice 4: Patient reads a grocery list prepared by the counselor.

b. Objective: The patient will classify an assortment of foods into the Exchange Lists.

_____ Possible Practice 1: Patient sees a movie about Exchange Lists.

_____ Possible Practice 2: Patient places food models, one by one, into appropriate groups.

_____ Possible Practice 3: Patient uses hospital menu to select a breakfast that fits the dietary modification.

_____ Possible Practice 4: Patient tells his spouse how important it is to follow the diet.

c. Objective: The patient will tell her physician how the prescribed diet affects her symptoms and disease.

_____ Possible Practice 1: The patient reads a pamphlet on the disease.

_____ Possible Practice 2: The patient talks with someone who has the same condition.

_____ Possible Practice 3: The patient plans a menu using the foods allowed on the diet.

_____ Possible Practice 4: The patient role-plays with the counselor what she will relate to the physician about her diet and symptoms.

PLANNING LEARNING ACTIVITIES

The counselor must keep in mind the question, What can the patient *do* with the information just presented that will provide practice using it? Similarly, the patient must be *doing* something to demonstrate successful acquisition of the behavior at each step of the instruction. This means that the counseling session consists of equal counselor-client interaction. No longer should an education session be 99 percent instructor and 1 percent learner. In fact, a successful session may become so interactive that the patient does most of the work!

In summary, it should be obvious by now that learners must *work* during instruction if they are to succeed. Perhaps the first benefit is the clear demonstration of learning which the counselor and learner share during an interactive session. When learners practice skills, either by verbalizing a response or by actually doing the behavior, the two partners in the process gain immense satisfaction from the activity. The learner's satisfaction gives him the competence to repeat the behaviors at home, and the counselor responds to the interaction by recognizing the uniqueness of this learner and his performance as compared with the last and the next learners. The process thus motivates both the practitioner and the recipient!

REINFORCEMENT

In Chapter 3, reinforcing statements were used to acknowledge the existing behaviors the patient identified during the interview. The same type of reinforcement can increase the learner's confidence about performance of a particular practice activity or overall performance during instruction. When the patient performs an activity well, the instructor is provided with an opportunity to respond with accolades about the success of the performance. Just as reinforcing words enhanced confidence during the interview process, these same recognizing statements build confidence to repeat successfully practiced behaviors. For example, when a patient has made a breakfast selection that meets the dietary modification, the counselor can stop at that time and say to the client, "That was well done. You have made selections that not only fit exactly with your diet, but also are items you said you enjoy eating." These statements of support become attached in the learner's mind to the successful behavior and thus reinforce the confidence the learner needs in order to repeat the behavior without the aid of the instructor.

TO TEST YOUR UNDERSTANDING

6. For each objective below, create an appropriate practice activity, describing what the patient will do to practice and what materials he will use to do it.

   a. Objective: The patient will select a well-balanced bedtime snack, using foods from at least three of the four basic food groups.

   b. Objective: The patient will select appropriate portion sizes for foods in the Bread Exchange.

   c. Objective: The patient will plan a holiday meal using foods allowed on the low-sodium diet.

7. Create a reinforcing statement for each of the following actions. Use words that are comforting and reassuring.

   a. The patient successfully places ten food items into the allowed and not-allowed categories.

   b. The patient verbalizes the key concept of the diet modification and asks a very relevant question about the diet.

   c. The patient tells her spouse why it is important for her to modify her diet and includes the relief of symptoms in her explanation.

ORGANIZING COUNSELING

Counseling endeavors should proceed according to a planned sequence of activities. The plan might look like the one presented in Table 6-3. Note that by proceeding through each activity, the counselor is reminded to incorporate those techniques that enhance motivation and increase adherence. The techniques described in the table should by now be familiar to you.

SUMMARY

Counseling is interacting. The counselor presents only essential information and organizes activities that enable the learner to perform the required skills. Counseling asks learners to be involved, as opposed to teaching in the traditional sense, which expects learners to absorb as much information as possible in the allotted time. Counseling calls for the instructor to be very clear about expected outcomes and to share those outcomes with the learner. Counseling produces *successful, competent* patients who know how to modify their diets because they have practiced the behaviors during their counseling sessions.

TABLE 6-3. Counseling Steps

1. Interview patient. (see Chapter 3)
2. Chart. (see Chapter 2)
   a. Identify problem(s).
   b. Prepare care plan; state objectives.
3. Counsel patient.
   a. State objectives for diet prescription.
   b. Control input (need-to-know only).
   c. Conduct performance activities.
   d. Reinforce patient performances and responses.
4. Chart progress.

TO TEST YOUR UNDERSTANDING

8. For each core objective, identify the need-to-know information necessary for the patient to complete the objective. Then create a practice activity that is appropriate to the behavior in the objective.

   a. The patient will explain the relationship between his 1-g-sodium diet and his hypertensive condition.

   b. The patient will classify an assortment of foods into appropriate groups as defined by the 1-g-sodium diet.

   c. The patient will identify foods allowed and not allowed on a 1-g-sodium diet.

   d. The patient will select portion sizes from each group based on allowances of the 1-g-sodium diet.

   e. The patient will plan a diet menu taking into account her preferred foods and foods allowed on the 1-g-sodium diet.

9. With the aid of the sequentially planned steps in Table 6-3, prepare a counseling session for a 33-year-old, 5-foot, 10-inch, 275-pound hypertensive male with a diet prescription of 1,800 kcal. The client tells you that he works as a traveling salesman, has minimal knowledge of the energy content of foods, lives alone, and eats lunch and dinner out almost every day.

   a. Identify two problems that will need special attention in counseling the client on this diet.

   b. State three behavioral objectives that will be part of your care plan. Include a practice activity for each objective.

   c. Now summarize your subjective and objective observations, assessment, and care plan in a SOAP note.

ADDITIONAL SOURCES OF INFORMATION

Bloom, B.S. *All Our Children Learning*. New York: McGraw-Hill, 1981.

Burks, H.M. and B. Stefflre. *Theories of Counseling* (3d ed.). New York: McGraw-Hill, 1979.

DiMatteo, M.R. *Achieving Patient Compliance: The Psychology of the Medical Practitioner's Role*. New York: Pergamon Press, 1982.

Gagne, R.M. and L.J. Briggs. *Principles of Instructional Design* (2d ed.). New York: Holt, Rinehart and Winston, 1979.

Compliance in Health Care, ed. R.F. Haynes. Baltimore: Johns Hopkins University Press, 1979.

Shortridge, R. *The Precepteur* (rev. ed.). Sacramento, Calif.: Dairy Council of California, 1982.

Snetselaar, L.G. *Nutrition Counseling Skills*. Rockville, Md.: Aspen Publications, 1983.

CASE STUDY I   NUTRITIONAL ASSESSMENT

TO THE LEARNER

This case study provides you with an opportunity to integrate and summarize the material and skills you learned in Chapters 1 through 6. Read the material given here carefully and use only the information given when forming your answers.

Mrs. C. is a 74-year-old woman who lives alone in a walk-up apartment. She has been a widow for two years and has no children. She has a very limited income. Mrs. C. was visited by the police when a neighbor reported that she had not been seen for several days. Finding her weak, bedridden, and unattended, the police brought Mrs. C. to the hospital emergency room, from which she was admitted to the Internal Medicine service.

For your initial nutritional assessment, the patient's medical record provided the following information:

Height	5 ft, 4 in
Present weight	100#
Serum albumin, g/dl	2.6
Total leukocyte count	4,000
Differential: Lymphocytes, %	25
Neutrophils, %	70
Eosinophils, %	1
Basophils, %	0.5
Monocytes, %	3.5
Total RBC count, × 10⁶/mm³	4.6
Hct, %	25
Hgb, g/dl	7.6

The in-depth nutritional assessment yielded the following additional information:

Triceps skinfold, mm	10.2
Midarm circumference, cm	20.4
Wrist measurement, in	6
Cell-mediated immunity in 48 hrs:	
SK/SD, mm	3.0

Mumps, mm	4.0
Candida, mm	2.5
Urinary urea nitrogen, g/24 hrs	6
Total iron-binding capacity, µg/dl	170

Mrs. C. has arthritis and poorly fitting dentures. She stated that she does not have "enough money to buy more food." In addition, she said she is afraid to walk alone to the supermarket, which is a mile away, and has no other means of transportation. Instead, she sometimes shops at a small convenience store nearby, where prices are higher. A neighbor occasionally brings her groceries. Mrs. C. further states that she has no allergies. She likes and is willing to eat any food except those that are too hard to chew, because of her ill-fitting dentures. She says that she weighed "about 125 pounds" for many years, but has been losing weight since her husband died.

Her typical intake, which you obtained in an interview, is represented by a 24-hour recall:

Breakfast	4 oz canned orange juice
	½ c oatmeal, 1 t sugar
	½ c evaporated whole milk
	Coffee, 1 t sugar
Lunch	1 c chicken broth with ½ c rice
	6 saltines
	1 oz sliced cold cuts
	1 slice white bread, enriched
	1 t butter
	Tea with 1 t sugar
	1 T evaporated whole milk
Supper	2 oz ground-beef patty
	½ c macaroni
	1 small banana
	Tea with 1 t sugar
	1 T evaporated whole milk

Mrs. C. said that she does not eat between meals and that food "doesn't have much taste any more." She reported that she takes one "multivitamin-with-iron tablet" daily, and takes "a lot" of aspirin for her arthritis. She denied taking any other medication, drinking alcoholic beverages, or smoking. There is no evidence of disease to account for her condition.

QUESTIONS

1. Using Form E, summarize Mrs. C.'s protein, fat, carbohydrate and caloric intake from the 24-hour recall. On the lower part of Form E indicate with an X the major vitamin and mineral content of foods listed in the 24-hr. recall. What nutrients are likely to be deficient in Mrs. C.'s diet?

FORM E

University Medical Center
Summary of Daily Nutrient Intake

Food Group	No. of Exchanges	PRO g	FAT g	CHO g
Starch/bread exchanges				
Milk exchanges (Circle non-fat, low-fat, or whole)				
Fruit exchanges				
Vegetable exchanges				
Meat exchanges (Circle low, medium, high fat)				
Fat exchanges				

Other

Total g _____   _____   _____

Kcal = _____ g protein   × 4 = _____
         _____ g fat   × 9 = _____
         _____ g carbohydrate × 4 = _____

_____ Total kcal

Food	Serving Size	Vit. A	Vit. C	Thiamin	Riboflavin	Niacin	Calcium	Iron

2. Your hospital uses Form F for recording the results of nutritional assessments. Fill in the form for Mrs. C.'s assessment, using the information given and *performing any necessary calculations*.

3. Explain the basis for your evaluation of nutritional status given at the end of Form F.

FORM F

University Medical Center Nutritional Assessment

Patient's Name _____

Sex (Circle one)   M   F   Date of Admission _____

Age: _____ Years   Date of Assessment _____

Height and Weight:

Height: _____ ft.   _____ in.   _____ cm

Body weight: On admission: _____ #   _____ kg

                        Current   _____ #   _____ kg

                        Usual   _____ #   _____ kg

                        Ideal   _____ #   _____ kg

                        Recent loss   _____ #   in _____ mos   _____ kg

                        % weight change _____ gain   or   _____ loss

Interpretation: Severely underweight   (20% < ideal)   _____
(Mark X where   Severely overweight (+20% > ideal)   _____
appropriate)   Unplanned weight change, > 10%   _____
                   Stable and within limits   _____

| *Somatic Protein* | | | *Mark X for interpretation* | | | |
Value Measured	Standard Value	Patient's Value	50th %ile	50th–15th %ile	15th–5th %ile	<5th %ile
TSF, mm						
MAC, cm						
MAMC, cm						

| *Visceral Protein:* | | | *Mark X for interpretation* | | | |
| | | | | *Deficit* | | |
Value Measured	Standard Value	Patient's Value	None	Mild	Moderate	Severe
Albumin, g/dl						
TIBC, ug/dl						
Total lymphocytes mm^3						

Cellular immunity, 48 hrs

    SK/SD _____   Interpretation:

    Mumps _____   Normal Reactivity _____

                                         Subnormal Reactivity _____

    Candida _____   Anergy _____

| *Hematological:* | | | *Mark X for interpretation* | | |
Value Measured	Standard Value	Patient's Value	Acceptable	Marginal	Deficient
RBC, × 10^6/mm^3					
Hct, %					
Hgb, g/dl					
MCV, FL					
MCH, pg					
MCHC, g/dl (%)					

Nutritional Status: (Mark X where appropriate)

_____ Normal

_____ Marasmus

_____ Kwashiorkor-like syndrome

_____ Combined Marasmus-kwashiorkor

_____

Diet Evaluation

Intake _____ kcal/24 hrs

_____ g protein/24 hrs

Nitrogen Balance: Positive _____ g

Negative _____ g

BEE = _____ kcal

Total Daily Energy Expenditure for Maintenance assuming patient is ambulatory = _____ × BEE = _____ kcal.

Recommended Intake

Energy: Oral anabolic requirement

BEE × _____ = _____ kcal

Protein: Oral anabolic requirement

kg actual body weight × _____ to _____ = _____ to _____ g protein.

kcal; g N = _____ ; N required = _____ g;

g N × 6.25 = _____ g.

---

4. a. Hematological data suggest that the patient has anemia which is (circle all that apply)

microcytic, normocytic, macrocytic

hypochromic, normochromic, hyperchromic.

b. Based on your calculations of hematological data in form F, a deficiency of _____ is suggested by depressed _____ and normal _____. The deficiency could be made more severe by _____ 2° to the high aspirin intake.

5. List 5 factors, *other than* the height, weight, and laboratory data, that suggest the patient is at nutritional risk.

6. For 3 of the factors listed in question 5, identify a goal and at least one measurable objective for each.

7. According to the problem list, problem 1 is primary malnutrition and problem 2 is degenerative arthritis. The attending physician has ordered "Diet as tolerated" and has asked for the dietitian's recommendation both for in-hospital feeding and for diet after discharge. Write the SOAP note you would record in the patient's medical record.

7

Nutrition During Pregnancy and Lactation

Adequate nutrition during pregnancy and lactation is extremely important to both maternal and fetal health (1). In this chapter we will discuss the monitoring of pregnancy, nutritional requirements for pregnancy and lactation, maternal nutritional assessment, and nutritional complications of pregnancy. You may wish to use one of the suggested references to provide additional background information.

MONITORING PREGNANCY

The normal human gestation period is approximately 40 weeks. Gestational age, or the maturity of a pregnancy, is calculated from the first day of the last menstrual period (LMP). The estimated date of delivery (EDD), ± 2 weeks, can be arrived at by using the following equation (2):

$$\text{EDD} = \text{1st day of LMP} - 3 \text{ months} + (1 \text{ year} + 7 \text{ days}) \qquad \textbf{(7-1)}$$

Detection of human chorionic gonadotropin (HCG) in urine is considered indicative of pregnancy. Commonly used urine tests for pregnancy are sensitive enough to detect HCG at levels normally found at 4 weeks from the LMP, or approximately 2 weeks after conception. A blood test is also available.

TERMINOLOGY

In obtaining information from the medical record, you will need to become familiar with specific terminology that is used to describe obstetrical history. *Gravidity* refers to the total number of pregnancies. A *primigravida* is a woman who is pregnant for the first time, and a *multigravida* is a woman who has been pregnant more than once. These may be written in the medical records as *gravida I* or *gravida II* for increasing numbers of pregnancies, or abbreviated as G_1 or G_2. *Parity* is the state of having given birth to an infant or

infants weighing at least 500 g or having an estimated gestational age of at least 24 weeks. A woman who has been pregnant 3 times, has 2 living children, and had a miscarriage at 12 weeks is described as G_3P_2, whereas a woman who has been pregnant 3 times and has 2 living children and one stillborn is G_3P_3. A current pregnancy is also included, so a woman pregnant for the first time is G_1P_0.

In addition to gravidity and parity, the number of *abortions* (Ab), either spontaneous or therapeutic, and *living children* (LC) are summarized in a woman's obstetrical history. An abortion or miscarriage occurs when a baby is lost prior to 24 weeks of gestation. A stillborn infant is born after 24 weeks of gestation. A nonpregnant woman who is $G_5P_4Ab_1LC_3$ has been pregnant 5 times, delivered 4 children weighing at least 500 g, lost 1 baby prior to 24 weeks gestation, either through miscarriage or abortion, lost another child in some way, such as accident or illness, and has 3 living children. The number of premature births, if any, is usually also noted.

ROUTINE PRENATAL CARE

For low-risk gravidas, the usual frequency of visits for prenatal care is monthly until 28 to 30 weeks, every two weeks until 36 weeks, and then weekly. Clinical data routinely obtained and recorded at these visits include gestational age, blood pressure, weight, presence of glucose or protein in urine, fetal heart sounds and movement, fetal presentation, and presence or absence of edema (3). In addition to these parameters, *fundal height,* or the distance from the top of the symphysis pubis to the top of the uterine fundus, is measured at prenatal visits. Fundal height in centimeters demonstrates a one-to-one correlation with gestational age after 16 weeks gestation and helps to confirm the EDD.

Nutritional education is a routine part of prenatal care, and, in general, pregnant women are highly motivated to follow health care advice. The setting and organization of prenatal nutritional education programs vary. Counseling may take place on an individual basis, in a classroom or group setting, using closed-circuit television or an interactive computer program, or via printed education materials. The nutritional care specialist should view maternal nutritional counseling as a special opportunity to impart nutritional information.

WEIGHT GAIN

The amount of weight gained, the components of that gain, and the general pattern of gain during gestation are important in nutritional assessment during pregnancy.

Amount

A 24- to 28-pound (11 to 13 kg) weight gain is recommended for the woman entering pregnancy at a normal weight. Improved pregnancy outcome is associated with a weight gain of 30 pounds in the underweight woman and a weight gain of 15 pounds in the obese woman (4). Table 7-1 summarizes recommendations for ranges of optimal weight gain for women who enter pregnancy underweight, overweight, or at a normal weight.

Components

Weight gain during pregnancy consists of the weight of the fetus and associated tissue, including the placenta, enlarged uterus, and amniotic fluid, plus the increase in weight of maternal tissue. The average weight gain is outlined in Table 7-2. Note that approximately half of the weight gain can be attributed to fetal tissue and half to maternal tissue. The increase in weight of various maternal tissues is needed for maintenance of pregnancy. Weight gain labeled as maternal stores is largely composed of increases in subcutaneous body fat, which is distributed over the abdomen, back, and upper thighs (5). The action of progesterone in the pregnant woman mediates the formation of this fat pad to serve as a calorie reserve for fetal growth and lactation. The pregnant woman can restrict weight gain to avoid development of the

TABLE 7-1. Weight Gains Associated with the Best Obstetrical Outcomes for Normal Weight, Underweight, and Overweight Pregnant Women

Weight Status at Conception	Weight Gain for Best Obstetrical Outcome	Range of Variation from Normal 27-Pound Gain
Normal weight	27 pounds	80% to 120%
Underweight	30 pounds	80% to 120%
Overweight	15 pounds	24% to 54%

Based on data from Naeye, R.L. *Am. J. Obstet. Gynecol.* 135:3, 1979.

TABLE 7-2. Average Composition of Pregnancy Weight Gain

Tissue	Weight (pounds)	
Fetus	7.5	
Placenta	1.0	Fetal = 13 pounds
Amniotic fluid	2.0	
Uterus*	2.5	
Breast tissue*	3.0	
Blood volume*	4.0 (1,500 ml)	Maternal = 11–15
Maternal stores	4.0–8.0	pounds
Total		24–28lb

Adapted from: Maternal nutrition and the course of pregnancy. NAS, 1970.

*Weight increase

fat pad, but this may also affect to some degree the normal development of the fetus.

Pattern of Weight Gain

The pattern of weight gain during pregnancy should be closely monitored by plotting the woman's incremental weights on a prenatal weight-gain grid, as shown in Figure 7-1. (The use of Figure 7-1 will be discussed in detail in the nutritional assessment section of this chapter.) The pattern of weight gain depicted

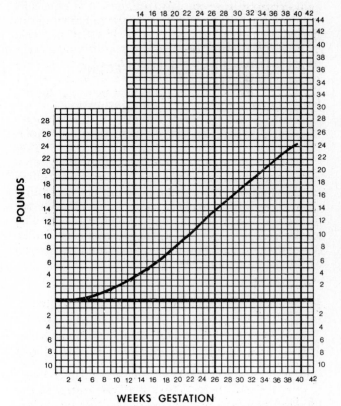

Figure 7-1 Pattern of normal prenatal weight gain.
(Adapted from *Clinical Obstetrics*. Philadelphia: Lippincott, 1953.)

TO TEST YOUR UNDERSTANDING

1. Define the following terms:
   a. Primipara
   b. Postpartum
   c. Antenatal
   d. Puerperium
2. You are working in a prenatal program associated with a clinic. You prepare to speak with a woman who has just received the results of a positive pregnancy test. The following information is noted in the medical record:
   $G_3P_1Ab_1LC_0$
   first day of LMP = 7/1/87
   present date = 9/1/87
   a. Describe the woman's obstetrical history.
   b. What is the approximate gestational age in weeks?
   c. What is the EDD?
3. A primigravida at 25 weeks gestation tells you that she is concerned about the extra fat around her thighs and back. She has decided to reduce her food intake because this extra fat has nothing to do with her baby's growth. How would you counsel this woman?

in Figure 7-1 is associated with the lowest incidence of preeclampsia, low birth weight, and perinatal mortality. This optimal pattern consists of little weight gain in the first trimester, usually a total of 2 to 4 pounds (1 to 2 kg), and then, during the second and third trimesters, a steady weight gain averaging 0.9 pounds (0.4 kg) per week. Because most of the fetal weight gain occurs during the last trimester, it is especially important to avoid restricting weight gain during this period.

FOOD-RELATED SUBSTANCES AFFECTING PREGNANCY OUTCOME

Excessive consumption of alcohol during pregnancy is associated with adverse effects on fetal development. Based on present data, total abstinence from alcohol is recommended during pregnancy (6).

Heavy caffeine intake (600 mg caffeine daily) during pregnancy is associated with increased reproductive loss and pregnancy complications, but there is no convincing human data to suggest that a moderate intake of caffeine affects pregnancy outcome (1). The current recommendation is for pregnant women to use caffeine in moderation (no more than 2 cups of a caffeine-containing beverage per day).

NUTRITIONAL REQUIREMENTS

Nutrient intake recommendations for pregnant, lactating, and nonpregnant adult women are given in the 1980 edition of the Recommended Dietary Allowances (7). The RDAs are listed in Appendix A.

PREGNANCY

The total energy cost of pregnancy is estimated to be approximately 80,000 kcal, which breaks down to an addition of 300 extra kcal per day above nonpregnant needs (7). Energy requirements increase minimally in the first trimester, but then increase and remain constant until term. Additional energy is required during the second trimester for expansion of maternal tissues—increase in blood volume, growth of uterus and breasts, and accumulation of fat stores. Additional energy needs in the third trimester reflect the growth of the fetus and placenta. Because of these differences in energy needs over the course of a pregnancy, the World Health Organization (WHO) recommends that energy intake be increased by 150 kcal per day during the first trimester and by 350 kcal per day during the second and third trimesters of pregnancy.

Requirements for protein, vitamins, and minerals substantially increase during pregnancy. Increased needs for protein (68 percent increase), folate (100 percent), calcium (50 percent) and iron (200 to 300 percent) deserve special attention when counseling pregnant women. The increase in energy needs is not large in comparison to requirements for other nutrients during pregnancy. Consequently, the *quality* of the diet must be very high during pregnancy. (Information on the vitamin and mineral content of foods can be found in Table B-1 and in Table 9-3.)

LACTATION

The production of high-quality milk is a major physiological priority during lactation. Women who consume diets that are inadequate in various nutrients or who have prolonged lactation still produce breast milk of *quality* similar to that of well-nourished women, although the *quantity* of milk may be small.

The fat and water-soluble vitamin content of human milk may vary depending on the mother's dietary intake. Consumption of a diet rich in vegetable oils will result in milk which contains a higher content of unsaturated fatty acids. Maternal dietary adequacy or inadequacy of the water-soluble vitamins is reflected in similar levels of these vitamins in the milk.

The lactating woman requires some nutrients at the same level recommended during pregnancy, others at a higher level because of energy needs and content of these nutrients in the milk being produced, and others at a lower level. Energy and fluid needs are increased to the greatest extent with lactation, compared to pregnancy. Fluid intake should increase by approximately one quart per day, to a total of 3 to 3.5 quarts of fluid per day, to provide for the production of approximately one quart of breast milk per day.

An additional 500 kcal per day is recommended during the first 3 months of lactation. This increase reflects average values for volume and efficiency of milk production. The 500-kcal-per-day recommendation is also based on the assumption that the pregnant woman will have stored 2 to 4 kg of body fat during pregnancy, and that during the first 3 months of lactation, these fat stores will provide 200 to 300 kcal per day, or about one-third of the energy cost of milk production. Thus, a gradual weight loss of 2 to 4 kg will occur after 3 months of lactation, permitting the mother to return to her prepregnant weight. Once prepregnant weight has been attained, 700 to 800 additional kcal per day may be needed to maintain weight during lactation. While these energy recommendations are based on sound data, recent observations suggest that current energy guidelines may overestimate energy needs during lactation (1, 8).

Because most compounds that enter the mother's body are secreted into breast milk, attention should be given to the mother's intake of drugs and alcohol and to her smoking habits (9).

PLANNING TO MEET NUTRITIONAL REQUIREMENTS

The Daily Food Guide (10) forms the basis for planning and evaluating adequate maternal dietary intakes (see Table 7-3). The Daily Food Guide was developed as a modification of the Basic Four Food Guide. In comparison with the 1980 RDAs, the Basic Four do not provide recommended amounts of magnesium, iron, zinc, vitamin B_6, and vitamin E. The Daily Food Guide encourages intakes of vegetable protein, especially legumes, dark green vegetables, and whole-grain breads and cereals, which are good sources of the nutrients shown to be limited in the Basic Four food groups.

The Daily Food Guide includes the following six food groups: (1) protein foods—animal and vegetable, (2) milk and milk products, (3) breads and cereals, (4) vitamin C–rich fruits and vegetables, (5) dark green vegetables, and (6) other fruits and vegetables. The content and portion sizes specified for these food groups differ from the ADA Exchange Lists and are shown in Appendix I. The Daily Food Guide empha-

TABLE 7-3. Daily Food Guide for Pregnancy and Lactation*

Food Group	Number of Servings		
	Nonpregnant Women	Pregnant Women	Lactating Women
Protein foods	2	4	4
Animal†	(1)	(2)	(2)
Vegetable‡	(1)	(2)	(2)
Milk and milk products	2	4	4–5
Breads and cereals§	4	4	4
Fruits and vegetables	4	4	4
Vitamin C-rich fruits and vegetables	(1)	(1)	(1)
Dark green vegetables	(1)	(1)	(1)
Other fruits and vegetables	(2)	(2)	(2)

*The Daily Food Guide meets the RDA for pregnancy for all nutrients except iron, folacin, and energy. Approximately 400 additional kcal are needed to meet energy needs. Daily supplementation of 30–60 mg iron and 400–800 µg folacin are recommended during pregnancy. In addition to the Daily Food Guide, 2 T (30 ml) of fats or oils should be included each day.

†One serving is 2 oz (60 g).

‡Should include at least 1 serving legumes.

§Whole-grain products should be emphasized to provide additional magnesium, zinc, folacin, and vitamin B_6.

sizes vitamin and mineral content within a food group rather than carbohydrate, protein, and fat content, which is a primary feature of the ADA Exchange Lists.

The Daily Food Guide meets the RDA for pregnancy for all nutrients except iron, folacin, and energy. In addition to the specified number of servings from the food groups, it is assumed that the dietary intake will also include at least 2 tablespoons of fats and oils daily. To achieve recommended energy intakes, approximately 400 additional kcal are needed daily.

NUTRIENT SUPPLEMENTATION

In order to meet the RDA for increased folacin and iron, daily supplementation of 400 to 800 µg folacin and 30 to 60 mg iron is recommended throughout pregnancy (7). For the first 3 months of lactation, supplementation with 30 to 60 mg iron should be continued to replete iron stores. A prenatal vitamin-mineral complex is usually recommended for pregnancy and lactation. Several brands of prenatal vitamin-mineral supplements are available. Most contain 30 to 60 mg iron as ferrous fumarate, 400 to 800 µg folacin, 200 mg calcium, and close to 100 percent of the pregnancy RDA for all other vitamins and minerals. Supplements containing only iron, folacin, or calcium are also available. Women with an intolerance to milk may benefit from calcium supplementation, especially in the last trimester, when the majority of the fetal skeleton is calcified. Iron supplementation is suggested for all pregnant women.

TO TEST YOUR UNDERSTANDING

4. a. Using the RDAs in Appendix A, list nutrients that are needed in increased and decreased amounts during lactation compared to pregnancy.

    b. Suggest why these changes in nutrient requirements occur when comparing lactation to pregnancy.

5. A woman has been exclusively breast-feeding her infant for 4 months. She has attained her prepregnancy weight and is continuing to lose weight.

    a. Explain the nature of the weight loss.

    b. What would you recommend to maintain present body weight?

6. The following questions refer to use of the Daily Food Guide.

    a. If a woman did not include any servings of vegetable protein in her diet, which nutrients would be likely to be available in marginal amounts?

    b. If vegetable protein foods were not included, how should the servings of animal protein be adjusted to provide the nutrients listed in question A?

7. Provide a list of foods that could supply a total daily intake of the following nutrients. (Use a handbook of food composition or consult Table B-1.)

    Iron—30 mg

    Calcium—1,200 mg

    Folacin—800 µg

NUTRITIONAL ASSESSMENT

Nutritional assessment during pregnancy includes an evaluation of pertinent clinical risk factors, and consideration of dietary, anthropometric, and biochemical data.

RISK FACTORS

Every pregnant woman needs an individual assessment of nutritional status. The assessment should begin with an examination of certain key nutritional risk factors, which will help to identify those women in need of in-depth nutritional guidance. These risk factors include a consideration of age, body weight, parity, previous reproductive performance, economic status, weight gain during pregnancy, preconception nutrition and social habits, and medical history (11). Table 7-4 gives an outline of the nutritional risk factors whose consideration will assist with the nutritional assessment of the pregnant patient. Form G is a sample nutrition questionnaire designed to elicit risk-factor information from the client (12).

Next, we will consider in more detail those dietary, anthropometric, and biochemical aspects of nutritional assessment that are pertinent to determining nutritional status during pregnancy.

DIETARY ASSESSMENT

The Pregnancy Diet Intake form (Form H) (10) is a tool by which to identify a patient's dietary pattern and to evaluate its nutritional adequacy by comparison to the Daily Food Guide. It should be completed, in addition to the Nutrition Questionnaire (Form G), during the initial prenatal visit.

The form has three major sections: daily food intake, influences on diet, and summary. In completing the daily food intake section, the interviewer may use either the 24-hour recall or the diet history. A description of how the food was prepared and served should be noted in the column headed "Food Eaten." Specific religious, social, or ethnic influences that may affect diet should be recorded under "Influences on Diet." In the "Summary" section, food eaten is transposed into serving(s) of the food groups as described in the Food Group Lists in Table I-1. The "servings eaten" are then totaled and compared with "servings needed"

TABLE 7-4. Nutritional Risk Factors During Pregnancy

Nutritional Risk Factors at the Onset of Pregnancy:
1. 18 years of age or less
2. Economically deprived (an income less than the poverty line or a recipient of local, state, or federal assistance, such as Medicaid or the USDA Food Programs, such as WIC)
3. Food faddism (ingestion of a bizarre or nutritionally restrictive diet)
4. Heavy smoking
5. Drug addiction
6. Alcoholism
7. Prepartum weight at first prenatal visit of <85% or >120% of standard weight
8. Multiple pregnancies (3 or more during the past 2 years)
9. History of poor obstetrical or fetal performance
10. Use of a therapeutic diet for chronic systemic disease

Risk Factors During Prenatal Care
11. Inadequate weight gain (any weight loss during pregnancy or gain <2 pounds (1kg) per month)
12. Excessive weight gain during pregnancy (>2 pounds, or 1kg, per week)
13. Low or deficient hgb/hct (low = hgb <11.0 gm, hct <33; deficient = hgb <9.5 gm, hct <30)

FORM G

Nutrition Questionnaire

Name _____ Date _____

Please answer the following by checking the appropriate box or filling in the blank. Answer only those questions which apply to you. All information is confidential.

			For Office Use Only

1. a. During your last pregnancy, how much weight did you gain?
   _____ # ☐ don't know
   b. How much weight do you expect to gain during this pregnancy?
   _____ # ☐ don't know
   c. Have you ever had any problems with your weight?
   ☐ yes ☐ no If yes, what? _____

2. a. How would you describe your appetite?
   ☐ hearty ☐ moderate ☐ poor
   b. With this pregnancy, have you experienced the following?
   ☐ nausea ☐ vomiting ☐ constipation
   ☐ diarrhea

3. How would you describe your eating habits?
   ☐ regular ☐ irregular

4. a. Indicate the person who does the following in your household:
   plans the meals _____
   buys the food _____
   prepares the food _____
   b. How much is spent on food each week for your household?
   $ _____ ☐ don't know

5. a. Are you now taking any vitamin or mineral supplement?
   ☐ yes ☐ no
   b. Do you take any pills to control your weight?
   ☐ yes ☐ no
   c. Do you take diuretic (water) pills?
   ☐ yes ☐ no

6. a. Are you now on a diet (low salt, diabetic, gallbladder, weight reduction, etc.)?
   ☐ yes ☐ no
   If yes, what kind of diet? _____
   b. If you have been on a special diet in the past, indicate what kind and when. _____
   _____
   _____

7. a. Is there any food you can't eat?
   ☐ yes ☐ no
   If yes, what food? _____
   What happens when you eat this food? _____

   b. Do you have any cravings for things such as
   ☐ cornstarch
   ☐ plaster
   ☐ dirt or clay
   ☐ ice
   ☐ other _____

8. a. Do you smoke?
   ☐ yes ☐ no
   If yes, how much each day? _____
   b. Do you drink alcoholic beverages (liquor, wine, beer)?
   ☐ yes ☐ no
   If yes, how much and how often? _____

9. Are you receiving either of the following?
   ☐ food stamps
   ☐ WIC voucher

10. How do you want to feed your baby?
    ☐ breast feed ☐ commercial formula
    ☐ evaporated milk formula ☐ undecided

Reproduced with permission from *Nutrition During Pregnancy and Lactation.* Maternal and Child Health Branch, California Department of Health Services, 1977.

FORM H

Pregnancy Diet Intake

Interviewer _____

Patient's name _____   Date _____

Time	Place	Food eaten	Amount	Animal protein	Vegetable protein	Milk and milk products	Breads & cereals	Vitamin C products	Dark green vegetables	Other fruits & vegetables	Fats & oils	Extra foods
Influences on Diet:			**Summary:** Svgs. eaten									
			Svgs. needed	2	2	4	4	1	1	2	2	—
			Difference									

Reproduced with permission from *Nutrition During Pregnancy and Lactation.* Maternal and Child Health Branch, California Department of Health Services, 1977.

based on the Revised Daily Food Guide. The difference between servings eaten and needed will identify changes that need to be made in the diet.

Those foods which do not fit into any of the food groups should be recorded in the "Extra Foods" column. Such foods provide mainly energy, with very few nutrients; they include desserts, candy, sauces, liquor, and soft drinks. A consideration of the intake of these foods provides a more complete picture of an individual's dietary habits. Dietary improvements evidenced by a decrease in intake of high calorie–low nutrient density foods, as noted in the "Extra Foods" column, will be apparent with repeated evaluation of dietary intake.

ANTHROPOMETRIC ASSESSMENT

Weight gain during pregnancy should be carefully followed. Use of the Prenatal Weight Gain Grid (Figure 7-1) allows comparison of an individual's weight gain with the normal pattern of prenatal weight gain for a woman of standard weight, for height. Another chart has been suggested for following weight gain in women who enter pregnancy under or overweight (13).

During the first prenatal visit, the patient's weight and height should be measured and recorded. Optimal weight and immediate pregravid weight should also be noted. A comparison of the standard and pregravid weight will help determine if the woman was under- or overweight prior to this pregnancy, thereby influencing recommended weight gain. The total recommended weight gain for women entering pregnancy under- or overweight will differ from that shown on Figure 7-1; however, the rate of weight gain as identified by the general shape of the curve in Figure 7-1 should be similar. The pregravid weight also serves as the reference for all prenatal weight gain. It is represented on Figure 7-1 by the wide horizontal line.

Plotting the patient's weight gain at every visit on the Prenatal Weight Gain Grid will alert the health professional to potential problems, including inadequate weight gain, weight loss, or sharp increase in weight. Inadequate weight gain should be carefully explored in terms of overall dietary intake, and specific suggestions for increasing calorie intake should be offered. A sudden sharp increase in weight after the twentieth week of pregnancy may indicate water retention and the onset of preeclampsia, as will be discussed later.

BIOCHEMICAL ASSESSMENT

Normal gestation is associated with changes from the nonpregnant state in various laboratory indices of nutritional metabolic status. Whenever possible, values for pregnant women should be compared with "normal" values derived from pregnant women (14). For example, expansion of the plasma volume during pregnancy results in dilution of the plasma proteins. A

serum albumin level of 3.0 g/100 ml and a total serum protein value of 6.0 g/100 ml are normal for pregnancy, but would be considered low-normal for the nonpregnant state. Another example relates to changes in glucose tolerance which normally accompany pregnancy. (See Chapter 18.)

Since anemia is the most common nutritional complication of pregnancy, hematological values, such as hemoglobin and hematocrit, are usually checked at the beginning of pregnancy and repeated if necessary. Again, it is important to use normal-pregnancy values, not nonpregnant values, when evaluating anemia in pregnancy because of hemodilution. Acceptable hemoglobin and hematocrit values during pregnancy are >11.0 g/dl and >33 percent, respectively. A marginal hemoglobin value is 9.5 to 10.9 g/dl, and a value indicating deficiency is <9.5 g/dl. A marginal hematocrit value is 30 to 32 percent, and one indicating deficiency is <30% (15). A reduction in erythrocyte cell size, mean corpuscular volume (MCV) is an early and sensitive indicator of iron deficiency in pregnancy. MCV is one parameter of iron status which is unaffected by the state of pregnancy (16). An MCV of 82 FL or less may indicate insufficient iron intake. Other useful measurements for evaluating iron status more fully include examination of a stained erythrocyte smear and measurement of serum iron, serum ferritin, and total iron-binding capacity. Serum folacin and vitamin B_{12} levels should be determined if megaloblastic anemia is suspected. Normal hematological values for pregnancy are included in Table F-15.

NUTRITIONAL COUNSELING

The nutritional care specialist should view maternal nutritional counseling as a special opportunity to impart nutritional information. One effective approach to maternal nutritional education uses the learning concept of "building" (1). The pregnant woman can easily visualize the building of a new human life and the need for building materials or nutrients. When using the building concept, the woman has a framework on which to base an understanding of the need for specific nutrients during pregnancy.

When counseling a woman regarding her food habits, it is important to provide positive reinforcement. If completion of the Pregnancy Diet Intake form reveals that food intake is adequate, then verbal recognition, such as "You're doing a good job with your diet," should be given. This might also be an opportunity to further reinforce good food habits by guiding the woman to see *why* it is important to consume specific quantities from each food group during pregnancy. If food intake is not optimal, then the counselor should provide positive teaching rather than using a threatening approach. The counselor should attempt to identify the *reasons* underlying the woman's poor dietary intake so that improvements in intake can be achieved.

Nutritional assessment and educational considerations for prenatal nutritional counseling are outlined in Table 7-5.

CULTURAL FACTORS AFFECTING FOOD INTAKE

Cultural factors may substantially influence a woman's food intake and need to be taken into consideration when giving nutritional advice. A summary of general dietary patterns for Chinese, Japanese, Filipino, American Indian, and black ethnic groups according to the Daily Food Guide food groups is given in Appendix J. Vegetarian diets are discussed in Chapter 9, and Table 9-6 outlines a daily vegetarian food guide for pregnancy.

Many cultural food patterns provide marginal levels of the nutrients needed in increased amounts during pregnancy and lactation. Calcium intake appears to be a particular problem. The Mexican-American, black, Chinese, Japanese, and Filipino diets all include small amounts of dairy products. In addition, lactose intolerance is common in these racial groups (see Tables 16-6 and 16-7). A vitamin-mineral supplement may need to be included (see Nutritional Supplements) to provide adequate intakes of calcium, vitamin D, and riboflavin. In addition, appropriate lactose-free high-calcium foods should be encouraged. Be-

TABLE 7-5. Considerations in Prenatal Nutritional Counseling

INITIAL VISIT
Assessment
1. Screen for risk factors with Nutrition Questionnaire.
2. Evaluate adequacy of dietary intake with Pregnancy Diet Intake.
3. Obtain height and pregravid weight to determine % IBW prior to conception and recommendation for weight gain during gestation.
4. Obtain present weight and week of gestation to begin plot of weight gain on Prenatal Weight Gain Grid.

Education
1. Discuss importance of nutrition during pregnancy and lactation; stress key increases in nutrients—protein, iron, folacin, calcium, and energy.
2. Use Revised Daily Food Guide for meal planning.
3. Counsel about nutritional supplements.
4. Discuss pattern of weight gain during pregnancy.
5. Describe common nutritional problems associated with pregnancy.

FOLLOW-UP CARE
Assessment
1. Plot weight on Prenatal Weight Gain Grid.
2. Reevaluate dietary intake with Pregnancy Diet Intake form.
3. Check hgb and hct values.

Education
1. Discuss diet-related problems.
2. Give feedback on dietary intake in relation to Revised Daily Food Guide.
3. Discuss diet and lactation.
4. Discuss infant feeding.

TO TEST YOUR UNDERSTANDING

8. A pregnant Mexican-American patient tells you that she will not drink milk. What suggestions would you make to her to improve the calcium content of her diet?

9. A woman who is 5 feet, 4 inches tall has the following pattern of weight gain throughout her pregnancy.

Week of gestation	Weight (#)
0	110
12	111
18	113
22	114
24	116
26	118
28	125
30	130
32	133

a. Suggest an optimal pregnancy weight gain for this woman.
b. How does the above rate of gain compare with the normal pattern?
c. What problems are suggested by the pattern of gain after 26 weeks?

10. A lacto-ovo-vegetarian patient who has not taken a prenatal supplement has a Hgb value of 9.0 g/100 ml, a transferrin saturation of < 15 percent, an MCV of 80 FL, and a serum folacin value of 6 ng/ml at 30 weeks gestation.
a. Suggest what nutrient might be deficient in her diet.
b. How could her intake of this nutrient be improved?

cause milk provides protein in the diet, a low intake of milk will reduce total protein intake. When using the Daily Food Guide, a 2 oz. serving of a protein food should be substituted for 2 servings from the Milk and Milk Products Group in order to meet protein needs.

Obesity is a common nutritional problem among Mexican-Americans and blacks. Excessive consumption of carbonated beverages, fruit drinks, and pastries and an emphasis on fried foods are common. In order to improve the energy-to-nutrient ratio of the diet, the intake of "empty calorie" foods and fried foods often needs to be discouraged.

Other dietary practices resulting in reduced nutrient intake include a limited variety of vegetables in the Mexican-American diet; overcooking of vegetables in an excess of water in the black diet; and use of nonenriched rice, washing of enriched rice before cooking, and small intakes of protein foods in the Asian diet. When giving nutritional advice to these ethnic groups, you should be aware of various dietary and cooking practices and counsel appropriately.

COMPLICATIONS OF PREGNANCY

Complications of pregnancy may occur if the pregnant woman is obese, is an adolescent, or demonstrates an elevation in blood pressure. Common problems during pregnancy often involve functional alterations in the gastrointestinal tract.

COMMON PROBLEMS

The more common problems include nausea, constipation, and heartburn. General nutritional guidance may be needed during pregnancy to help alleviate these common problems.

Nausea

Nausea and vomiting usually occur during the first trimester of pregnancy. Because these symptoms occur on arising, the term "morning sickness" is often used. Simple dietary practices will often improve food tolerance during this time. Small, frequent, dry meals consisting chiefly of high-carbohydrate foods are more readily tolerated. Other suggestions for the management of nausea are presented in Table 7-6. Occasionally, *hyperemesis,* or severe, prolonged, and persistent vomiting, will develop. Hyperemesis requires medical attention to prevent dehydration.

The medication doxylamine succinate (Bendectin) was previously used to treat morning sickness. This drug has been taken off the market because of controversy concerning its teratogenic potential. Alteration of dietary practices is the safest way to treat the temporary nausea of early pregnancy.

Constipation

Constipation is common during pregnancy due both to hormonal changes which tend to increase relaxation

TABLE 7-6. Morning Sickness or Nausea

Suggestions to Alleviate Morning Sickness
Before Going to Bed
Be sure to have plenty of fresh air in the room where you sleep. The odor of soiled clothes and other household odors in the room where you sleep may upset your stomach.
Place some dry cereal, toast, or crackers within reach of your bed.
Before Getting Up in the Morning
Eat some of the toast or dry cereal. A little jelly on the bread may make it taste better, but do not use butter or margarine.
When Getting Up
Get up very slowly; take five or six minutes. Avoid sudden movements when getting out of bed. Then, before cooking breakfast, eat some more toast or cereal shortly after you get up.
Suggestions to Alleviate Nausea During the Day
Because you are more likely to feel nauseated when your stomach is empty, eat several small meals a day instead of three large ones. Eating small amounts of the following foods may be helpful when you feel nauseated: dry cereal without milk, popcorn, carbonated beverages, fruit juice.
Do not drink fluids or eat soups at mealtimes. If you are thirsty, try eating ice chips. Drink small sips of liquid frequently between meals.
Some time during the day you will find you can eat a regular meal. Be sure not to overeat at this time.
Foods to Avoid
Fats and greasy foods tend to upset the stomach. For this reason, avoid fried foods and foods cooked with grease, oils, or fat meats. Eat very little of the following foods: butter, margarine, gravy, bacon, fat back, oils, mayonnaise, salad dressings, pie crusts, pastries.
Highly seasoned foods, such as those cooked with garlic, onion, pepper, chili and other spices, may upset your stomach and should be avoided.
Avoid foods that may give you gas while you are nauseated. Some of these foods may be the following: cabbage, broccoli, Brussels sprouts, collard greens, onions, turnips, radishes, cucumbers, and dried beans.

Adapted from materials used in the Southern California Kaiser-Permanente Medical Care Program.

of the gastrointestinal muscles and to the pressure of the enlarging uterus on the colon. Iron supplementation is also associated with constipation in pregnancy. Increased fluid intake and use of naturally laxative foods such as whole grains with added bran, fibrous fruits and vegetables, dried fruits, and other fruits and juices generally help maintain regularity.

Heartburn

Heartburn may occur after meals, especially during the later stages of pregnancy, due to crowding of the stomach by the enlarging uterus. The symptoms of heartburn are usually reduced by eating smaller, more frequent meals. Wearing loose-fitting clothing, eating slowly, avoiding reclining after meals, and elevating the head of the bed may also help.

THE OVERWEIGHT PREGNANT WOMAN

Women who are overweight at the beginning of pregnancy need individual nutritional attention. These women are the most likely to develop gestational diabetes, the most common medical complication of pregnancy. The diagnosis and nutritional management of gestational diabetes is discussed in Chapter 18. Another consideration is that a lower total weight gain (15 pounds) is suggested for the obese pregnant woman (4). However, severe weight restriction or reduction is never recommended during pregnancy.

A minimum energy intake of 36 kcal per kg of current maternal body weight is recommended for optimum protein utilization during pregnancy (7). This energy intake may result in excessive weight gain for the overweight pregnant woman and may more accurately reflect energy needs when calculated using ideal, rather than actual, body weight. In counseling the obese pregnant woman, the best approach to assessment of energy needs is to monitor the pattern of pregnancy weight gain. Because overweight women often have poor eating habits, careful instruction in the nutrient quality of the food groups and in elimination of empty-calorie foods may be needed when counseling these women.

HYPERTENSIVE DISORDERS ASSOCIATED WITH PREGNANCY

Hypertensive disorders adversely affect both maternal and fetal health and are a common complication of pregnancy. Hypertensive disorders which are associated with pregnancy include the presence of chronic hypertension prior to pregnancy and the development of a specific condition referred to as *pregnancy-induced hypertension* (PIH).

Chronic Hypertension

Chronic hypertension prior to pregnancy is demonstrated by a persistent blood pressure of 140/90 mm Hg or more. Women with chronic hypertension often experience a drop in blood pressure during the early weeks of pregnancy, a small rise after the twentieth week which accompanies the expansion of plasma volume, and a persistent elevation in blood pressure after delivery. Women with a documented record of chronic hypertension prior to pregnancy often develop preeclampsia, which may progress to eclampsia before the thirtieth week of pregnancy if untreated.

Pregnancy-Induced Hypertension

PIH refers to a unique hypertensive syndrome characterized by the progression of symptoms from preeclampsia to eclampsia. The term *PIH* has been adopted by the American College of Obstetricians and Gynecologists to replace the terms *preeclampsia* and *eclampsia* (17). While preeclampsia and eclampsia have previously been used as diagnostic labels, they actually refer to the nature and degree of symptoms associated with PIH. Preeclampsia usually develops after the twentieth week of pregnancy and is characterized by hypertension with proteinuria and/or

edema. *Eclampsia* comes from the Greek word *eclampsis,* meaning a "sudden flash" or a "sudden development." Eclampsia is considered an extension of preeclampsia and diagnosis is based on the presence of convulsions.

The term *toxemia* was previously used to denote PIH, but it is actually a misnomer. *Toxemia* means "toxins in the blood," which doesn't apply to PIH.

Incidence and Etiology The etiology of PIH is poorly understood, but it is felt to involve interaction between nutritional intake and the physiologic adjustments associated with pregnancy. PIH occurs most commonly in primigravidae and in women under 20 or over 35 years of age. The incidence of PIH is higher among women from low-income groups, suggesting that nutritional status and quality of prenatal care are related to the development of this disorder.

It was previously felt that excess weight gain during pregnancy contributes to the development of PIH, but the incidence of PIH is actually greater among *underweight* women who fail to gain weight normally during pregnancy (1). The nutritional value of the diet and the pattern of weight gain throughout pregnancy, *not* the total weight gain, seem to be important factors in the development of PIH.

Symptoms: The symptoms of PIH, or those associated with preeclampsia, usually occur after the twentieth week of gestation and include hypertension, proteinuria, and edema. Table 7-7 summarizes the symptoms associated with the progression from preeclampsia to eclampsia.

Hypertension: A blood pressure greater than 140/90 is used to diagnose hypertension in the nonpregnant population. This value is not useful during pregnancy because many younger females have normal blood pressures of less than 120/80, and use of the 140/90 diagnostic value will often miss their hypertension. Hypertension associated with pregnancy is best assessed by comparison with individuals' usual blood pressure levels (18). The diagnosis of hypertension in pregnancy is indicated by repeated blood pressure measurements of 140/90 or by an elevation of 30 mm Hg systolic or 15 mm Hg diastolic from previous blood pressure measurements during pregnancy.

Proteinuria: Proteinuria usually develops late in the course of PIH. The degree of proteinuria varies with the progression from preeclampsia to eclampsia. With preeclampsia, a 24-hour urine collection may include 300 mg of protein; with progression to severe preeclampsia, the collection may contain at least 5 g of protein.

Edema: The majority of pregnant women develop a certain amount of edema in the extremities during the last trimester of pregnancy. This is a normal consequence of the expansion of the plasma volume, decrease in plasma albumin, and the pressure exerted on the venous vasculature by an enlarging uterus. The edema associated with PIH is much more severe. It is usually evident in the hands, face, feet, and legs and may be associated with dizziness, headache, visual disturbances, nausea, and vomiting.

TABLE 7-7. Symptoms of Pregnancy-Induced Hypertension

Stage	Symptom
Preeclampsia	*Hypertension:* 140/90 or increase of 30 mm Hg systolic or 15 mm Hg diastolic above woman's usual baseline; at least two observations 6 or more hours apart *Proteinuria:* 300 mg or more in 24-hour urine collection or random 2+ protein; develops late in course of PIH *Edema:* significant; usually in face and hands
Severe preeclampsia	One or more of the following symptoms: *Hypertension:* systolic pressure 160 mm Hg or diastolic 110 mm Hg on two observations 6 or more hours apart at bed rest. *Proteinuria:* 5 g or more of protein per 24-hours or random 3+ to 4+ protein *Edema:* pulmonary edema *Clinical:* blurred vision, headache, altered consciousness *Advancing disease:* epigastric or upper-quadrant pain, impaired liver function, thrombocytopenia
Eclampsia	Extension of preeclampsia with grand mal seizure occurring near time of labor

Treatment. Medical therapy for hypertension during pregnancy is similar to that for hypertension in the absence of pregnancy. Bed rest in the lateral recumbent position is usually recommended. Use of diuretic therapy during pregnancy is controversial and usually avoided. A no-added-salt or 4–5 g Na diet may be used (see Chapter 19), but severe sodium restriction is generally not appropriate for the treatment of PIH.

THE PREGNANT ADOLESCENT

Adolescent pregnancy refers to gestation which occurs between the maternal ages of 11 to 18 years. These young girls are viewed as a high-risk population which is susceptible to suboptimal pregnancy outcome. Biologic immaturity and a variety of psychosocial circumstances contribute to the problems experienced by the pregnant adolescent. Adolescence is a time of tremendous physical growth and development. For the pregnant adolescent, the nutritional demands of pregnancy are thus superimposed on those required for growth.

Gynecological Age

Gynecological age is defined as the number of years which have passed since menarche, or the onset of menses. For example, a 16-year-old who started menstruating at 11 years of age would have a gynecological age of 5 years. The average age of menarche in the United States is now 12.5 to 13 years of age (19). While the adolescent growth spurt usually occurs in females between the ages of 10½ to 13 years, complete linear growth is usually not achieved until 4 years postmenarche. Because of this growth pattern, a consideration of gynecological age is more useful than chronological age in evaluating the nutritional needs of the pregnant adolescent. Those girls who become pregnant at a gynecological age of less than 2 to 3 years have greater nutritional needs and are at greater risk because they are more biologically immature. In general, a young woman with a gynecological age of 5 years or more has reproductive risks similar to those of women in the prime reproductive years.

Associated Problems

The outcome of pregnancy is viewed in terms of both maternal and fetal health. The two problems most commonly associated with adolescent pregnancy are maternal PIH and fetal prematurity. The rates of both these conditions are highest in the youngest adolescent patients, and both may occur in the same patient. Prematurity is a leading cause of perinatal mortality and morbidity, and PIH may lead to maternal problems with chronic cardiovascular and renal disease later in life. Nutrition is felt to play a role in the etiology of both these disorders. Evidence suggests that comprehensive, individualized prenatal care for the pregnant adolescent improves the outcome of pregnancy.

Nutritional Requirements

The RDAs for the pregnant adolescent are derived by adding the pregnancy RDAs for adult women to the RDA specifications for nonpregnant teenagers from 11 to 14 and from 15 to 18 years of age, as outlined in Table A-1. This approach may overestimate total pregnancy requirements for the adolescent; in general, however, it seems the most rational method since little information is available on the nutritional needs of pregnant adolescents.

Nutritional Counseling

Establishing a good rapport with the pregnant adolescent is a key part of effective nutritional counseling. Once an open atmosphere has been established, a careful evaluation of dietary intake, along with suggestions for improvement, can be made. Attention to individual needs, awareness of adolescent eating habits (see Chapter 8), and willingness to listen are especially important when working with pregnant teenagers.

Prenatal Weight Gain

Optimal prenatal weight gain is higher for many adolescents compared to adults. Optimal weight gain for the pregnant adolescent should include usual pregnancy gain (Table 7-1), gain to bring weight to normal for height, and gain for the 9-month postmenarcheal interval corresponding to gynecological age (1). The normal weight range for an adolescent of a given height can be found in percentile height and weight tables for age provided by the National Center for Health Statistics (20). A weight falling between the 25th and 75th percentiles for a given height is considered to be normal. Weight gain associated with gynecological age is as follows: 10.1 pounds for the first postmenarcheal year, 6.2 pounds for the second year, 2.4 pounds for the third year, and 1.8 pounds for years 4 to 5 (1).

As an example, we will calculate the optimal prenatal weight gain for a 17-year-old, at gynecological age 3 years, who weighs 103 pounds (10th percentile) and is 5 feet, 3 inches tall.

Optimal weight gain equals the sum of

27	#	usual pregnancy gain
9	#	to bring weight to 25th percentile
2.4	#	to achieve gain associated with gynecological age

Total gain = 38.4 #

TO TEST YOUR UNDERSTANDING

11. A young pregnant woman tells you that her mother has suggested that she avoid salt and carefully watch her weight gain during pregnancy in order to prevent the development of "toxemia." How would you advise the young woman?

12. Compare the RDAs for the pregnant adolescent (Table A-1) to those for the adult woman:

    a. Which nutrients relevant to mineral metabolism are needed in increased amounts by the pregnant adolescent?

    b. How could the Daily Food Guide be altered to provide the nutrients listed in part A?

13. Amy, a 14-year-old girl, is referred to you for prenatal nutrition counseling. Amy is three months pregnant and is still experiencing fairly severe morning sickness. She resides with her grandmother, who lives on Social Security. Amy now weighs 116 pounds and is 5 feet, 8 inches tall. Her usual weight is 120 pounds, and she began menstruating at age 12.

    a. Describe how you would initiate counseling with Amy. What kind of information would be important to obtain from Amy in your initial interview?

    b. What suggestions could you make for treating the morning sickness?

    c. Estimate Amy's optimal prenatal weight gain. For Amy's age and height percentile, weights are as follows: 5th percentile = 111#, 10th percentile = 116#, 25th percentile = 122#, 50th percentile = 132#.

TOPICS FOR FURTHER DISCUSSION

1. Discuss the nutritional implications of pica during pregnancy.

2. What are the recommendations for exercise during pregnancy? Discuss some of the advantages of an exercise program during pregnancy.

3. What are some of the nutritional effects associated with the use of oral contraceptive agents?

4. A nutritional care specialist, you present an informal prenatal class on breast-feeding. Briefly outline the main topics that you will discuss.

5. Discuss the various supplemental feeding programs available for the maternal-infant population.

6. Discuss recommendations for the use of alcohol and caffeine during pregnancy. What is fetal alcohol syndrome?

REFERENCES

1. WORTHINGTON-ROBERTS, B., J. VERMEERSCH, AND S.R. WILLIAMS. *Nutrition in Pregnancy and Lactation*. St. Louis: Times Mirror/Mosby, 1985.

2. ESKIN, B.A. Diagnosis of pregnancy. In *Principles and Practice of Obstetrics and Perinatology*, Vol. 1, eds. L. Iffy and H.A. Kaminetzley. New York: John Wiley, 1981, p. 707.

3. FRITZ-ZAVACKI, S. AND L.E. BRUNEL. Prenatal care. In *Manual of Obstetrics*, ed. K.R. Niswander. Boston: Little, Brown, 1983, p. 27.

4. NAEYE, R.L. Weight gain and the outcome of pregnancy. *Am. J. Obstet. Gynecol.* 135:(1979)3.

5. TAGGART, N.R. ET AL. Changes in skinfolds during pregnancy. *Br. J. Nutr.* 21:(1967)439.

6. COUNCIL ON SCIENTIFIC AFFAIRS. Fetal effects of maternal alcohol use. *J.A.M.A.* 249:(1983)2517.

7. FOOD AND NUTRITION BOARD, NATIONAL RESEARCH COUNCIL, NATIONAL ACADEMY OF SCIENCES. *Recommended Dietary Allowances*, 9th ed. Washington, D.C.: U.S. Government Printing Office, 1980.

8. WORTHINGTON-ROBERTS, B. Nutrition and maternal health. *Nutrition Today*, Nov./Dec. 1984, p. 6.

9. COMMITTEE ON DRUGS, AMERICAN ACADEMY OF PEDIATRICS. The transfer of drugs and other chemicals into human breast milk. *Pediatrics* 72:(1983)375.

10. *Food Guides: Their development, use and specific changes suggested for Nutrition During Pregnancy and Lactation*. Sacramento Calif.: Maternal and Child Health Branch, California Department of Health Services, 1977.

11. THE AMERICAN DIETETIC ASSOCIATION AND THE AMERICAN COLLEGE OF OBSTETRICIANS AND GYNECOLOGISTS. *Assessment of Maternal Nutrition*, 1978.

12. *Nutrition During Pregnancy and Lactation.* Maternal and Child Health Branch, California State Department of Public Health, rev. 1975.

13. ROSSO, P. A new chart to monitor weight gain during pregnancy. *Am. J. Clin. Nutr.* 41:(1985)644–652.

14. COMMITTEE ON NUTRITION OF THE MOTHER AND PRESCHOOL CHILD, FOOD AND NUTRITION BOARD, NATIONAL RESEARCH COUNCIL, NATIONAL ACADEMY OF SCIENCES. *Laboratory Indices of Nutritional Status in Pregnancy: Summary Report.* Washington, D.C., 1977.

15. U.S. DEPARTMENT OF HEALTH, EDUCATION, AND WELFARE: *Ten-State Nutrition Survey, 1968–1970.* DHEW Pub. No. (HSM) 72-8130. Atlanta: Center for Disease Control, 1972.

16. KING, J.C. Nutrition during pregnancy. In *Frontiers of Clinical Nutrition*, ed. N. Kretchmer. Rockville, Md.: Aspen, 1986, pp. 3–13.

17. WILLIS, S.E. Hypertension in pregnancy. *Am. J. Nurs.* 82:(1982)792.

18. FERRIS, T.F. AND L.L. FRANCISCO. Toxemia and hypertension during pregnancy, *Bull. N.Y. Acad. Med.* 58:(1982)178.

19. COMMITTEE ON MATERNAL NUTRITION, FOOD AND NUTRITION BOARD, NATIONAL RESEARCH COUNCIL, NATIONAL ACADEMY OF SCIENCES. *Maternal Nutrition and the Course of Pregnancy.* Washington, D.C.: U.S. Government Printing Office, 1970.

20. NATIONAL CENTER FOR HEALTH STATISTICS. *Height and Weight of Youths 12–17 years, United States.* Washington, D.C., Department of Health, Education and Welfare, Vital and Health Statistics, Series 11. No. 124, 1973.

ADDITIONAL SOURCES OF INFORMATION

AMERICAN ACADEMY OF PEDIATRICS. The promotion of breastfeeding. *Pediatrics* 69:(1982)65.

BURROW, G.N. AND T.F. FERRIS. *Medical Complications During Pregnancy.* Philadelphia: Saunders, 1982.

HURLEY, L.S. *Developmental Nutrition.* Englewood Cliffs, N.J.: Prentice-Hall, 1980.

LAWRENCE, R. *Breastfeeding: A Guide for the Medical Profession* (2d ed.). St. Louis: C. V. Mosby, 1985.

Nutrition During Pregnancy and Lactation. Maternal and Child Health Branch, California State Department of Public Health, rev. 1975.

CASE STUDY II   NUTRITION IN PREGNANCY AND LACTATION

Part I: Presentation

Present Illness: Juanita is a 32 y.o., G_8P_6, Mexican-American mother of five who requests a pregnancy test at the local Public Health Clinic (LMP = 4/1, approximately 12 weeks ago). The pregnancy test is positive (G_9P_6).

Previous Obstetrical History: $G_9P_6Ab_9LC_5$. She has had two early spontaneous abortions and delivered one stillborn. Her living children are ages 14, 12, 5, 2, and about 1. Her last two liveborn children were born 1 and 2 years ago and weighed 8½ pounds and 9 pounds, respectively, at birth. All her children were breast-fed, and Juanita plans to nurse this child. She gained 35 pounds with her last pregnancy and lost about 25 pounds before this conception.

Family History: Her mother died of influenza and her father died at age 55 from complications resulting from diabetes.

Social History: Lives with husband who works as a gardener; does housekeeping work to earn extra money. The family receives $150 per month in Food Stamps.

Physical Exam: Ht 5 ft, 2 in, usual wt 160#, present wt 163#, BP = 120/80

Laboratory: Hct 35%, Hgb 11 g/100 ml

Impression: Intrauterine pregnancy at 12 weeks

QUESTIONS

You speak with Juanita at the Public Health Clinic after she receives the positive results of her pregnancy test. The results of a brief diet history indicate that the family diet consists mainly of rice, beans, tortillas, chilies, eggs, and occasionally meat. Juanita likes milk but usually drinks soft drinks with her meals. You help Juanita apply for the Special Supplementary Food Program for Women, Infants, and Children (WIC). The WIC program provides vouchers for the purchase of foods high in those nutrients needed in increased amounts during pregnancy. These foods may include eggs, fruit and vegetable juices, milk, cheese, iron-fortified cereals, or infant formulas. You also schedule Juanita to attend the Clinic's prenatal nutrition class, which is held once a month for an hour.

1. List five nutritional risk factors for pregnancy which this patient displays (see Table 7-4 and Form G).

2. In what nutrients is her diet likely to be deficient?

3. Assuming that Juanita is eligible for the WIC program, suggest four changes that she could make in her diet.

4. You are responsible for teaching the Public Health Clinic Prenatal Nutrition class. Describe four areas that you will cover in your class.

Part II: Excessive Weight Gain in the First Two Trimesters

Juanita's pregnancy progresses without difficulty, but at 30 weeks the physician becomes concerned because Juanita has already gained 30 pounds and the fetus appears to be large. The physician suspects that the EDD may have been incorrectly calculated because the fundal height is consistent with a gestational age of closer to 34 weeks. An ultrasound test is performed to get a better idea of gestational age; the results suggest an age of 33 weeks.

Because of Juanita's history of delivering large infants and family history of diabetes, gestational diabetes is another concern. An oral, nonfasting, loading test for gestational diabetes, using a 50 g glucose load, is given. The 1-hour plasma glucose value is 130 mg/dl, which is also within normal limits (WNL), suggesting normal gestational carbohydrate tolerance.

Laboratory determinations at 33 weeks are as follows: BP 125/85, wt 195#, Hgb 10 g/100 ml, Hct 30%, MCV 82 FL, serum albumin 3 g/100 ml, and urine is negative for protein and sugar.

The physical examination indicates a fundal height of 34 cm, a trace of edema, the presence of fetal heart sounds, and a vertex fetal position.

The physician asks you to counsel Juanita regarding her dietary intake.

QUESTIONS

5. a. Fill in, on Form I—Prenatal Weight Gain Grid—Juanita's pregravid weight, height, optimal body weight for height, and hematological values.

Form I Prenatal Weight-Gain Grid

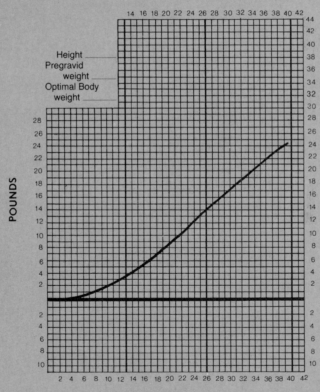

Hematologic Values				
Test	Desirable Value	Patient's Values		
		Date	Date	Date
Hematocrit	>33%			
Hemoglobin	>11 mg/dl			
MCV	>82 FL			

b. Plot Juanita's weight gain on the prenatal weight-gain grid using the values given here.

Weeks of gestation	Weight (#)
0	160
12	163
18	173
24	185
33	195

c. What does the pattern of weight gain suggest?

d. Under ideal conditions, what would be an optimal total pregnancy weight gain for this patient?

e. Would you recommend holding weight stable for the remainder of pregnancy? Explain why. If not, what pattern of weight gain would you recommend for the remainder of pregnancy?

f. What is suggested by the change in hematological values?

6. You obtain a 24-hour recall from Juanita as follows:

1 c nonfat milk	1 c refried beans	1 c nonfat milk
2 fried eggs	2 oz cheese	1 c refried beans
2 doughnuts	2 c rice	2 flour tortillas
2 c orange juice	2 flour tortillas	2 c vegetable soup with 1 oz meat
3 slices bacon	12 oz cola	
		1 2-oz candy bar

She also comments that she takes her prenatal vitamin-mineral supplement whenever she remembers it—maybe three times a week.

a. Using the Pregnancy Diet Intake form (Form H in Chapter 7), evaluate the diet. In the following columns, list the food groups being consumed in inadequate amounts and the nutrients that are limiting in the diet due to this eating pattern. Also, suggest appropriate foods to include in the diet from the food groups that are being consumed in inadequate amounts.

Food Group   *Limiting Nutrients*   *Foods to Include*

b. What correlations can you make between dietary intake and hematological status?

c. Using the ADA exchange system and Form J, list the number of exchanges consumed and estimate the daily caloric intake.

FORM J

University Medical Center
Summary of Daily Nutrient Intake

Food Group	No. of Exchanges	PRO g	FAT g	CHO g
Starch/bread exchanges				
Milk exchanges (Circle NF, LF, or who.)				
Fruit exchanges				
Vegetable exchanges				
Meat exchanges (Circle lo, med, hi fat)				
Fat exchanges				
Other				
TOTAL g		_____	_____	_____

Kcal = _____ g protein   × 4 = _____
_____ g fat   × 9 = _____
_____ g carbohydrate × 4 = _____
_____ TOTAL Kcal

d. How many kcal per day are coming from empty-calorie foods, which provide energy but are low in proteins, vitamins, and minerals?

e. What daily calorie intake would you estimate is required for Juanita to achieve an optimal weight gain for the remainder of pregnancy (see question 5e)? Explain your answer.

7. Assume that you will use the Pregnancy Diet Intake form as a teaching tool to show Juanita how she should modify her diet.
    a. List those foods that she should eliminate from her diet.

b. Explain why she should eliminate these foods.

c. Suggest alterations in food preparation that could reduce Juanita's calorie intake.

8

Pediatric Nutrition

The pediatric population comprises individuals who are from newborn to 18 years of age. The population can be divided into the following age groups: infants (0–12 months), preschoolers (1–5 years), school-age children (5–11 years), and adolescents (11–18 years). This chapter will focus on nutritional requirements, feeding patterns, and nutritional assessment for the pediatric population. A knowledge of normal pediatric feeding patterns forms the basis of diet modification for specific pediatric disease states.

NUTRITIONAL REQUIREMENTS

Nutritional requirements for the pediatric population are a function of the child's age, size, activity, and rate of growth. Because there is considerable individual variation in growth rate and size, the RDAs are expressed per kg of body weight for the infant. In general, nutritional requirements are the greatest during the two periods of peak growth rate—infancy and adolescence. (The RDAs for the pediatric population can be found in Table A-1. Daily fluid requirements are discussed in Table 12-2 of the chapter on tube feeding and Table 13-9 in the chapter on parenteral feeding.)

INFANT FEEDING

Breast milk or infant formula is the basis of an infant's diet. For developmental and nutritional reasons, solid foods are usually not needed in the diet until 4 to 6 months of age. The need for supplementation of specific vitamins and minerals during infancy depends on whether the infant receives human milk or other milk feeding. This section reviews breast feeding, bottle feeding, introduction of solid food to the diet, and infant formulas.

The guidelines for normal infant feeding presented in this chapter represent the opinions of various well-regarded pediatric nutrition groups (1–3), including the American Academy of Pediatrics (4). You should be aware that there are no firm data to support specific infant feeding recommendations and that a wide variety of feeding practices have been shown to result in healthy babies.

Breast Feeding

Human milk is considered the optimal sole food for an infant's first 4 to 6 months of life. It is currently estimated that 61.4 percent of new mothers in the United States leave the hospital breast feeding (5). The decision to breast feed should be made during the prenatal period. Because breast feeding is a learned skill, health professionals need to be prepared to assist new mothers in the techniques of successful breast feeding. Several useful references on this topic are listed at the end of this chapter.

Advantages. Breast feeding has advantages for both mother and infant (2,4). Breast milk provides the infant with immunological protection from gastroenteritis, respiratory infection and allergic reactions. Many feel that breast-fed infants have fewer problems with colic than do bottle-fed infants. Breast feeding also promotes facial and muscular development and thus assists with the development of speech patterns. Breast feeding helps the mother lose weight gained during pregnancy and also helps the uterus return to its normal size. It is the most economical method of feeding, even though the current recommendations provide an additional 500 kcal and 20 g protein daily for lactation (see Chapter 7).

The adequately breast-fed infant of a well-nourished mother does not require vitamin and mineral supplementation, with the possible exception of fluoride, and vitamin D in those areas where the infant may not receive sufficient sunlight (4).

Frequency and Duration of Feedings. Breast feeding should be initiated as soon after delivery as possible. During the first weeks of life, infants usually require feeding every 2 to 3 hours, with a minimum of 8 to 10 feedings every 24 hours. The infant should nurse from both breasts at each feeding to empty the initial side and stimulate production in the alternate breast. Generally, 15 minutes on the first breast plus 5 to 15 minutes on the other side are appropriate.

A baby is usually getting enough breast milk if he is sleeping 2 to 3 hours between feedings, has 6 to 8 wet diapers each day, has frequent bowel movements during the first 6 weeks of life, and is gaining weight. Failure to regain birth weight by 3 weeks of age or continued weight loss after 10 days of life suggests that the intake of breast milk is inadequate.

Supplemental Feedings. Routine supplemental feedings of water or formula should be discouraged during the first 4 to 6 weeks of breast feeding. Adequate breast feeding provides the infant's fluid needs. An infant given water or supplements is less likely to provide adequate suckling stimulation for the mother to produce an appropriate quantity of milk. Also, bottle feeding may result in nipple confusion, as standard nipples promote a sucking action different from that needed for successful breast feeding.

Once lactation is well established, generally after 4 to 6 weeks, replacement bottles of breast milk or formula can occasionally be used. For the working mother who wishes to continue to feed her infant breast milk, it is suggested that the separated mother pump her breast at about the same time the infant feeds and then store the milk in the refrigerator to use as a replacement feeding within 24 to 48 hours. If she does this in addition to frequent feedings when they are together, she should maintain her milk supply. Alternatively, the mother may wish to nurse her child when she is not at work and then use commercial formula for the remainder of the day's feedings. This will result in reduction of the mother's milk volume but may allow the working mother to partially breast feed her infant.

Cup Introduction and Weaning. The breast-fed infant can be weaned directly to a cup, omitting the use of a bottle. The infant can usually begin drinking from a cup at 5 to 6 months of age. A small plastic cup with a top and spout works well to start. To accomplish weaning, the quantity of fluid consumed by cup should be gradually increased as the number of breast feedings is reduced. While drinking from a cup should be introduced between 5 and 6 months, breast feeding may continue until 12 months of age or longer.

Bottle Feeding

Bottle feeding of infant formulas provides the best alternative to breast feeding to meet nutritional needs during the first year. Because there is increasing social pressure to breast feed, it is important to avoid making a woman feel guilty if she decides to bottle feed. Various aspects of good bottle-feeding techniques are discussed in this section.

Number and Volume of Bottle Feedings. At birth, the full-term infant's stomach holds between 30 and 90 ml. As the infant grows, the stomach enlarges and its rate of emptying slows. During the first week of life, an infant usually consumes 6 to 10 feedings of 30 to 90 ml each per day. Recommendations for number and volume of bottle feedings for a normal infant are shown in Table 8-1. Fifteen or twenty minutes is an adequate bottle-feeding time for most infants.

Good Feeding Technique. Infants should be held when bottle fed; the bottle should never be propped up. Putting an infant to bed with a bottle should be discouraged because the practice can cause dental caries and may be associated with a high incidence of otitis media and a psychological dependence on the bottle.

The bottle should be held and tilted so that the nipple is always filled with formula, not air. Many styles of bottles are available. The disposable plastic-bag bottles generally decrease the amount of air that is swallowed during feedings. Bottles should only be used for formula or water feeding, not for introduction of juices or solids such as cereal.

Weaning from the Bottle. Weaning from the bottle is usually started between 5 and 8 months of age. At this age, the infant usually receives four 8-oz bottles per day, often corresponding to three bottles during the day and one before bedtime. Weaning is usually accomplished by eliminating one bottle feeding at a time and substituting a cup. During this time, the infant is also being offered an increased amount and variety of solid foods. This makes it practical to plan a three-meal-a-day-plus-snacks pattern with the rest of the family. Usually, the infant can take 3 to 4 oz of fluid by cup with a meal and the same amount between meals.

Children 1 to 2 years of age or older should not be taking a daily or nightly bottle. Bottle feeding in the toddler can lead to an excessive intake of milk or other sweetened liquids, which may interfere with recommended nutrient intake or lead to excessive calorie intake.

Introduction of Cow's Milk. Breast milk or commercial formula is the recommended feeding from birth through 6 to 12 months of age (2,3). For many families, it may be impractical or too expensive to provide formula for their child through 12 months of age. In these cases, the nutritional care specialist should determine the infant's age, weight, and intake of solid foods. If the infant is at least 6 months old, weighs 6 to 7 kg, and eats both iron-fortified cereal and 1½ jars of baby food daily, then whole, fresh cow's milk or homogenized, vitamin D–fortified, evaporated whole milk with equal parts of water may be recommended (2). The feeding of skim or low fat milk during infancy is not recommended because the lower calorie density of these milks encourages excess milk consumption to meet energy needs.

TABLE 8-1. Dietary Evaluation Guidelines for Infants (0–12 months)

Age (months)	0	1	2	3	4	5	6	7	8	9	10	11	12
50th percentile of weight in kg (#)	3.3 (7.3)	4.1 (9.0)	5.0 (11.0)	5.7 (12.5)	6.4 (14.1)	7.0 (15.4)	7.5 (16.5)	8.0 (17.6)	8.5 (18.7)	8.9 (19.6)	9.2 (20.2)	9.6 (21.1)	9.9 (21.8)
kcal per 24 hr (range)	115 kcal/kg (95–145 kcal/kg) 52 kcal/# (43–66 kcal/#)							105 kcal/kg (80–135 kcal/kg) 48 kcal/# (36–61 kcal/#)					
Fluid per 24 hr (oz)	125–145 ml/kg (4.2–4.8 oz. kg; 2–2½ oz/#)												
No. of milk* feedings per 24 hr	8 or more		6 or 7		4 or 5				3 or 4			3	
Oz formula per feeding†	2½–4	3½–5	4–6	5–7				6–8				6–7	
Solids‡							Strained (pureed) foods		Junior (chopped) foods		Table foods‡		
Breads and cereals					Iron-fortified cereal, rice		Teething biscuit			Iron-fortified mixed-grain cereals			
Vegetables						Carrots, squash, beans, peas							
Fruits§							Applesauce, pears, peaches, bananas						
Meat Group and meat alternates									Strained meats, cheese, yogurt, cooked beans, egg yolk				
Age (months)	0	1	2	3	4	5	6	7	8	9	10	11	12

*Milk is breast milk or formula, with the possible introduction of whole cow's milk after 6–7 months of age. See footnote †.

†Formula is preferred to whole milk during the first year of life. However, if the infant is consuming the equivalent of 2 jars (1 cup) of beikost (pureed or chopped foods) and is 6–7 months of age, whole milk may be given.

‡No solid foods should be introduced until the infant is 4–6 months of age or has reached 6–7 kg of weight.

§Whole eggs, orange juice, and citrus fruits should not be introduced until the infant is 12 months old.

Copyright 1983 Denise Ney, RD and Elizabeth G. Jones RD.

Solid Foods, or Beikost

The introduction of beikost, or foods other than milk, into an infant's diet should be withheld until 4 to 6 months of age. The rationale for this recommendation is based on the developmental readiness of the infant to consume solids, the increased probability of the infant's developing allergies with early introduction of solids, the lack of sound data to suggest that early feeding of solids helps the infant sleep through the night, and the fact that, until 4 to 6 months of age, breast milk or formula best meets the infant's nutritional needs. The order of introduction of solid foods is usually iron-fortified cereal, followed by vegetables, fruit, meat, and egg yolk. Table 8-2 summarizes recommen-

dations for the introduction of solid foods, including the rationale and the stage of feeding development.

As the infant starts eating greater amounts of solid foods, the volume of formula or milk consumed will decrease. After 9 months of age, infants generally do not need more than 32 oz of formula per day. By the age of one year, most babies take approximately 16 to 24 oz of formula per day plus solids equal to 2 to 4 jars (2 to 3 cups) of baby food. Portion sizes for solid foods in the infant aged 4 to 12 months are summarized in Table 8-3.

Foods to Avoid in Infancy

It is wise to avoid feeding certain foods to infants. Nuts, potato chips, fruits with seeds, popcorn, celery,

TABLE 8-2.   Introduction to Solid Foods (Beikost)

Age	Introduction of New Foods	Reasons for Introduction	Development
Birth–12 months	Breast milk or formula	Meets the infant's nutritional needs for the first 4–6 months or 6–7 kg of weight.	Rooting reflex, suck-swallow pattern, extension tongue movement.
4–6 months (6–7 kg)	Iron-fortified cereal (rice, oats, barley).	Provides a dietary source of iron at the age when body stores from birth are depleting. Cereal is hypoallergenic.	Lips have muscular control to seal oral cavity. Tongue can move back and forth. Infant can begin to draw in lower lip as spoon is removed.
5–7 months	Strained or pureed vegetables and fruits. Unsweetened fruit juice (except orange juice) may be introduced by cup.	Provides dietary sources of vitamins, minerals, and calories. Introduces new food flavors. Starts setting basis for good eating habits. Introduce vegetables first to reduce the tendency to develop a taste for sweets.	Up-and-down movement begins (beginning of chewing process). (This does not begin until the biting reflex fades at 3 to 5 months.) Controls sucking impulse. Opens mouth to accept spoon. Turns head freely.
6–8 months	Cottage cheese, plain yogurt, egg yolk, strained meats (start with lamb), poultry, and meat alternates (purees of beans and lentils), dried breads.	Provides additional protein, vitamins, and iron for rapid growth. Encourages chewing when teeth erupt. (Note: To avoid allergies, egg white is not suggested until 12 months.)	Infant has ability to grasp and route food from hand to mouth, and can sit with support. Teeth begin to come in.
7–9 months	Junior meats, poultry, or cooked fish, mashed vegetables and fruits, mild cheese, other infant cereals (wheat, mixed grain, and high protein).	Adds variety and additional protein, minerals, and vitamins for rapid growth.	Infant can sit alone, has mobility of shoulders, can reach, grasp, and transfer items. Infant has more tongue maturity for spoon feeding. Can suck from a cup. Can tolerate harder-to-masticate foods (junior types).
8–10 months	Chewy finger foods, bite-size meat, poultry, and fish. Soft-cooked vegetables in strips or slices.	Encourages the development of hand-to-mouth coordination and proper chewing.	Infant has concept of spoon and its use. Has increased hand and eye control, and can drink from a cup.
9–12 months	Variety of regular table foods. Meat, poultry, fish, and cheese. Mild casserole dishes, beans, fruits, vegetables, cereal and breads.	Infant can feed self.	Infant develops pincer grasp. Has rotary chewing movements, holds, and transfers food to mouth. Tries to feed self.
12 months	Whole egg, orange juice, cow's milk.	Infant can drink from a cup. Infant should be weaned from a bottle, and may be weaned from the breast.	Infant is able to spit and stick out tongue. Is more interested in feeding self and is quieter at meals.

Adapted from material developed by Elizabeth G. Jones, Pediatric Nutrition Consultant, San Diego, California.

TABLE 8-3. Portion Sizes for the Infant Aged 4–12 Months

4–6 months	6–8 months	8–10 months	10–12 months
Breast milk or formula			
24–32 oz in 5–6 feedings	24–32 oz in 4–5 feedings in a cup	24–32 oz in 3–4 feedings in a cup	24 oz in 3 feedings in a cup
Cereal (dry)			
2–4 T	4 T	4 T or more	4 T or more
Vegetables			
—	4 T or 1/2 jar	4 T or more	4 T bite-size pieces
Fruit			
—	4 T or 1/2 jar	4 T or more	4 T bite-size pieces
Meat			
—	Strained—up to 4 T or 1/2 jar	Junior—up to 4 T or 1/2 jar	4–6 T bite-size pieces
Water			
—	3–4 oz, if desired	As needed	As needed
Other			
Dilute cereal with breast milk or formula and feed with a spoon.	Teething foods—dry toast, crackers, cottage cheese, and plain yogurt—2–4 T	Fruit juice, 3–4 oz/day, teething foods; start introducing finger and table foods	Fruit juice, 4 oz/day, teething foods, variety of table foods, including mild casserole dishes.

grapes, wieners, carrots, fish with bones, tough meat, and small or hard candies may cause choking in children until 3 years of age. Daily intake of cookies, pastry, sugar-coated cereals, candy, soft drinks, and artificially flavored fruit drinks may replace more nutritious foods and encourage a desire for sweets. Honey and corn syrup should be avoided in the child under one year of age. Evidence shows that these sweeteners may be contaminated with *Clostridium botulinum* spores. Chapter 14 discusses the foods most likely to cause allergic reactions in atopic children. Sensitization can sometimes be prevented in atopic children by introducing these foods only after one year of age.

Infant Formulas

There are three broad categories of infant formulas: standard commercial infant formulas, evaporated whole-milk formulas, and specialized infant formulas (6).

Standard Commercial Infant Formula. The standard commercial formulas are designed to mimic the nutritional composition of human milk. The American Academy of Pediatrics has developed standards for infant formulas designed as breast-milk substitutes for the normal full-term infant from birth to 1 year of age (2.5 to 4.0 kg through 8 to 10 kg) (7). These stand-

ards include a calorie density of 20 kcal/oz (0.67 kcal/ml), an osmolality of 300 to 400 mOsm/L, and a calorie distribution of 7.2 to 18 percent protein, 30 to 54 percent fat, and 40 to 50 percent carbohydrate. The formulas are supplemented to provide adequate levels of vitamins and minerals. Some of the formulas are fortified with iron (12 mg/L), while others are not and require that the infant receive an additional iron source by 4 to 6 months of age, when iron stores may be depleted. Fluoride may need to be supplemented, depending on the water supply and the method of formula preparation. Composition of commonly available formulas is given in Table 8-4.

Three forms of formula are available:

1. *Powder*—The powder comes in 1-pound cans and requires dilution with water. The usual dilution is 1 T or 1 measure (included in each can) to 2 oz water. The formula should be refrigerated and prepared fresh daily. Powder is the least expensive form of formula.
2. *Liquid concentrate*—Concentrates come in 13-oz cans and are prepared by diluting 1 oz water to 1 oz concentrate.
3. *Ready-to-Feed*—This form comes in various size cans and needs no dilution. It is the most expensive type of formula.

The standard commercial formulas fall into two groups—those which are based on cow's milk protein and those which are soy protein based and are also lactose-free. The most commonly used commercial infant formulas are the cow's milk–based formulas Enfamil (Mead Johnson), Similac (Ross), and SMA (Wyeth). These proprietary, or exclusively manufacturer-protected, formulas are prepared by one of two methods. The first includes a blending of nonfat cow's milk, a mixture of vegetable oils (soy, coconut, corn, and safflower) and added carbohydrate, which yields a whey-to-casein ratio of 20:80. The other method blends nonfat cow's milk, sodium caseinate, demineralized whey, a blend of oils, and added carbohydrate to achieve a whey-to-casein ratio of 60:40, which approaches the 70:30 to 80:20 whey-to-casein ratio of human milk.

The soy protein–based formulas are recommended for those infants who have lactose intolerance or galactosemia, or who are allergic to cow's milk protein. They include the following products: Prosobee (Mead Johnson), Isomil (Ross), Nursoy (Wyeth), Soyalac (Loma Linda), and Neo-Mull-Soy (Syntex). These formulas are composed of soy-protein isolate with added methionine, sucrose, or corn syrup solids or both as a carbohydrate source, vegetable oil, and added vitamins and minerals, including iron. When consumed in appropriate quantities, they do not require additional supplementation other than, possibly, fluoride.

Evaporated Whole-Milk Formula. Evaporated whole-milk formula can be prepared at home and is less expensive than commercial formulas. It is not recommended as frequently as is commercial formula,

TABLE 8-4. Infant Formula Composition

Formula	Manufacturer	kcal/ml	Protein (%)	Fat (%)	CHO (%)	Protein source	Fat source	CHO source	Nutrients per 100 ml		
									Protein (g)	Fat (g)	CHO (g)
Mature human milk	—	0.71	7	51	42	Whey:casein (80:20)	Butterfat	Lactose glycoproteins	1.05	3.9	7.2
Cow's milk	—	0.70	20	51	29	Whey:casein (18:82)	Butterfat	Lactose	3.5	3.7	4.9
Goat's milk	—	0.67	14	53	28	—	Butterfat	Lactose	3.7	4.3	4.6
Evaporated milk	—		16	38	46	Whey:casein (18:82)	Butterfat	Lactose	2.9	3.3	8.8
Standard Infant Formulas											
Cow's milk based											
Enfamil	Mead Johnson	0.67	9	50	41	Reduced mineral whey, nonfat milk	Soy, coconut	Lactose	1.5	3.8	6.9
Similac	Ross	0.68	9	48	43	Nonfat milk	Coconut, soy	Lactose	1.5	3.6	7.2
SMA Infant Formula	Wyeth	0.67	9	48	43	Nonfat milk, demineralized whey solids	Coconut, soy safflower, oleo	Lactose	1.5	3.6	7.2
Soy based											
Isomil	Ross	0.68	12	48	40	Soy	Coconut, soy	Corn syrup, sucrose	2.0	3.6	6.8
Isomil SF	Ross	0.68	12	48	40	Soy	Soy, coconut	Glucose, polymers	2.0	3.6	6.8
I-Soyalac	Loma Linda	0.68	13	49	38	Soy with L-methionine	Soy	Sucrose, tapioca starch	2.2	3.8	6.7
Nursoy	Wyeth	0.67	12	48	40	Soy isolate	Oleo, safflower, coconut	Sucrose in fluid formula only	2.1	3.6	6.9
ProSobee	Mead Johnson	0.67	12	48	40	Soy with L-methionine	Soy, coconut	Corn syrup solids	2.0	3.6	6.9
Soyalac	Loma Linda	0.67	13	49	38	Soy	Soy	Corn syrup, sucrose	2.2	3.8	6.7
Special Infant Formulas											
LBW and premature infant formulas											
Enfamil Premature 20	Mead Johnson	0.67	12	44	44	Nonfat milk, whey	MCT: corn, coconut	Lactose corn syrup solids	2.0	3.4	7.4
Enfamil Premature 24	Mead Johnson	0.81	12	44	44	Nonfat milk, whey	MCT: corn, coconut	Lactose, corn syrup solids	2.4	4.1	8.9

Formula	Manufacturer					Fat source	Protein source	Carbohydrate source			
Similac Special Care 20	Ross	41	48	11	0.67	MCT: corn, coconut	Nonfat milk, whey	Lactose, glucose, polymers	2.2	4.4	8.6
Similac Special Care 24	Ross	42	47	11	0.81	MCT: corn, coconut	Nonfat milk, whey	Lactose, glucose, polymers	2.2	4.4	8.6
SMA Preemie	Wyeth	42	48	10	0.81	MCT: oleo, safflower, coconut, soy	Nonfat milk, demineralized whey solids	Lactose, glucose, polymers	2.0	4.4	8.6
Special Indication											
Nutramigen	Mead Johnson	52	35	13	0.67	Corn	Casein hydrolysate	Sucrose, tapioca	2.2	2.6	8.8
Pregestimil	Mead Johnson	54	35	11	0.67	MCT corn	Casein hydrolysate + amino acids	Corn syrup solids, tapioca	1.9	2.7	9.1
Portagen	Mead Johnson	46	40	14	0.67	MCT corn	Casein	Corn syrup solids, sucrose	2.4	3.2	7.8
Similac PM 60/40	Ross	41	50	9	0.68	Coconut, corn	Nonfat milk, whey	Lactose	1.6	3.8	6.9

Vitamins per 100 ml

Formula	Manufacturer	A(IU)	D(IU)	E(IU)	K(μg)	C(mg)	Folic acid (μg)	B₁ (μg)	B₂ (μg)	B₆ (μg)	B₁₂ (μg)	Niacin (mg)	Choline (mg)	Biotin (μg)	Pantothenic acid (μg)
Mature human milk	—	190	2.2	0.20	1.5	4.3	0.5	16	36	10	0.03	1.47	—	—	200
Cow's milk	—	103	1.4	0.04	6.0	1.1	5.5	44	175	—	0.04	0.94	—	—	350
Goat's milk	—	280	2.4	—	1.2	1.5	0.6	40	184	70	0.19	—	—	—	340
Evaporated milk	—	185	4.0	0.01	—	0.5	5.5	28	190	37	—	0.10	—	—	350
Standard Infant Formulas															
Cow's milk based															
Enfamil	Mead Johnson	210	42.0	2.10	5.8	5.5	10.6	53	110	42	0.16	0.85	10.6	1.58	320
Similac	Ross	200	40.0	2.00	5.5	5.5	10.0	65	100	40	0.15	0.70	—	1.00	300
SMA	Wyeth	265	42.0	0.95	5.8	5.8	5.3	71	106	42	0.11	0.53	11.0	1.50	210
Soy based															
Isomil	Ross	200	40	2.0	10.0	5.5	10.0	40	60	40	0.30	0.90	5.3	3.0	500
Isomil SF	Ross	200	40	2.0	10.0	5.5	10.0	40	60	40	0.30	0.90	5.3	3.0	500
I-Soyalac	Loma Linda	205	40	—	—	6.6	—	33	66	—	—	1.00	9.0	—	320
Nursoy	Wyeth	264	42	1.0	10.6	5.8	5.3	71	105	42	0.21	0.50	5.3	3.7	320
ProSobee	Mead Johnson	210	42	2.1	10.6	5.5	10.6	53	63	42	0.21	0.85	5.3	5.3	320
Soyalac	Loma Linda Johnson	211	42	0.5	—	6.3	11.0	55	60	40	0.02	0.80	11.0	5.5	300

(continued)

TABLE 8-4. *(Continued)*

Vitamins per 100 ml

Formula	Manufacturer	A(IU)	D(IU)	E(IU)	K(μg)	C (mg)	Folic acid (μg)	B_1 (μg)	B_2 (μg)	B_6 (μg)	B_{12} (μg)	Niacin (mg)	Choline (mg)	Biotin (μg)	Pantothenic acid (μg)
Special Infant Formulas															
LBW and premature infant formula															
Enfamil Premature 20	Mead Johnson	210	42.0	1.32	6.3	5.7	20.0	50	60	42	0.21	0.85	4.8	1.59	320
Enfamil Premature 24	Mead Johnson	250	51.0	1.59	7.6	6.9	24.0	60	70	50	0.25	1.01	5.7	1.90	380
Similac Special Care 20	Ross	458	100.0	2.50	8.0	25.0	25.0	170	420	170	0.37	3.40	—	25.00	1250
Similac Special Care 24	Ross	550	120.0	3.00	10.0	30.0	30.0	200	500	200	0.45	4.00	8.0	30.00	1500
SMA Preemie	Wyeth	320	51.0	1.50	7.0	7.0	10.0	80	130	50	0.20	0.63	12.7	1.80	360
Special indications															
Nutramigen	Mead Johnson	169	42	1.1	10.6	5.5	10.6	50	60	40	0.21	0.85	9.0	5.3	320
Pregestimil	Mead Johnson	210	42	1.6	10.6	5.5	10.6	50	60	40	0.21	0.85	9.0	5.3	320
Portagen	Mead Johnson	530	53	2.1	10.6	5.5	10.6	110	130	140	0.42	1.37	9.0	5.3	710
Similac PM 60/40	Ross	250	40.0	0.90	—	5.5	—	60	30	30	0.15	0.73	—	—	—

Minerals

Formula	Manufacturer	Na (mEq)	K (mEq)	Cl (mg)	Ca (mg)	P (mg)	Mg (mg)	I (μg)	Mn (mg)	Cu (mg)	Z (mg)	Fe (mg)	Intestinal osmolality	Estimated renal solute load
Mature human milk		0.5	1.3	39.6	34.0	14.0	4.0	3.0	1.10	0.04	0.4	0.50	300	—
Cow's milk		2.2	3.5	108.0	117.0	92.0	12.0	4.7	0.02	0.10	0.4	0.05	270	—
Goat's milk		1.4	4.5	—	129.0	106.0	—	—	—	—	—	0.01	—	—
Evaporated milk		2.6	3.9	—	126.0	102.5	—	—	—	—	—	0.05	300	—
Standard Infant Formulas														
Cow's milk based														
Enfamil	Mead Johnson	0.9	1.8	42.0	46.0	32.0	5.3	10.6	0.01	0.06	0.5	0.11*	300	10
Similac	Ross	1.1	2.1	50.0	51.0	39.0	4.1	10.0	0.003	0.06	0.5	0.15*	290	105
SMA	Wyeth	0.7	1.4	37.5	44.3	33.0	5.3	6.9	0.016	0.05	0.4	1.27	300	91
Soy based														
Isomil	Ross	1.4	1.9	59.0	70.0	50.0	5.0	10.0	0.02	0.05	0.50	1.20	250	126
Isomil SF	Ross	1.4	1.9	59.0	70.0	50.0	5.0	10.0	0.02	0.05	0.50	1.20	150	126
I-Soyalac	Loma Linda	1.6	1.8	—	62.7	52.8	6.6	—	—	—	—	1.60	230	—
Nursoy	Wyeth	0.9	1.9	37.0	63.4	44.4	6.9	6.9	0.02	0.05	0.37	1.30	296	122
ProSobee	Mead Johnson	1.3	2.0	55.0	63.0	50.0	7.4	6.9	0.02	0.06	0.53	1.27	200	130
Soyalac	Loma Linda	1.5	2.0	—	63.0	53.0	8.0	5.0	0.10	0.07	0.50	1.60	203	140

TABLE 8-4. (Continued)

Formula	Manufacturer	kcal/ml	Protein (%)	Fat (%)	CHO (%)	Protein source		Fat source		CHO source			Protein (g)	Fat (g)	CHO (g)
														Nutrients per 100 ml	
Special Infant Formulas															
LBW and premature infant formulas															
Enfamil Premature 20	Mead Johnson	1.1	1.9	57.0	79.0	40.0	7.1	5.4	0.02	0.06	0.7	0.11	244		17
Enfamil Premature 24	Mead Johnson	1.4	2.3	69.0	95.0	48.0	8.5	6.4	0.02	0.07	0.8	0.13	300		21
Similac Special Care 20	Ross	1.5	2.6	65.0	144.0	72.0	10.0	15.0	0.02	0.20	1.2	0.30	300		154
Similac Special Care 24	Ross	1.7	2.9	71.0	144.0	72.0	10.0	15.0	0.01	0.17	1.0	0.25	240		122
SMA Preemie	Wyeth	1.4	1.9	53.0	75.0	40.0	7.0	8.3	0.02	0.07	0.5	0.30	268		128
Special indication															
Nutramigen	Mead Johnson	1.4	1.8	48.0	63.0	48.0	7.4	4.8	0.11	0.06	0.42	1.27	480		13
Pregestimil	Mead Johnson	1.4	2.2	58.0	63.0	42.0	7.4	4.8	0.02	0.06	0.42	1.27	350		12
Portagen	Mead Johnson	1.4	2.1	58.0	63.0	48.0	13.7	4.8	0.08	0.11	0.63	1.27	220		15
Similac PM 60/40	Ross	0.7	1.5	40.0	40.0	20.0	4.2	4.2	0.003	0.06	0.5	0.15	260		96

*Enfamil with Iron and Similac with Iron have 1.2 mg Fe per 100 ml.

but it is superior to unmodified whole milk. The protein content and renal solute load of evaporated whole-milk formula are higher, and the fat is not as well absorbed compared with breast milk or commercial infant formula. Supplemental vitamin C and iron must be provided when feeding this formula. Fluoride supplementation is recommended if the formula is prepared with nonfluoridated water.

A commonly used formula consists of one can of vitamin D–fortified evaporated whole milk (13 oz), 1½ cans of water (19 oz), and 2 T of sugar.

Specialized Infant Formulas.   The specialized infant formulas include those for premature or low-birth-weight infants; those with a modified protein, carbohydrate, or fat source; those with a modified amino acid content for inborn errors of amino acid metabolism; and Protein Modular Formula (Ross), which is a "base" formula composed of casein and minerals for infants with complex malabsorption syndromes. Their composition is also listed in Table 8-4.

The formulas for low-birth-weight infants include Enfamil Premature (Mead Johnson), Special Care (Ross), and SMA "Preemie" (Wyeth). These cow's milk–based formulas are manufactured containing 20 or 24 kcal per oz, with a 60:40 whey-to-casein ratio. The calcium-to-phosphorus ratio is approximately 2:1, similar to that of human milk. The fat is a blend of medium-chain triglycerides (MCT) and vegetable oils, and the lactose content is reduced by addition of glucose polymers. The formulas are designed to be fed at 120 kcal per kg, which usually provides a fluid intake of 150 ml per kg. These formulas are available only by prescription.

Nutramigen and Pregestimil (Mead Johnson) are lactose-free and formulated from a casein hydrolysate. They are used for infants who have a sensitivity to cow's milk or soy protein, or who have severe or chronic malabsorption. Pregestimil contains MCT and

glucose polymers and is both lactose- and sucrose-free. It may be useful for infants with intractable diarrhea.

Vitamin and Mineral Supplementation

Guidelines for vitamin and mineral supplementation in healthy, full-term infants are summarized in Table 8-5. In addition, infants usually receive 1 mg of vitamin K at birth. Supplementation with most nutrients is not generally needed for full-term infants fed breast milk or commercial formula supplemented with iron. Nutrients that *may* need to be supplemented include both vitamin D in the breast-fed infant not exposed to sunlight, and fluoride. The American Academy of Pediatrics (8) recommends that supplementation with fluoride in the breast-fed infant be initiated shortly after birth or at least by 6 months of age, since fluoride is not thought to pass into breast milk in significant amounts. If powdered or concentrated commercial formulas are used, fluoride supplements should be administered only if the community water supply contains less than 0.3 parts per million (ppm) of fluoride. Ready-to-use formulas contain little fluoride, so fluoride supplementation should begin shortly after birth. Recommendations for fluoride supplementation are included in Table 8-6.

Iron stores for the term infant may be depleted by 4 to 6 months of age. Infants fed breast milk or infant formula not fortified with iron should start to receive an iron supplement by 6 months of age. This may be in the form of iron-fortified infant cereal, which provides 1.6 mg iron per T of dry cereal, multivitamins with iron (10 mg Fe per dose), or iron sulfate drops.

Liquid multivitamin preparations given by the drop are available with or without iron or fluoride for infants. Generally, they contain either (1) vitamins A, C, and D, with or without iron, (2) vitamins A, C, D, E, thiamine, riboflavin, and niacin, or (3) vitamins A, C, D, E, thiamin, riboflavin, niacin, and vitamin B_6, with or without iron.

Folic acid is omitted from liquid dietary supplements because it is relatively unstable in liquid preparations. Preparations with fluoride are available only with a prescription.

TABLE 8-5.   Guidelines for Vitamin-Mineral Supplementation in Healthy Full-term Infants

Alimentation	A	C	D	E	Folic acid	Iron	Fluoride
Human milk	−	−	±	−	−	−	±
Commercial formula without iron	−	−	−	−	−	+	±
Commercial formula, iron-fortified	−	−	−	−	−	−	±
Cow's milk, evaporated	±	+	±	−	−	+	±
Cow's milk, whole homogenized	−	+	−	−	−	+	±
Goat's milk, evaporated	±	+	±	−	++	+	±
Goat's milk, fresh fluid	±	+	±	−	++	+	±

++ = Supplementation strongly recommended; + = supplementation recommended; − = supplementation not recommended; ± = Supplementation may be required.

Reproduced with permission from *Manual of Pediatric Nutrition,* eds. D. G. Kelts and E. G. Jones. Boston: Little, Brown, 1984.

TABLE 8-6.   Recommended Daily Fluoride Supplementation (mg/day) as Influenced by Fluoride Concentration in the Drinking Water

Fluoride concentration in drinking water (ppm)	Age		
	2 weeks–2 years	2–3 years	3–16 years
<0.3	0.25	0.50	1.00
0.3–0.7	0	0.25	0.50
>0.7	0	0	0

Adapted from Committee on Nutrition, American Academy of Pediatrics. Fluoride supplementation: Revised dosage schedule. *Pediatrics* 63:150–155, 1979.

TO TEST YOUR UNDERSTANDING

1. a. A new mother is concerned that her baby may not be receiving enough breast milk. What clues can you tell her to watch for?

   b. Another new mother is concerned that her 2-day-old baby does not consume much of the 4-oz bottle of formula which the nurses on the obstetrics floor give her at each feeding. How would you advise the mother?

2. Patty is exclusively breast-fed until 3 months of age. At this point her mother returns to work and weans Patty to Enfamil with Iron formula.

   a. Outline a feeding program for Patty's first year including age in months, number of feedings per day, amount of milk per feeding, solid foods, and stage of feeding development.

   b. Write a typical menu for Patty at 1 year of age.

3. How would you respond to the following question from a young mother? "My baby is 2 months old, and I'm nursing him, but my mother tells me that I need to start giving him solids. The nurse who gave my baby his immunizations said not to start any solid food until the baby is 4 months old. Why should I wait to start solid foods for so long?"

4. Indicate the usually recommended vitamin supplementation for the following infant formulas, assuming that the child is not consuming solid foods. Place a (−) in the appropriate column if the nutrient is not needed in extra amounts, a (+) if the nutrient is usually supplemented, and a (+ / −) if the nutrient is supplemented under specific conditions. For the (+ / −) cases, explain the circumstances affecting supplementation.

	Iron	Vitamin D	Fluoride	Vitamin C	Folate
Breast milk					
Evaporated milk formula					
Infant formula, Iron fortified					
Goat's milk					

5. A list of snacks for infants ranging in age from 6 to 12 months follows. Circle those snacks that would *not* be a good choice for an infant and explain why these snacks should be avoided.

Snack	Reason to Avoid
Cooked egg white	
Cheerios	
Popcorn	
Donut	
Fruit juice in a bottle	
Fruit juice in a cup	
Raw celery and carrot sticks	
Hard candy	
Banana	
Toast with honey	
Yogurt	
Bacon	

6. Suggest appropriate specific infant formula(s) for the following situations.

Infant Description	Recommended Formula
Allergy to cow's milk protein	
Infant has cystic fibrosis, which affects fat digestion and absorption	
Lactose intolerance without fat malabsorption	
Persistent diarrhea with tolerance to fat but intolerance to intact protein-containing formulas	
Normal full-term infant	

The Low-Birth-Weight Infant

The normal, full-term infant is born between 37 and 42 weeks' gestation and weighs approximately 3,500 g (7.7 pounds). Infants weighing less than 2,500 g (5½ pounds) are defined as low birth weight (LBW), and those weighing less than 1,500 g (3½ pounds), as very low birth weight (VLBW) (9). Infants have low birth weights, most commonly, for one of two reasons. Either they may be born before 37 weeks' gestation, in which case they are *premature,* or they may exhibit a retarded rate of intrauterine growth, which makes them *small for gestational age* (SGA).

Because LBW infants may have a variety of clinical problems in the postnatal period, their management frequently involves care in tertiary-care hospitals with neonatal intensive care units (NICUs). Recent advances in neonatology are increasing the survival rate of LBW infants, although those born before 25 weeks' gestation still rarely survive. This increase in survival rate has resulted in a great interest in providing optimal nutritional support for these infants and, consequently, in an increased use of the nutritional care specialist in the NICU.

Nutrient Requirements. Nutritional requirements and optimal growth rate for the LBW infant are poorly understood and are the subject of current research. One commonly used approach is to estimate nutritional requirements based on the goal of having the LBW infant continue a rate of growth similar to that which would have occurred in utero (4). The nutritional requirements of preterm and SGA, LBW infants are higher per kg of body weight than those of normal-weight, full-term infants. This is because maintenance energy needs are increased due to a greater body surface area relative to weight and because of an accelerated rate of growth. Premature birth, in particular, increases energy, protein, and mineral needs for growth. During the last 10 weeks of gestation, infant weight doubles, length increases by 25 percent, and two-thirds of the mineral deposition in the fetal skeleton occurs (10).

If an infant is born between 26 and 34 weeks' gestation, the ability to digest, absorb, and metabolize carbohydrate, protein, and fat is only partially developed, resulting in a need to provide modified forms of these nutrients. Lactase activity is greatly reduced in the preterm infant, so glucose polymers supplemented with smaller amounts of lactose are more easily digested and absorbed. Decreased levels of bile acids and pancreatic lipase impair fat absorption in LBW infants, and polyunsaturated fats supplemented with MCT are generally better absorbed. In infants born after 26 weeks' gestation, protein digestion is generally adequate, although several enzymes of amino acid metabolism are not mature, and cystine and taurine need to be provided. Table 8-7 summarizes specific recommendations for the LBW infant (4,10).

TABLE 8-7. Recommendations for Feeding the Low-Birth-Weight (LBW) Infant

Nutrient	Recommendation	Nutritional Considerations
Energy	110–150 (mean = 120) kcal/kg/day	Formulas providing 24 kcal/oz are recommended. Intakes of 150–200 ml/kg/day of these formulas provide for sufficient water and adequate weight gain.
Protein	2.25–5.0 (mean = 3.5–4.0) g/kg/day from cow's milk–based formula.	Consumption of breast milk at 120 kcal/kg provides a marginal intake. Improved growth rates are observed with feeding of special LBW formulas which provide at least 2.0 gm pro/100 ml.
Carbohydrate	Formulas providing a mixture of lactose and either glucose polymers or sucrose are preferred.	Maltase and sucrase reach full activity by the 6th–8th month of gestation, while lactase activity is not usually fully developed until the end of a full-term gestation.
Fat	40%–50% of formula calories as fat, with 4% of total calories as linoleic acid.	LBW formulas providing polyunsaturated vegetable oils supplemented with MCT are well absorbed. Human milk fat is especially well absorbed by the LBW infant.
Minerals		
Calcium	Ca = 200–250 mg/kg/day	LBW formulas provide for increased mineralization of the skeleton compared to human milk.
Phosphorus (6)	P = 110–125 mg/kg/day 2:1 Ca:P ratio	
Copper	90 µg/100 kcal	
Zinc	0.5 mg/100 kcal	
Manganese	5 µg/100 kcal	
Iron	2–3 mg Fe/kg/day by 2 months of age or at 2 kg body weight. Formulas to provide 0.1–1.5 mg iron per 100 kcal.	LBW infants have low iron stores and are susceptible to the development of iron-deficiency anemia.
Vitamin E	0.7 IU vitamin E/100 kcal and at least 1.0 IU vitamin E/g linoleic acid plus 5–25 IU supplement of vitamin E/day.	LBW infants fed formulas high in polyunsaturated fatty acids and iron are prone to the development of hemolytic anemia with inadequate Vitamin E intake. Vitamin E stores and absorption are reduced in the preterm infant.

Constructed with information from Committee on Nutrition. Pediatric Nutrition Handbook (2d ed.). Elk Grove Village, Ill.: American Academy of Pediatrics, 1985.

Methods of Feeding.   Most infants of less than 32 to 34 weeks' gestational age have poor coordination of sucking, swallowing, and respiration and immature development of the gastrointestinal and respiratory systems. Both these factors result in the preterm infant's frequently being unable to nipple feed. Enteral tube feeding, parenteral nutrition, or a combination of these methods of feeding are frequently necessary (see Chapters 12 and 13). Important advantages of tube and parenteral feeding in the LBW infant are that these feeding methods decrease the risk of aspiration and reduce energy expenditure compared with that required for nipple feeding. Parenteral feedings are usually needed in infants weighing less than 1,600 g. When the infant gains weight and the gastrointestinal tract develops more fully, enteral feedings can be begun, although the transition from parenteral to enteral feedings should occur very slowly. Continuous orogastric or orojejunal feeding is usually used in LBW infants who are unable to suck because most newborns are obligate nosebreathers, and orogastric feeding interferes less with breathing than does nasogastric feeding. Continuous, rather than bolus or intermittent, tube feeding is preferred because gastric capacity is very small in these infants, and continuous feeding reduces the risk of aspiration.

The choice of formula for an LBW infant is controversial. There are several options: (1) human milk from a mother who has given birth to a full-term infant; (2) human milk from the infant's mother (preterm human milk, or PTHM), as is or fortified; (3) standard infant formula; or (4) special formulas designed for LBW infants (LBW formula). PTHM has several advantages compared with mature human milk for feeding the LBW infant. It has a similar calorie content but a greater concentration of protein, sodium, chloride, magnesium, and iron compared with mature human milk (11). The LBW formulas are thought to be superior in promoting growth compared with the standard infant formulas because the LBW formulas contain a higher nutrient density and are more easily digested and absorbed by the premature infant. Soy protein formulas are not recommended because of reports of hypophosphatemia and rickets in very-low-birth-weight infants receiving soy based formulas (4). The two preferred feeding methods for LBW infants are PTHM or a specialized LBW formula. Each of these approaches has advantages, and many centers choose to use a combination of PTHM and LBW formulas. While PTHM offers some immunological advantages if given fresh, it may not provide an optimal level of protein and calcium. Weight gain and bone mineralization are, in general, better in those LBW infants receiving special formulas compared with PTHM (12). Supplementation with additional protein, carbohydrate, vitamins, and minerals has been suggested, but there have been no published studies on the nutritional effects of human milk fortified in this manner. The use of human milk as a sole food for the LBW infant is, at present, a subject of intense investigation.

TO TEST YOUR UNDERSTANDING

7. a. Compare the composition of mature human milk, Enfamil, and Enfamil Premature 24 in terms of the following nutrients (per 100 ml):
Kcal
Protein
Fat
Folate
Vitamin A
Sodium
Calcium
Iron

b. Compare the energy, protein, and fluid requirements for a term (3.5 kg) infant and an LBW (1.8 kg) infant.

c. How much of the formulas listed in part (a) of this question would the LBW infant (1.8 kg) have to consume to meet her protein needs?

	ml/day
Mature human milk	_____
Enfamil	_____
Enfamil Premature 24	_____

d. Discuss the reason for the differences in energy, protein, and calcium content between Enfamil and Enfamil Premature 24.

THE PRESCHOOL CHILD

The growth rate slows after the first year of life, resulting in both a decrease in nutrient requirements per unit of body weight and a decrease in appetite. Irregular weight gain is not unusual for the preschool child. Average growth for this group is 12 cm during the second year, 8 to 9 cm during the third year, and 7 cm per year thereafter. The average weight gain during those years is 2 to 2½ kg per year.

During these years, children learn to walk and speak; they also develop the fine motor skills which allow them to learn to feed themselves. Children learn to feed themselves independently between 1 and 2 years of age. Messiness is common between 10 and 18 months, but by 2 years of age most children spill very little (13).

Feeding the preschool child can be frustrating. At this age, food jags and rituals are common, as are strong food preferences and dislikes and, at times, an apparent lack of interest in eating. It is important to realize that a decrease in appetite is expected during these years because of the decreased growth rate; in addition, many of the food behaviors common in this age group are related to the child's developing sense of independence. Children should not be forced to eat, nor should food be used as a reward. The development of good eating patterns in a child should allow the child to stop eating whenever satiety is reached.

It is important to be familiar with the appropriate portion sizes for the preschool child (see Table 8-8). In general, it is better to offer a child less to eat, and thus to allow for success, than to overwhelm the child with large portions. Most children in this age group eat 5 to 6 small meals per day.

Several generalizations can be made about the food preferences of the preschool child (13). Fibrous meats are not well accepted because rotary chewing motion is not well established until 2½ years of age. Before this age, fish, chicken, ground meats, and cheese are usually preferred. Single foods are more popular than combination dishes. Finger foods are especially popular because children are interested in the texture of food. Color and variety are also important. Raw vegetables are often more popular than cooked ones. Dry foods are usually hard for a preschool child to swallow and should be combined with moister foods. A final consideration is the ease with which a food can be manipulated. For example, soup or peas might not be good choices for a 2-year-old child. Warm, rather than hot, foods are usually preferred.

THE SCHOOL-AGE CHILD

Growth of the school-age child tends to be more stable, and there are generally fewer apparent feeding problems compared with the preschool child. Height usually increases by 5 to 6 cm each year, and the average weight increase is 2 kg each year for the first 2 to 3

years and 4.0 to 4.5 kg per year as the child approaches puberty.

School-age children usually eat four to five times per day on school days and generally eat after-school snacks which they prepare themselves. Sugar makes a significant contribution to the daily calorie intake in school-age children (13). This is of concern in terms of dental health and potential obesity.

THE ADOLESCENT

After a slow rate of growth during the childhood years, adolescence is characterized by an increase in the velocity of physical growth similar to that seen during infancy. Up to the age of approximately 9 years, males and females grow in height and weight at about the same rate. The growth spurt preceding puberty, or the initial ability to reproduce, begins between 10 and 12 years of age in girls and about 2 years later in boys. The ages at which average peak growth velocity is achieved in males is 14.1 years for height and 14.3 years for weight (14). In females, average peak velocities of height and weight increases are observed at 12.1 and 12.9 years, respectively (14). Menarche occurs at the end of the growth spurt, approximately 9 to 12 months after peak height velocity is attained (13).

Nutrient requirements in the adolescent population parallel the growth rate, with the greatest need occurring at the peak velocity of growth. The RDAs for energy in the adolescent population are expressed as ranges of kcals for two age periods—11 to 14 years and 15 to 18 years of age. Ranges are used because the individual rate of growth is quite variable during adolescence. Most of the allowances for nutrients are extrapolations from data on young children and adults, and are therefore only estimates of nutritional needs. Rate of growth, as determined by rate of increase in height, and activity level are key factors in estimating energy needs for adolescents.

There are several general nutritional concerns in the adolescent population. Eating patterns tend to be erratic, with frequent skipping of meals, adherence to various fad weight-reduction diets, snacking, and reliance on "fast foods." Nutrients that are frequently limiting in the diet include zinc, iron, and vitamins A, D, B_6, and folate (15). Many females become preoccupied with slimness during the adolescent years, resulting in marginally adequate dietary intakes and a high incidence of eating disorders such as bulimia and anorexia nervosa. Pregnancy in adolescence is also of nutritional relevance, as discussed in Chapter 8. Males involved in athletic programs during these years may become preoccupied with nutrition in relation to body building and athletic performance.

NUTRITIONAL ASSESSMENT

Nutritional assessment for the pediatric population, as for adults, includes an evaluation of pertinent dietary,

TABLE 8-8. Dietary Evaluation Guidelines for Children 1–15 Years Old

Food Group	Recommended Number of Servings per Day	Average Size of Servings					
		1 yr (1,000 kcal/day)	2–3 yr (1,300 kcal/day)	4–5 yr (1,700 kcal/day)	6–9 yr (2,100 kcal/day)	10–12 yr (2,500 kcal/day)	13–15 yr (2,600–3,000 kcal/day)
Milk and cheese	4						
Milk		½ c	½–¾ c	½–¾ c	¾–1 c	1 c	1 c
Cheese		¾ oz	¾–1⅛ oz	¾–1⅛ oz	¾–1½ oz	1½ oz	1½
Ice cream		¾ c	¾–1⅛ c	¾–1⅛ c	¾–1½ c	1½ c	1½ c
Yogurt		½ c	½–¾ c	½–¾ c	¾–1 c	1 c	1 c
Meat and meat alternatives	2 or 3						
Egg		1	1	1	1	1	1 or more
Meat, poultry, fish		2 T	2 T	4 T (2 oz)	2–3 oz	3–4 oz	4–5 oz
Peanut butter		—	1 T	2 T	2–3 T	3 T	3 T
Dried beans, peas		4 T	4 T	½ c	¾ c	1 c	1–1½ c
Fruits and vegetables	4						
Vitamin C sources (citrus fruits, berries, tomatoes etc.)	1	4 T (¼ c)	8 T (½ c)	½ c	1 c	1 c	1 c
Vitamin A sources (e.g., green or yellow fruits and vegetables)	1	2 T	3 T	¼ c	¼ c	¼ c	½ c
Others	2	2 T	3 T	½ c	½ c	½ c	¾ c
Breads and cereals	4						
Bread		½ slice	1 slice	1–1½ slices	1 or 2 slices	2 slices	2 slices
Cold cereal		½ c	¾ c	1 c	1 c	1–1½ c	1–1½ c
Cooked cereal or pasta		4 T (⅓ c)	5 T	½ c	½ c	¾ c	1 c or more
Fats and carbohydrates	To meet caloric needs						
Butter, margarine, mayonnaise, or oil (100 kcal/T)		1 T	1 T	1 T	2 T	2 T	2–4 T

Reproduced with permission from *Manual of Pediatric Nutrition*, eds. D. G. Kelts and E. G. Jones. Boston: Little, Brown, 1984.

biochemical, and anthropometric data. Evaluation of the progress of physical growth is a unique and powerful additional tool for the assessment of nutritional status in children.

DIETARY

Evaluation of the adequacy of dietary intake in the pediatric population requires a knowledge of nutritional requirements, normal feeding patterns, including appropriate portion sizes, and normal development of feeding skills (16). Tables 8-1, 8-2, and 8-3 provide a summary of information needed to evaluate the diet of an infant, and Table 8-8 provides a summary of information relevant to assessing dietary intake in the older child.

BIOCHEMICAL

Determination of various biochemical parameters is a useful part of nutritional status assessment in the pediatric population. The procedures and calculations necessary to assess these parameters are similar for children and adults, and are discussed in detail in Chapter 4. Normal laboratory values for both children and adults can be found in Appendix Tables E-1 through E-4, and also in Appendix F.

The calculation of nitrogen balance differs slightly in children compared to the method used for adults (16). Instead of a value of 4 g to account for nonurinary nitrogen losses, a value of 1.2 g is more appropriate for children. The adjusted equation is

$$\Delta N \text{ (g/day)} = \frac{\text{protein intake}}{6.25} - (\text{UUN} + 1.2) \quad \textbf{(8-1)}$$

where UUN is urinary urea nitrogen and all values are given in g. Total urinary nitrogen excretion is more accurate than UUN and should be used if available.

Normal children are in positive nitrogen balance which reflects growth. Values for ranges of nitrogen balance in healthy children include:

0–4 months	+180 to +90 mg N/kg body weight
4–17 months	+90 mg N/kg body weight
17 months–3 years	+70 mg N/kg body weight
3–7 years	+40 mg N/kg body weight

EVALUATION OF GROWTH

Growth standards for height (or length), weight, and head circumference make it possible to evaluate a child's growth. Evaluation of growth using *growth charts* is considered the most useful nutritional assessment tool for children. If the growth chart indicates that growth is not proceeding normally, additional assessment methods, such as measurement of skinfold thickness and determination of bone age, may be useful. Determinations of skinfold thickness and arm

circumference provide a basis for assessing adiposity, as discussed in Chapter 4. Standards for bone age permit an estimate of a child's physiologic maturity.

Growth Charts

Growth charts have been constructed from repeated measurements of height and weight obtained from large-scale studies of healthy children from a cross-section of ethnic and economic backgrounds. The height and weight measurements are ranked in percentiles based on a scale of 100. For example, if a child is at the 30th percentile for height, 70 percent of children of the same age and sex are taller, and 29 percent are shorter. At a specific age, 95 percent of the population of children, or the mean ± 2 standard deviations, are between the 2.5th and 97.5th percentile. The most commonly used growth charts are those provided by the National Center for Health Statistics (NCHS) (18).

NCHS growth charts for the pediatric population appear in subsequent pages. Separate grids are available for boys and girls from birth to 36 months of age (Figs. 8-1 to 8-4). These growth charts allow both determination of age-specific percentiles for length, weight, and head circumference and evaluation of weight for length. The NCHS growth charts include data on head circumference only from birth to 36 months of age. Head circumference in children over 36 months of age can be evaluated using graphs prepared by Nellhaus (19). For children aged 2 to 18 years, NCHS graphs are available to evaluate height and weight and weight for stature (Figs. 8-5 and 8-8).

Weight gain can be evaluated in the LBW infant by using a growth chart which estimates intrauterine growth in weight based on live birth weights in infants from 26 to 42 weeks' gestational age (Fig. 8-9). This graph is used by plotting daily infant weights and comparing the pattern of weight gain to average rates of gain associated with a specific birth weight.

Measurement Techniques. Weight values for the child of less than 36 months of age should be obtained while the child is nude, using calibrated beam-balance scales. Stature is measured as recumbent length, not height, when using the birth-to-36-month chart. Recumbent length can be determined using a wooden length board. The charts for children between 2 and 18 years of age use measurements of children in stocking feet and standard clothing worn during examination. Weight is recorded to the nearest 0.1 kg or 1.0 oz and length to the nearest 0.5 cm or 0.125 in.

Interpretation. When undernutrition exists, gain in weight is affected earlier and to a greater degree than gain in height. If malnutrition persists, height will eventually be retarded or halted and/or pubertal maturation and epiphyseal closure will be delayed. In general, weight gain is decreased when energy intake is deficient, while linear growth is more delayed when protein intake is inadequate. Overnutrition usually re-

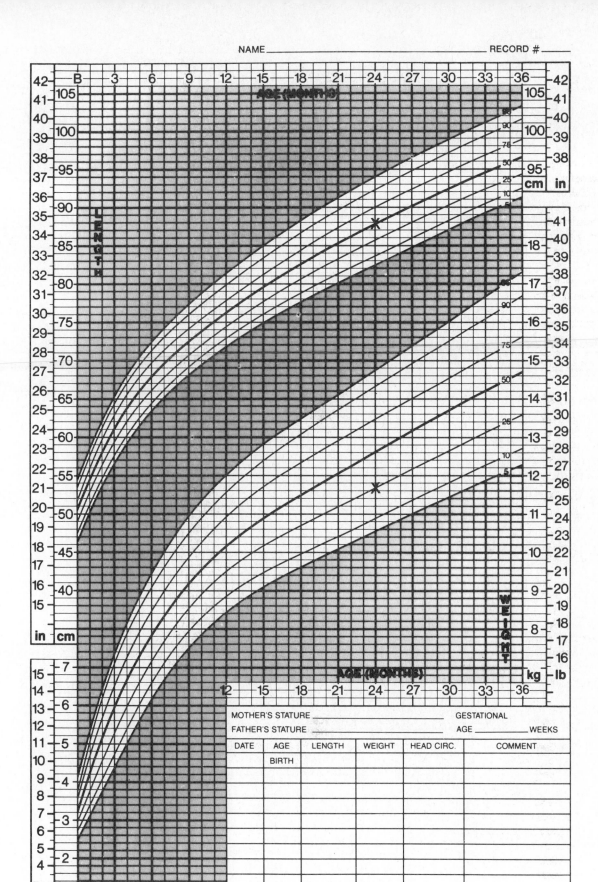

DATE	AGE	LENGTH	WEIGHT	HEAD CIRC.	COMMENT
	BIRTH				

MOTHER'S STATURE _____ GESTATIONAL

FATHER'S STATURE _____ AGE _____ WEEKS

Figure 8-1 Boys: Birth to 36 months physical growth, NCHS percentiles. (Adapted with permission from Hamill, P.V.V., T.A. Drizd, C.L. Johnson, R.B. Reed, A.F. Roche, and W.M. Moore. Physical growth: National Center for Health Statistics percentiles. *Am. J. Clin. Nutr.* 32:(1979)607–629. Data from the Fels Research Institute, Wright State University School of Medicine, Yellow Springs, Ohio.)

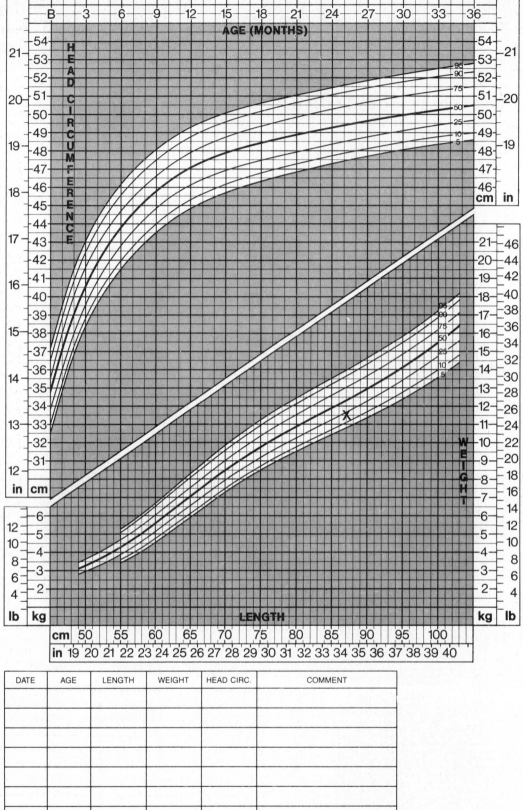

DATE	AGE	LENGTH	WEIGHT	HEAD CIRC.	COMMENT

Figure 8-2 Boys: Birth to 36 months physical growth, NCHS percentiles. (Adapted with permission from Hamill, P.V.V., T.A. Drizd, C.L. Johnson, R.B. Reed, A.F. Roche, and W.M. Moore. Physical growth: National Center for Health Statistics percentiles. *Am. J. Clin. Nutr.* 32:(1979)607–629. Data from the Fels Research Institute, Wright State University School of Medicine, Yellow Springs, Ohio.)

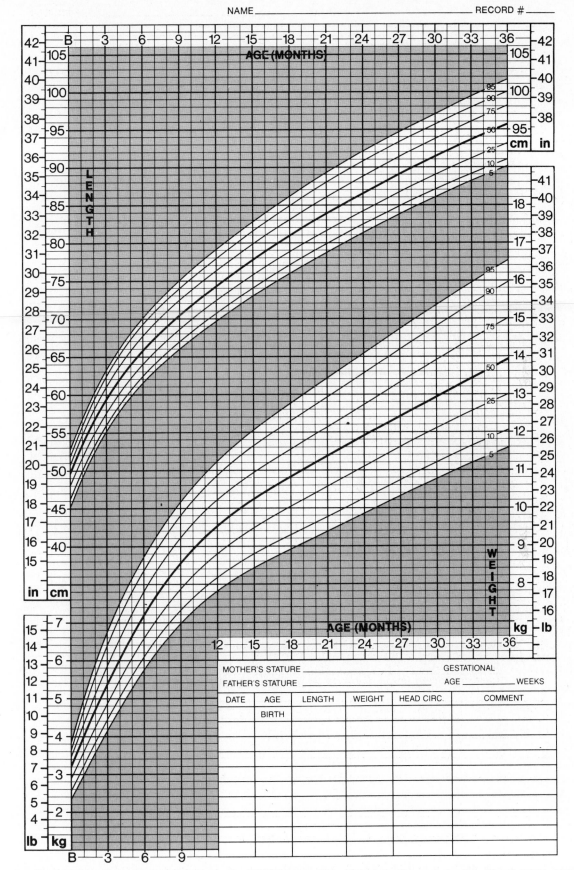

Figure 8-3 Girls: Birth to 36 months physical growth, NCHS percentiles. (Adapted with permission from Hamill, P.V.V., T.A. Drizd, C.L. Johnson, R.B. Reed, A.F. Roche, and W.M. Moore. Physical growth: National Center for Health Statistics percentiles. *Am. J. Clin. Nutr.* 32:(1979)607–629. Data from the Fels Research Institute, Wright State University School of Medicine, Yellow Springs, Ohio.)

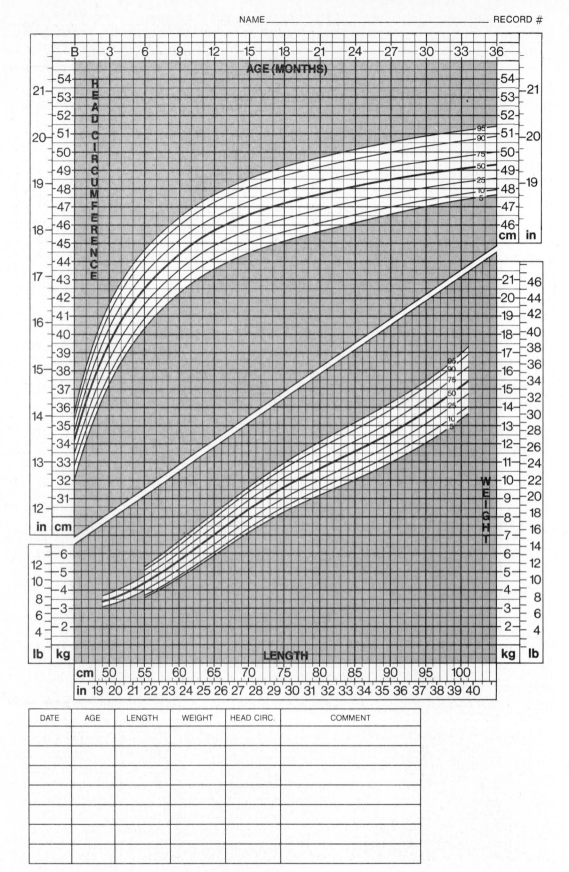

DATE	AGE	LENGTH	WEIGHT	HEAD CIRC.	COMMENT

Figure 8-4 Girls: Birth to 36 months physical growth, NCHS percentiles. (Adapted with permission from Hamill, P.V.V., T.A. Drizd, C.L. Johnson, R.B. Reed, A.F. Roche, and W.M. Moore. Physical growth: National Center for Health Statistics percentiles. *Am. J. Clin. Nutr.* 32:(1979)607–629. Data from the Fels Research Institute, Wright State University School of Medicine, Yellow Springs, Ohio.)

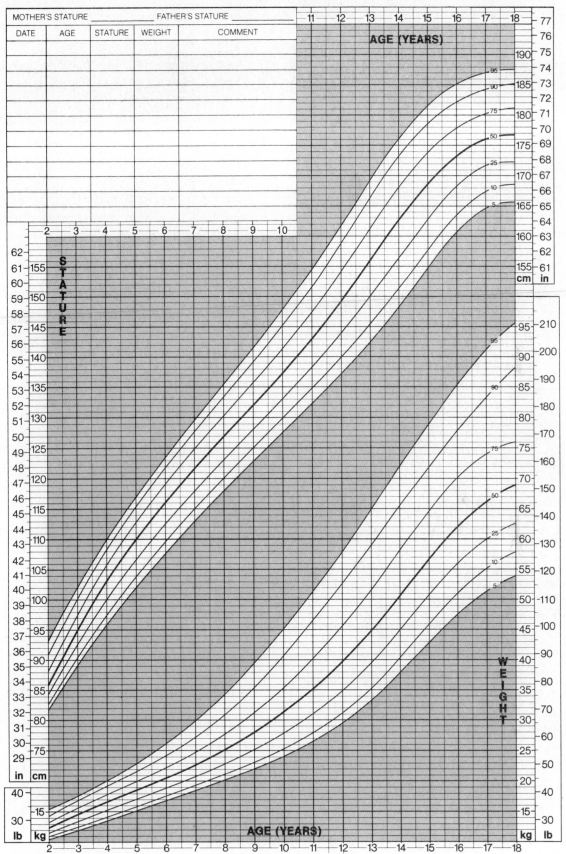

Figure 8-5 Boys: 2 to 18 years physical growth, NCHS percentiles. (Adapted with permission from Hamill, P.V.V., T.A. Drizd, C.L. Johnson, R.B. Reed, A.F. Roche, and W.M. Moore. Physical growth: National Center for Health Statistics percentiles. *Am. J. Clin. Nutr.* 32:(1979)607–629. Data from the National Center for Health Statistics (NCHS), Hyattsville, Maryland.)

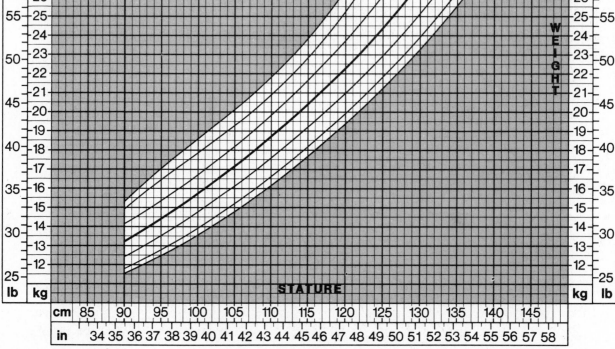

Figure 8-6 Boys: Prepubescent physical growth, NCHS percentiles. (Adapted with permission from Hamill, P.V.V., T.A. Drizd, C.L. Johnson, R.B. Reed, A.F. Roche, and W.M. Moore. Physical growth: National Center for Health Statistics percentiles. *Am. J. Clin. Nutr.* 32:(1979)607–629. Data from the National Center for Health Statistics (NCHS), Hyattsville, Maryland.)

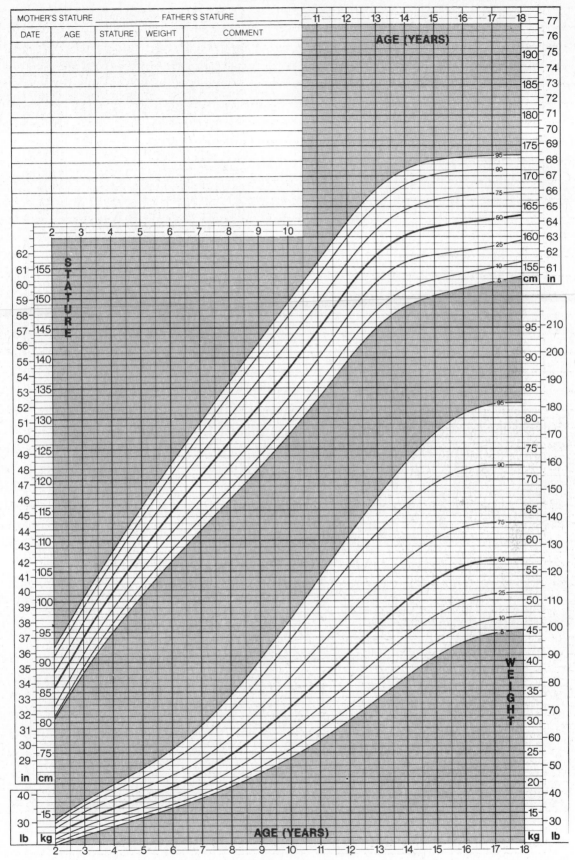

Figure 8-7 Girls: 2 to 18 years physical growth, NCHS percentiles. (Adapted with permission from Hamill, P.V.V., T.A. Drizd, C.L. Johnson, R.B. Reed, A.F. Roche, and W.M. Moore. Physical growth: National Center for Health Statistics percentiles. *Am. J. Clin. Nutr.* 32:(1979)607–629. Data from the National Center for Health Statistics (NCHS), Hyattsville, Maryland.)

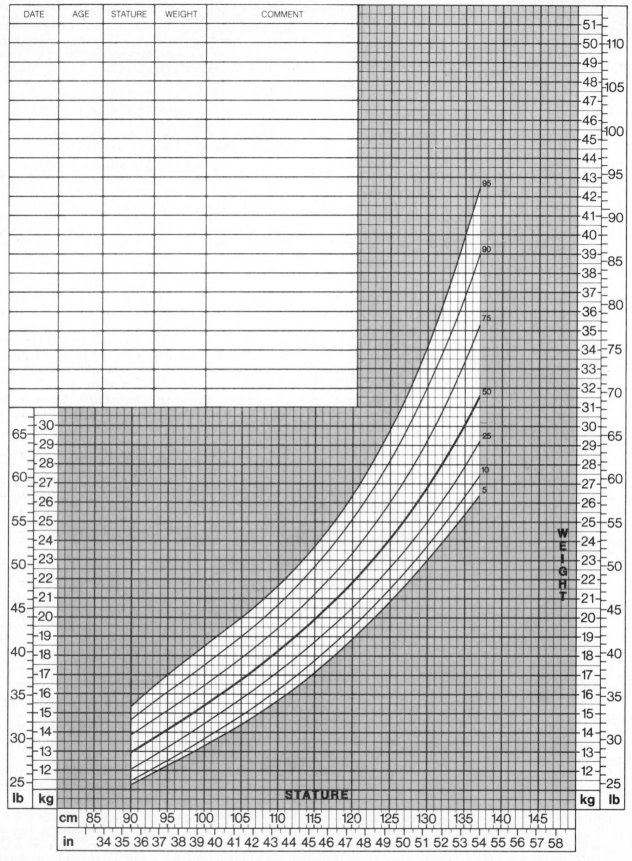

Figure 8-8 Girls: Prepubescent physical growth, NCHS percentiles. (Adapted with permission from Hamill, P.V.V., T.A. Drizd, C.L. Johnson, R.B. Reed, A.F. Roche, and W.M. Moore. Physical growth: National Center for Health Statistics percentiles. *Am. J. Clin. Nutr.* 32:(1979)607–629. Data from the National Center for Health Statistics (NCHS), Hyattsville, Maryland.)

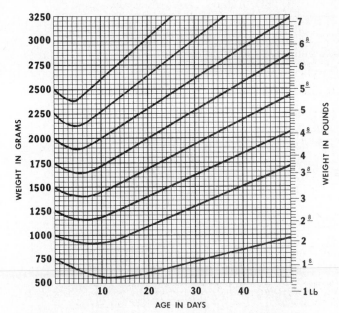

Figure 8-9 Live birth weights of infants of gestational age 26–42 Weeks (Reproduced with permission from Dancis, J. and J.R. O'Connell. A grid for recording the weight of premature infants. *J. Pediatr.* 33:(1948)570–572.)

sults in taller, heavier, more physically mature children.

Growth charts are used to evaluate growth in height and weight by determination of either single or repeated measurements. Plotting of height and weight for a child at a *single age* gives information on the relationship of weight to height compared with other children of the same age and sex. Alternatively, *repeated* measurements of height and weight plotted on a growth grid at different ages in the same child allow determination of the pattern of growth in comparison with that of healthy children. An evaluation of weight without comparison to length has little meaning other than in a statistical sense.

Single measurements: Single measurements of weight and height can be interpreted in two ways: (1) percentile for weight compared to percentile for height, and (2) weight for length or height. These approaches give the same information—that is, weight relative to height—but use different growth charts.

We will use an example of a single measurement of height and weight in one child to illustrate how these data can be interpreted in each of the two ways just described. Consider a boy who is 24 months old and weighs 25 pounds, 8 ounces and measures 34.5 inches in length. Figure 8-1 demonstrates that the child is at the 25th percentile for weight and at the 50th percentile for length. Figure 8-2 demonstrates that the child is at approximately the 25th percentile *weight for length* We can interpret these single measurements using the two methods as follows:

1. Compared to children his age, the child's weight at the 25th percentile does not correlate with the weight of other children who are his length. In other words, 50th percentile for weight and 50th percentile for length are the usual values observed. This suggests that calorie intake may be low or that the child is genetically leaner in comparison to his height than the majority of children his age. If the child is healthy and eating an adequate diet, it probably indicates normal growth.

2. A 25th percentile *weight for length* indicates the same information as the weight-for-height method but uses a different growth chart. Measurements that fall within the 50th percentile of weight for length indicate median weight for height. Values over the 50th percentile suggest above-average weight for stature and values under the 50th percentile suggest below-average weight for stature.

Since both methods actually give the same information, you may choose to use the growth chart you find easiest to work with. However, it is important to understand the terminology used in both approaches.

An evaluation of *weight for stature* in adolescents (males taller than 145 cm and females taller than 138 cm) using growth charts is not useful because of individual variation in the rate of maturation. If single measurements are used in adolescents, it is most useful to evaluate body weight and height by comparison with age-specific height and weight values.

Repeated measurements: If possible, it is generally better to evaluate growth by plotting repeated measures of height, weight, and head circumference on an appropriate growth chart. This allows one to visualize how a child's growth is proceeding and also highlights certain growth patterns. In evaluating growth curves, it should be recognized that growth does not always proceed in a smooth curve, as the charts depict. In general, however, children will grow along approximately the same percentile track and, if there is a substantial change in the percentile of growth, nutritional or clinical factors need to be further evaluated.

For example, consider the pattern of growth shown in Figure 8-10, curve A. The child is near the 75th percentile for both length and weight at birth. Weight drops to the 50th percentile by 3 months of age and continues along the 50th percentile until about 9 months of age, when the rate of weight gain again falls off. By 24 months of age, weight has dropped to the 25th percentile. Length also drops from the 75th percentile from birth but lags behind the drop in weight percentile. By 24 months, length is at the 50th percentile. One would project that this child would normally grow along a curve between the 75th and 50th percentiles for both weight and length. The drop in percentile growth may suggest interference with growth potential due to poor food intake secondary to irregular eating habits, which are particularly common in the second year of life, increased activity, a disease process, or any combination of these factors. A clinical evaluation if the child is symptomatic or a careful di-

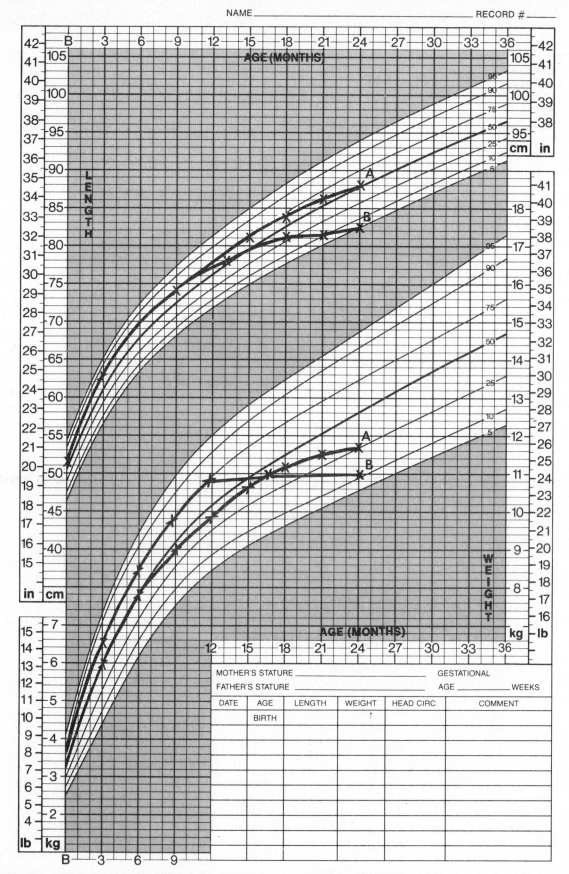

Figure 8-10 Boys: Birth to 36 months physical growth, NCHS percentiles. (Adapted with permission from Hamill, P.V.V., T.A. Drizd, C.L. Johnson, R.B. Reed, A.F. Roche, and W.M. Moore. Physical growth: National Center for Health Statistics percentiles. *Am. J. Clin. Nutr.* 32:(1979)607–629. Data from the Fels Research Institute, Wright State University School of Medicine, Yellow Springs, Ohio.)

etary evaluation if the child is asymptomatic will help clarify the nature of the growth pattern. In the asymptomatic child, this growth pattern is most likely to be a temporary result of poor eating habits, which will probably improve as the child ages.

As an example of a clearly abnormal growth curve, consider Figure 8-10, curve B. Growth in weight and length practically ceases, or flattens, between 12 and 24 months of age. This type of curve indicates interference in growth potential due to a disease process or inadequate nutrition, or both. A child with this type of growth curve would need a careful clinical evaluation to rule out an underlying disease process. Children with conditions such as chronic renal failure commonly display growth patterns similar to curve B.

During adolescence, growth patterns may change in percentiles due to differences in maturation rates. The early maturer may jump to a higher percentile, and the late maturer may be at a lower percentile at the same age point. Both patterns usually return to the original percentiles by the time growth is completed.

Head Circumference

Changes in head circumference reflect brain growth but are not a sensitive indicator of nutritional status. After 36 months of age, there is little relationship between nutrition and head circumference because maximum head circumference is usually attained by this age.

Bone Age

Bone, or skeletal, age can be determined by evaluation of the degree of fusion of the epiphyses using roentgenographic studies. Epiphyseal closure is a measure of how far the bones have progressed toward maturity. Once the epiphyses have closed, there is no further growth in height. Estimation of bone age, or degree of epiphyseal closure, allows for an estimation of the potential for catch-up growth in children with growth retardation. Bone age is generally retarded in any condition in which growth in height is slowed secondary to malnutrition, but the percent of retardation may be less for epiphyseal closure than for height. As an example, consider a 10-year-old child who is growth retarded and of a height comparable with that of a 6-year-old. The bone age would also most likely be retarded and fall somewhere between 6 and 10 years. Knowing the bone age would thus give an indication of how many years remained for promotion of "catch-up growth" before epiphyseal closure. Roentgenograms of the hand and wrist are generally used to assess epiphyseal closure, or bone age, in comparison to standards (20).

TO TEST YOUR UNDERSTANDING

8. Evaluate the following dietary intakes:

    a. An 11-month-old infant who consumes 40 oz formula and 2 T of dry iron-fortified cereal each day.

    b. A 1½-year-old child who takes juice in a bottle, consumes 1 cup of whole milk per day in a bottle, and eats only peanut butter and jelly sandwiches.

    c. A 10-year-old boy who eats cereal with juice for breakfast, consumes a school-lunch-program meal, eats a sandwich with milk after school, and has a balanced dinner with his family in the evening.

9. The following nutritional assessment data is obtained from a 5-year-old girl who has a history of multiple allergies, chronic emesis and diarrhea:

At birth:	Weight	3.6 kg
	Length	51.0 cm
	Head circumference	34.5 cm
At 5 years:	Weight	15.0 kg
	Length	105.0 cm
	Head circumference	50.0 cm
	MAC	15.7 cm
	TSF	7.0 mm
	Average daily protein intake	35.0 g
	24-hr urine volume	700.0 ml
	Urine total N	0.61 g/dl

    a. What are the patient's percentiles for age at birth and at 5 years for the following parameters?

	Birth	5 years
Weight	_____	_____
Length/height	_____	_____
Head circumference	_____	_____
Weight for length	_____	_____

Provide an interpretation of the child's growth pattern.
b. Determine the percentiles for TSF _____ and MAC _____.
   Calculate MAMC _____ mm and percentile for MAMC _____
c. Calculate N balance (mg/N/kg) using Equation **8-1**.
   _____ mg N/kg

d. Discuss how the information in parts b and c of this question relates to the parameters of growth that were evaluated in part a.

e. Assume that the child is referred to you for dietary counseling for a milk-free, wheat-free diet. Her usual dietary intake is as follows: 6 oz Isomil formula, 1 egg, 1 c rice, 3 oz meat, 1 c juice, ½ c vegetables, and one 3.5 oz bag of corn chips. Write a SOAP note summarizing her nutritional status and your recommendations for energy and protein intake.

TOPICS FOR FURTHER DISCUSSION

1. Discuss proper breast-feeding techniques, including positioning and latching on.

2. Assume that you are planning a class on infant feeding to be given to women who are in their last trimester of pregnancy. List the major topics you might include in your class and outline the major points you would discuss in relation to each topic.

3. Discuss the incidence, etiology, and treatment of bulimia and anorexia nervosa.

4. Visit a grocery store and observe the variety, cost, and content of the various baby foods. Outline how you would instruct mothers to prepare their own baby foods.

5. Compare the cost of the various forms of infant formulas.

6. What are important aspects to consider for nutrition of adolescent athletes?

7. Discuss the evidence for a dietary role in relation to hyperactive behavior in children.

REFERENCES

1. FOMAN, S.J., L.J. FILER, T.A. ANDERSON, AND E.E. ZIEGLER. Recommendations for feeding normal infants. *Pediatrics* 63:(1979)52–59.

2. JONES, E.G. Normal infant feeding. In *Manual of Pediatric Nutrition*, eds. D.G. Kelts and E.G. Jones. Boston: Little, Brown, 1985, pp. 21–48.

3. MATERNAL AND CHILD HEALTH BRANCH. *Recommendations for Infant Feeding Practices.* Sacramento: California Department of Health Services, 1979.

4. COMMITTEE ON NUTRITION. *Pediatric Nutrition Handbook* (2d ed.). Elk Grove Village, Ill.: American Academy of Pediatrics, 1985.

5. WORTHINGTON-ROBERTS, B. Nutrition and maternal health. *Nutrition Today* 19:(1984)6–19.

6. SARETT, H.P. The modern infant formula. In *Infant and Child Feeding*, eds. J.T. Bond, L.J. Filer, and G.A. Leveille. New York: Academic Press, 1981, pp. 99–117.

7. COMMITTEE ON NUTRITION, AMERICAN ACADEMY OF PEDIATRICS. Commentary on breast feeding and infant formulas, including proposed standards for formulas. *Pediatrics* 57:(1976)278–285.

8. COMMITTEE ON NUTRITION, AMERICAN ACADEMY OF PEDIATRICS. Fluoride supplementation: Revised dosage schedule. *Pediatrics* 63:150–152, 1979.

9. O'LEARY, M.J. Nourishing the premature and low-birth-weight infant. In *Nutrition in Infancy and Childhood*, ed. P. Pipes. St. Louis: Times Mirror/Mosby, 1985, pp. 122–174.

10. ZIEGLER, E.E., R.L. BIGRA, AND S.J. FOMON. Nutritional requirements of the premature infant. In *Textbook of Pediatric Nutrition*, ed. R.M. Suskind. New York: Raven Press, 1981, pp. 29–39.

11. LEMONS, J.A., L. MOYE, D. HALL, AND M. SIMMONS. Differences in the composition of preterm and term human milk during early lactation. *Pediat. Res.* 16:(1983)113–117.

12. OWEN, G.M. Nutrition of low-birth-weight infants: Enteral feeding. *Clinical Nutrition* 2:(1983)9–13.

13. PIPES, P.L. *Nutrition in Infancy and Childhood* (3d ed.). St. Louis: Times Mirror/Mosby, 1985.

14. TANNER, J.M., R.H. WHITEHOUSE, AND M. TAKAISHI. *Arch. Dis. Child.* 41:(1966)454–471.

15. GREGER, J.L., M.M. HIGGINS, R.P. ABERNATHY, A. KIRKSEY, M.B. DECORSO, AND P. BALIGAR. Nutritional status of adolescent girls in regard to zinc, copper, and iron. *Am. J. Clin. Nutr.* 31:(1978)269–275.

16. NEY, D.M. Nutritional assessment. In *Manual of Pediatric Nutrition*, eds. D.G. Kelts and E.G. Jones. Boston: Little, Brown, 1984, pp. 99–104.

17. NEY, D., C. BAY, J.-M. SAUDUBRAY, D.G. KELTS, S. KULOVICH, L. SWEETMAN, AND W.L. NYHAN. An evaluation of protein requirements in methylmalonic acidaemia. *J. Inher. Metab. Dis.* 8:(1985)132–142.

18. HAMILL, P.V.V., T.A. DRIZD, C.L. JOHNSON, ET AL. NCHS Growth Charts, 1976. Rockville, Md.: *Monthly Vital Statistics Report* (HBS) 25(3):(1976)76–1120 (Suppl.).

19. NELLHAUS, G. Head circumference from birth to 18 years. *Pediatrics* 41:(1968)106–.

20. GREULICH, W.W. AND S.I. PYLE. *Radiographic Atlas of Skeletal*

Development of the Hand and Wrist (2d ed.). Stanford: Stanford University Press, 1959.

ADDITIONAL SOURCES OF INFORMATION

FOMON, S.J. *Infant Nutrition.* Philadelphia: Saunders, 1974.

JONES, E.G. *Good Nutrition for Your Baby.* San Diego: Slawson Communications, 1985.

SUSKIND, R.M. *Textbook of Pediatric Nutrition.* New York: Raven Press, 1981.

Vitamin and Mineral Requirements in Preterm Infants, ed. R.C. Tsang. New York: Marcel Dekker, 1985.

The Womanly Art of Breast Feeding. Franklin Park, Ill.: La Leche League International, 1970.

9

Nutritional Care of the Vegetarian Patient

The number of people who adhere to some form of vegetarian diet has grown in recent years. Vegetarians now number about 7 million in the United States. In addition to their increased numbers, their motivations and the types of vegetarian diets they follow are more varied. A person may become a vegetarian because of religion (Seventh-Day Adventists and adherents to various Eastern religions and philosophical groups follow vegetarian diets) or because of opposition to killing animals. Others cite concern about the purity of the food supply and a desire to maintain and improve health. In many parts of the world, populations are wholly or partially vegetarian because of poverty and unavailability of animal foods. In the more prosperous, developed countries, this is less often the case. Instead, people *choose* to be vegetarians. The cost of a vegetarian diet is not markedly different from the cost of a diet containing meat.

Vegetarians are widely distributed geographically; it is highly probable, therefore, that you will have opportunities to provide nutritional care to vegetarians. It is thus important to understand the types of vegetarian diets and their advantages and disadvantages, and to be skilled in planning diets for, and counseling, these patients.

TYPES OF VEGETARIANS

Vegetarians are often classified according to either the extent of restriction of meat products in their diets or, conversely, the types of meat products they are willing to eat. A person whose diet includes plant foods and all categories of animal foods is an *omnivore*. However, most, if not all, societies refuse to eat some animal foods. In the United States and Canada, for example, insects, dogs, cats, and horses are generally not considered acceptable food, although these are prized in some societies. *Partial vegetarians*, or semivegetarians, avoid some animal foods but not others. For example,

some avoid red meats only. The *pollovegetarian* will eat poultry in addition to plant foods, while the *pescovegetarian* eats fish plus plant foods. *Lacto-ovo-vegetarians* accept milk, milk products, and eggs; more restricted versions are lactovegetarians (milk and milk products, but no eggs or meat) and *ovo-vegetarians* (eggs, but no milk or milk products or meat.) The *total, pure, or strict vegetarian*, or *vegan*, will not accept any animal products, but eats only plant foods. The *fruitarian*, who eats a diet largely composed of fruits, nuts, honey, and olive oil, is rare (1, 2).

Vegetarians can also be categorized into traditional and new vegetarians. *Traditional vegetarians* are members of religions or cultures traditionally associated with vegetarian diets. Seventh-Day Adventists, one of the traditional vegetarian groups, are a denomination with about a half million members. The church recommends a lacto-ovo-vegetarian diet, and about half of the members adhere to this diet. Most members abstain from eating pork products, caffeine-containing products, hot condiments and spices, and alcoholic beverages. Some abstain from highly refined foods. Most do not smoke.

The *new vegetarians* are a heterogeneous group whose diets often include avoidance of other foods and are accompanied by life-styles and philosophical beliefs different from those previously followed (3). Some groups among the new vegetarians can be identified; there are other individuals whose diets can be described only after obtaining a careful diet history.

The *Zen macrobiotic philosophy,* described in the 1960s by Ohsawa (4), advanced the concept that the path to health and happiness consisted of four parts: no medicine, no surgery, no inactivity, and a diet of natural food. The stated objective was to maintain a good balance of *yin* and *yang*.

The "yin-yang" theory goes by different names in other cultural groups, such as the Chinese and some Spanish-speaking groups, but the basic beliefs are similar. Adherents to this theory believe that their health depends on a balance between opposing forces known as yin and yang. *Yin* (or *lyang*) is described as "female," negative, introverted, empty, dark, or cold while *yang* (or *bou*) is "male," positive, extroverted, full, warm, or light. The classification applies to other aspects of life as well as to food.

Foods may be classified as yin or yang depending on the effects that a food is believed to have on the body. The classification is not dependent upon color, texture, flavor, or temperature. Rather, foods are classified according to five "flavors"—acid, salt, sweet, bitter, or pungent—and according to seasons and other factors. Meat is a yang food and its use is discouraged.

Too much or too little yin or yang is believed by adherents to be the cause of certain diseases. In groups that adhere to these beliefs, a folk healer might use yang foods or herbs to treat a disease caused by an overabundance of yin. Nutritional counseling of patients with these beliefs may be more effective if suggestions are in accordance with the yin-yang classification.

In the macrobiotic diet, there are ten levels of diets, numbered from −3 to +7, with progressively greater restriction (4). Avoidance of preservatives and processed foods is emphasized, in addition to maintenance of the balance of yin and yang. Fluid intake is restricted. Diets from −3 to +3 may be made nutritionally adequate with care, but may be deficient in calcium, iron, ascorbic acid, and vitamin B_{12}. The more restricted diets have resulted in cases of scurvy, hypocalcemia, hypoproteinemia, anemia, and emaciation. The final level (+7) consists only of grain, usually brown rice, and boiled herb tea. This diet was believed to have the proper balance of yin and yang, but several deaths have resulted from its use. More recently, adherents to this philosophy have been encouraged to "eat more widely"—that is, to eat a greater variety of foods, including dairy products, eggs, and fish (5).

RISKS AND BENEFITS OF VEGETARIAN DIETS

Certain groups who may be particularly at risk are pregnant and lactating women, infants, children, and those with problems such as lactose intolerance and diabetes. For any person, the risks of malnutrition from poorly planned vegetarian diets increase with greater restrictions on varieties of foods eaten. Thus, the risk of malnutrition is greater for a vegan than for a lacto-ovo-vegetarian. The vegan may risk inadequacies in protein, calcium, iron, zinc, and vitamins B_{12}, D, and riboflavin. The nutritional care specialist must develop expertise in diet planning and counseling for these high-risk groups.

Studies of various vegetarian groups have indicated some health benefits. The extent to which differences in habits of smoking, alcohol and caffeine consumption, and exercise affect the health benefits varies in different groups. Among the suggested benefits are decreases in body weight, hypertension, blood lipid levels, coronary heart disease, osteoporosis, and some cancers.

SPECIAL FOODS USED IN VEGETARIAN DIETS

When interviewing patients, you may encounter references to unfamiliar foods. Some foods used by vegetarians, often unfamiliar to omnivores, are described here.

SOY PRODUCTS

Soy flour contains about 40 percent protein, or 50 percent if defatted. *Soy protein concentrate (SPC)* is 60 percent protein, while *isolated soy protein (IPC, or isolated protein concentrate)* is 90 percent protein. *Soy grits* are partially cooked and cracked soy beans. All soy products should be cooked or roasted. This process destroys the enzyme *phytohemagglutinin*, which impairs intestinal protein digestion.

Tofu, a curd, or "cheese," prepared from fresh soybeans, and *miso*, a paste of soybeans, wheat or barley, salt, and water, have been common ingredients in oriental foods. They are now used as a source of protein in Western diets. Miso is high in sodium and cannot be used by patients requiring a low-sodium diet. Tofu may be a good source of calcium, depending upon the coagulant used. Sea salt as a coagulant is high in magnesium.

Tempeh (pronounced *tem-pay*) is an Indonesian dish which is growing in popularity. It is usually made from soybeans, but may be prepared from other beans or from grains or seeds. It is prepared by culturing with *Rhizopus oblgosporus* by a method analogous to those used to prepare cheese or yogurt. It may be steamed, fried, grated, or mixed in salads, appetizers, and main dishes.

Four ounces of tempeh contain 169 kcal, 21 g protein, 4.5 g fat, 9.5 g carbohydrate, 1,471 mg calcium, 175 mg phosphorus, and 11 mg iron. The culture is reported to synthesize niacin, riboflavin, and vitamin B_6 as it grows. These vitamins are thus increased, while thiamine decreases. Vitamin B_{12} may be present in tempeh. The bacteria *Klebsiella*, found on many plant materials, grows during the culturing of tempeh. *Klebsiella* produces vitamin B_{12}, but the amount produced depends on the number of bacteria. Since the amount is variable, tempeh should not be relied upon as the sole source of the vitamin (6).

TEXTURED VEGETABLE PROTEINS

Textured vegetable proteins, often called *TVP*, are usually made from beans and are available in dried form. Some are made from soy flour and are available in dehydrated form. They are used in casseroles, stews, sausages, and hamburger-type dishes. Other

TVPs are made of soy spun protein and textured to resemble meat.

MEAT ANALOGS

Meat analogs are foods designed to look and taste like meat. They are made primarily of plant foods, usually soy, wheat gluten, or nuts, and then canned or frozen. Many are made from soy spun protein. They may be flavored to resemble beef, poultry, bacon, or sausage. The vitamin and mineral contents often vary from those of the meats they resemble, and labels should be read carefully. Since these products are processed foods, they are not acceptable to individuals who eat only unprocessed foods. Some of these products contain egg albumin or dried milk; these are not acceptable to vegans.

Recipes, catalogs, and nutritional analyses of meat analogs may be obtained from the manufacturers. As the number of vegetarians has increased, these products have become available in larger supermarkets. Detailed information on their contents is contained in the diet manual from the Seventh-Day Adventist Dietetic Association (7).

NUTRITIONAL, OR FOOD, YEAST

Nutritional yeast is grown on a vitamin B_{12}–enriched medium so that it has a relatively high vitamin B_{12} content. Many are high in phosphorus and low in calcium. Labels should be checked for an acceptable calcium-to-phosphorus ratio (1:1) for patients who do not obtain an appreciable amount of calcium from other dietary sources. Brewer's yeast may serve as a good source of B vitamins, particularly thiamine and folate.

MILK SUBSTITUTES

Milk substitutes may be commercially prepared or homemade. Most commercially prepared products have soy protein as a base. Sesame seeds and almonds may also be used. These milks are usually fortified with calcium and vitamins A, D, B_{12}, and sometimes K.

Homemade products are usually soy-based and not fortified. If they are not heated to destroy the antitrypsin factor in raw soybean, their available protein can be highly variable. Homemade soy milk may be fortified by the addition of a scant teaspoon of calcium carbonate per quart and a ground 25-mg vitamin B_{12} tablet in each 2 quarts.

Kokkoh is sometimes prepared and used by vegans as an infant formula. It is prepared with 30 percent brown rice, 30 percent sesame seeds, 20 percent sweet brown rice, and 10 percent azuki beans. The remaining 10 percent consists of equal parts by weight of soybeans, wheat, and oats. It has been used in infant feeding, with unfortunate results. The protein is of high quality, but kokkoh has been used in very dilute form, and the total volume necessary to meet infants' energy and protein needs exceeds their intake capacity.

SELECTED CHEESES

Rennin, the enzyme used in processing many hard or semihard cheeses, is an animal product. It is thus unacceptable to some vegetarians. Among domestic cheeses, only ricotta cheese is never made with rennin. Rennin is not used in all cottage cheeses; the processor can identify those in which rennin is not used.

SEAWEED AND ALGAE PRODUCTS

Sea products are sometimes used as food by vegetarians. *Agar-agar,* for example, is a gelatin which has been used in puddings and soups. Seaweed and algae may have some vitamin B_{12} from contamination with plankton, but the amount is variable and thus unreliable. *Kombu* is a seaweed found in deep sea water.

MISCELLANEOUS PRODUCTS

Several other products, not usually familiar to an omnivore, are sometimes encountered when interviewing vegetarian patients:

gosamasio—roasted sesame seeds ground with sea salt, high in sodium, and used as a condiment on grains

---

TO TEST YOUR UNDERSTANDING

1. List the nutrients that are provided in important amounts in the following foods:

   a. Fortified soy milk
   b. Tofu
   c. Miso
   d. Meat analogs
   e. Textured vegetable proteins

2. Why might some meat analogs be unacceptable to a vegan? to a lactovegetarian?
3. Why might some cheeses be unacceptable to a lacto- or lacto-ovo-vegetarian?
4. Compare and contrast unsupplemented homemade and commercial soy milk.

mochi—a glutinous rice

hummus—a spread for bread made from chick peas and sesame seeds

tahini—a paste made from sesame seeds

CONSIDERATIONS RELATIVE TO SPECIFIC NUTRIENTS

PROTEIN

Vegetarian diets which contain a source of complete protein, such as milk or eggs, can be planned for nutritional adequacy with relative ease. In contrast, diets containing only plant proteins must be planned with great care to ensure nutritional adequacy.

The plant proteins, which are sources of protein in the diet of vegans, are *incomplete*—that is, deficient in one or more essential amino acids. The essential amino acid that is present in least amount in proportion to the requirement is the *limiting amino acid*. The most limiting amino acids from plant proteins are lysine, methionine, and tryptophan. In general, grains are low in lysine and high in methionine, while legumes are low in methionine and tryptophan and high in lysine. Most nuts and seeds are lysine-deficient. Thus, if a high-lysine, low-methionine food is combined with a high-methionine, low-lysine food, the two sources will compensate for each other's deficiencies. Adequate amounts of all amino acids may be obtained by including a combination of different foods that provide all the necessary amino acids. This process, called *mutual supplementation*, is effective only if the foods providing all the essential amino acids are provided at the same meal or within about 4 hours. For your assistance in planning, Table 9-1 gives the limiting and abundant amino acids in foods that are especially useful in planning for protein intake on vegetarian diets (8).

Three types of combinations have been described to provide the essential amino acids: (1) grains and legumes, (2) grains and a small amount of milk products, and (3) seeds and legumes; however, not all items in each group contribute equally. Examples of complementary proteins are given in Table 9-2. In counseling, you need to advise patients to use plant foods in combinations as indicated in the table. In addition, the quantities used must provide the necessary proportions of amino acids. Some useful proportions, given as dry measures, are as follows (6):

1 c grain + 1/8 c soy grits (granules)

1 c grain + 1/3 c sesame or sunflower seeds + 2 T soy

1 1/3 c grain + 1/2 c beans

1/2 c seeds + 1/3 c beans

1 c seeds + 3/4 c peanuts

It is also important to ensure adequate energy supplies so that protein is not used for energy.

TABLE 9-1. Limiting and Abundant Amino Acids in Selected Foods

	Limiting Amino Acids	Abundant Amino Acids
Corn	Lysine, tryptophan, threonine	
Millet	Lysine, threonine	
Oats	Lysine, threonine	
Rice	Lysine, threonine	Methionine
Flour, white	Lysine	
Legumes		
Beans, mature	Methionine, valine	
Beans, immature	Methionine, isoleucine	
Peas	Methionine, tryptophan	
Oil Seeds and Nuts		
Soybeans	Methionine	Lysine, threonine
Sesame seeds	Lysine	Tryptophan, methionine, cystine, cysteine
Sunflower seeds	Lysine	Tryptophan, methionine, cystine, cysteine
Peanuts	Lysine, methionine, threonine	Tryptophan, methionine
Cottonseed	Lysine	
Coconut	Lysine	
Vegetables		
Green peas	Methionine	Lysine
Green leafy	Methionine	All others
Gelatin	Methionine, lysine, tryptophan	
Yeast	Phenylalanine	Threonine, tryptophan

IRON

Iron exists in foods as easily absorbed heme iron and as nonheme iron. *Heme iron* constitutes 40 percent of the total iron in animal foods. *Nonheme iron* is 60 percent of the iron in animal foods and all the iron in plant foods, iron-fortified foods, and eggs. Absorption of nonheme iron is reduced by phytic and oxalic acid and large amounts of fiber in plants, tannic acid in tea, and phosvitin in egg yolk. Absorption is increased by ascorbic acid. In counseling and menu planning for vegetarians, foods high in iron and ascorbic acid should be recommended to be included in *each meal*. In general, foods high in iron are dark green, leafy vegetables, winter squash, sweet potatoes, beans, whole-grain or enriched cereal products, dried fruits, and eggs (if accepted). The iron content of selected plant foods useful for this purpose is given in Table 9-3.

ZINC

Selected food sources of zinc are whole-grain cereals, peas, oatmeal, dried yeast, and wheat germ. Specific values are shown in Table 9-3. Absorption is decreased by phytates and fiber. Therefore, vegetarians may become deficient in zinc. The phytate in whole wheat is reduced by yeast fermentation. The zinc in leavened

TABLE 9-2. Complementary Proteins

Grains	+	Legumes	+	Nuts & seeds	+	Other
Wheat		Legumes				
Corn		Legumes				
Rice		Legumes				
Rice & wheat		Soy				
Rice						Milk
Wheat		Soy		Sesame seeds		
Wheat						Milk
Wheat				Peanuts		Milk
Wheat		Beans				
Cornmeal		Beans				
		Beans				Milk
				Peanuts		Milk
Wheat & corn		Soy Soy		Peanuts & sesame		
Wheat & rice		Soy Beans		Peanuts Sesame		
Rice						Brewer's yeast

Compiled from: Goodwin, M. T. *Better Living Through Better Eating* (2d ed.) Montgomery County Health Dept., Maryland, 1974, 19, Lappe, F. M. *Diet for a Small Planet.* New York: Friends of the Earth/Ballantine, 1971.

bread may therefore be more available than the average of 10 percent availability from plant sources.

CALCIUM

Calcium intake is easily provided for lactovegetarians. Vegans, however, must plan carefully to select plant foods high in calcium, such as dark green, leafy vegetables, broccoli, brussels sprouts, okra, rutabagas, legumes, dried fruits, and almonds. Specific values are given in Table 9-3. Again, bioavailability is reduced by the oxalic acid and fiber in spinach, chard, and beet greens. Calcium may also be obtained from calcium-fortified soy milk and calcium-precipitated tofu. Calcium supplementation may be needed, in ad-

TABLE 9-3. Calcium, Iron, and Zinc Contents of Selected Plant Foods

	Serving Size	Calcium (mg)	Iron (mg)	Zinc (mg)
Legumes, Cooked				
Blackeyed peas	1 c	43	3.5	6.7
Black beans	1 c		7.9	1.8
Garbanzo beans	1 c		6.9	2.0
Great Northern beans	1 c	90		
Green split peas	1 c		3.4	2.1
Lentils	1 c		4.2	2.0
Lima beans	1 c		4.3	2.0
Navy beans	1 c	95	5.0	
Peanut butter	4 T		1.2	2.0
Peanuts, roasted	½ c		2.7	2.2
Pinto beans	1 c		6.4	N/A*

(continued)

TABLE 9-3. *(Continued)*

	Serving Size	Calcium (mg)	Iron (mg)	Zinc (mg)
Red kidney beans	1 c		3.6	
Soy beans	1 c		4.9	N/A
Soy milk	1 c	60	1.8	N/A
Tofu	4 oz		2.3	N/A
Cereals and Cereal Products				
Corn, cooked	1 c		0.7	1.0
Rice, brown, cooked	1 c	7	1.0	1.2
Rice, white, cooked	1 c		1.8	0.8
Oatmeal, cooked	1 c	22	1.7	1.2
Wheat germ, toasted	¼ c 18	18	2.0	3.6
Bread, whole-wheat	1 slice	25	0.8	0.5
Bread, white	1 slice		0.6	0.2
Nuts (Shelled, Whole)				
Almonds	½ c	166	3.5	1.9
Brazil nuts	4 med			0.76
Cashews	6–8			
Filberts	½ c	146		
Pecans	½ c		1.2	2.0
Seeds				
Sesame, whole	½ c	1160	10.5	
Sesame, hulled	½ c	110	2.4	
Soy, mature, cooked	½ c	37	1.3	
Soy, milk	1 c	60	1.5	
Sunflower seed kernels	½ c	87	4.2	
Vegetables, cooked				
Broccoli	1 c	136–2882	1.6	0.2
Cabbage	1 c			0.6
Carrots	1 c			0.05
Kale	¾ c	111–206†	1.2	N/A
Spinach	1 c	—*	4.0	1.3
Greens, beet	1 c	—‡		2.8
collard	1 c	220–2522	1.6	
dandelion	1 c	252	3.6	
mustard	1 c	194	2.6	
turnip	1 c	267	1.5	
Peas, green	½ c	19	1.5	
Potato, baked with skin	1 med			0.96
Sweet potato	1 small	44	1.0	
Dried Fruits				
Apricots, cooked	½ c	25	2.0	
Dates, pitted	½ c		1.9	0.4
Figs, uncooked	1 lg.	26	0.6	0.4
Peaches, raw	1		0.5	0.2
Prunes, cooked	½ c	28	2.3	0.4
Raisins	½ c	48	2.7	0.2
Other Fruit and Juice				
Banana	1 med			0.3
Mango	½ med			0.47
Cranberry-apple juice	8 oz			0.62
Pineapple juice	8 oz			0.38

*N/A = information not available.

†Range of values available from various sources

‡Present as soluble calcium oxalate and not available

Compiled from: Fanelli, M. T. and R. J. Kuczarski Food selection for vegetarians. *Dietetic Currents.* 10(1):(1983) 1–6; Williams, E. R. Making vegetarian diets nutritious. *American Journal of Nursing.* 75:(1975) 2168–70; Pennington, J. A. T. and H. N. Church. *Food Values of Portions Commonly Used* (13th ed.). Philadelphia: Lippincott, 1980.

dition to food sources, for children and pregnant or lactating women.

RIBOFLAVIN

Milk products are important sources of riboflavin. Those vegetarians who eliminate milk should include in their daily diets two servings of alternative sources —that is, whole or enriched grains, dark green leafy vegetables, asparagus, brussels sprouts, okra, winter squash, mushrooms, dried yeast, legumes and nuts, broccoli, or avocado.

VITAMIN B$_{12}$

Vitamin B$_{12}$ is not found in plant foods; therefore, it may present a problem in the vegan diet. Vegans must obtain vitamin B$_{12}$ by using a supplement or eating B$_{12}$–fortified foods, including nutritional yeast, soy milk, cereals, and meat analogs. Cheerios, Total, Product 19, and Raisin Bran are fortified with vitamin B$_{12}$ but are not acceptable to all vegans. Seaweed and plankton are not reliable sources because their B$_{12}$ content is highly variable. Although adults may take 7 to 8 years to develop a vitamin B$_{12}$ deficiency, infants of vegan mothers have smaller stores and a deficiency may develop rapidly (9).

VITAMIN D

Vitamin D may be obtained from fortified cow's milk or fortified soy milk. Sunlight for endogenous synthesis is not always a sufficiently reliable source in many geographical areas. Vitamin D is not present in plant foods. Supplementation should be provided for children and pregnant or lactating women.

TO TEST YOUR UNDERSTANDING

5. List those nutrients that are likely to be deficient in the diets listed here. Then, for each deficient nutrient, recommend three food sources that are appropriate for the type of vegetarianism given.

   a. Vegan
   b. Ovovegetarian

6. If a lacto-ovo-vegetarian asked you if he needed injections of vitamin B$_{12}$, what would you answer? Why? If a vegan asked you the same question, what would you reply?

7. Explain specifically, but succinctly, why the ingredients in each of the following foods complement each other. Use your knowledge of amino acid composition to justify your answer.

   a. Cream of split pea soup
   b. Macaroni and cheese casserole
   c. Rice and beans
   d. Baked beans and whole-wheat bread
   e. Whole-wheat bread with sesame-seed and chick-pea spread (hummus)

MENU PLANNING FOR VEGETARIANS

"Food guides," which suggest menu patterns somewhat on the order of the Daily Food Guide described in Chapter 5, have been established for ease of planning adequate diets. Given the variations in the degree of diet restriction in vegetarian diets, coupled with the variation in nutrient requirements, several patterns are necessary. The nutrient content of major food groups considered in planning vegetarian diets may be summarized as follows:

Meat, poultry, and fish: protein; kcal; EFA; Fe, Zn; vitamins B$_1$, B$_{12}$, folate
Milk: protein; kcal; Ca; vitamins A, D, B$_{12}$, riboflavin
Grains: protein; kcal; riboflavin, niacin
Legumes: protein; Ca, Fe, Zn
Vegetables and fruits: vitamins A, C; fiber

The following principles can be followed in vegetarian meal planning (1,5):

1. Reduce high-calorie foods that are not important sources of other nutrients.
2. Use a variety of nutrient-dense foods and plant foods.
3. Replace meat with other animal foods, meat analogs, or complementary proteins from legumes, cereals, seeds, and nuts.
4. If milk is not accepted, replace with dark green, leafy vegetables, legumes, nuts, seeds, and fortified soy milk.
5. Increase intake of breads and cereals, legumes, nuts, seeds, and dried fruits as necessary to meet energy needs.
6. Replace fruits that are not accepted; increase vegetables and grains.
7. Include a food high in ascorbic acid at each meal to improve iron absorption.

TABLE 9-4. Food Guide for Lacto-Ovo Diets

	Food Group	1–3 yr Both sexes	4–6 yr Both sexes	7–9 yr Both sexes	10–12 yr Both sexes	13–17 yr M	13–17 yr F	18–19 yr M	18–19 yr F	20+ yr M	20+ yr F	Standard Serving
		Minimum Number of Servings Daily										
I.	Cereals, whole grains, breads	3	3–4	4	5	7	5	9	5	8	6	1 slice whole-grain or enriched bread or ¾ c cooked cereal or 1 oz dry cereal
II.	Legumes, meat analogs, textured vegetable protein (TVP)	⅛	¼	½	½	¾	½	1½	1	1	¾	1 c cooked legume or 2–3 oz meat analog or 20–30 g TVP
	Nuts, seeds	⅛	¼	½	¾	1	¾	2	1	1	1	1½ oz or 3 T
III.	Milk, milk products	2–3	2–3	3	4	4	4	2–3	2–3	1½	1½	1 c milk*
	Eggs	1	1	1	1½	1½	1½	1½	1½	1½	1½	1 medium egg
IV.	Fruits, vegetables	2–3	3–4	4	5	5	5	6	5	6	5	½ c juice or 1 medium piece or 1 c raw or ½ c cooked
V.	Oils	⅓–1	⅔–1	⅔–1	1	1	1	1	1	1	1	1 T

*Common portions of dairy foods and their milk equivalents in calcium: 1-in. cube cheddar-type cheese = ½ c milk; ½ c yogurt = ½ c milk; ½ c cottage cheese = ¼ c milk; 2 T cream cheese = 1 T milk; ½ c ice cream or ice milk = ⅓ c milk.

Reprinted with permission of Ross Laboratories, Columbus, Ohio 43216.

8. If vegetables are not accepted, increase fruits and grains.
9. If milk is not used, use a fortified soy milk drink and increase the intake of green, leafy vegetables that are low in oxalate.
10. If goat's milk, low in methionine, is used, recommend intake of a food abundant in methionine *at the same meal.*
11. For vegans, use nutritional yeast or foods fortified with vitamin B$_{12}$, or provide a vitamin B$_{12}$ supplement.

A good guide for lacto-ovo-vegetarian children and adults is given in Table 9-4. The serving sizes appropriate for children of various ages are given in Tables 8-3 and 8-8.

As stated previously, planning an adequate diet becomes more difficult as more groups of foods are excluded from the diet. A suggested food guide for adult vegans is shown in Table 9-5, and guides for use in pregnancy are given in Table 9-6.

Providing nutritionally adequate diets for infants and children of vegans can present special problems. Their diets may be inadequate in energy, calcium, zinc, and vitamins B$_{12}$ and D, as well as, possibly, protein, riboflavin, and iron (10). Some suggestions have been made to overcome these deficiencies (10):

1. To increase energy intake,
   • increase intake of legumes, and legume spreads, nuts, and nut butters in favor of vegetables with lower caloric density.
   • use avocadoes (remove strings for infants) and dried fruit spreads (puree ½ c uncooked dried fruit with 2 t fruit juice).

• do not use honey or corn syrup for infants because of the danger of botulism.
• encourage intake of foods high in complex carbohydrates.
• allow children to eat frequently.

2. Recommend the use of fortified cow's milk or *fortified* soy milk. Commercial soy formulas are Soyalac, Prosobee, Nursoy, and Isomil.
3. Zinc may be provided from legumes, nuts, miso, and tofu.
4. Calcium is contained in soy, navy and pinto beans, tofu, some drinking water, almonds, molasses, and baking powder.

TABLE 9-5. Food Guide for Adult Vegan Diets

	Food Group	Minimum Number of Servings Daily*	Estimated Protein (g) per Serving†
I.	Bread	4	2
	Whole grains	3–5	4
II.	Legumes	2	10
	Nuts or seeds	1	5
IV.	Fruits	1–4	—
	Vegetables	4	2
V.	Oils	1	—

*A serving = 1 slice whole-grain or enriched bread; 1 c cooked cereal or whole grains; 1 c cooked legumes; 3 T nuts or seeds; ½ c fruit juice; ½ c cooked or 1 c raw vegetables; and 1 T oil.

†Vegan protein balance formula: 60% of protein from grains; 35% of protein from legumes; 5% of protein from leafy, green vegetables (D. Calloway, Professor of Nutrition, University of California, Berkeley).

Reprinted with permission of Ross Laboratories, Columbus, Ohio 43216.

TABLE 9-6. Daily Food Guide for Pregnancy

Food Group	Lacto-Ovo-Vegetarian Pattern	Strict Vegetarian Pattern
Milk and milk products	4	—*
Protein foods		
Animal source	1 (2 egg)	—
Dried beans/peas	2	3
Nuts	1	1
Fruits and vegetables		
Vitamin C–rich	1	1
Dark green/deep yellow	2	2
Other	2	2
Whole-grain or enriched cereal products	6	6
Fats and oils (T)	2	2†

*4 c fortified soy milk should be recommended.

†More fats and oils may be needed for palatability and energy.

5. Because of their limited capacity, an increase in bulky plant foods of low caloric density is not advisable. In addition, beets, carrots, collard greens, spinach, and turnips are high in nitrates and may need to be limited.

6. Yeast is high in purine content and is not recommended for infants or toddlers.

Suggested diet plans for vegan children to the age of 6 years are given in Table 9-7.

Those who depends on nuts and seeds for a large portion of their protein must remember that these products can become contaminated with aflatoxins. These toxins are produced by the *Aspergillus flavus* mold, which grows on nuts or seeds stored at humidities above 70 percent. Aflatoxins are a cause of liver cancer in some countries, but are not usually a problem in the United States. Aflatoxins grow well on peanuts but the level may be reduced by roasting. Vege-

---

TO TEST YOUR UNDERSTANDING

8. Examine the following sample menus.

   Menu 1:   Greek-style skillet (1 c brown rice, ¼ c soy grits, eggplant, green beans, seasonings)
   Sliced tomato salad
   Carrot cake
   Tea

   Menu 2:   Cooked bulgur with blackstrap molasses
   Cooked green cabbage
   Carrot-raisin salad
   Banana
   Lemonade

   Menu 3:   Sesame-rice fritters
   Citrus salad on romaine lettuce
   Oatmeal bread
   Cheese cake
   Fruit juice

   Assuming average size servings, explain the following for each menu:
       a. Does it contain a balanced protein (all essential amino acids)?
       b. If so, what foods contribute to the protein?

9. The following menu was written for nonvegetarian patients. Modify the menu so that it is acceptable for the diet indicated in the column heading. Be sure to provide for adequacy of *all* nutrients.

Omnivore menu	Lacto-ovo-vegetarian	Vegan
Consommé		
Broiled chicken		
Rice pilaf		
Buttered broccoli		
Citrus sections in gelatin on lettuce		
Blueberry crepe		

10. What are sources of ascorbic acid which can be included in a menu to improve iron absorption?

TABLE 9-7. Food Guide for Vegan Children

Food Group	Serving Size*	Minimum number of Servings Daily†		
		½–1 yr	1–3 yr	4–6 yr
Cereal (enriched or whole grains); breads	1–5 T / 1 slice	1	3	4
Protein sources‡	1–6 T	2	3	3
Soy milk (fortified)§	1 c	3	3	3
Fruits, citrus	4–8 T	0	2	2
other	2–6 T	3	2	3
Vegetables, Green or yellow	4–6 T	¼	½	1
Other	4–6 T	½	1	1
Fats	1 t	0	3	4
Brewer's yeast	1 T	0	1	1
Molasses	1 T	0	1	1

*Detailed information on serving sizes appropriate for age is contained in Table 8–7.

†Foods should be strained or chopped as necessary for age.

‡Includes legumes, miso, tofu, seeds, seed butters, nuts, nut butters.

§Isomil[R], Nursoy[R], Prosobee[R], or Soyalac[R].

tarians who use large quantities of nuts and seeds should avoid long-term storage at high humidity. Peanuts should be roasted before eating.

Some vegetarians, particularly those who avoid caffeine, use herb teas. Many of these substances can be hazardous, however. A list of these is given in Table 9-8.

TABLE 9-8. Toxic Effects of Herbal Teas

Effect	Herb
Diuretic, mild patent	Bucker, quack grass, dandelion, green tea
	Juniper berries, shave grass, horsetail
Cathartic	Buckthorn, senna; dock; aloe
Anticholinergic or psychotogenic	Burdock, catnip, juniper, hydrangea, lobelia, jimson weed, wormwood, shave grass, horsetail
Allergenic	Camomile, goldenrod, marigold, yarrow, St. John's wart
Abortifacients	Devil's claw root (South African imported), pennyroyal
Cardiovascular toxicity	St. John's wart
Possible carcinogen	Sassafras oil
Poisons	Mistletoe leaves, stems, berries; Indian tobacco; pokeweed
Gastrointestinal irritant	Juniper, mistletoe, pokeweed
Hormonal effects	Gensing, mandrake, snakeroot

Compiled from Dwyer, J. Vegetarian and other alternative dietary practices. In *Manual of Clinical Nutrition.* Pleasantville, N.J.: NPT, 1983. Anonymous. Toxic reactions to herbal teas. *Nutrition and the M.D.* 5(8):(1983)4.

THERAPEUTIC MODIFICATIONS OF VEGETARIAN DIETS

Most therapeutic diets can be planned as vegetarian diets. The *Diet Manual Utilizing a Vegetarian Diet Plan* (7) is a useful resource for those who plan diets for vegetarian patients or counsel lacto-ovo-vegetarians willing to accept meat analogs in the diet. You will be given an opportunity to modify for the vegetarian patient the therapeutic diets studied in later chapters.

TOPICS FOR FURTHER DISCUSSION

1. Do some students in the class use some form of vegetarian diet? What proportion of the class does so? What are their reasons for adopting their type of diet? Ask selected students to describe their meal pattern.

2. How do meat analogs compare in cost to the meat products they resemble?

REFERENCES

1. AMERICAN DIETETIC ASSOCIATION. Position paper on the vegetarian approach to eating. *J. Am. Dietet. Assoc.* 77:(1980)61–69.
2. VYHMEISTER, I.B. Vegetarian diets: Issues and concerns. *Nutrition and the M.D.* 10(5):(1984)1–3.
3. ERHARD, D. The new vegetarians. Parts 1 and 2. *Nutrition Today.* 8(6):(1973)4–12 and 9(1):(1974)20–25.
4. OHSAWA, G. *Zen Macrobiotics.* Los Angeles: Ignoramus Press, 1965.
5. TRAHMS, C.M. Vegetarianism as a way of life. In *Contemporary Developments in Nutrition,* ed. B. Worthington-Roberts. St. Louis: C.V. Mosby, 1981.
6. PRIDE, C. *Tempeh Cookery.* Summertown, Tenn.: Book Publishing Company, 1984.
7. *Diet Manual Utilizing a Vegetarian Diet Plan.* Loma Linda, Calif.: The Seventh-Day Adventist Dietetic Association, 1975.
8. LAPPE, F.M. *Diet for a Small Planet* (rev. ed.). New York: Ballantine Books, 1975.
9. HIGGENBOTTOM, M.C., L. SWEETMAN, AND W.L. NYHAN. A syndrome of methylmalonic acidemia, homocystinuria, megaloblastic anemia, and neurologic abnormalities in a vitamin B_{12}–deficient breast-fed infant of a strict vegetarian. *New Eng. J. Med.* 299:(1978)317.
10. TRUESDELL, D.D. AND P.B. ACOSTA. Feeding the vegan infant and child. *J. Am. Diet. Assoc.* 85:(1985)837–840.

ADDITIONAL SOURCES OF INFORMATION

ACOSTA, P.B. A view of vegetarianism by a lacto-ovo vegetarian. In *Nutrition and Vegetarianism,* ed. J.J.B. Anderson. Proceedings of Public Health Nutrition Update, May 1981. Chapel Hill: Health Sciences Consortium, 1981.

DWYER, J. Wonderful world of vegetarianism: Benefits and disadvantages. In *Nutrition and Vegetarianism,* ed. J.J.B. Anderson. Proceedings of Public Health Nutrition Update, May 1981. Chapel Hill: Sciences Consortium, 1981.

FANELLI, M.T. AND R.J. KUCZMARSKI. Food selection for vegetarians. *Dietetic Currents* 10(1):(1983)1–6.

FANELLI, M.T. AND R.J. KUCZMARSKI. Guidelines for lacto-ovo vegetarian and vegan diets. In *Nutrition and Vegetarianism,* ed. J.J.B. Anderson. Proceedings of Public Health Nutrition Update, May 1981. Chapel Hill: Health Sciences Consortium, 1981.

FARTHING, M.C. Prenatal nutritional guidance for the vegetarian mother. In *Nutrition and Vegetarianism,* ed. J.J.B. Anderson. Proceedings of Public Health Nutrition Update, May 1981. Chapel Hill: Health Sciences Consortium, 1981.

KRAMER, L.B., D. OSIS, J. COFFEY, AND H. SPENCER. Mineral and trace-element content of vegetarian diets. *J. Am. Coll. Nutr.* 3:(1984)3–11.

MACMILLIAN, J.B. AND E.B. SMITH. Development of a food guide for lacto-ovo vegetarians. *J. Canad. Dietetic Assoc.* 36:(1975)1110.

ROBERTSON, L., C. FLINDERS, AND B. GODFREY. *Laurel's Kitchen.* New York: Bantam Books, 1978.

SMITH, E.B. A guide to good eating the vegetarian way. *J. Nutr. Ed.* 7:(1975)109–111.

VYHMEISTER, I.B., U.D. REGISTER, AND L.B. SONNENBERG. Safe vegetarian diets for children. *Ped. Clinics N. Am.* 24:(1977)203–210.

10

Cultural Factors in Nutritional Care

The nutritional care specialist must keep in mind that it is not sufficient merely to provide quantity of food; the food provided must also be acceptable to the patient. The acceptability of food is influenced by economic, environmental, cultural, and social factors. Personal habits and preferences may be particularly pronounced in the elderly and ill. If preferred foods can be provided, it is more likely that the patient's diet will be adequate. It is also important to realize that a person eats for reasons in addition to avoidance of hunger. Food is important in cultural identification and has many symbolic meanings related to family traditions and feelings of security, expressions of friendship, religious observances, and demonstrations of status and prestige. Acceptance of meals and compliance with diet will be improved if the symbolic meanings of foods and other factors affecting acceptance of foods are taken into account in nutritional care.

LEARNING ABOUT THE FOOD HABITS OF OTHER CULTURES

It is important to realize that other cultures have nutritionally adequate diets, even though their food patterns may differ from those common to this country. In the process of becoming familiar with the food habits of other cultures, you will need to be able to identify characteristic foods and use every opportunity to learn about others from friends, from travel, from patients, and from visits to restaurants serving ethnic foods.

In addition, you must understand the interrelationships between food and other aspects of a culture. As you try to learn about these relationships from your patients, you should consider the following variables (1):

1. *The social unit.* What kind of family unit is typical of the culture? What are the roles of various family members? Is there a hierarchy of availability of foods? Is the breadwinner favored, or children, or pregnant women? How permissive is the family in relation to child feeding? Is a child allowed to eat as desired, or is food intake structured?

2. *Social status.* How do food habits and status interrelate? Are specific foods associated with high or low status? What is their nutritional value? Are high-status foods available at reasonable prices? If not, is an equally nutritious substitute available and acceptable? Are these high-status foods an important part of the diet?

3. *Special events and celebrations.* Are celebrations or special observances that involve food an integral part of the culture? What are these events? When and how frequently do they occur? How long do they last? What foods are served? How much? Is there a tradition of fasting? How long and how often? What is the extent of the limitations on food and fluid intake?

4. *Economic factors.* Is desired food affordable? Is it available with reasonable convenience? Are preparation methods compatible with employment schedules and time available?

5. *Relationship to health.* How is *health* defined, and what importance is put on good health? Is optimal health a valued objective, or is a low level of functioning considered adequate? Does the group use traditional scientific medical services? To what extent does the group adhere to the beliefs and practices of folk medicine? Does the group relate good or poor health to the supernatural or to natural processes? Are there food-related taboos?

    Are some foods considered harmful? Conversely, are some foods believed to have special, beneficial properties? Are there certain combinations or groups of foods which are believed to have special properties? Are herbs and tonics used for special purposes? What items are used and what are their properties and effects?

    Do the food habits characteristic of the culture conflict with the requirements of nutritional care? For example, is there a large intake of salt, alcohol, caffeine, or saturated fat?

REGIONAL FOOD HABITS IN THE UNITED STATES

The variable climate and geographical features of North America have supported great variety in the food supply. Modern food processing, storage, transportation, and the increasing tendency to "eat out" have, to some extent, moderated the regional differences which once existed. Nevertheless, some regional differences persist. It is important for you to be familiar with foods that may be reflected in the food preferences of a particular population. Information on the identity of unfamiliar foods and methods of preparation may be obtained from American recipe books that contain regional recipes.

SOUTHERN BLACK DIET

One type of regional food habit deserves particular mention. The typical diet of southern blacks and poor whites has been known for years, but only recently has it been called "soul food." As the black population has migrated to other parts of the country, it is increasingly likely that you will see some patients who prefer this type of food regardless of your location.

The diet dates back to the days of slavery and consists largely of foods that were available to the slaves. It has evolved since that time, of course, but the main ingredients include greens of all kinds, peas, beans, sweet potatoes, molasses, chicken, pork, and catfish. All parts of the pig are used. The liquid in which the greens are cooked, known as pot liquor, is also used. Table J-1 classifies commonly used foods into the four food groups. One must be careful not to assume, however, that every black patient prefers this type of diet.

NATIVE AMERICAN FOOD HABITS

Native Americans include Eskimos as well as American Indians, and their diets will vary with the geographic area, and perhaps also with the tribe. There are only limited studies of the Indian diet. Table J-1 lists the types of foods seen in the diets of Indians in the Southwest.

TO TEST YOUR UNDERSTANDING

1. a. Name some locally available foods or categories of foods that are considered specialties of the area in which you live.
   b. In what meal(s) are these foods usually used? What place do these foods have in the meal?
   c. What are their nutrient contributions?
2. Are there foods that are rare and expensive in your area? If so, name some less expensive substitutes of approximately equal nutritional value.

FOOD HABITS OF SELECTED FOREIGN CULTURES

As a nation whose population is primarily composed of immigrants or descendents of immigrants, our food habits are heavily influenced by those of foreign cultures. These cultural influences may be divided into three categories. There are those which are of such long standing, or universal acceptance, or both, that they have become integrated into the dominant culture. A second category includes those cultural factors characteristic of population groups who have maintained, to some extent, their ethnic identity, despite the fact that they may already be integrated into the larger culture. Third, there are newly arrived immigrant groups, who are still in the process of adjusting to their new environment. This last group may be in particular need of nutritional counseling.

It is often difficult for the nutritionist to obtain food values of unfamiliar foods for diet evaluation. Some sources of these are given in tables of composition of foreign foods (2–4).

A belief common to many ethnic groups, particularly Latin American and Asian cultures, is the classification of food, beverages, herbs, and drugs as "hot" or "cold." The terms may be *caliente* (hot) and *fresco* or *frio* (cold) in Latin America, or *yang* and *yin* in Eastern cultures. Some foods are considered neutral. It is

important to keep in mind that the classification is unrelated to the temperature of the food. Although the philosophy of the adherent groups is basically similar, the beliefs vary in detail. Differences between Latin American and Eastern forms of these beliefs are discussed later in this chapter. Similar beliefs are found among some vegetarians (see Chapter 9).

In nutritional counseling, it is important to discover the beliefs of the individual patient. If patients can be counseled in terms of their individual beliefs, compliance may be enhanced.

ETHNIC FOODS INTEGRATED INTO AMERICAN CULTURE

All food habits except those relating to the original diets of American Indians may be considered to be derived from foreign cultures. Some of these are now so ingrained in the dominant culture that they need no further discussion. Some examples of recent additions of ethnic foods to the dominant culture include Italian pizza, and, in the Southwest, the Mexican taco.

FOODS AND FOOD HABITS OF ESTABLISHED ETHNIC GROUPS

In various parts of the country are groups who have retained, to varying degrees, their ethnic identity even though they have been in this country for many years.

When members of these groups are elderly and ill, ethnic food preferences often become stronger and more important, and it then becomes particularly important for you to understand these food habits. At the same time, persons from ethnic minorities may adopt into their diets some foods characteristic of other ethnic minorities. You might find, for example, a Chinese who eats tacos or enchiladas (5).

Some established ethnic groups in the United States include the following: Scandinavians in Minnesota and the Dakotas, Finns in upper Michigan, Portuguese in New England and California, Armenians in California, Greeks in Florida, groups of most central and eastern European cultures in large cities of the East and Middle West, and some Asian and Mexican-American groups in Western cities. The food habits of four of the larger European groups are shown in Table J-2.

Although many long-established groups are citizens of Mexican origin, there has recently been a large influx of new immigrants from Mexico and other countries of Latin America; therefore, food habits of this group are discussed in the next section describing new immigrant groups.

Characteristics of Chinese Foods and Food Habits

There are five main regions of China, each with a distinctive cuisine. North China, including Peking, was influenced by the Moslems and Manchurians. The resulting Mandarin cuisine contains wheat as the staple grain. The cuisines of Szechwan-Hunan in west and central China, Fukien and coastal China, and Eastern China, including Shanghai, are less common. The cuisine of South China and Canton is most commonly found in this country since this is the source of most immigrants to North America.

Foods that are indigenous to East Asia and are common in southern Chinese foods include the following:

Cereals: wheat, corn, and millet (north); rice (south)
Fruits and vegetables: bananas, coconuts, mangoes, cucumbers, eggplants, yams, daikon, winter melon, bok choy, bean sprouts, bamboo shoots, water chestnuts, and snow peas
Protein foods: pork, chicken, duck, tofu
Flavoring: ginger, sugar cane
Beverages: tea

Raw vegetable consumption is limited, possibly related to the use of human excreta for fertilization. Milk products are minimally used, except by immigrants from south China. Tofu is extensively used and is a good source of protein and iron, and of calcium when the protein is precipitated with calcium salts. The use of sweet or sugar products is limited. Rapidly cooked mixtures of vegetables with fish, pork, and chicken are popular.

A belief in the "hot-cold" system may be encountered, particularly among the elderly. "*Chi,*" or air, breath, or wind, is believed to be energy, which is broken down, when food is metabolized, into categories of yin (cold, female) or yang (hot, male). The elderly believe that yin, or "cold," foods must not be eaten because they contribute to the development of "weak blood" as one ages. Among avoided foods are *white turnips,* believed to cause indigestion and shortness of breath, *seaweed,* believed to cause an increase in urination and a decrease in blood pressure, and *bean sprouts* (6). Many yin foods are also believed to cause cancer. The desire to limit the use of "weak foods" and disease-causing foods must be considered when counseling these elderly patients.

Pregnant and lactating women may also require special consideration. Some patients may believe that foods eaten by the mother will not have an immediate effect on the child, but will, instead, have effects that will become evident years later. Food avoidances include the following for the reasons given (6):

Food	Belief
Soy sauce	Causes baby to be too dark
Shrimp and shellfish	Causes allergies in adolescence
Watermelon	Causes abortion
Persimmon	Causes "chills"
Deep-fat-fried foods	Causes large birth size
Rice noodles	Causes mother's intestines to twist into the shape of the noodles
Mangoes	Causes severe dermatitis
Mung beans	Causes abortions and glossitis

Other taboos for pregnant and lactating women include lamb and foods considered yin (or lyang). These include bananas, apples, pineapple, pumpkin, bean sprouts, asparagus, string beans, bamboo shoots, mustard greens, spinach, cucumber, grapefruit, beer, cold juice, tea, bitter melon, and winter melon (7).

Dietary intake is reduced during pregnancy, in the belief that the size of the fetus will be reduced and delivery will be easier. Tonics high in iron are used during the last trimester, and *ginseng* tonic is used to "increase strength for labor." Iron or potassium supplements in capsule form are avoided in order to reduce the "hardening of the bones" of the mother and fetus to allow an easier labor (6).

In the postpartum period, the woman is believed to have shifted from yang during labor to yin. Therefore, yin foods are avoided. This has the effects of increasing calories, but decreasing the number of fruits and vegetables eaten. The traditional Chinese belief is that the pores are open following delivery, and cold air enters. Yang foods, such as rice, eggs, vinegar, ginger, peanuts, rice wine, and a soup from chicken and pig knuckles are used during this period.

The meal pattern commonly consists of the following.

Breakfast: Eggs and fresh milk
Lunch: Rice, eggs, chicken, ginger
Snack: Wine
Dinner: Chicken–pigs' knuckles soup, vinegar, alcohol

Specific rejected foods include the following (7).

During First 30 Days

of Lactation	Reason
Turnips and carrots	Cause drying up of mother's milk
Taro root	Prolongs vaginal infection
Ice cream	Causes digestive disorders in infants
Sugar cane	Causes periods of sterility in offspring

After 30 Days of Lactation

Fresh fish	Causes fever in infants
Melons	Cause diarrhea or measles in infants
Frog legs	Cause leg cramps in infants
Tomatoes	Cause a red face in older infants
Oranges	Cause diarrhea in old age

Problems resulting from these food habits result in an increased incidence of deficiencies of B vitamins, ascorbic acid, and some minerals. Constipation is also a frequent problem. Categorization into the four food groups of foods particularly characteristic of the Chinese diet is given in Table J-1.

Characteristics of Japanese Foods and Food Habits

The Japanese have been quite persistent in retaining their own cultural food habits through several generations (8). These generations are called *Issei,* those born in Japan who have immigrated to the United States; *Nisei,* or first-generation Americans; and *Sansei,* or second-generation Americans. Some characteristics of the *traditional* Japanese diet include the following:

Rice is the center of the diet; other foods are side dishes.
A largely vegetarian diet is common following the adoption of Buddhism.
A number of "pickled or soured" foods are used—indicated by the suffix "bishio."
Soybean products and fish are frequently used. A number of these products are described in Chapter 9.
Seaweeds and a variety of vegetables are included.
Green tea (*ocha*) is the common beverage.
Seasonings are miso, soy sauce, sugar, and vinegar.

A traditional Japanese breakfast consists of rice, miso soup, a pickled vegetable, and tea. Other meals, not markedly different, may contain rice, fish, vegetables, miso, and tea. Beef, pork, chicken, or eggs may be substituted for fish. A distribution of these foods among the four food groups is shown in Table J-1.

TO TEST YOUR UNDERSTANDING

3. You have a young Chinese patient who is pregnant. During counseling, she tells you that she does not, and will not, drink milk. What alternative high-calcium foods can you suggest?
   Choose the two best sources and calculate the amounts necessary to provide the amount of calcium in 1 quart of milk. Assume that you would provide some of each food each day.

FOOD HABITS OF NEW IMMIGRANT GROUPS

Among the most recent immigrants are those from Southeast Asia and from Latin America. These groups may be in particular need of nutritional counseling. Their food habits will therefore be considered in greater detail.

Latin-American Food Habits

There are many groups with different food habits in the Southwest United States, Mexico, Central and South America, and the Caribbean. They have been referred to by various terms, not all of which are interchangeable, including *Mexican-American; Chicano,* with its political connotations; *Latino; Hispanic;* and *Spanish-American,* the original settlers of the Southwest who did not intermarry with the Indians. Many, but not all, of the areas from which most of the immigration occurs are Spanish-speaking. Nevertheless, food habits vary widely and cannot be stereotyped.

Mexican-American Foods and Food Habits. Mexican-American food habits are a composite of those of the Aztecs, Spanish, French, and Anglo-Americans. The diet of Mexican-Americans in the United States has been found to vary somewhat with the number of generations since the family left Mexico. The first generation of immigrants and Mexican nationals are very familiar with the indigenous Mexican diet; second- and third-generation Mexican-Americans may be at various stages of acculturation and usually retain some, but not all, of their parents' and grandparents' culture. Generally, the speed of acculturation is also proportional to the distance to the United States–Mexico border. Middle- and upper-class Mexican-Americans may not differ from Americans of other ethnic origins. When counseling Mexican-American patients, therefore, it is important for you to establish the level of acculturation to Anglo-American food habits and the degree to which Mexican food habits are retained.

Another group that deserves mention are the migrant farm workers. Many of them are of Mexican origin in the Southwest, in Texas, New Mexico, Arizona, and California, and in the states to the north of these border states. Their food habits are similar, largely for economic reasons. Migrant farm workers on the East coast who migrate from Florida to New England may consist mostly of members of other groups, including those from the Caribbean.

The total number of Mexican nationals and Mexican-Americans in the United States is large and is increasing daily. Therefore, it is important to be familiar with the details of their food habits.

Many Anglo-Americans are familiar with the dishes served in Mexican restaurants. However, dishes requiring long preparation time, such as tamales and enchiladas, are prepared primarily for Sundays, holidays, and special occasions in Mexican-American homes. Most everyday dishes are easier to prepare and include soups (*caldos*), rice and macaroni dishes (*sopas*), and stews (*guisados*). The staple foods of low-income families are beans and tortillas. Beans are often eaten for more than one meal a day, fried at first and then refried for succeeding meals. Tortillas, made from cornmeal or wheat flour, or purchased ready-made, are used instead of bread. As income improves, meat, eggs, fruits, and vegetables are used in greater quantities (9).

Milk is scarce in Mexico, and refrigeration is a problem. Immigrant families are thus unaccustomed to using milk and often use it in inadequate amounts. Evaporated milk is sometimes used since it does not require refrigeration before opening. Cheese is more commonly used. The native cheese resembles a fine-curd, dry cottage cheese, and American and Monterey Jack cheeses are popular (9).

Pork, beef, and chicken are well liked. Because meat is expensive, the native Mexican diet includes many parts of the animal not frequently used in the United States, such as hogs' heads, and the tongue, brains, tripe, liver, kidney, and intestines of beef. These are still used, highly seasoned, by the older generation and new immigrants. Fish is often eaten on Friday and during Lent. Eggs are popular in mixed dishes and as extenders (9).

Corn, green beans, peas, potatoes, and summer squash are eaten cooked, and carrots, spinach, and sweet potatoes are included in stew. Lettuce and tomatoes may be eaten in salads. Chile peppers are commonly used, usually in a sauce containing onion and garlic plus other seasonings, with or without tomatoes. The nutritional value depends on the method of preparation and, of course, the amount (9).

Chiles belong to the pepper family. They may be green, yellow, or red and vary in shape from large and round to small and pointed. As a rule of thumb, the smaller and more pointed they are, the "hotter" they are. The heat is greatest in the interior "ribs" (9).

Mexican-Americans may make their own chile sauce from fresh peppers, but various commercial products are available, including pickled peppers, chile sauce, dried chiles, and a chile powder consisting of dried, ground chiles plus red pepper and other seasonings (9).

Chile, if eaten raw or home cooked, is a good source of ascorbic acid. A fourth-cup of green chile contains about the same amount of ascorbic acid as a serving of cabbage. Commercial red chile sauce is highly variable in vitamin content. Dried chiles and chile powder are poor vitamin sources.

Many fruits are popular and are eaten if income permits. Oranges are popular, as are some tropical fruits such as guavas, mangos, sapates, and tuna, the fruit of the prickly pear cactus.

Desserts are not usually included in the native culture. *Pan de dulce* (sweet rolls) may be eaten for breakfast. American foods added to the diet often include ice cream, pie, doughnuts, and preserves.

The most common cooking methods are simmering, boiling, frying, and a small amount of baking. Commonly used fats in food preparation are lard, salt pork, and bacon fat. Broiling is seldom used in families with the more traditional food habits. This fact may present a compliance problem with some diet modifications.

A typical meal pattern in the Los Angeles area is as follows (9).

Breakfast: Cooked or dry cereal with evaporated milk, coffee, bacon and eggs if income is not limited, and sweet rolls occasionally.

Lunch: Soup, canned or homemade, sandwich, coffee or soft drink, and fruit.

Dinner: Stew or other dish with meat, fish, or chicken, a rice or macaroni dish, refried beans, bread or tortillas, lettuce and tomato salad, and beverage.

Attention must be called to the belief in the hot-cold (*caliente-frio* in Spanish) system among Mexican-Americans and other Latin Americans. The classification varies among individuals, among generations, and from one village of origin to another; therefore, individualized counseling is necessary.

In the *Hippocratic system*, treatment is with opposites, and "hot" diseases require "cold" treatment. In the *homeopathic* system, by contrast, treatment is with like items, so a "hot" disease requires a "hot" treatment.

In general, "cold" foods are most fresh vegetables, tropical fruits, dairy products, and low-prestige meats such as goat, fish, and chicken. "Hot" foods are chili, temperate-zone fruits, cereals, goat's milk, cooking oils, alcoholic beverages, and high-prestige meats such as mutton and water fowl. "Neutral" foods are beans, legumes, rice, pork, and peaches. Some "hot" or "cold" foods may be neutralized by preparation methods.

Water is considered a strong "cold" food. A problem may arise when a patient with a "hot" disease such as a fever is believed to need only hot food and may be forbidden to drink water.

In Mexico, cold foods are linked with sterility, and the diet is based on "hot" foods. In menstruation, a "hot" condition, homeopathy predominates and the woman eats only "hot" foods. "Hot" foods are consumed during pregnancy lest the fetus be harmed, and "hot" foods are considered to increase milk production. On the other hand, an excess of "hot" foods is believed to cause *enlechado,* curdling of milk in the stomach of the child. An iron supplement is considered "hot," as is the mother. It may therefore be necessary to dissolve the iron supplement in fruit juice to neutralize it before the mother will take it. This will help ensure that an excess of hot foods is not consumed.

Puerto Rican Foods and Food Habits. The Spanish-speaking population in the east and midwest is more likely to be from Puerto Rico or other areas of the Caribbean. Again food habits may vary with the degree of acculturation over the years, and may also be affected by income limitations.

The food habits may have the Spanish influence in common with Mexican-Americans, but the different climate, the island environment, and the absence of Aztec influence result in major differences. For example, while beans are used by both groups, corn is not much used in Puerto Rican foods, nor is chile. Puerto Rican foods are not as highly spiced. Rice and red kidney beans are the Puerto Rican staples.

Beef, chicken, and pork, either fresh, smoked, or in sausage are often used in small pieces in stews and to flavor vegetables. A frequently used seasoning mix is known as *refrito.* Chicken is eaten with red kidney beans or as *arroz con pollo* (rice with chicken). Fish is accepted either fresh or dried and salted and served as a salad with hard-cooked eggs and onions. *Serenata* is a staple dish containing salted cod (*baculao*), avocado, *vianda* (a starchy vegetable such as plantain, green banana, or cassava), onion, and sometimes egg. Other protein sources are the various legumes, lima, navy, pinto, and red beans, and chick peas or garbanzo beans, which are a basic food.

Commonly used cereals are rice, wheat (including white bread), oatmeal as a breakfast cereal, and cornmeal. A common staple, used several times weekly, is a stewed mixture of beans and rice with lard or olive oil, flavored with refrito; tomatoes are sometimes added. Spaghetti and noodles are also widely used. A native white cheese, *queso blanco,* is popular but expensive. It is used with pasta. Boiled fresh milk is used, when income permits, as a beverage for children and in *cafe con leche* (half each coffee and milk) for adults. It is also used in chocolate or cocoa drinks.

Vegetables are used in stews or salads of tubers and onions with an oil- and vinegar-dressing. Acceptable vegetables include eggplant (chayote), green peppers, beets, tomatoes, green beans, carrots, and okra. In addition, the vegetables known as *viandas* are eaten as such or used in fritters, turnovers, pies, and desserts; viandas include *batata, name, yautia, platano* (plantain), *panapin, malanga,* and *apio. Sofrito,* a tomato sauce, is used with many foods. Popular fruits include plantain, or banana, mashed and mixed with onion, or raw oranges, acerola, mango, guava, papaya, and pineapple.

Common seasonings are garlic, onion, and vinegar and flavorings from lard, ham fat, and olive oil. *Malta* is a common beverage of caramel, malt extract, and sugar. Other beverages are fruit juices and drinks, coffee, beer and rum (10). Some Puerto Ricans believe in the *caliente-frio* system, which must be considered during counseling.

Cuban Foods and Food Habits. Cubans have tended to eat in restaurants and have adapted American eating habits more than have Puerto Ricans (10). At home, however, main staples are rice and beans; black beans, rather than kidney beans, are the most popular. These are cooked in a sauce similar to sofrito but with more pork. Beef, lamb, veal, poultry, sausages, all types of fish, and eggs are accepted. The most popular rice dish is *arroz con qui,* rice and black beans. Vegetables in the typical diet include native tubers (yucca, name, malanga, *boniato* (white yams), *berenjena,* plantain, and potatoes) and tomatoes and carrots. Accepted cereals include rice, cornmeal, and dry breakfast cereals.

Fresh cow's milk is used for a beverage for children, in coffee for adults, and in sauces and desserts. Native cheese is hard cheese eaten with guava paste.

Lard is popular for cooking. Oil—olive, peanut, or soy—is used on salads and beans. Butter, margarine, and hydrogenated shortenings are also used. Foods are seasoned with vinegar, oregano, garlic, onion, and green peppers.

Desserts are eaten at each meal and as a snack. Ice cream, cake, pie, custard, and pudding are popular. Other sweets are those made from fruit and viandas. Another is *panetelas,* a coconut candy-like dish (10). In general, tropical fruits are well liked. Native dessert names are *raspadura, terrejas, boniatillo, bunuelos,* and *cafiroleta.* Coffee, tea, wine, beer, and soft drinks are commonly used beverages.

Indochinese Foods and Food Habits

A large, somewhat heterogeneous, recent immigrant group consists of those from southeast Asia. Many arrived in poor physical, emotional, and financial condition. Their educational level varies from near illiteracy to completion of postgraduate education. Their social customs vary to a great extent from those common in North America. These factors, in addition to language barriers, and the unfamiliar dietary habits of this population, greatly impeded nutritional counseling, as well as the provision of other social services, when the first of these refugees arrived.

TO TEST YOUR UNDERSTANDING

4. An impoverished Mexican-American family cannot afford citrus fruit, and no one in the family will drink milk. The family consists of two parents, aged 30; a grandmother, 50 years old; and three children, ages 7, 9, and 11. What sources of the following nutrients are available to them in a low-cost, traditional Mexican diet?

   Protein
   Calcium
   Riboflavin
   Ascorbic acid

5. If the family followed a typical Puerto Rican diet, what would be the best sources of these same nutrients?

   Protein
   Calcium
   Riboflavin
   Ascorbic acid

6. A pregnant Mexican-American patient tells you that she will not drink milk, and that she buys ready-made wheat tortillas. What suggestions would you make to her to improve the calcium content of her diet?

7. Visit a retail store that specializes in Mexican or Puerto Rican foods. List the fresh fruits and vegetables that are not sold in most supermarkets. (Ask the grocer their names if necessary.) List each, describe its use in a typical meal pattern, and comment on its nutritional value and cost.

8. In the same store, scan the shelves of canned goods. List items not commonly seen in most supermarkets, describe the use of each in the meal pattern, state its primary nutritional value, and comment on cost.

The information that follows is detailed, in order to provide you with examples of the types of information you will have to seek and the methods you might use when counseling these kinds of patients. You can then apply these methods to other groups with similar problems.

The Indochinese comprise three distinct groups: the Vietnamese, the Cambodians, and the Laotians. The population of Laos is sometimes further classified into three subgroups, based principally on language, but with other cultural differences. One group consists of the *Tai*, which has a number of subgroups, the largest of which are the *Thai/Lao*. There are also minority Tai tribes who lived in mountain valleys, growing rice, corn, millet, sweet potatoes, and beans. The second group are the *Mon-Khmer*, or *Lao Theung*, who lived on the hillsides. Third are the *Hmong* and *Yao*, mostly mountain dwellers, who used slash-and-burn agriculture and raised livestock. (They are sometimes called *Meo*, but this is a pejorative term in Chinese and should not be used.) There are some Hmong among the refugees. Their food habits are sufficiently different that they are often considered a separate group.

The Cambodians tend to be the most culturally homogeneous group. Many are highly educated and familiar with urban living. Some Vietnamese and Cambodian refugees are ethnic Chinese and tend to follow Chinese food habits, rather than those which will be described here.

The Vietnamese.   The Vietnamese are the largest of the refugee groups; most now reside in California and Florida, with smaller numbers on the Gulf coast and elsewhere. Some diet changes have occurred, but most still prefer the typical Vietnamese diet (11, 12).

A typical meal pattern is shown in Table J-3. Foods are generally highly spiced with hot chili, ginger root, pepper, onion, garlic, herbs, spices, and fish sauce. Most cooked food is boiled, stir-fried, or steamed.

Rice is the staple food. Long-grain rice is preferred, served with fresh or dried fish or shellfish, or sometimes meat. Accepted meats are pork (most common), including the heart, liver, stomach, intestines, tongue and coagulated blood, Chinese sausage, chicken and giblets (on special occasions), and some beef. Fish may be fresh, dried, salted, or fermented, but the preferred method of preparation is fried and dipped in fish sauce. A spicy fish sauce, *nuoc mam*, is used extensively for seasoning and is rich in protein and calcium. It is available in Asian grocery stores as "Filipino fish sauce." Other protein foods are soy milk, tofu, peanuts, and legumes in desserts. Milk and dairy products are not typically part of the diet, but small children are sometimes given evaporated milk.

Favorite fruits are banana, mango, melon, orange, pineapple, and papaya. A wide variety of vegetables are acceptable if fresh or frozen, including many vegetables commonly available in North America, plus bamboo shoots, bean sprouts, bok choy, snow peas, bittermelon, dried lily flowers, lotus root, and wintermelon. Bok choy, snow peas, and lotus root are good sources of ascorbic acid. Canned vegetables, which are considered too soft, are not popular.

Among cereal products, besides rice, bean thread

and noodles are used. French bread is accepted, a legacy of French colonialism. Other foods in the diet are lard for frying, gluten flour, and seeds. Tea is the main beverage, but coffee, soft drinks, soy milk, sugar cane drink, beer, and wine are accepted. Condensed milk is used in coffee and on bread, and is sometimes given to infants in formula. Soft drink intake has increased markedly in Vietnamese families.

During pregnancy, the Vietnamese woman is expected to eat nourishing food and avoid "unclean" food, such as beef. After delivery, preferred foods are salty foods, pork stew, rice, and chicken. All foods must be hot to "keep the stomach warm and avoid heat loss." Cold foods and cold water are not used because they are thought to be bad for the teeth and stomach. Sour foods, which include salads, beef, and all seafood, are forbidden for 6 months (13).

The Laotians. Laotian food habits differ in a few ways from those of the Vietnamese. Meat, fish, fruit, and vegetables are similar. Laotians prefer glutinous rice. Soybean products are eaten by the Hmong, but not by the Lao. A major seasoning is a fermented fish paste called *padek*. Others are chili, fish sauce, coconut milk, tamarind, and curry. Tea, coconut juice, fruit and vegetable juices, a soy bean drink, sugar cane drink, beer, and wine serve as beverages. Diluted condensed milk is used as a beverage for adults and sometimes as an infant formula. Typical meal plans for Laotians and Hmong are shown in Table J-3.

The Cambodians. Cambodian food habits also do not differ markedly from those of the Vietnamese. Fish—fresh, smoked, or dried—is common. *Prahoc*, a salted, fermented fish paste is popular. Soybeans are not eaten, except by Chinese Cambodians, but various legumes are made into desserts. Rice may be long- or short-grain, or black, sweet rice, which is used as a dessert. Seasonings include prahoc as well as those used by Laotians and Vietnamese. Beverages are also similar. Sweetened, condensed milk is spread on bread and used for infant formula. The Cambodian meal pattern is also shown in Table J-3.

TO TEST YOUR UNDERSTANDING

9. Consult a table of food values and compare the food value of evaporated and condensed milk. If an Indochinese mother told you she was using condensed milk to feed her infant, what would you recommend? Why?

CONSIDERATIONS IN COMMUNICATING WITH REFUGEE PATIENTS

When you are interviewing or counseling a patient from another ethnic group, it is important to have some appreciation of that group's customs. If your behavior is not acceptable, communication may be blocked. Some of the difficulties in working with the Indochinese can serve as an example (14).

Often, one of the first problems is a language barrier. Pantomime is limited, and an interpreter must often be found. A member of the family can sometimes serve as an interpreter. In any case, it is usually helpful to find an interpreter of the same sex and same social class. When working with an interpreter, it is important to talk to the *patient,* not to the interpreter. Speak slowly and distinctly, emphasizing gestures and facial expressions.

Whether speaking through an interpreter or directly with a patient who knows some English, there are some policies which should be kept in mind:

1. A soft-spoken, pleasant approach should be adopted. When language is not understood, do not shout; it does not help in any language.
2. Indochinese are accustomed to a slow pace. Be careful not to appear rushed.
3. Indochinese are accustomed to a degree of formality. A very casual manner will be regarded as rude.
4. Do not beckon with an upturned finger; this gesture is regarded as insulting by the Vietnamese. Beckoning, if unavoidable, should be done with the whole hand with fingers down. Pointing with your toe is regarded by Laotians as very rude. Never cross your legs: If your toe is pointed at the patient, he will be insulted.
5. The eldest male is considered the head of the family and should be addressed first, even if he is not the patient. Elders are highly respected. Show respect by using both hands to give anything to elderly patients. Bow the head slightly in greeting.
6. Many Indochinese believe the soul resides in the head and are disturbed if the head is touched. Do not touch a patient's head unless absolutely necessary, and always explain first. *Never* pat children on the head.
7. Southeast Asians are used to fleeting eye contact. Do not try to maintain eye contact.
8. If it is necessary to deny a patient's request, do so indirectly by saying that you "will see what can be done."
9. When making home visits, do not sit down until invited to do so, and always accept offers of refreshments. Preliminary small talk is regarded as good manners.
10. Do not assume you have established rapport with a patient if he is polite. It may indicate he does not understand or is rejecting what you have said.

You will need similar types of information when you wish to communicate with patients of any other culture. The more you can learn about the cultures of your patients, the more effective you will be.

RELIGIOUS INFLUENCES IN PATIENT CARE

In addition to national and racial influences, religion may also influence a patient's food habits. It is not only necessary to consider the religion of any individual patient if that affects food habits, but it is also important to understand policies based on religious beliefs in church-operated hospitals.

The effects on food habits of beliefs of the world's five major religions—Christianity, Judaism, Islam, Hinduism, and Buddhism—will be discussed. Emphasis is on those religions followed by larger groups in North America.

In many religions, there are *feasts*, *fasts*, and *food taboos* which may affect nutritional status. Feasts and fasts may be *fixed*, occurring on the same day each year, or *movable*, occurring at different times yearly, often varying with the lunar cycle. Specific foods, seating arrangements, menus, and eating customs may be associated with certain festivals and serve to maintain the ethnic traditions.

CHRISTIANITY

In the United States and Canada, Christianity has the most adherents of the five major religions. They may be broadly subdivided into Roman Catholic, Protestant, and Eastern Orthodox.

Roman Catholic Dietary Regulations

The regulations vary somewhat with geographical location; therefore, it is wise to inquire at the office of the local diocese if there is any doubt. The following regulations are typical:*

1. The law of *fast* obliges only on Ash Wednesday and Good Friday. On fast days, one full meal and two other partial meals, which together would not equal a full meal, are allowed. Eating between meals is not permitted, but liquids, including milk and fruit juices, are allowed. *When people are ill or their ability to work would be seriously affected, the laws of fast and abstinence do not oblige.* Fasting is observed by all those between the ages of 21 and 59.

2. The law of *abstinence*, which prescribed the abstention from meat, and soup or gravy made from meat, no longer obliges on Fridays in general. It does, however, oblige on Ash Wednesday, Good Friday, and on all Fridays of Lent besides Good Friday. Abstinence is observed by all those beyond the age of 14 years.

It is important to note the difference between *fast*, in which less food is eaten, and *abstinence*, in which meat and meat products are not eaten. Ash Wednesday and Good Friday are days of both fast and abstinence. Patients may need to be reminded that these obligations do *not* apply when they are ill.

*These regulations were obtained from the Roman Catholic Diocese of Sacramento, California.

Seventh-Day Adventists

The beliefs of Seventh-Day Adventists are discussed in Chapter 9, since many are vegetarians. They usually do not use caffeine-containing beverages, such as coffee, tea, or cola drinks, nor alcoholic beverages. Meat is not served in Seventh-Day Adventist–operated hospitals, except on prescription by a physician (15).

Mormons

The Church of Jesus Christ of Latter-Day Saints, also known as the Mormon church, disapproves of alcoholic and caffeine-containing beverages. Although the church is centered in the state of Utah, members are found throughout the United States and Canada, particularly in the West, and also in many foreign countries.

Other Protestant Denominations

The Protestant denominations generally do not emphasize fast days or food taboos. They share some holidays (feast days) and fast days with Roman Catholics, but the degree of observance varies greatly with the denomination and individual choice.

Orthodox Christians

Members of the Eastern Orthodox church were originally the Christians of the Balkan states in Europe, the area northeast of the Mediterranean Sea, Greece, and Russia. Each state church is independent, and is thus called, for example, Greek Orthodox and Russian Orthodox. The head of the state church is the patriarch or archbishop. The patriarch at Istanbul is the spiritual leader.

The Greek Orthodox religion has many fast days—every Wednesday and Friday in the year except two, the 40 days of Lent, the 40 days of Advent (before Christmas), and two shorter fasts in July and August. The requirements are more severe than in Roman Catholicism. On fast days, no meat, animal products such as dairy products, or fish, with the exception of shellfish, are eaten. The more devout members also abstain from olive oil. A soup of dried beans and lentils is commonly served on fast days.

Easter is the most important event in the Orthodox church calendar. It is preceded by 40 days of Lent. Since the Orthodox calendar is not identical to the Gregorian calendar used by the Roman Catholic and Protestant churches, Easter falls on a different day. Other dates vary in similar fashion.

Lent is preceded by several weeks of preparation. This period includes *Apokreos*, or *Meat-fare Sunday*, 10 days before Ash Wednesday, the first day of Lent. On this day and during the ensuing week, all meat in the house is eaten. A week later is *Cheese-fare Sunday*, the Sunday before Ash Wednesday, when all cheese, eggs, and butter are eaten. As a result, this is a period of feasting.

During Lent, adherents abstain from all animal foods; the only exception is fish, which is allowed on Palm Sunday and on the Day of Annunciation. Lentil soup is eaten on Good Friday. Lamb is traditionally eaten on Easter Sunday.

JUDAISM

Adherents to Judaism constitute the second largest religious group in North America. You will be called upon to see Jewish patients in almost every hospital, and their diets may have to be modified to conform to their religious beliefs. In addition, Jewish hospitals in large cities may have policies which are based on Jewish religious beliefs.

The adherence to the Dietary Laws varies among Jews. There are four groups. *Orthodox* Jews observe the laws strictly; and because of difficulties in obtaining acceptable food elsewhere, Orthodox Jews eat away from home only in restaurants or homes with kosher kitchens. The *Conservative* Jews generally observe the Dietary Laws in their own homes, but accept more variations when eating elsewhere. *Reform* Jews may conform to few of the Dietary Laws, and sometimes none. The last group is the *Reconstructionists*, for whom observance varies from very strict to none at all, based on individual conscience.

In institutions that are not equipped to prepare kosher meals on the premises, frozen meals may be purchased in many large cities. When instructing patients for use of diets at home, their beliefs must be kept in mind. The practices of Orthodox Jews will be described in some detail.

The Jewish Dietary Laws are known as *Kashruth,* or *Kashrus.* They originate in the Torah, were interpreted in the Talmud, and specify the foods that are "fit and proper" (*kosher,* or *kasher*) for Jewish people to eat. The term *glatt kosher* means that the food satisfies even the strictest kosher standards.

The Dietary Laws divide all foods into three categories (1):

1. Those foods which are inherently kosher—that is, they are "neutral," or *pareve,* and may be eaten in their natural state. Such foods include grains, fruits, vegetables, eggs, tea, coffee, and other foods free of meat, poultry, or dairy products.
2. Foods that require processing in order to be kosher—that is, meat, poultry, and cheese;
3. Foods that are inherently nonkosher, or *trayf*—that is, pork products, fish without scales and fins, and shellfish.

In order to be kosher, meat must come only from "clean" animals—those that chew their cud and have divided (cloven) hooves. Cows, sheep, oxen, goats, and deer are considered clean. Liver, chicken, and turkey are also acceptable, as well as most species of ducks, geese, pigeon, squab; pork is not acceptable. Other forbidden foods are winged insects, reptiles, creeping animals, and birds of prey. The latter restrictions are, of course, of little consequence in North America. It is not permissible to eat blood because it is "the life of the animal."

The slaughter of animals must be supervised by a rabbi. The actual slaughter, however, is done by a trained person called a *schochet,* and the animal is killed in such a way as to allow the draining away of a maximum amount of blood. The meat must then be further treated to remove the remaining blood. It is soaked in water for 30 minutes, then salted on all surfaces with a medium-coarse salt, allowed to drain for almost an hour, and then washed three times to remove the salt (16). Iron and B vitamins are probably lost in the process (17). Since the blood cannot be removed from liver by this process, liver must be broiled on a rack designed so that the blood can drip from it as it cooks. Usually, only the forequarter of quadrupeds may be used, so the cuts available in kosher meats are the less-tender cuts. Hind-quarter cuts are usable only if the hip sinew of the thigh vein is removed.

Many dairy products are not kosher because meat derivatives are used in their manufacture. These include rennin in some cheeses and the gelatin used in making some yogurts, ice creams, and other frozen desserts. Many Orthodox Jews will only eat *cholov yisroel* dairy products or those whose total preparation is supervised by reliable Jewish authorities.

Fish must have fins and scales to be fit to eat. Therefore, shellfish, eels, and shark meat are prohibited. The roe of nonkosher fish are also forbidden. Other taboo foods are animals which died of disease or natural causes, blood, and the internal fat of an animal. Because of this last stricture, soaps made from animal fats are forbidden, and detergents are used instead for dishwashing. For cooking, vegetable fats and oils are permitted.

Another practice important to Orthodox Jews is the prohibition of eating meat and milk in the same meal. In addition, meat and milk cannot be prepared or served with the same dishes and utensils. After meat is eaten, some time must pass before dairy may be consumed. The time required may vary with the customs of the national ancestry. Eastern European Jews wait 6 hours; German and West European Jews, 3 hours; and Dutch Jews, 72 minutes (18). On the other hand, milk may be consumed just before eating meat, but not with it (16). Commonly, breakfast and lunch are milk meals, and dinner is a meat meal.

In order to keep meat and milk separate, Orthodox Jewish homes must keep two completely separate sets of cooking utensils, dishes, and silverware. The separation also applies to dishwashing and towel drying. An electric dishwasher can be used for both milk and meat dishes only if it can be properly koshered between washing separate loads of milk and meat dishes.

Meals are therefore meat (*fleischig*) meals or dairy (*milchig*) meals. Allowable fish are eaten with either, as are eggs; however, an egg with a blood spot cannot be used. Pareve foods may be eaten with either type of meal. Some foods are not acceptable on a kosher diet or are considered to be waste products; one of the latter is cream of tartar, made from the sediment remaining after wine is filtered.

Prepared products may be acceptable as kosher if produced within kosher standards, which is indicated by emblems on the *sealed* package. There are many of these emblems (19). The symbol Ⓤ is used by the Union of Orthodox Jewish Congregations of America, while the symbol Ⓚ is the emblem of the Organized Kashrus Laboratories. Two emblems are common in Canada—ⓂⓀ from the Montreal Vaad-Harabonim, and ⓒⓄⓇ from the Council of Orthodox Rabbis of Toronto.

Food plays an important role in the observance of Jewish festivals and holy days. No food may be cooked on the Sabbath, which extends from sundown Friday to sundown Saturday. Food is cooked in advance on Thursday or Friday, so that the Sabbath can be a day of rest.

The Sabbath dinner on Friday evening is often the most substantial of the week. At that dinner, two loaves of bread (*challah*) are on the table. These two loaves are in remembrance of the double portion of manna provided on Fridays during the 40 years that Jews wandered in the wilderness (20).

Food also has symbolic meanings on other Jewish holy days. The most solemn of these are the ten days in September or October of each year, which begin with *Rosh Hashanah*, the Day of Judgment, and end with *Yom Kippur*, the Day of Atonement. The challah for Rosh Hashanah, which is the Jewish New Year, is commonly made round, to symbolize the desire for a well-rounded year. It may be made with ladders or birds baked on top to symbolize the carrying of family

prayers to heaven. The wish for sweetness in the New Year is symbolized by bread and apple slices dipped in honey. Yom Kippur is a day of complete fast for all except children younger than 13 years, people who are ill, and pregnant women (17).

The eight-day *Festival of Pesach*, or *Passover*, occurs in the spring and commemorates the flight of the Israelites from Egypt. This festival requires many preparations in Orthodox Jewish homes. None of the foods in daily use can be used during Passover. Prepared foods that are purchased must be labeled *Kasher L'Pesach* (Kosher for Passover) and certified for use by rabbinical authority. The Kasher L'Pesach label alone is insufficient (16).

The home is thoroughly cleaned and all leaven is removed. All leavened products in the home are eaten or disposed of prior to Passover, and no leavened bread or other leavened food can be eaten during Passover. An unleavened wheat cracker-like bread known as *matzo* has been used by Jews for many centuries. It is now prepared commercially under rabbinical supervision.

Flour and grain cannot be used for cooking during Passover since either may become naturally leavened very quickly. The result of this process is called *hametz*. Other hametz foods forbidden for use during Passover include coffee-like materials derived from cereals, dry peas, dry beans, and all liquids that contain ingredients or flavors made from grain alcohol. No malt liquors may be used during Passover, including malt vinegar. Matzo which is finely ground to make *matzo meal* may be used in food preparation in place of flour. No salt is used in traditional Passover matzo.

If certified for Passover use by rabbinical authority, Passover noodles, candies, cakes, beverages, canned and processed foods, milk, butter, jams, jellies, cheese,

Table 10-1. Summary of Jewish Holidays

Holiday	Approximate Date	Observation	Traditional Foods
Rosh Hashanah (New Year)	September/October	Beginning of Jewish New Year	Carrot tzimmes, honey, honey cakes
Yom Kippur	September/October	Day of Atonement	Fast all day
Sukkoth	October	Harvest festival and Feast of Booths (Booth or shelter in which the Jews lived during flight from Egypt)	Kreplach or holishkes (chopped meat rolled in cabbage leaves); strudel
Hanukkah	December	Festival of Lights; celebrates battle of Maccabees for Jewish independence	Grated potato latkes and potato kugel
Tu b'Shevat	January	Festival of Trees (Arbor Day); the blossoming time of trees in Palestine	Bokser (St. John's Bread), cakes, raisins, fruits, nuts
Purim	March	Feast of Esther; celebrates fall of Haman and deliverance of Hebrews by influence of Queen Esther on King Xerxes	Hamantaschen (3-cornered cookie), apples, nuts, raisins
Passover	April	Festival of Freedom; celebrates escapes of Israelites from slavery in Egypt	Seder meal, matzoth, nuts, wine
Shavuoth	May/June	Feast of Weeks; celebrates Moses' receiving the Ten Commandments on Mt. Sinai	Cheese blintzes, cheese kreplach, dairy foods
Tisha b'Av	August	Fast day; commemorates destruction of the First and Second Temples	Meat not eaten on Tisha b'Av or the 9 days preceding it. Blintzes and dairy foods are traditional

relishes, dried fruits, vegetable oils, vegetable gelatin, vinegar, wines, and liquors are acceptable (16). Fresh fruits and vegetables, except peas and beans, are acceptable without certification. Coffee, tea, sugar, salt, and pepper are permitted if the container has not been previously opened (16).

The *seder* meal is a special feast which occurs the evening of the first day of Passover. In Orthodox homes outside of Israel, the seder is repeated the second night.

Nearly all Orthodox Jewish homes have separate dishes for use during Passover. An Orthodox Jewish home may thus have four sets of dishes—milk dishes and meat dishes for daily use, and milk dishes and meat dishes for Passover. This may present a financial burden; however, there is a ritual for purifying the everyday dishes for Passover use if the family cannot afford the extra sets. Another alternative is to use disposable tableware during Passover. In Jewish hospitals, patients wishing to have kosher foods are often

TO TEST YOUR UNDERSTANDING

10. In the following table, mark an X in the column in which the food would be included by an Orthodox Jew:

Food	Pareve	Fleischig	Milchig	During Passover	Trayf
Orange juice					
Oatmeal					
Poached egg					
Whole-wheat toast					
Cereal coffee					
Cream					
Oxtail soup (from kosher-killed beef, with vegetables)					
Salmon salad					
Sliced tomato					
Breaded shrimp					
Roast lamb					
Carrots					
Harvard beets					
Molded fruit salad					
Fried liver and onions					
Angel food cake					

11. An elderly Conservative Jew has been admitted to your hospital. He is willing to make some adjustments for the fact that you do not have a kosher kitchen. You plan to order some commercial frozen kosher meals for him and serve them with disposable tableware. It will take two days to get delivery. In the meantime, how would you adjust the following hospital menus to satisfy as many of his expectations as possible? Write the menu as you would modify it in the space to the right.

Breakfast:
½ grapefruit
Cornflakes/milk/sugar
Soft-cooked egg
Salt and pepper
White toast/butter/jam
Coffee/cream/sugar

Dinner:
Lamb chops, broiled
Mint jelly
Baked potato/butter
Buttered peas
Fruit salad (melon, strawberries, banana, grapes)
Maple-nut ice cream

served with disposable tableware. Special frozen meals are available for use during Passover.

Passover and other Jewish festivals are listed in Table 10-1. It is important to realize that foods preferred by individual Jews may be strongly influenced also by their country of origin.

ISLAM

Adherents to the *Islamic* (*Muslim* or *Moslem*) religion reside primarily in the Middle East, North Africa, and across Asia as far as the Philippines. There are also Muslims in the Balkan nations of Europe and in Russia. Several million Muslims reside in North America, and there are a great many Muslim visitors, such as students. Therefore, although Islam is not a major religion in North America in terms of numbers, it is quite possible that you will encounter Muslim patients in need of nutritional counseling. Detailed information on Muslim customs has been published (21, 22).

HINDUISM

Hinduism originated in India and is still the dominant religion in that country. The number of Hindus in North America is quite small, but you may encounter some. It is important to realize that a Hindu's adherence to dietary strictures will depend somewhat on his or her caste. These castes, from high to low, are as follows: the *Brahmins,* currently a large portion of the professional class and those in the universities and government; the *Ksatriyas,* the soldier class; the *Vaisyas;* and the *Sudras,* or Untouchables. Although the caste system, and untouchability in particular, is legally prohibited in India, it is still alive and well in the society. Hindus who come to North America may be imbued with its provisions.

Devout Hindus, particularly of the Brahmin caste, are usually vegetarians. The practice of avoiding meat results from the fundamental tenets of Hinduism regarding reincarnation and reverence for life. Some also do not eat eggs since eggs are a form of life, but milk and milk products are acceptable. All Hindus regard the cow as sacred and will not eat beef or beef products, such as gelatin. Lower castes may eat other meats, but those who wish to identify themselves with a higher caste are likely to follow the diet of that caste. Some Hindus, but not all, eat fish. The higher castes are forbidden to eat onions, garlic, turnips, mushrooms, salted pork, and fowl. Even in those lower castes which eat meat, eating of pork and chicken may be eliminated because the animals are regarded as scavengers and therefore unclean. *Ghee* (clarified butter), cow's milk, and coconut are sacred foods.

Days of fasting and prayer are called *Vratas.* On these days, the Hindu is expected either to observe a complete fast or to abstain from eating cooked foods (1).

BUDDHISM

Buddhism is the predominant religion in Ceylon, Burma, Thailand, Japan, Laos, and Cambodia. Although there are relatively few Buddhists in North America, the number has risen in recent years, partly because the religion has been adopted by many of those involved in the "counterculture" movement. In addition, some of the Indochinese refugees are Buddhists.

The taking of any life is contrary to the tenets of Buddhism. Some Buddhists, however, do eat fish. Intoxicating beverages are forbidden.

SUMMARY

Religion is likely to assume greater importance for patients who are ill. To provide proper nutritional care, it is necessary to plan a diet that is acceptable to the patient's religious beliefs. At the same time, racial and ethnic preferences must be considered, and all must be integrated with the physiological requirements for diet modification. You will have an opportunity in subsequent chapters to modify diets for patients of various ethnic and religious groups.

TOPICS FOR FURTHER DISCUSSION

1. Name some foods, acceptable elsewhere, that are universally considered unacceptable in this country.

2. If there are students in the class from other regions of the country, ask them to describe differences that they have observed in availability of foods and in food habits of the population.

3. Students in the class will have varying ethnic backgrounds. Ask for volunteers to describe how their ethnic background has affected family food habits.

4. Assume that a group of refugees from a culture not previously found in this country begins arriving here in large numbers. The group consists of whole families who are destitute. Few speak English. You are a nutritionist in a public clinic in a large city to which this group has come. List some of the information you will need in order to be able to provide effective nutrition counseling to these refugees. Discuss some of the methods you could use to acquire this information.

5. Class members of various religions can volunteer to describe food habits related to religious observances in their families. How do their religious practices involving food compare to the practices of their grandparents?

REFERENCES

1. SUITOR, C.J.W. AND M.F. CRAWLEY. *Nutrition Principles and Application in Health Promotion* (2d ed.). Philadelphia: Lippincott, 1984.

2. HERNANDEZ, M., A. CHAVEZ, AND H. BOURGES. *Valor Nutritivo de Los Alimentos Mexicanos.* Mexico: Instituto Nacional de la Nutricion, 1977.

3. LEUNG, W.-T.W. AND M. FLORES. *Food Composition Tables for Use in Latin America*. Bethesda, Md.: National Institutes of Health, 1977.

4. LEUNG, W.-T.W., R.R. BUTRUM, AND F.H. CHANG. *Food Composition Table for Use in East Asia*. Bethesda, Md.: National Institutes of Health, 1973.

5. GRIVETTI, L.E. AND M.B. PAQUETTE. Nontraditional ethnic food choices among first-generation Chinese in California. *J. Nutr. Educ.* 10:(1978)109–112.

6. CHANG, B. Some dietary beliefs in Chinese folk culture. *J. Amer. Dietet. Assoc.* 65:(1974)436–438.

7. LING, S., J. KING, AND V. LEUNG. Diet, growth and cultural food habits in Chinese-American infants. *Am. J. Chinese Med.* 3:(1975)125–132.

8. ABIAKA, M.H. Japanese-American food equivalents for calculating exchange diets. *J. Amer. Dietet. Assoc.* 62:(1973)173–180.

9. GLADNEY, V.M. *Food Practices of the Mexican-American in Los Angeles County.* Los Angeles: Los Angeles County Health Department, 1966.

10. YOHAI, F. Dietary patterns of Spanish-speaking people living in the Boston area. *J. Amer. Dietet. Assoc.* 71:(1977)273–275.

11. CRANE, N.T. AND N.R. GREEN. Food habits and food preferences of Vietnamese refugees living in northern Florida. *J. Amer. Dietet. Assoc.* 76:(1980)591–593.

12. *Asian Food Guide for Teachers.* Sacramento, Calif.: Dairy Council of California, 1980.

13. HOLLINGSWORTH, A.O., L.P. BROWN, AND D.A. BROOTEN. The refugees and childbearing: What to expect. *RN:* November 1980, 45–48.

14. SANPIETRO, M.-C.S. How to get through to a refugee patient. *RN:* January 1981, 43–46.

15. *Diet Manual Utilizing a Vegetarian Diet Plan.* Loma Linda, California: The Seventh-Day Adventist Dietetic Association, 1975.

16. DRESNER, S.H. AND S. SIEGEL. *The Jewish Dietary Laws: Their Meaning For Our Time; A Guide to Observance.* New York: Burning Bush Press, 1966.

17. KAUFMAN, M. Adapting therapeutic diets to Jewish food customs. *Am. J. Clin. Nutr.* 5:(1957)676–682.

18. ANONYMOUS. Cultural food practices of elderly observant Jews. *Nutrition and the M.D.* 9(12):(1983)4.

19. NATOW, A.B., J. HESLIN, AND B.C. RABEN. Integrating Jewish Dietary Laws into a dietetics program. *J. Amer. Dietet. Assoc.* 67:(1975)13–16.

20. LOWENBERG, M.E., E.N. TODHUNTER, E.D. WILSON, M.C. FEENEY, AND J.R. SAVAGE. *Food and Man.* New York: John Wiley, 1968.

21. SAKR, A.H. Dietary regulations and food habits of Muslims. *J. Amer. Dietet. Assoc.* 58:(1971)123–126.

22. SAKR, A.H. Fasting in Islam. *J. Amer. Dietet. Assoc.* 67:(1975)17–21.

ADDITIONAL SOURCES OF INFORMATION

HOANG, G.N. Cultural barriers to effective medical care among Indochinese patients. *Ann. Rev. Med.* 36:(1985) 229–239.

PANGBORN, R.M. and C.M. BRUHN. Concepts of food habits of "other" ethnic groups. *J. Nutr. Educ.* 2:(1971)106–110.

RUIZ, P. Cultural barriers to effective medical care among Hispanic-American patients. *Ann. Rev. Med.* 36:(1985)63–71.

SANJUR, F. *Puerto Rican Food Habits: A Sociocultural Approach.* Ithaca, N.Y.: Cornell University, 1970.

11

ROUTINE AND TRANSITIONAL DIETS

Patients' voluntary food intake may vary in quantity from large amounts to little or none. Some patients have voracious appetites; at the other extreme are those who are unable or unwilling to take any food. The nutrient needs of patients may also vary greatly. Some patients need to have their intakes of one or more nutrients reduced, while others have increased needs.

For patients who are willing and able to make the necessary alterations in their diets, the function of the nutritional care specialist involves providing the necessary foods when they are hospitalized and providing the necessary education when they are to be discharged or when they are outpatients. For the patient who is having difficulty complying with the diet or is unable to do so, however, nutritional care becomes more challenging.

In providing nutritional care, consideration must be given not only to the nutrient content of the diet, but also to the methods of feeding. Patients may obtain food in the usual manner, eating at meals from trays or at the table. For some patients, however, the usual manner of eating does not meet their needs, and they must be given formula feedings directly into the gastrointestinal tract via *tube feedings*. Still others do not have a functional digestive system and take nutrients directly into the circulatory system via *parenteral feeding*.

These methods are introduced in this and the next two chapters without reference to specific diagnoses. This chapter will discuss some procedures for feeding patients by traditional methods of oral feeding and several of the more common methods for increasing intake. As you proceed, you may wish to refer to background material in your text.

ROUTINE HOSPITAL DIETS

The *regular*, or *house*, diet is given to a large number of patients who do not require any modification of in-take. The house diet is not individualized, although in some institutions patients may express preferences from a menu. The diets classified as "routine" include the house diet and modifications in consistency, usually called *soft* and *liquid* diets; these may differ slightly among institutions, but they are generally similar.

In most institutions, the house diet is planned by the administrative dietitians, but the clinical staff may have responsibility for planning the routine modifications. These modifications are often used as a basis for planning other diets. It is important, therefore, that the clinical nutritionist be familiar with the foods included on these diets, the nutrient content of the diets, and the circumstances in which they are used. A table of routine diets typical of those used in many general hospitals is reproduced in Table 11-1.

The *house*, or *general*, diet is intended for adult patients who do not require diet modifications. Many hospitals provide a restaurant-like "selective" menu from which the patient makes choices. In other institutions, a single, set menu is planned. It is important that the menu be planned so that it is nutritionally adequate or so that the patient is able to select a nutritionally adequate diet. The menu should also be planned to provide foods most patients are willing to eat. It may be used, in addition, to teach principles of good nutrition by example.

In some institutions, other diets are used as the general house diet. In a hospital in which most patients are vegetarians, for example, the house diet might be a vegetarian diet.

The *soft* diet serves as a transition diet between the liquid diet and the house diet. It varies from one institution to another in minor ways. Many institutions have several soft diets which vary in consistency. For instance, the *soft diet* or *whole soft diet* generally contains tender cuts of meats and whole, cooked vegetables and fruits, usually without skin or seeds. The *mechanical soft diet* uses chopped, ground, or pureed meats with gravies as necessary, and also casseroles. It is usually

TABLE 11-1. Summary of Routine Hospital Diets

Food Group	Clear Liquid*	Full Liquid	Pureed†	Soft	House
Soup	Broth, bouillon (fat-free)	Broth, bouillon (fat-free), and strained cream soups	Broth, bouillon (fat-free), and strained cream soups	Broth, bouillon (fat-free), and strained cream soups	All
Cereal	None	Refined or strained in gruels	Refined or strained	Refined, cooked cornflakes, rice, paste products	All
Bread	None	None	White or refined wheat; seedless rye; toast	Foods from preceding column; rolls; crackers	All
Meat and substitutes	None	Pasteurized or dried eggs in milk drinks, eggs in custards; strained meat or poultry in soup	Eggs, ground, or blenderized meats or poultry, white fish (not fried); no pork; small-curd cottage cheese; other cheeses in sauces	Eggs, milk, cheese, tender whole or ground beef, lamb, veal, bacon, poultry (not fried)	All
Vegetables	Tomato juice (in some institutions)	In strained cream soups only; vegetable juices	Potatoes (not fried); strained or pureed bland cooked vegetables	Potatoes (not fried); whole tender or chopped bland cooked vegetables	All
Miscellaneous	Sugar, honey; hard candy; salt	Foods from preceding column; butter, margarine, oil, cream in cream soups; honey, syrup; cocoa, chocolate syrup; mild spices, Mocha mix	Foods from preceding columns, plus pepper, jelly, and jam without seeds; well-cooked pasta, rice	Foods from preceding columns, mayonnaise or similar dressing	All

*Adjust to patient's capacity. Meal size is usually small. If patient is nauseated, it may be helpful to avoid fruit and tomato juice. Avoid any food not listed.

†Avoid fried foods, any foods containing nuts, seeds, pickles and pickle relish, whole meats, fruit and vegetables.

intended to minimize the amount of chewing necessary. The diet is individualized to provide the required consistency for each patient. The *pureed diet* commonly includes pureed-consistency foods. The *soft* and *pureed* diets given in Table 11-1 are typical examples. They should be planned to be nutritionally adequate.

These diets may be the basis for other modifications. In many institutions, the soft diet is also used when a "bland" diet or low-residue diet is ordered, since the soft diet is "bland" according to most definitions and is also reasonably low in residue. Therefore, they do not usually contain highly spiced foods, fried foods, or "strong-flavored" or "gas-forming" vegetables. The latter terms usually refer to cabbage-family, or *cruciferous,* vegetables (cabbage, cauliflower, broccoli and brussels sprouts) and onion-family vegetables (onions, leeks). Vegetables are not served raw, and those with large amounts of indigestible material, such as corn, are eliminated.

The liquid diets include the *full liquid* and *clear liquid* diets, similar to those shown in Table 11-1. The clear liquid diet, as usually served, contains 600 to 900 kcal per day. It comprises mostly carbohydrate, with some protein, largely of low biological value, and little fat. Obviously, it is nutritionally inadequate and should be used only for a short period. In some institutions, use of the clear liquid diet for more than 3 days is considered to place the patient at nutritional risk and indicates the need for nutritional support.

The full liquid diet is more adequate, but is often inadequate in niacin, folacin, and iron. With its high water content, however, its caloric density is low. Patients are often given between-meal snacks to increase their intake. Vitamin and mineral supplements should be ordered if the diet is used for more than a few days. This diet may be further modified for special purposes. The milk or fruit juices are sometimes eliminated to adjust to patients' tolerances. These diets may be given special titles, such as the *surgical liquid* diet.

Another variation is the "cold semiliquid," or "T and A" (*tonsils* and *adenoids*), diet, which is used following throat surgery. Foods on this diet are soft, smooth, and either cold or lukewarm. Acid juices and very hot soups and beverages must be used carefully. Some patients produce copious mucus if large amounts of milk are given; milk may thus need to be eliminated. Chocolate products are not used because they interfere with the detection of hemoptysis (blood in sputum). This diet is inadequate in ascorbic acid, thiamin, niacin, folacin, and iron.

Some patients require a liquid diet containing higher levels of nutrients. These are variously referred to as "high-calorie, high-protein," "fortified," and "wired-jaw" diets. The latter title refers to the fact that wiring the jaws is often required following broken-jaw injuries.

The full liquid diet can also be modified to be low in fat or restricted in sodium content.

TO TEST YOUR UNDERSTANDING

1. A sample house diet menu is given on Form K (p. 129). Assume that this is a menu for the general hospital in which you are a clinical nutritionist and that it is your responsibility to modify this menu to plan the remaining routine diets. Your modifications should be based on the diets listed in your diet manual or on those given in Table 11-1. Your instructor will specify which to use. If your diet manual has diets with titles other than those given on the menu, you will need to change the titles at the top of the columns. When planning this menu, be sure to abide by the following policies:

   a. Use as many items from the house diet as possible, and limit the number of separate items that must be prepared by using the same item if possible. For example, if the house diet said "fried chicken," you could write baked chicken in the soft-diet column. Be sure to make a choice of one only when there are two usable items on the house menu. In other words, do not make a "selective menu" for the soft, pureed, and liquid diets.

   b. Make all menus as nutritionally adequate as possible.

   c. Take care to apply the usual principles of menu planning so that diets are acceptable to patients. Try, for example, to provide for a variety of colors and flavors, and follow a commonly accepted meal plan.

2. Standard accompaniments are not usually written on the menu plan. Instead, institutional policies state which items are to be automatically included in the patient's meal. The items listed on Form L (p. 130) are those which are usually available for inclusion with the diets you have just planned. Put an X in each column for each item that would be acceptable on the diet specified in the column heading.

INCREASING NUTRIENT INTAKE

Persons who are ill often have depressed appetites, and many simultaneously have increased nutrient needs. Under these circumstances, the nutritional care specialist may use some of the following techniques for increasing nutrient intake.

ENCOURAGE EATING AT MEALTIME

When sufficient food is provided in three regular meals but the patient does not eat, it is sometimes sufficient to undertake the following adjustments:

Use a selective menu if this is not in routine use, and cater to the patient's preferences.

Ensure an environment conducive to eating, including absence of offensive odors, provision of comfortable temperature, and acceptable light and ventilation.

Provide assistance as necessary for self-feeding, or arrange for the patient to be fed.

Schedule meals adequately so that appetite can return.

Relieve pain.

Review drug intake as a source of food intake problems.

Many of these interventions require the cooperation of the attending physician and the nursing staff.

INCREASE NUMBER AND SIZE OF SERVINGS

If a patient has an increased appetite as well as increased requirements, it is occasionally sufficient to increase the sizes of servings. For example, patients may be given larger glasses of juice and milk, extra bread and rolls, two pork chops instead of one, or two eggs at breakfast instead of one.

In addition, foods may be added to the menu. Here are some examples:

Add appetizers and salads to menus on which they do not already appear.

Give both fruit and juice at breakfast.

Provide both jelly and honey for bread and rolls at all meals.

Add mayonnaise to sandwiches, and mayonnaise or other salad dressings to salads.

Use sour cream or yogurt as a topping on vegetables and fruit, and whipped cream on desserts and hot chocolate.

Add ice cream to milk drinks.

Add peanut butter to crackers and fruit.

INCREASE NUTRIENT DENSITY

A patient may be limited in the total volume of food which can be tolerated. If nutrient needs cannot be met within that volume, the total nutrient density can sometimes be successfully increased. These steps are specifically intended to increase intake of protein and energy, since vitamins and minerals will accompany properly chosen protein- and energy-containing foods or can be given as supplements.

The energy content of the diet can be increased by taking some of the following steps (1, 2):

Stir butter or margarine into hot cereals, soups, rice, mashed potatoes, gravies, and casseroles.

Fry foods rather than baking, broiling, or boiling.

Substitute half-and-half for milk in cooking.

Add dried fruits to baked goods.

Add less water when reconstituting beverages.

FORM K

	Menu Plan				
General	Soft	Pureed	Full Liquid	Clear Liquid

Breakfast
Orange juice
Stewed prunes
Farina
Bran flakes
Fried egg
Bacon
Waffles

Lunch
Beef-vegetable soup
Saltines
Lamb patty
Tuna salad (w/onions,
  celery, pickles) on bed of
  lettuce
Potato chips
Buttered peas
Spiced canned peach half
Sliced tomato salad with
  French dressing
Blueberry muffins
Baked caramel custard

Dinner
Tomato juice/lemon wedge
Breaded shrimp
Roast beef/gravy
Mashed potatoes
Buttered broccoli
Buttered carrots
Fresh fruit salad (Orange
  sections, sliced banana,
  diced pineapple) on lettuce
  leaf
Maple-nut ice cream
Sugar cookies

The following steps will increase the protein content of the diet:

Stir skim-milk powder into milk beverages and milk used in cooked dishes, such as cereals, scrambled eggs, mashed potatoes, casserole dishes, meat balls, patties, or loaf, soups, gravies, and baked goods.
Substitute milk or half-and-half for water in recipes for cereals, soups, puddings, and canned soups.
Add ground or diced meats to soups and casseroles.
Sprinkle grated cheese on vegetables and salads.
Substitute instant breakfast mix for milk beverages.

As well as these additions of familiar foods, some special concentrated sources are available that can be added to foods:

Protein sources: Maxipro HBV, High Fat Supplement, Nutrisource Protein Powder, Pro-Mix, ProMod, Propac.

(See Table G-2 for specific content.) These can be added to other foods.
Lipid sources: Calogen, High Fat Supplement, Liquigen, Lipomul, Microlipid, MCT Oil, Nutrisource Lipids. (See Table G-2.) For rationale for use of these products, see Chapters 12 and 15.
Carbohydrate sources: Cal Power, Hy-Cal, Liquid Carbohydrate Supplement, Maxijul, Moducal, Polycose, Sumacal.

In addition, there are protein-energy supplements, such as

Delmark Eggnog, Delmark Milkshake, Dietene, and Gevral, used as beverages (see Table G-1).
Sustacal Pudding and Forta Pudding—high calorie, high-protein puddings (see Table G-1).

The clear-liquid diet presents a special problem in increasing nutrient intake. If the patient cannot be

FORM L

Food	Standard Menu Accompaniments: House	Soft	Pureed	Full Liquid	Clear Liquid
Bread, white					
wheat					
rye					
Butter					
Margarine					
Jelly					
Milk, whole					
skim					
Coffee					
Cream					
Sugar					
Tea					
Lemon					
Salt					
Pepper					

advanced to a more adequate diet, the following procedures may be useful:

Add Polycose powder (6 oz contains 170 g carbohydrate and 680 kcal). (See Table G-2.)

Add 6 oz Citrotein (Table G-1) as a drink t.i.d. in standard dilution (provides 65.5 g carbohydrate, 21.5 g protein, and 1 g fat, for a total of 354 kcal).

Combining the two procedures just listed will provide 235.5 g carbohydrate, 21.5 g protein, 1 g fat, and 1,034 kcal.

Substitute Ross SLD (see Table G-1) for the clear-liquid diet, or add the product to the clear-liquid diet.

INCREASE FREQUENCY OF FEEDING

Some patients must be fed at more frequent intervals. If this procedure is not carried out carefully, however, it may be self-defeating. It is a common practice for patients to be given additional feedings in the midmorning (10:00 or 10:30 AM), midafternoon (2:00 or 3:00 PM), and evening ("HS feeding"), usually at about 8:00 PM. The midmorning and midafternoon snacks, in particular, may reduce the appetite for the next meal.

Some patients are given the usual diet divided into six meals instead of three. A typical diet order might read "small, frequent feedings," with hot foods served at the regular meal times and cold foods, such as salad and desserts, served with a beverage at the between-meal feedings. This procedure reduces the volume of individual feedings, promoting intake in the patient with limited capacity.

An increase in nutrient intake may be provided by adding between-meal snacks *in addition to* the full meals on the menu served at the usual time. There are two broad categories of between-meal snacks. Some consist of the usual types of foods and beverages served at other meals, such as fruit, juice, milk beverages, sandwiches, and dessert items. Other useful foods are nuts, dried fruits, candy, popcorn, cheese, crackers, and granola.

Commercially available liquid-formula products are alternatives for adding energy and protein to the patient's intake. Many of these are listed in Table G-1. It is important to note that these formulas may not be nutritionally complete. Other formulas for oral supplementation are included in Table G-3, with the notation that they can be used for either oral or tube feeding. Most of these formulas are nutritionally complete.

Several questions must be kept in mind when choosing a supplement:

1. Is the patient lactose intolerant, so that a lactose-free formula must be chosen?
2. Is the patient capable of digesting and absorbing fat?
3. Does the patient need a supplement low in residue, protein, sodium, or potassium, separately or in combination?
4. Does the supplement have an acceptable taste, odor, and consistency?

TO TEST YOUR UNDERSTANDING

3. You have a patient who is capable of eating any food, but who needs an increased protein and calorie intake. The patient has a large appetite. Modify the menu for _____ (day to be assigned by your instructor) to provide an intake of about 3,500 kcal in three meals plus an evening snack.

4. You have a patient who requires three between-meal formula feedings to supplement his regular meals. The patient is unable to digest lactose.

   a. How are your choices of formula limited for this patient?
   b. Name some formula products you might choose to give this patient.

5. You are planning to mix a protein supplement into the food of a protein-depleted, anorexic patient. The patient is lactose intolerant and has shown some evidence of mild fat malabsorption.

   a. What protein source would you use and why?
   b. What other nutrient is it important to supplement?

6. A patient is receiving, in addition to her three meals, 240 ml of Sustacal Liquid at midmorning, 240 ml of Meritene Liquid in mid-afternoon, and 240 ml of Delmark Milkshake at bedtime. How much protein and energy are added to the patient's daily intake by providing each of these supplements? (The information necessary for your calculations is given in Appendix G.)

TOPICS FOR FURTHER DISCUSSION

1. Assume you have a patient who is 6 feet, 3 inches tall and of normal body weight. His digestive system is intact, but he will require a liquid diet for several weeks because his jaws are wired. Enough space has been left between his teeth to admit a large-caliber straw. How could you modify the routine full-liquid diet to make it higher in protein and calories to more nearly meet his needs? How could you provide greater variety in his diet?

2. Some institutions list routine diets other than those shown in Table 11-1. Survey other diet manuals to which you have access and list the routine diets they contain. Explain the purpose of each one that differs from those in Table 11-1.

3. Some diet manuals list soft, bland, and low-residue diets. If your diet manual is one of these, compare and contrast the content of these diets.

REFERENCES

1. Escott-Stump, S. *Nutrition and Diagnosis-Related Care.* Philadelphia: Lea & Febiger, 1985.
2. Walker, W.A. and K.M. Hendricks. *Manual of Pediatric Nutrition.* Philadelphia: W.B. Saunders, 1985.

12

Tube Feeding

Some patients are unable to eat enough food in familiar forms to maintain or restore good nutritional status, even though they have a functioning gastrointestinal (GI) tract. Under these circumstances, one of the alternatives is to feed the patient through a tube into the gastrointestinal tract, either as a supplement to other food intake or as the sole source of nutrition.

This chapter will explain, without reference to specific diagnoses, the characteristics of formulas used for, and the procedures involved in administering, tube feedings. Before proceeding, you should review the information on tube feeding in your text.

PRINCIPLES OF FLUID BALANCE

In order to provide good nutritional care of the patient who is being tube fed, it is essential that you understand some basic principles of *fluid balance*, its relationship to osmotic pressure, and its significance in pathological conditions.

BODY WATER CONTENT AND DISTRIBUTION

The water in the body serves as a carrier of nutrients and waste materials and as a medium for chemical reactions. It is thus important that the appropriate amounts of fluids be present in the proper compartments.

Approximately 60 percent of the body weight of an average adult male is water. Water content varies, however, with age, sex, and body fat content. The adult female body, for example, is about 50 percent water. Children's bodies have higher proportions of body fluid; a newborn's body at term is composed of about 75 percent water. This amount decreases progressively with age.

Of the total fluid, about two-thirds, or 40 percent, of body weight is within the cells (*intracellular fluid*, or *ICF*). In dehydration, fluid shifts out of the cells, and total ICF is decreased. The remaining one-third of total fluid, or 20 percent of body weight—the *extracellular fluid (ECF)*—is divided between the 3 to 5 percent within the blood vessels (*intravascular*) and the 12 to 15 percent in the intercellular space (*interstitial fluid*, or *ISF*). In some conditions, the ISF increases, resulting in edema. A small quantity, 1 to 5 percent, is categorized as *transcellular*, which includes water in cerebrospinal and intraocular fluids, and water in the glands, excretory portion of the kidney, secretions of the gastrointestinal tract, bone, and "potential spaces."

Potential spaces, also called "third spaces," are important in that they can expand to hold large quantities of fluid in some disease states. They include the pericardial and peritoneal cavities, joint space and bursae, and the thoracic cavity. In the burned patient, for example, a fluid shift to "third space" can result in shock and circulatory collapse as blood volume decreases. Fluid can also shift to the peritoneal cavity and accumulate in large amounts, a condition known as *ascites*. Potential spaces communicate easily with the intercellular space. The intravascular and intercellular fluids mix freely through the highly porous capillary walls, but the intracellular fluid is separated from extracellular fluid by semipermeable membranes—that is, cell membranes. Table 12-1 summarizes values for these fluid compartments.

FLUID REQUIREMENTS

Estimates of water requirements for normal persons have been based on calorie intake, body surface area, or body weight. Methods of estimation are shown in Table 12-2. These methods vary in their results, but the differences are within the range of the compensatory ability of the normal kidney. The estimates are not applicable to patients with diarrhea, renal disease, fever, or catabolic diseases. These will be discussed in later chapters.

TABLE 12-1. Water Compartments in the Adult Male Human Body

Water Compartment	% Total Body Weight	Volume in 70 kg Man, L
Extracellular fluid	20–23	14
Intravascular	3–5	3.0
Intercellular (Interstitial)	12–15	10.0
Transcellular	1–5	1.0
Intracellular fluid	35–40	28
Total	~55–60	42

FLUID INTAKE

Fluid is supplied to the body via three routes (Table 12-3):

1. by ingestion of liquids
2. from preformed fluid in solid foods such as meats, fruits, and vegetables
3. from the production of water from the metabolism of proteins, fats, and carbohydrates.

In metabolism to carbon dioxide and water, 100 g of fat produce 107 g of water; 100 g of carbohydrate yield 55 g of water; and 100 g of protein produce 41 g of water. In some pathological conditions, human muscle is catabolized and contributes water. This is not calculated into the fluid balance since the exact amount of muscle catabolized is not accurately measurable in clinical situations.

TABLE 12-2. Methods of Estimation of Daily Fluid Requirements

Basis of Estimation	Calculation
Body weight	
Adults:	
Young active, 16–30 years	40 ml/kg
Average, 25–55 years	32
Older, 55–65 years	30
Elderly, >65 years	25
Children:	
1–10 kg	100 ml/kg
11–20 kg	an additional 50 ml/each kg > 10
21 kg or more	an additional 25 ml/each kg > 20
Energy intake	1 ml/kcal
Nitrogen plus energy intake	100 ml/g nitrogen intake PLUS 1 ml/kcal*
Body surface area	1,500 ml/M²†‡

*Especially useful with high protein feedings

†Body surface area may be calculated from the following formula:
$S = W^{0.425} \times H^{0.725} \times 71.84$ or
$\log X = (\log W \times 0.425) + (\log H \times 0.725) + 1.8564$
where X = cm² body surface area, W = kg body weight, and H = cm height.

‡Body surface area often used for "average" adult is 1.73 M².

TABLE 12-3. Representative Fluid Balance

Water Intake	(ml)	Water Loss	(ml)
Sensible		*Sensible*	
Oral fluids	1,500	Urine	1,500
Solid foods	700	Intestinal	250
Insensible		*Insensible*	
Metabolic water	250	Lungs and skin	700
Total	2,450	Total	2,450

From Wolfe, B.M. and W.I. Yamahata, "Nutrition in hypermetabolic conditions," in Zeman, F.J., *Clinical Nutrition and Dietetics.* New York: Macmillan, 1983. Used by permission of the publisher.

FLUID TRANSFER

There are two processes by which transfer of water and some solutes from one fluid compartment to another can occur without expenditure of energy.

Diffusion

Diffusion refers to the movement of a substance from an area of high concentration to an area of low concentration. If a membrane is permeable to a substance, diffusion can take place across the membrane.

Osmosis

Some membranes in the body are semipermeable—that is, water and some solutes, *but not all,* will pass through freely. *Osmosis* is the movement of *solvent* molecules across a semipermeable membrane. The solvent (water) moves from the area of low concentration of solute to an area of high concentration of solutes *that cannot cross the membrane.* The movement of the water equalizes the concentration of the solute on the two sides of the membrane.

The force that pulls the water through the semipermeable membrane toward the concentrated solution is called *osmotic pressure.* It is directly proportional to the *number* of particles in the solution and inversely proportional to their molecular weights. In biological materials, the osmotic pressure of a solution is measured in *milliosmols* (*mOsm*). One millimole (mmol) of a substance that does not dissociate in solution, such as glucose, exerts an osmotic pressure of 1 mOsm. One mmol of a substance that dissociates into two particles, such as sodium chloride, has an osmotic pressure of 2 mOsm. In substances producing three ions, 1 mmol = 3 mOsm. In clinical practice, the most commonly used term is *osmolality,* defined as the number of osmotic particles per *kilogram* of solvent, which, in biological systems, is water. *Osmolarity,* less commonly used, is measured per *liter* of solution. In tissue fluids that are very dilute, the difference between osmolality and osmolarity is small and can be ignored. In feeding solutions, which contain large amounts of solute, the values are significantly different, with osmolarity as low as 80 percent of osmolality. *Osmolality* is the preferred term for liquid formulas.

When sufficient water has moved across the semipermeable membrane so that the concentration of particles is equal on both sides of the membrane, the solutions are called *isotonic*. For clinical purposes, examples of isotonic solutions are 0.85 percent sodium chloride (NaCl)—also known as *normal saline*—or 5 percent glucose. A *hypotonic* saline solution has less NaCl than does an isotonic solution, while a *hypertonic* saline solution has a higher NaCl concentration. It is important to remember that, in clinical usage, a 10 percent solution consists of 10 g of a material in 100 ml of solution.

The normal osmolality of plasma is usually given as 280 to 294 mOsm/kg. However, a range of 280 to 320 mOsm/kg is generally considered acceptable and not of clinical concern.

Serum osmolality can be calculated from values found in a patient's chart, using Equation 4-35. Osmotic pressure is dependent upon the number of particles. Large amounts of small molecules, such as glucose and electrolytes, exert the greatest osmotic pressure while small amounts of large molecules, such as proteins, exert little osmotic pressure in most body fluids. The electrolyte sodium is the source of 90 to 95 percent of the osmotic pressure of the *extracellular* fluid. This is reflected in the calculation of serum osmolality using Equation 4-35 where the Na^+ concentration is multiplied by 2. The remainder of the osmotic pressure is provided by potassium (K), calcium (Ca), and magnesium (Mg) cations. To maintain electrical neutrality in body fluids, there must be an equal number of anion charges, commonly Cl^- or HCO_3^-.

Intracellular osmotic pressure is provided mainly by potassium as the cation, with small contributions by magnesium and sodium. The major anion is phosphate. Even though it is not measured, we assume that the total intracellular osmotic pressure is equal to that in the extracellular fluid.

In tube feeding, one concern is the osmotic effect of the tube feeding in the gastrointestinal tract. We can visualize two compartments: One is the intestinal lumen, while the other is the fluid in the tissue and circulatory system. A comparison of the osmolality of the tube feeding with serum osmolality will tell you in which direction the fluid will move.

TO TEST YOUR UNDERSTANDING

1. a. Estimate the total water available to the following patient.
   20 y.o. active adult male. 75 kg total body weight.
   Diet: 100 g protein, 80 g fat, 250 g carbohydrate, and containing 1,550 ml preformed water.
   Fluids: 1,500 ml in water, fruit juice, soup, and soft drinks.
   b. Estimate this man's normal fluid needs. Show your calculations.
2. In the list below, number the substances in order of their osmolality when mixed with equal quantities of water. Number the most osmotically active material as 1 and the least active as 7.

   _____ NaCl, 1 mmol

   _____ MgCl$_2$, 1 mmol

   _____ Glucose, 180 mg

   _____ Sucrose, 180 mg

   _____ Dextrin, 180 mg

   _____ Glycine, 100 mg

   _____ Casein, 100 mg
3. Calculate the osmolality of a solution consisting of 1 g NaCl in 100 g H_2O. Show your calculations.
4. A patient has a serum Na level of 142 mEq/L, a BUN of 28 mg/dl, and a blood glucose level of 100 mg/dl. Estimate the serum osmolality. Show your calculations. Compare the values given and your results with normal values.
5. If tube-feeding solutions with the following osmolalities are fed into the jejunum, give the net direction of fluid movement:
   a. 600 mOsm/kg _____
   b. 294 mOsm/kg _____
   c. 176 mOsm/kg _____

FLUID EXCRETION

Routes of fluid excretion, summarized in Table 12-3, are urine, feces, respiratory water loss (via the lungs), and perspiration (via the skin). Urinary fluid excretion may be divided into two parts. *Obligatory* fluid represents the minimum necessary to remove the waste materials to be excreted in the urine. The amount of obligatory excretion is dependent upon the concentrating ability of the kidneys. *Facultative* excretion depends on the tubular resorption rate and fluctuating body needs.

One of the materials that must be excreted in largest amount by the kidney are products of protein metabolism, mainly *urea*. In addition, sodium, potassium, and chloride must be excreted. These materials, which together constitute the *renal solute load (RSL),* determine the volume of fluid needed for excretion. The carbohydrate in a feeding solution normally does not contribute to the RSL because it is metabolized and does not appear in the urine. Fat also does not contribute to RSL since fat is not excreted in the urine.

The kidneys of a normal adult are able to concentrate urine to 1,200 to 1,400 mOsm/L. The immature kidneys of infants, or diseased kidneys with low concentrating ability, are not able to do so. They require more fluid for an equivalent amount of load. Diets producing a large solute load—high-protein or high-salt diets, for example—result in a higher fluid requirement.

To calculate the RSL, the following values are useful. Each g of protein (or amino acids) yields an RSL of 5.7 mOsm in adults. On the other hand, in young children, each g of protein yields only 4.0 mOsm, since it is estimated that only about 70 percent of the protein in growing children is excreted (1). Ana-bolic patients would also excrete less urea. Conversely, the catabolic patient would have an increased RSL as a result of catabolism of body protein. In all patients, in addition to the osmolality of the nitrogen compounds, each mEq of electrolyte yields 1 mOsm.

The total renal solute load from a tube feeding, infant formula, or other diet for an adult may be estimated from a simplified equation (2):

$$\text{mOsm in formula} = (\text{g protein} \times 5.7) + \text{mEq} \atop (\text{Na} + \text{K} + \text{Cl}) \qquad \textbf{(12-1)}$$

Recall that when using this formula for infants and anabolic patients, the factor 5.7 should, instead, be 4.0. The catabolized protein is assumed to be excreted as urea. Total RSL is calculated as mOsm per day and all values used in the formula refer to the amount per day.

The kidney works most efficiently when urine output (ml) is 1.5–2 × RSL, justifying additional water intake. This does not apply if mild dehydration is desired, as in the case of head injury. In the unfed patient, the dietary RSL is zero, but we do not expect urine output to cease. Obligatory urine output for these patients is estimated to be 700 ml per day, or 30 ml per hour.

TO TEST YOUR UNDERSTANDING

6. Estimate the renal solute load of 2,000 ml of a tube-feeding formula for an adult, providing 1 kcal/ml, 4.6 g crystalline amino acids/dl, and 20.3 g carbohydrate/dl. The formula contains, in addition, the following electrolytes: 3.3 mEq Na/100 ml, 1.79 mEq K/100 ml, and 5.24 mEq Cl/100 ml of formula. Show your calculations.

7. a. Calculate the obligatory fluid necessary to excrete 92.6 g dietary protein and 2,320 mg NaCl. Show your calculations.
   b. What fluid volume would provide maximum renal excretory efficiency?

8. The items in the list which follows may be found in tube feedings. In the spaces provided,
   —Write the letter *O* for any material that would have a significant effect on the osmolality of a tube feeding.
   —Write an *R* before any material that would contribute significantly to renal solute load.

   _____ a. Casein
   _____ b. Hydrolyzed casein
   _____ c. Crystalline amino acids
   _____ d. Cornstarch
   _____ e. Tapioca starch
   _____ f. Starch hydrolysates
   _____ g. Disaccharides
   _____ h. Monosaccharides
   _____ i. Triglycerides
   _____ j. NaCl
   _____ k. $NaHCO_3$
   _____ l. KCl

CHARACTERISTICS OF TUBE FEEDING FORMULAS

A familiarity with the nutritional and physical characteristics of tube-feeding formulas is essential in planning for tube feeding. The formula composition and concentration, physical properties, rate of feeding, and delivery systems must be carefully integrated.

NUTRIENT CONTENT OF FORMULAS

An understanding of the nutritional composition of tube-feeding formulas is needed in order to evaluate different formulas.

Caloric Density

Caloric density is defined as the amount of energy per unit volume of food. For tube feedings, it is usually expressed in kcal/ml. Most tube feedings contain 1 kcal/ml, but some are more concentrated—1.5–2 kcal/ml. Patients whose caloric needs are high, whose appetites are depressed, or whose tolerance to volume is limited are candidates for feeding with more calorically dense formulas. The patient must, however, be able to tolerate the higher osmolality of such formulas and must also receive adequate fluid for excretion of the high RSL. Another consideration is that greater density delays gastric emptying. In particular, a high fat content has a significant effect.

Protein

Various methods are used to express protein quality. *Protein efficiency ratio (PER)* is obtained by measuring the growth of rats in relation to protein intake:

$$PER = \frac{\text{weight gain in g}}{\text{protein intake in g}} \qquad (12\text{-}2)$$

Casein, the reference protein, has a PER of 2.5. Low-quality proteins have a lower PER. When PER is 2.5 or more, 45 g of the material will provide the adult RDA for protein.

Biological value (BV) indicates the amino acid ratio in the protein. Specifically, it measures the retention of absorbed nitrogen:

$$BV = \frac{\text{N retained}}{\text{N absorbed}} \times 100 \qquad (12\text{-}3)$$

Amino acid profile consists of a list of the specific amino acids and their amounts. The list is usually available from the manufacturer of the product.

Patients must receive sufficient total protein to meet their normal needs plus the increased needs resulting from illness. The protein must also be of high biological value in order to provide the required amino acids. On the other hand, excessive amounts of protein in the diet will markedly increase the RSL. The amount of fluid necessary for excretion of the load must be provided in the formula or as added free water. It is generally recommended that the protein portion of formulas provide no more than 15 percent of the calories.

Protein-to-Calorie Ratio

The composition of the formula must be such that sufficient energy from nonprotein sources is available so that protein is not used for energy. A useful technique for evaluating a tube-feeding formula is the calculation of the *calorie-to-nitrogen (C:N)* ratio. The nitrogen content is calculated from the protein content, assuming that nitrogen is 16 percent of the protein. The C:N ratio is then calculated by using the following equation:

$$\text{C:N ratio} = \frac{\text{kcal per day}}{\text{g N per day}} \qquad (12\text{-}4)$$

The kcal/day may represent total energy intake or may indicate energy from carbohydrate and fat, but not protein—that is, nonprotein kcal (nonpro kcal). An acceptable ratio of kcal per g of N in a normal adult male may be 300 if *nonprotein* kilocalories are used as the basis for calculation:

$$\text{Nonprotein kcal/g N} = \frac{\text{total kcal} - \text{kcal from protein}}{\text{g N}}$$
$$(12\text{-}5)$$

For the critically ill patient, the nonpro kcal:N ratio often needs to be in the range of 100 to 200, providing a greater proportion of protein. Ratios greater than 200 may be inadequate in protein, while those less than 100 usually provide a formula that requires the use of protein as a source of energy. Recommended C:N ratios to provide for anabolism in a patient are about 150, based on nonprotein kcal (3), or 120 to 180, based on total kcal (4), within the same range. It appears, therefore, that a ratio of 150 is a useful guideline.

Carbohydrate

Carbohydrates commonly provide about 55 percent of the energy in tube-feeding formulas. Some formulas contain milk and thus contain lactose, but many patients are deficient in lactase (a problem discussed in more detail later). These patients, if tube fed, need a formula that is lactose-free.

Vitamins and Minerals

The majority of ready-to-use tube-feeding formulas are nutritionally complete. They provide NRC RDA of vitamins and minerals when caloric requirements are satisfied. Two precautions must be observed, however:

1. Some patients have disorders that increase the need for one or more vitamins or minerals. As the specialist in nutritional care, it is your responsibility to monitor these requirements and recommend supplements when indicated.
2. Some formulas that are otherwise complete do not contain vitamin K. A weekly supplement has been recommended as a precaution (5). Such a supplement may be particularly important for patients with fat malabsorption.

PHYSICAL PROPERTIES OF FORMULAS

Physical properties must also be considered in choosing a tube-feeding formula for an individual patient.

Osmolality

Osmolality has an important effect on the patient's tolerance to the formula. Gastric emptying is delayed by hypertonic solutions and may result in gastric retention, nausea, and vomiting. In the duodenum, solutions in the lumen are adjusted to isotonicity by

TO TEST YOUR UNDERSTANDING

9. a. How many grams of protein would be contained in 2,000 ml of a formula with a caloric density of 1 kcal/ml, 15% of which are from protein?

   b. What is the nonpro kcal:N ratio?

10. A proposed tube feeding intended for weight maintenance contains 30% carbohydrate, 2% fat, and 20% protein (W/V) per L. For this formula, calculate the following. Show your calculations.

    a. Caloric density

    b. Nonpro kcal:N ratio

    c. Would you expect 1,000 ml of this formula to meet the protein needs of a normal adult male? Why?

adding or removing water. If a solution is very hypertonic and is delivered into the duodenum, a large fluid shift into the lumen of the gut will follow, since the membranes of the enterocytes are semipermeable. Severe diarrhea and dehydration can result.

It is important, therefore, to be aware of the osmolality of feeding formulas that you recommend for patients. Information on osmolality of unflavored formulas and the effects of the use of the flavor packets is provided by the manufacturers.

Renal Solute Load

Renal solute load is a major consideration in pediatric feeding. Recall that, for any patient, if the solute load is excessive, a larger quantity of water will be required to excrete it. If sufficient water is not given, the patient may become dehydrated, hypernatremic (having a high serum Na), and azotemic (having a high serum N), with weight loss, oliguria, fever, cyanosis, and irritability. Convulsions, brain damage, and coma may ensue. At the same time, the ill tube-fed patient, adult or child, may have other conditions that add to the fluid requirement. These include impaired urine concentrating ability and excessive water losses from fever, diarrhea, vomiting, or burns. Protein catabolism will also add to the load.

In summary, in choosing a formula, you must carefully consider the osmotic pressure and renal solute load in relation to the patient's disease, renal concentrating ability, and ability to ingest liquids. A frequent problem occurs as a consequence of the administration of a high-protein formula with a volume of fluid insufficient to excrete the resulting high RSL. Under these conditions, the patient may develop a dehydration which can be life-threatening if not corrected.

Residue

In a healthy adult, the feces may weigh 75 to 175 g per day, about 70 percent of which is water (6). The composition of the solid material varies with the diet, as do the total mass of stool and the transit time. Many tube-feeding formulas are low in *residue,* the material re-

maining in the intestine after digestion and absorption. In the tube-fed patient, residue could consist of fat, intestinal cells, mucus, and the residue of intestinal bacteria. Recently, a formula containing fiber to increase residue has become available (see Table G-3).

In some circumstances, a reduction in, or absence of, intestinal content is desirable. Formulas low in residue may be useful in some diagnostic procedures, in feeding preoperative or postoperative patients, for those being weaned from parenteral feeding, and for patients with specific gastrointestinal disorders such as colitis or Crohn's disease. On the other hand, a patient who becomes constipated may be helped with a formula containing fiber if it is not contraindicated.

Viscosity

The *viscosity* of the formula is determined by its composition. In general, larger molecules increase viscosity; more calorically dense formulas are also more viscous. Viscosity, in turn, will determine the size of the feeding tube that must be used. More viscous formulas require a larger tube.

FORMULA INGREDIENTS

In order to use tube feedings, you must have a thorough knowledge of the content of the formula and be able to relate that content to the patient's ability to tolerate the feeding. A major consideration is the molecular size of the substrates, which relates to osmolality, and the patient's ability to digest the substrates. Digestive ability varies with the area of the gastrointestinal tract that lies below the end of the feeding tube. For example, if the tip of the tube lies in the jejunum below the site of action of pancreatic enzymes, the content of the tube feeding cannot consist of materials which require pancreatic enzymes for digestion.

Carbohydrate

Carbohydrates used in tube feedings are listed in Table 12-4. They may vary considerably in molecular size. The larger molecules are less sweet and exert less

TO TEST YOUR UNDERSTANDING

11. Number the formulas below in terms of viscosity from 1 (most viscous) to 3 (least viscous).

    _____   a. Compleat B

    _____   b. Osmolite

    _____   c. Vivonex

12. A patient is receiving a tube feeding that contains the following: 1,000 ml, 2 kcal/ml, 20% of energy from crystalline amino acids, 5.0 mEq Na$^+$/100 ml, 2.5 mEq K$^+$/100 ml, and 7.8 mEq Cl$^-$/100 ml.

    a. What is his renal solute load? (Show your calculations.)

    b. If the patient had a renal disease in which his maximum renal concentrating ability were 200 mOsm/L, what would be the consequences of giving this formula? Why?

    c. What would you recommend for this patient?

---

osmotic pressure. They also require more digestion, but most patients have sufficient amylase to digest starch. Starch may consist of 400 to several thousand glucose units and thus contributes very little to formula osmolality. It has limited use because it is relatively insoluble.

Starch molecules can be made smaller by hydrolysis to molecules of shorter lengths. These "glucose polymers" are more soluble and more osmotically active than starch, but less osmotically active than glucose. They are rapidly hydrolyzed and absorbed in the intestine. Some confusion arises because of inconsistent terminology. The terms *hydrolyzed cornstarch, glucose oligosaccharides, glucose polymers, glucose polysaccharides,* and *maltodextrin* are often used interchangeably.

Sucrose, lactose, and maltose, plus smaller dextrin molecules from starch hydrolysis, may be used in formulas, but their use increases the formula's osmolality.

TABLE 12-4.   Sources of Ingredients in Commercial Formulas

CARBOHYDRATES

Polysaccharides: Hydrolyzed cereal solids, pureed vegtables, modified food starch, tapioca starch

Glucose polymers: Glucose polysaccharides (> 100 glucose units), glucose oligosaccharides (2–10 glucose units), glucose polymers (partial hydrolysis of cornstarch), maltodextrins, corn syrup, corn syrup solids

Disaccharides: Lactose (from milk), sucrose, maltose (by-product of oligosaccharide or starch digestion)

Monosaccharides: Glucose (dextrose), fructose

PROTEIN

Intact: pureed beef, egg white solids, soy protein isolates, casein, lactalbumin, dry milk, caseinate of sodium or calcium

Partially hydrolyzed: from casein whey, soy, or meat protein, lactalbumin, collagen

Crystalline amino acids: L-amino acids

FAT

Long chain triglycerides: butterfat, corn oil, safflower oil, soy oil, sunflower oil

Medium chain triglycerides: MCT

Lecithin

Diglyceride

Monoglycerides

In addition, they require specific disaccharidases for digestion and are therefore not tolerated by patients with deficiencies of these enzymes.

Glucose may be used in formulas but will markedly increase osmolality and is very sweet. It does not require any digestion, however. In clinical situations, glucose is commonly called *dextrose.*

The carbohydrate content of a formula is sometimes expressed in *dextrose equivalents (DE).* The DE indicates the reducing action of sugars and syrups. Dextrose is the same as D-glucose and is used as the standard. It has a DE of 100. In a dextrose polymer, one end will have a free reducing group. The number of these groups in relation to the total weight of the polymer is used to calculate DE. DE values of some carbohydrates commonly used in tube feedings are as follows:

liquid corn syrup	36–60
corn syrup solids	20
maltodextrins	20

Substances with higher DE are sweeter and have a higher osmotic load.

A list of the carbohydrates contained in a formula is called a *saccharide profile.* It may contain the exact sugar, such as glucose or sucrose. Alternatively, it may list categories, such as mono-, di-, and polysaccharides.

Protein

Three major categories of protein are used in tube-feeding formulas (see Table 12-4). They differ in the amount of digestion that is required prior to absorption.

Intact Proteins.   Intact proteins are in their original, natural form and require complete digestion. Examples include milk, eggs, and pureed meat. Some intact proteins have been separated from the original food. These are sometimes called "isolates," such as "soy protein isolate." Lactalbumin and casein are isolates from milk with removal of lactose, and albumin may be isolated from egg white. Some are used in combinations. Caseinate, which is expensive, may be combined with the cheaper soy isolate. This reduces cost while still providing high-quality protein. All intact proteins require normal amounts of pancreatic enzymes for digestion. Since they are large molecules, they do not appreciably affect formula osmolality.

Hydrolyzed Proteins. These products may be made from some of the same proteins or from fish, whey, or meat, and then hydrolyzed with enzymes. The enzyme hydrolysis results in a mixture of peptides of various sizes and some free amino acids. Some formulas have added free amino acids to improve the protein quality of the formula. The smaller molecules, such as tripeptides and dipeptides, as well as amino acids, add to the osmotic load of the formulas. These formulas are useful for patients with problems of amino acid transport and reduced absorptive surface. There is some evidence that dipeptides in combination with amino acids are absorbed more easily than the equivalent amino acids alone.

Pure Crystalline Amino Acids. Amino acids require no digestion. The amino acids markedly add to the osmotic load, however. It is particularly important to examine the amino acid composition of these products since not all provide the necessary amino acids within the amount of protein provided in the feeding (7). Additional needs related to individual diagnoses must also be taken into consideration.

Fat

Most tube-feeding formulas contain lipid from a vegetable source such as soy, corn, safflower, or sunflower seed, or, in the case of milk-based formulas, from butterfat. The fatty-acid chains in these products are long—14 carbons or more—and the lipid is called *long-chain triglyceride (LCT)*.

The amount of essential fatty acid (EFA)—that is, linoleic acid—required has not been specifically determined, and recommendations vary. About 2 to 3 percent of total kcal intake is commonly recommended for adults (8, 9) but as much as 5 percent is occasionally recommended (10). For infants, it has been estimated that EFA requirements may be as low as 1 to 2 percent of total kcal to avoid symptoms of EFA deficiency (11),

TABLE 12-5. Linoleic Acid Content of Vegetable Oils

Source of Oil	Linoleic acid (%)
Corn	58
Safflower	74
Sesame	74
Soy (not hydrogenated)	51
(hydrogenated)	39
Sunflower	67

but optimum intake may be 4 percent of total kcal or 100 mg/kg body weight (12). LCT sources provide generous quantities of linoleic acid (13), as shown in Table 12-5.

For patients who are unable to digest and absorb LCT, feedings that contain medium-chain triglycerides (MCT) may be formulated. MCT is prepared by fractionating coconut oil and isolating fatty acids with 6 to 12 carbon atoms. The triglyceride prepared from these fatty acids provide 8.3 kcal/g. Each 15-ml tablespoon of oil weighs 14 g and thus contains about 115 kcal. Since the product is rapidly hydrolyzed in the intestinal lumen, it adds to the osmolality of a tube-feeding formula. MCT does not provide EFA, an important consideration if MCT is the only lipid. Other problems arise from the side effects sometimes produced. Nausea, vomiting, diarrhea, and abdominal distention occur. MCT is oxidized to ketone bodies and carbon dioxide in the liver and may result in excess ketogenesis. It should be added to formulas gradually to avoid the side effects.

Many ready-to-use formulas contain both LCT and MCT. The LCT provides essential fatty acids, while MCT improves the overall digestion and absorption of the formula. MCT adds appreciably to the cost of a formula.

TYPES OF COMMERCIAL FORMULAS

Two broad categories of commercial tube-feeding formulas are available—fixed ratio formulas and modular formulas.

Fixed-Ratio Formulas

Fixed-ratio formulas are those which contain protein, fat, and carbohydrate in "ready-to-use" form; they require only the addition of water. The ratio of the ingredients relative to each other is thus fixed, except if they are altered by further addition of ingredients.

There are five types of commercial fixed-ratio formulas (see Table G-3). You will need to be familiar with the properties of each. These formulas, besides the categories listed next, are also classified as polymeric and monomeric formulas. Those containing glucose and amino acids are *monomeric*, while those prepared with whole protein, starch, or other polymers of glucose and amino acids are *polymeric*.

Blenderized Formulas. Blenderized formulas are based on intact protein, starches, and long-chain triglycerides. This type of formula is available commercially and can also be made in the hospital from common ingredients such as pureed meat, strained fruits and vegetables, nonfat dry milk, and added carbohydrate, oil, vitamins, and minerals. They are moderate in osmolality, high in viscosity, and low in cost. They usully contain 25 to 35 g lactose per L. The most common caloric density is 1 kcal per ml. These feedings require intact digestion and absorption; therefore, patients need a normal, functioning gastrointestinal tract. Blenderized formulas are used for patients who have difficulty ingesting food. These include those who have esophageal disease, head or neck surgery, or sequelae of a cerebrovascular accident. They are placed via the feeding tube into the patient's stomach.

Isolates of Intact Protein: Milk-Based. Formulas containing milk are the most palatable types of tube-feeding preparations and may also be used as an oral supplement. They should be used with caution when administered by tube, because they have a high protein content and, thus, a high renal solute load. Osmolality is usually 500 to 700 mOsm per kg. They are best used in tubes into the stomach, but are contraindicated in lactose intolerance.

Isolates of Intact Protein: Non-Milk-Based. These lactose-free formulas are composed of protein isolates, oligosaccharides, oil, vitamins, and minerals. Some contain medium-chain triglycerides. Many are low in osmolality (300 to 400 mOsm per kg) compared to milk-based formulas. They are less viscous than those just listed and can thus be used with a smaller-diameter tube. Most commercial formulas yield 1 kcal per ml. A few are especially formulated to yield 2 kcal per ml for patients with high requirements but low volume tolerance.

Hydrolyzed Protein-Based "Chemically Defined" Feedings. These "defined formulas" are composed of amino acids or small peptides or both as a source of protein, glucose, or glucose oligosaccharides as a source of carbohydrate, and minimal amounts of triglycerides. They are used for patients with problems of malabsorption. They are hyperosmolar and must be used with caution.

Special-Purpose Formulas. Special-purpose formulas are available for patients with renal failure, hepatic failure, or severe metabolic stress (see Table G-3).

Modular Formulas

There are some patients whose needs are not met by standard, fixed-ratio formulas and who may benefit from an individualized modular formula. A module is a single nutrient, or combination of a few nutrients, that can be used to prepare an individualized formula suited to a patient's unique needs. Modules may be used to prepare the whole feeding or can be added to a fixed-ratio formula.

Several modules are available, providing various forms of carbohydrate, fat, and protein. Vitamin and mineral modules have only recently been developed and the choice is still limited. The modules available are listed in Table G-2. Modular-type feedings can be planned using these products.

Alternatively, a module-style tube feeding can be made by blenderizing regular foods. This is a simple and economical method of preparing a tube feeding, but it has definite disadvantages. The risk of contamination is high, and the mixture is viscous, necessitating a large-bore tube. Therefore, tube feedings are seldom formulated in this fashion. The planning of modular feeding requires greater expertise than that needed for the use of fixed-ratio feedings.

SELECTING A FORMULA

When you are asked to recommend a tube feeding for a patient, major considerations are the capacity of the patient for digestion and absorption, as well as the patient's fluid needs and renal function. Polymeric formulas must be administered only to patients who are physiologically capable of digestion and absorption of their ingredients.

Monomeric formulas are chosen for patients who need a feeding that is residue-free or fat-free, or for which no digestion is required. In general, they can be absorbed if the patient has 100 cm of functioning jejunum, an ileocecal valve, and 150 cm of ileum.

Here are some pointers to keep in mind in special circumstances:

1. A patient who was taking nothing by mouth (NPO) for a few days or who has gastroenteritis may best tolerate a low-osmolality, lactose-free formula.
2. It is commonly recommended that a patient who is in transition from total parenteral nutrition to tube feeding be given a low-residue formula. Most tube-feeding formulas are low in residue.

TO TEST YOUR UNDERSTANDING

13. Your instructor will provide some samples of supplementary feedings and tube feedings. Form M provides space for you to evaluate these formulas. Fill in the form after examining and tasting the products.
14. Suggest some formulas you might select for the following patients. Explain your answers.
    a. A patient who has been NPO for 4 days.
    b. An adult patient with severely decreased gastrointestinal function.
    c. An infant patient with severely decreased gastrointestinal function.
    d. A patient in transition from total parenteral nutrition (TPN) to tube feeding.
    e. A premature infant.

FORM M
Evaluation of Special Feeding Products

PRODUCT	Appearance (Check one)				Viscosity (Check one)			Taste & Acceptability (Check all that apply)			
	Clear	Cloudy	Opaque	Color	Watery	Syrupy	Semiliquid	Very acceptable	Marginally acceptable	Distasteful	Repulsive

3. Special guidelines may apply to children.
   a. Premature infants requiring tube feeding because of immature suck, swallow, or gag reflexes will often benefit from breast milk.
   b. If an infant is less than 6 months of age and has normal bowel function, an infant formula or breast milk may be given by tube.
   c. An older child with normal bowel function who needs a tube feeding can often be given the nutritionally complete formulas for adults. However, care must be taken that the formula has an appropriate C:N ratio and that sufficient vitamins and minerals are provided.

FORMULA DELIVERY

In designing a tube-feeding regimen, the choice of a formula must be integrated with both a delivery system and a protocol for administering the tube feeding.

TUBE PLACEMENT

It is essential that you know the location of the tube in the patient who is being tube fed. Some tubes can be placed without surgery, but surgical procedures are required for others. The tip of the tube lies either in the stomach or in the duodenum or jejunum of the small intestine.

Nonsurgical Tube Placement

In hospitalized patients, tubes are usually placed by nurses or physicians. Nutritional care specialists in outpatient settings, however, sometimes work with tube-fed patients and will insert tubes. They may also instruct patients, or parents of child patients, on tube insertion. If you are expected to do this, it is essential that you ask for detailed coaching on techniques. The procedure will not be described in detail here. In any setting, tubes should not be inserted until 3 hours after the patient's last intake of food or fluid. This precaution is observed because of the danger of vomiting and aspiration when the tube is inserted. Tubes are usually inserted via the nasal passages into the stomach (*nasogastric, or NG, tube*), into the duodenum (*nasoduodenal*) or into the jejunum (*nasojejunal* or *nasoenteric*). (See Fig. 12-1.) Vomiting and aspiration are hazards in ventilator-dependent patients, those who have depressed levels of consciousness or depressed gag reflexes, or those who are restrained. Feeding for such patients should be administered below the stomach with a weighted tip nasoduodenal tube. The nasal routes are used in tube placement if possible. Tubes

are relatively easy to insert, but there is a hazard of tube insertion into the trachea. Tubes are withdrawn if the patient is coughing. Rarely, an orogastric tube is placed in an adult. This tube is inserted through the mouth instead of the nasal passages and is usually removed after each feeding. In premature infants, orogastric tube placement is common since the nasal passages are too small to accommodate the tube.

In any case, position is confirmed after insertion by aspirating gastric contents with a syringe. Markings on the tube can also be helpful in indicating proper placement, although various manufacturers mark their tubes differently, and interpretation must be made accordingly. The normal distance from the mouth to the cardia of the stomach is about 45 cm, and from the cardia to the duodenum, 15 cm. Excessive length of tube insertion may indicate that the tube is coiled in the stomach. If the tip is pointed toward the head, vomiting and aspiration may result (14). Tube placement may also be confirmed radiologically. Many brands of tube are radiopaque to make them visible on X ray.

Tubes are well tolerated if the appropriate type is chosen. On the other hand, the nasogastric tube, in particular, is easily removed by a patient who is uncooperative or disoriented.

Surgically Placed Tubes

Surgical placement is necessary if an obstruction through the nasal passages or esophagus exists. It is also useful if very long-term tube feeding is anticipated since the opening for the tube (an *ostomy*) is not usually visible when the patient is clothed. Ostomies may be placed into the esophagus at the level of the cervical spine (cervical esophagostomy) or into the stomach (gastrostomy). (See Fig. 12-2.) These can be placed under local anesthesia. A tube may also be placed into the jejunum (jejunostomy), also shown in

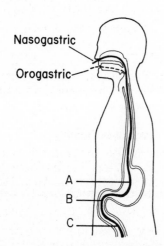

Figure 12-1   Location of non–surgically placed feeding tubes. Nasal and oral access sites are shown. A: End of nasogastric tube; B: End of nasoduodenal tube; C: End of nasojejunal tube.

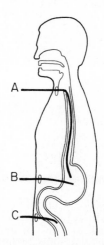

Figure 12-2   Location of surgically placed feeding tubes. A: Cervical esophagostomy; B: Gastrostomy; C: Jejunostomy.

Figure 12-2. A needle-catheter jejunostomy tube is a small polyethylene catheter introduced into the jejunum through a large-bore needle (trocar). This procedure is done during the patient's surgery. This type of tube requires a feeding of very low viscosity.

Duodenostomy is seldom used because the duodenum swings toward the back and is not easily available via the anterior abdominal wall. Also, there is danger of leakage into the abdominal cavity.

EQUIPMENT

Three types of equipment are required for tube feeding: feeding tubes, the container for the feeding, and, sometimes, a pump. This equipment is shown assembled for use in Figure 12-3.

Types of Feeding Tubes

For the comfort of the patient, the tube (1) should have the smallest diameter through which the formula will flow and (2) must be as pliable as possible. The diameter of feeding tubes is measured in *french* (F) units. One unit F = 0.33 mm.

Modern feeding tubes tend to be quite small in diameter, commonly 8F or 9.6F. They usually are made of polyurethane, silicone rubber (silastic), or a combination of these, and tend to remain relatively pliable for long periods, even if left in place. Tubes may be radiopaque and mercury-weighted or tungsten-weighted for ease of insertion and ease of determining location. Some brands contain a wire stylet in the lumen to stiffen it for easier insertion. When the tube is in place, the stylet is withdrawn. Some tubes are treated with a substance to provide lubrication when wet. Recommended tube sizes are given in Table 12-6, and some commercially available tubes are described in Table 12-7. Polyvinyl chloride (PVC) and polyethylene (PE) tend to become stiff and uncomfortable, and increase the danger of perforation. It is usually recommended that they not be used.

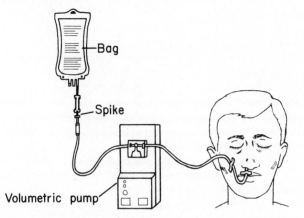

Figure 12-3 Combined setup for nasoduodenal feeding. A volumetric or peristaltic pump may be used. Correct taping of the tube will reduce pressure on the nares for greater patient comfort.

TABLE 12-6. Feeding Tube Sizes and Preferred Uses

Formula type	Size* Gravity	Size* Pump	Preferred use
Blenderized	12.0–18.0	8.0–9.6	Gastric feeding
Milk-based†	8.0–9.6	7.3	Gastric feeding
Lactose-free†	7.3–9.6	7.3–9.6	Gastric and duodenal feeding
Defined formula	5.0–6.0	5.0–6.0	Duodenal and jejunal feeding

*french units
†Protein isolates

Feeding Containers

A number of feeding containers and feeding sets are available. Many are available from the manufacturers of the formulas. You need to be knowledgeable about the advantages and limitations of each. Some of the factors for consideration include the following:

1. Container size must be considered. Volumes as large as 1 L are available. They are convenient for the nursing staff, but the formula they contain must be used within a limited time to control bacterial contamination. Sets that can attach to the manufacturer's bottle of formula can reduce contamination.
2. Some sets are designed to be used with pumps.
3. Accurate flow rates are essential.

Pumps

A pump is often needed to obtain more accurate control of the tube-feeding rate. Pumps are essential if the feeding is to go directly into the small intestine. They are also needed for the more viscous formulas. They make it possible to reduce the tube size and thus improve patient comfort. Two types of pumps are available: peristaltic and volumetric. Generally, peristaltic pumps are used for tube feedings since they are less expensive than the volumetric pumps.

PROTOCOLS FOR FEEDING

Protocols for administering a tube feeding must take into consideration the frequency, volume, and concentration of formula to be infused.

Frequency and Amount of Feeding

One protocol for delivery involves administration of a large volume (*bolus*) of formula at widely spaced intervals. For example, a patient receiving 2,400 ml per day might be given 400 ml of feeding every 4 hours. The entire feeding is given from a large syringe within a few minutes. This method is often poorly tolerated, leading to nausea, vomiting, diarrhea, distention, cramps, or aspiration. The advantages of this system are that it requires the least equipment and nursing time, and it does not limit the movement of an ambulatory patient.

TABLE 12-7.   Characteristics of Several Small-Caliber Tubes for Forced Enteral Feeding

Tube	Composition	Length	External Caliber (French)*	Tip	Comment
Dobbhoff (Biosearch)	Polyurethane	43 in	8	7 g mercury bolus weight (16 Fr)	Metal stylet available; bulbous tip promotes stable small bowel placement
Duo-Tube (Argyle)	Silicone elastomer	40 in	5, 6, 8	15–17 Fr mercury filled tip	Silicone tips also available; outside sleeve for tube placement
Entriflex (Biosearch)	Polyurethane	36 in 43 in	8	3-g mercury-filled tip (8 Fr)	Small-caliber tip allows placement through narrow stricture; stylet available
Keofeed (Hedeco)	Silicone rubber	36 in	7.3, 9.6	Mercury-filled tip without caliber change	Silicone tubes have lower I.D./O.D. ratio than similar-caliber polyurethane tubes
Keofeed (Hedeco)	Silicone rubber	43 in	7.3, 9.6	5-g mercury bolus weight (18 Fr)	
Vivonex Tungsten Tip (Norwich-Eaton)	Polyurethane	45 in	8	Flexible tungsten bolus weight (8 Fr)	Avoids any disposal problem of mercury-weighted tubes

*1 Fr = 0.33 mm outside diameter

Reproduced with permission from Alpers, D.H., R.E. Clouse and W.F. Stenson. *Manual of Nutritional Therapeutics.* Boston: Little, Brown, 1983.

An alternative to bolus feeding is the administration of the formula by *intermittent gravity drip* over a 20-to-30- or 60-to-90-minute period. Although tolerance may also be poor by this method, it is usually better than that produced by bolus feeding. This method can be quite successful if the patient is allowed to gradually adapt to it. It also does not confine the ambulatory patient.

Another alternative is the *continuous feeding,* whereby the formula is administered over 16 or 24 hours. A closed, sterile administration system can be used. This method should be chosen if hypertonic solutions are to be fed directly into the small intestine. It is the best tolerated of the three methods, but it requires a pump and is thus more expensive. The patient receiving 2,400 ml per day in 16 hours would receive 150 ml per hr, a volume more likely to be tolerated.

Volume and Concentration

As explained previously, a hypertonic solution may cause complications if it is too concentrated or if it is administered too rapidly. The volume and concentration fed, as well as the amount and rate, depend to a great extent on the location of the tube.

Nasogastric Feedings.   The stomach is often able to tolerate hyperosmolar feedings. Gravity feedings are well tolerated but demand a great deal of nursing time to administer. If gravity feedings are poorly tolerated, a pump may be used. In some institutions, pumps are not used at night as a precaution against aspiration. Bolus feeding should not be attempted unless the patient has first shown a tolerance to intermittent drip feeding.

In general, the most common recommendations are to begin with slow administration of 50 ml per hr or less of a formula diluted to isosmolar or hyposmolar concentration. The amount is then increased, followed by an increase in concentration, until the final rate, concentration, and total volume are reached. This may take several days.

It is important to note that adding a flavor packet to the formula increases the osmolality. If no untoward symptoms occur during the initial 8 to 12 hours, the feeding rate is increased. Formula volume is usually increased before concentration in nasogastric feeding, but there is some disagreement on this point. In any case, volume and concentration are never increased simultaneously.

Some maintain that it is not wise to dilute a fixed-ratio formula. Many fixed-ratio formulas are purchased in sterile packages which fit accompanying sterile feeding sets. Dilution of the formula may increase the possibility of contamination. Instead, it is recommended that the formula be given in lower volume (20 ml per hour), but at full strength, and then increased by 20-ml increments each 8 hours to a maximum of 200 ml per hour (15).

The feeding remaining in the stomach (gastric residual) should be measured every 4 to 6 hours if a pump is used, or before each feeding in intermittent gravity drip. This procedure consists of using a syringe to gently withdraw the stomach contents through the tube. Nasoduodenal feeding may be necessary if residuals remain high (>100 ml two hours after the last feeding). Feeding must be stopped if the patient vomits.

The measurement of gastric residuals is usually a

TABLE 12-8. Sample of a Nasoduodenal or Nasojejunal
Protocol*

Time	Concentration	Infusion Rate ml/hr	Volume ml	Kcal
Day 1				
8 hr	¼ strength	50	400	100
8 hr	¼ strength	75	600	150
8 hr	½ strength	75	600	300
Day 2				
12 hr	½ strength	100	1,200	600
12 hr	¾ strength	100	1,200	900
Day 3	¾ strength	125	3,000	2,250
Day 4	full strength	125	3,000	3,000

*Assume a commercial tube feeding containing 1 kcal/ml at full strength, 600 mOsm/L, administered by continuous infusion.

nursing responsibility. The resistance of very small-bore tubes makes them unpopular with nurses. More important, the residual volumes are unreliable when the small-bore tubes are used.

Nasoduodenal or Nasojejunal Feedings. Osmolality is a particularly important consideration in this feeding location. A common protocol is to begin feedings at 50 ml per hour and increase 25 to 50 ml/hour/day, or per 8-hour shift, as tolerated, until the desired volume is reached, provided there is no diarrhea, glycosuria, or intestinal obstruction. At first, feedings are usually diluted to about 150 mOsm/kg. Volume is increased before concentration. A pump for continuous administration is usually necessary. Residuals may be checked every 4 hours. With postpyloric feeding sites, there will usually be little or no residual. A sample tube-feeding protocol is shown in Table 12-8.

Other Considerations

To guard against dehydration or overhydration ("water intoxication"), particularly in the patient unable to communicate, the patient's total fluid requirements must be calculated and actual fluid intake must be determined. Fluid intake includes the water content of the tube feeding and of any food or liquid taken orally, the fluid used to flush the tube, and any fluid taken with oral medication. In estimating water content, total volume of the formula may be used if the patient is alert and can express thirst. For unconscious or incompetent patients, infants, and others who cannot express thirst, a more accurate calculation may be necessary. Free water in the tube feeding is estimated by subtracting the protein, fat, and carbohydrate content from the total volume. The difference between intake and need must be provided as free water in order to prevent dehydration.

Tubes may be flushed with water before and after each feeding. This prevents tube obstruction and also helps provide fluid to the patient. Alternatively, cranberry juice is sometimes used. It cleans out the tube effectively, but adds to the osmolality.

The temperature at which tube feedings are given is believed to affect formula tolerance. Although there is some disagreement on the question (16), cold formulas are generally believed to cause cramping and diarrhea, and tube feedings are usually given at room temperature.

The patient's head should be elevated during feeding and for 30 minutes after an intermittent feeding to reduce the risk of aspiration (see next section). A sample tube feeding order form is shown in Form N.

TO TEST YOUR UNDERSTANDING

15. A patient who had a traumatic injury to his head and neck, followed by major plastic surgery, has a feeding gastrostomy created by the surgeon. The end of the feeding tube lies immediately distal to the pyloric sphincter. The patient is underweight and is losing more weight. He is known to be lactose intolerant.
    a. What category of tube feedings would you recommend the patient be given?
    b. What diameter tube would be required?
    c. Name three tube feeding formulas that would serve the purpose.
16. A comatose patient is receiving 2,000 ml of a tube-feeding formula which provides 1 kcal/ml. Composition is as follows: carbohydrate 54.5% of kcal, protein 14% of kcal, and fat 31.5% of kcal. It is given in eight bolus feedings of 250 ml each. The tube is rinsed with 20 ml of water as previously described. How much *free water* does the patient receive in 24 hours? Show your calculations.

COMPLICATIONS OF TUBE FEEDING

The avoidance of complications demands that great care be taken in the process of tube feeding. In general, the complications may be categorized as those related to (1) the mechanical process, (2) the patient's gastrointestinal function, (3) the patient's metabolism, (4) infectious processes, and (5) psychological factors.

MECHANICAL COMPLICATIONS

Mechanical complications include nasopharyngeal discomfort such as erosions and abscesses, excessive gagging, esophageal ulceration or rupture of varices, and inability to withdraw the tube. These complications are usually related to the pliability and size of the feeding tube. Since small-lumen, mercury-weighted,

FORM N

University Medical Center Enteral Feeding Orders
(Check boxes, circle items, fill in blanks as needed.)
1. Formula _____
2. Vitamins _____
3. Insert _____ feeding tube.
   Location _____
   _____ Stomach
   _____ Begin feeding when tube is in place, confirmed by aspiration of gastric contents.
   _____ Continue to advance tube 1–2 cm/hr to duodenum.
   _____ Leave on right side 2 hrs. Leave 15–21 cm showing ABO, X-ray in 24 hrs to confirm placement.
   _____ Do not begin feeding until placement in duodenum is confirmed.
4. Head of patient elevated 30° during feeding + 30 min.
5. Fill container with feeding for _____ hrs. + ½ t blue food coloring.
6. No formula to hang more than _____ hrs.
7. Change feeding container and tubing q 24 hrs.
8. Start formula at _____ ml/hr, _____ strength.
9. Increase rate to _____ ml/hr in _____ hrs if there is no N & V, abdominal distention, or gastric residuals more than _____ ml.
   Then:

_____ ml/hr	_____ strength	_____ time	_____ date
_____	_____	_____	_____
_____	_____	_____	_____
_____	_____	_____	_____

10. If diarrhea occurs, administer _____ after checking for impaction.
11. Check gastric residuals every _____ hrs and record. If more than _____ ml, hold feeding.
    Flush tube with water.
    Recheck residual in 2 hrs.
    Restart feeding when residual less than _____ ml.
12. Flush tube with _____ ml water or cranberry juice q _____ hrs, following delivery of crushed medication and when tube is disconnected
13. Urine sugars q _____ hrs × _____ hrs, then _____ .
    Notify physician if > or = to 1%.
14. Record I & Os. Chart volume of feedings separately from water or other oral intake for each shift.
15. Measure height.
16. Weigh pt. now and Q.O.D. Chart on graph.
17. Blood sugars and 'lytes, now and q M,W,F.
18. Calorie count daily for _____ days and then _____ .
19. SMA-12,* CBC, TIBC, serum Fe, mg weekly.
20. SMA-6† every Mon and Thurs.
21. 24-hr. urine collections for urea to start 8:00 AM on _____ in conjunction with calorie count for nitrogen balance calculation.

*total protein, albumin, Ca, PO_4, cholesterol, creatinine, bilirubin, alkaline phosphatase, CPK, LDH, SGOT, and uric acid

†Na, K, Cl, HCO_3, glucose, BUN

polyurethane and silicon rubber tubes have been available, the incidence of complications of this type has decreased markedly. The viscosity of the formula, size of the tube, and other equipment must be carefully integrated, as described earlier in this chapter, to avoid complications.

An additional problem is obstruction of the tube.

Tubes should be flushed with water before and after any infusion to keep them open. If a tube becomes clogged, a small syringe can sometimes push the obstruction through. If this is not effective, a few milliliters of meat tenderizer or carbonated cola drink may loosen the clog. Tubes sometimes become clogged because a high-viscosity formula is put into a very small tube. A larger tube may be necessary. An additional precaution is to strain any formulas that are made in the institution.

GASTROINTESTINAL COMPLICATIONS

The most common gastrointestinal complications are nausea, vomiting, and diarrhea; on the other hand, some patients become constipated. Tables 12-9 and 12-10 describe the causes, diagnostic indicators, therapeutic measures for, and prevention of nausea, vomiting, and diarrhea in tube-fed patients. Examination of these tables demonstrates that many of the causes are within the responsibilities of the nutritional care specialist; therefore, you should study these tables carefully.

A number of pathogenic mechanisms unrelated to tube feeding can cause diarrhea; however, diarrhea can be produced in a tube-fed patient who does not have a diarrheal disease. An important etiologic factor is hyperosmolality of the feeding solution, particularly if the feeding is delivered directly into the small bowel. The hyperosmolar solution may delay the passive diffusion of water from the intestinal lumen, or it may even cause a net secretion of water into the lumen to correct the high osmolality. In the case of extremely hyperosmolar solutions delivered very rapidly, the movement of fluid from the vascular system into the intestinal lumen may be rapid enough to cause vas-

cular collapse. As indicated in Table 12-8, hyperosmolar tube feedings should be diluted at first so that they are approximately isosmotic, and they should be given slowly. If the tube feeding is isosmotic at full strength, further dilution is unlikely to be necessary, and the feeding is simply initiated at a slower rate. Concentration and rate can be increased as previously described until the patient's nutritional needs are met. If reduction of volume and osmolality do not help resolve the problem, an antidiarrheal agent—such as tincture of opium (paregoric), in a dose of 6 to 10 drops every 6 to 12 hours, kaolin, pectin, 30 mg codeine sulfate every 6 hours, diphenoxylate HCl (Lomotil), or loperamide (Imodium)—is sometimes ordered by the physician and added to the feeding. The intestinal flora of a patient who has been receiving antibiotics may be restored with buttermilk or Lactobacillus tablets.

Some tube-fed patients complain of constipation. The causes, therapy, and prevention are shown in Table 12-11. Of those therapeutic and preventive measures listed in the table, your responsibility will center on observing the patient's intake and output and providing additional free water as necessary. For some patients, it may be helpful to use a feeding with added fiber. You should keep in mind that patients on lactose-free feedings will have a markedly diminished stool volume, which is *not* constipation.

TABLE 12-9. Gastrointestinal Complications—Nausea and Vomiting

Cause	Diagnosis	Therapy	Prevention
Offensive smell	Patient complains of smell of formula	Add flavorings to enteral formula; be cautious of effect on osmolality	Use polymeric formulas whenever possible. Elemental formulas tend to have offensive odor.
High osmolality leading to gastric retention	Gastric residual more than 100 ml 4 hours after bolus feeding or greater than 115% of vol/hour with continuous feeding	Dilute hyperosmolar formulas to isotonic strength, then slowly increase concentration over several days	Dilute hyperosmolar formulas to isotonic strength, then slowly increase concentration over several days
		Switch to isotonic formula	Use isotonic formulas when possible
Rapid rate of infusion	Nausea and vomiting develop within a short time after a change in infusion rate	Return infusion rate to previous level, and then advance by 25 ml/hr every 12 to 24 hr (if tolerated by patient)	Start gastric feedings at 40–50 ml/hr and jejunal and duodenal feedings at 20–25 ml/hr and advance at 25 ml/hr every 12–24 hr depending on clinical tolerance. Bolus feedings at 30 ml/min.
Lactose intolerance	Review of past history to reveal lactose intolerance; lactose tolerance test; switch to lower lactose or non–lactose-containing formula with resolution of nausea and vomiting	Switch to lower lactose or non–lactose-containing formula	Use formulas with low lactose content (particularly in very ill patients with intestinal factors that predispose to relative lactose intolerance)
Excessive fat in diet	Review of past history to reveal fat intolerance or illness that predisposes to fat intolerance	Switch to lower fat diet	Maintain fat at no greater than 30%–40% of total calorie intake

Reproduced with permission from Bernard, M. and L. Forlow. Complications and their prevention. In *Enteral and Tube Feeding,* eds. J.L. Rombeau and M.D. Caldwell. Philadelphia: Saunders, 1984.

TABLE 12-10. Gastrointestinal Complications—Diarrhea

Cause	Diagnosis	Therapy	Prevention
Hyperosmolar solution	Osmolality of solution greater than 300 mOsm	Use isotonic solutions, or dilute hypertonic solutions to isotonic strength	Use isotonic solutions, or dilute hyperosmolar solutions to isotonic strength
	Increase in water content and frequency of stools without associated pain, blood, or pus in stool	Start at slow rate (40–50 ml/hr or less) and increase in 12–24 hr increments	Start at slow rate (40–50 ml/hr or less) and increase in 12–24 hr increments
		Increase caloric density with glucose polymers	Increase caloric density with glucose polymers
		Stop current formula for 12 hours—resume with isotonic formula at slow rate (40–50 ml per hour or less)	Stop current formula for 12 hr—resume with isotonic formula at slow rate of (40–50 ml/hr or less)
		Use Kaopectate or paregoric in appropriate dosage; Lomotil if necessary. Stop antidiarrheal medication at 2 days and monitor for impaction if required for longer	
Lactase deficiency	Review of past history to reveal lactose intolerance	Switch to lower lactose or non–lactose-containing formula	Use formulas with low lactose content (particularly in very ill patients with small bowel factors that predispose to relative lactose intolerance)
	Lactose tolerance test Switch to lower lactose or non–lactose-containing formula with resolution of diarrhea		
Fat malabsorption	Review of past history to reveal diarrhea associated with fat ingestion or illness predisposing to fat malabsorption	Pancreatic enzyme supplements in patients with true pancreatic insufficiency	Use products with low fat content in patients with pancreatic insufficiency or other known illnesses that predispose to fat malabsorption
	72-hour fecal fat assessment	Switch to product with lower fat content	
Cold feedings	Tubing cold to touch	Discontinue feedings until formula has warmed to room temperature	Start recently refrigerated formulas at a slow infusion rate (40 ml/hr) to allow for warming to room temperature
Protein malnutrition	Albumin less than 3 gm/dl	Use isotonic solutions, or dilute hypertonic solutions to isotonic strength	Use isotonic solutions, or dilute hypertonic solutions to isotonic strength
		Start at slow rate, 20–25 ml/hr or less, and increase in 12–24 hr increments, depending on patient response	Start at slow rate, 20–25 ml/hr or less, and increase in 12–24 hr increments, depending on patient response
		Give parenteral nutrition concomitantly or prior to start of enteral feedings	Give parenteral nutrition concomitantly or prior to start of enteral feedings
		Use antidiarrheal agent for 48-hr period, if necessary	Use antidiarrheal agent for 48-hr period, if necessary
Factors independent of enteral formula	Careful review of patient history, physical examination, and medications	Reverse primary factor, e.g., discontinue antibiotics causing pseudomembranous enterocolitis or bacterial overgrowth; or treat infectious diarrheal agents	
Unidentifiable factors	Careful review of patient history, physical, and medications	Discontinue feedings for 48 hr, then resume at lower flow rate and utilize peripheral TPN in interim; or, decrease flow rate to 25–50 ml/hr for	

(continued)

TABLE 12-10. *(Continued)*

Cause	Diagnosis	Therapy	Prevention
		at least 24 hr then increase by 25–50 ml/hr every 24 hours; or, dilute formula and then slowly increase concentration over several days; or add an antidiarrheal agent; or add a bulk forming agent	

Reproduced with permission from Bernard, M. and L. Forlow. Complications and their prevention. In *Enteral and Tube Feeding*, eds. J.L. Rombeau and M.D. Caldwell. Philadelphia: Saunders, 1984.

METABOLIC COMPLICATIONS

The metabolic complications common in tube-fed patients are overhydration, dehydration, and nutrient imbalances. These are usually avoidable if the patient is carefully monitored. The causes, therapy, and prevention of these complications are listed in Table 12-12, which should be studied carefully. Dehydration is a particular hazard for tube-fed patients, especially infants and patients who cannot express thirst, such as those who are confused or unconscious.

INFECTIOUS COMPLICATIONS

The most common infectious complications are the result of aspiration or contamination of formula.

Aspiration Pneumonia

Pneumonia can develop as a result of vomiting or regurgitation and aspiration of stomach contents. A major preventive measure is to keep the patient's head elevated 30 degrees at all times during continuous feeding and for 2 hours following intermittent feeding. Aspiration is more likely to occur in patients with decreased mental ability or with decreased ability to close the glottis. These include those with a tracheostomy, for example, patients after radical neck surgery, or those with an endotracheal tube, such as patients on respirators. Other patients at high risk are those with head or neck surgery or respiratory problems and those who have trouble swallowing their own saliva. It is helpful in those patients to use nasoduodenal, in preference to nasogastric, feeding and to elevate the patient's head 30 degrees if possible. The volume of gastric contents should be minimized. Since high osmolality retards gastric emptying, you will need to dilute hypertonic fluids and build up to concentrated forms slowly. High-fat formulas also retard gastric emptying, and reducing fat content may be helpful.

It is the responsibility of the nursing staff to check the gastric residual. The patient should not receive another bolus feeding if the stomach contents are greater than 100 to 150 ml. Patients receiving continuous feeding should have feeding discontinued if the residual is more than 10 to 20 percent of the flow rate for an hour.

Contaminated Formulas and Equipment

Commercially prepared formulas are generally preferred over those prepared in the hospital because they reduce the risk of contamination. Hospital-prepared formulas are prepared in the pharmacy in some institutions and by the Department of Dietetics in oth-

TABLE 12-11. Gastrointestinal Complications—Constipation

Cause	Diagnosis	Therapy	Prevention
Dehydration	Intake less than output, dry skin and mucous membranes, orthostatic hypotension; BUN: creatinine ratio > 10:1	Supplemental fluids in enteral formula or by parenteral route	Careful watch of intake and output, giving supplements of free water when intake is not greater than output by 500–1,000 ml (or more in febrile states)
Impaction	Rectal examination	Digital disimpaction	Careful watch of intake and output giving supplements of free water when intake is not greater than output by 500–1,000 ml (or more in febrile states)
Obstruction	Nausea, vomiting, flat plate of abdomen showing dilated bowel with air fluid levels	Possible decompression by Miller-Abbott tube; generally requires surgery	

Reproduced with permission from Bernard, M. and L. Forlow. Complications and their prevention. In *Enteral and Tube Feeding*, eds. J.L. Rombeau and M.D. Caldwell. Philadelphia: Saunders, 1984.

TABLE 12-12. Metabolic Complications

Complication	Incidence (Percent)	Cause	Therapy	Prevention
Overhydration	20–25	Severe malnutrition and refeeding	Decrease fluid flow rate	Careful monitoring of intake and output and clinical status
		Significant cardiac, renal, or hepatic disease	Occasional diuretics (particularly in patients with cardiac, renal, or hepatic disease)	
Hypertonic dehydration	5–10	Hypertonic formula given to a patient unable to communicate or respond to thirst	Supplemental water either in enteral formula or parenterally	Careful monitoring of intake and output and clinical status
Hyperosmolar, hyperglycemic, nonketotic coma	<1	Relative insulin lack	Discontinue feedings until blood sugar controlled, then restart at a slow rate, and slowly increase rate while titrating insulin	Careful monitoring of blood sugar on a daily basis as feedings are initiated; at least twice daily in patient with known diabetes
			Vigorous hydration Small doses IV or IM insulin	
Hyperglycemia	10–30	Insulin lack	Slow enteral fluid administration rate initially; slow increase in Insulin or an oral hypoglycemic flow rate	Give formulas with higher percent fat; calories contributed by fat may require use of modular formula
Hypoglycemia	2	Sudden cessation of feedings in patients on medication for hyperglycemia	Taper feedings	Taper feedings
			Decrease fluid flow rate	Decrease fluid flow rate
Hyperkalemia	40	High potassium content of enteral formulas	Switch to formula with lower potassium content	Check electrolytes daily as flow rate is being increased; at least weekly once rate is established
		Renal insufficiency	Keyexalate, insulin and glucose	
Hepatic encephalopathy		Liver disease	Decrease protein	Limit protein content
Renal failure		Renal disease or pre-renal conditions	Decrease Mg, K, protein, phosphate; give feeding with essential amino acids	Limit Mg, K, protein, phosphate
Cardiac failure		Cardiovascular disease Acidosis	Reduce sodium, fluid	Limit sodium, fluid
Hypokalemia	8	Insulin administration Diarrhea Marked malnutrition	Potassium supplements in enteral formula or parenterally	Check electrolytes daily as flow rate is being increased; at least weekly once rate is established
Hypophosphatemia	30	Insulin administration Severe malnutrition	Phosphate supplements in enteral formula or parenterally	Check electrolytes daily as flow rate is being increased; at least weekly once rate is established
Hyponatremia	31	See overhydration Prolonged enteral therapy	Water restriction	Same as above
Hyperphosphatemia	14	Renal insufficiency	Switch to product with lower phosphate content	Same as above
Hypomagnesemia	3	Decreased carrier protein levels	Continued therapy	
Hypocupremia	3	Inadequate delivery	Supplement formula, as necessary	Check serum levels
Elevated transaminases	Unknown	Activation of hepatic enzymes	If progressively abnormal, discontinue formula, though there are reports of reversal of the abnormality in spite of continued enteral therapy	

(continued)

TABLE 12-12. *(Continued)*

Complication	Incidence (Percent)	Cause	Therapy	Prevention
Vitamin K deficiency	Unknown	Low vitamin K content of elemental formulas	Vitamin K replacement	Adequate provision of vitamin K
Essential fatty acid deficiency	Unknown	Low linoleic acid content of diet	Modular fat product added to enteral formula Daily 5 ml of safflower oil orally Parenteral fat administration	Adequate provision of essential fatty acids

Reproduced with permission from Bernard, M. and L. Forlow. Complications and their prevention. In *Enteral and Tube Feeding*, eds. J.L. Rombeau and M.D. Caldwell. Philadelphia: Saunders, 1984.

ers. In any case, clean technique should be used during preparation. You may need to be familiar with this technique in order to instruct employees in formula preparation.

Policies regarding the length of time a formula can be left hanging vary among institutions. In some hospitals, it is believed that enteral formulas can be hung for 8 to 12 hours at room temperature without clinically significant contamination. Feeding equipment, except for the tube, should be changed every 24 hours. Formula preparation should be limited to the amount used in 24 hours.

PSYCHOSENSORY COMPLICATIONS

You may be able to assist the patient with the psychosensory deprivation which accompanies tube feeding. Some patients are distressed by the lack of the taste of food. If they are cooperative, they may be allowed to chew, and then spit out, food. Other patients have considerable discomfort from dryness of the mouth and nasal passages. Depending on the specific condition, the patient might be given additional water, ice, chewing gum, or hard candy. Some patients are particularly in need of reassurance.

TO TEST YOUR UNDERSTANDING

17. Describe the type of complications you might expect in the following situations and describe preventive measures.

   a. Compleat B given through an 8F tube into the stomach.
   b. 2,000 ml of formula, 900 mOsm/kg, containing 30% intact protein.

18. A patient in a coma is being fed by tube a lactose-free formula containing soy protein isolate. The protocol includes 100 ml of water to follow each feeding. What purpose(s) does this water serve?

19. What change in a tube-feeding protocol might be indicated by the following developments?

   a. Elevated temperature (fever) in the patient
   b. Large amount of exudate from a wound
   c. Warm environment
   d. Loss of ability to concentrate urine

20. List possible actions that might be taken to correct the following in the tube-fed patient.

   a. Dehydration
   b. Constipation
   c. Hyperglycemia

MONITORING THE TUBE-FED PATIENT

All patients receiving tube feeding must be carefully monitored by the Nutrition Support Service. Usually, the nursing staff will monitor gastric residuals, flow rate, and vital signs and will record the intake and output of fluid and formula. Patients should be monitored by a nutritionist for indicators in three areas (17): tolerance to the formula, state of hydration, and nutritional response. It is important to use these indicators, as well as routine nutritional assessment methods (see Chapter 4), not only to establish the patient's original status, but also to monitor the effects of treatment; therefore, repeated measurements are made. The laboratory test panels commonly used in monitoring the tube-fed patient are those listed as Preliminary Screening and Broad Spectrum Screening in Table E-5. You should be familiar with normal values (see Tables E-1 to E-10) and the significance of abnormal values in the tube-fed patient.

INDICATORS OF FORMULA TOLERANCE

Stool frequency and consistency will be noted in the medical record by the nursing staff, who will also note any vomiting that occurs. The patient can be questioned concerning untoward symptoms such as abdominal distention and bloating. When these occur, it may be necessary to stop the feedings until symptoms subside and then restart them on a more conservative schedule.

Urine is tested for glucose and acetone when feedings begin as an indication of carbohydrate tolerance, and then daily for 3 to 14 days, depending on institution policy. Some protocols require urine tests for glucose twice daily. These tests are discontinued in the nondiabetic patient if consistently negative for 3 days. Blood sugar is sometimes screened in place of urinalysis.

If the diabetic, septic, or severely stressed patient cannot metabolize the carbohydrate, insulin is sometimes given, rather than reducing the carbohydrate content, and thus the energy level, of the formula. The use of a continuous feeding to replace intermittent feeding is also helpful.

INDICATORS OF HYDRATION STATUS

The patient should be weighed initially and at frequent intervals thereafter. Some protocols require daily weighing, while others require weights three times per week. Daily measurements of input and output of formula and of water, recorded separately, are essential. This is generally a nursing responsibility. If the patient suddenly gains or loses weight, a disturbance in hydration status should be investigated. In addition, the dehydrated patient will show evidence of dry mucous membrane, poor skin turgor, decreased blood volume with low blood pressure, and increased levels of serum protein, hematocrit, and blood cells.

Overhydration may be indicated by weight gain, elevated blood pressure, edema, and jugular vein distention.

In a typical protocol, laboratory values available in the patient's chart are BUN, serum glucose, serum sodium, serum potassium, serum chloride, serum albumin (done twice a week), Broad-Spectrum Screening (done weekly), and a CBC with red-cell indices (done weekly). (See Table E-11 and Chapter 4.). Urine specific gravity should also be measured every 8 or 12 hours. Indicators of dehydration will include hypernatremia, azotemia, hyperchloridemia, hyperglycemia, elevated hematocrit, and high urine specific gravity.

Dehydration can be prevented by supplying the patient's fluid requirements. Water can be supplied through the tube. Precautions are important since dehydration can be life-threatening. Severe dehydration in these patients has been called "tube-feeding syndome." If dehydration does occur, feeding must be stopped. The physician may order intravenous 5-percent glucose in water to rehydrate the patient.

EVALUATION OF NUTRITIONAL RESPONSE

Nutritional assessment of the tube-fed patient must be more detailed than is the case for many orally fed patients. Body weights and the selected laboratory values just described are useful. In addition, the following are necessary for evaluation of nutritional response:

1. Calorie count daily for 5 to 7 days, and then weekly. Monitor the amount actually administered compared to the amount ordered.

2. Urinary urea nitrogen and urine creatinine for original nutritional assessment and weekly thereafter for assessment and calculation of nitrogen balance.

3. Determination of nitrogen intake to calculate nitrogen balance.

4. Estimation of energy expenditure initially and repeated any time a change is likely to have occurred.

TO TEST YOUR UNDERSTANDING

21. For each item listed, give the normal value and the possible significance of an elevation in the value indicated in the tube-fed patient.

    a. BUN
    b. Serum glucose
    c. Serum sodium
    d. Serum albumin
    e. Hematocrit
    f. Serum potassium
    g. Serum acetone

22. What categories of tube-fed patients are at particular risk of dehydration?

5. Serum albumin every 2 to 3 weeks.
6. Serum iron and transferrin or TIBC every 2 to 4 weeks.
7. Serum magnesium biweekly in the severely malnourished patient.

DOCUMENTATION OF THE TUBE FEEDING

The medical record is an essential tool in communicating information on the tube feeding to other members of the health care team. The information documented by the nutritionist varies with the division of responsibility. You may be expected to include the following:

1. Recommendations on the type of feeding tube, if not surgically placed
2. Recommended formula
3. Recommended method and rate of delivery
4. Actual formula intake, with kcal and protein content
5. Patient's tolerance to tube feeding: complications
6. Recommended corrective action
7. Education about tube feeding provided to the patient

In most institutions, your recommendations for items 1 through 3 and 6 must be countersigned by the attending physician.

TOPICS FOR FURTHER DISCUSSION

1. New tube-feeding products are frequently developed, and changes are continually being made in existing formulations. What methods and sources of information could you use to keep up to date in this area?

2. Discuss the content and purpose of new products not listed in Appendix G.

3. Why are most tube-feeding formulas not recommended for use in newborn infants?

REFERENCES

1. BERGMAN, K.E., E.E. ZIEGLER, AND S.J. FOMON. Water and renal solute load. In *Infant Nutrition* (2d ed.), ed. S.J. Fomon. Philadelphia: Saunders, 1974, pp. 245–266.
2. ZIEGLER, E.E. AND S.J. FOMON. Fluid intake, renal solute load and water balance in infancy. *J. Pediatr.* 78:(1971)561–568.
3. BLACKBURN, G.L. AND B.R. BISTRIAN. Curative nutrition: Protein-calorie management. In *Nutritional Support of Medical Practice*, eds. H.A. Schneider, C.E. Anderson, and D.B. Coursin. Hagerstown, Md.: Harper & Row, Pub., 1977.
4. KINNEY, J.M. Energy requirements of the surgical patient. In *Manual of Surgical Nutrition*, eds. W.F. Ballinger, J.A. Collins, W.R. Drucker, S.J. Dudrick, and R. Zeppa. Philadelphia: Saunders, 1975.
5. SHILS, M.E., ET AL. *Liquid Formulas for Oral and Tube Feedings.* New York: Memorial Sloan-Kettering Cancer Institute, 1979.
6. ROTHMAN, M.M. AND A.B. KATZ. Analysis of feces. In *Gastroenterology* (2d ed.), Vol. 2, ed. H.S. Bockhus. Philadelphia: Saunders, 1964.
7. MARBLE, N.L., M.L. HINNERS, N.W. HARDISON, AND N.L. KEHMBERG. Protein quality of supplements and meal replacements. *J. Am. Diet. Assoc.* 77:(1980)270–276.
8. NATIONAL RESEARCH COUNCIL, FOOD AND NUTRITION BOARD. *Recommended Dietary Allowances* (9th ed.) Washington, D.C.: National Academy of Sciences, 1980.
9. NATIONAL RESEARCH COUNCIL. Publication No. 474. *The Role of Dietary Fat in Human Health.* Washington, D.C.: National Academy of Sciences, 1966.
10. FISCHER, J.E. Nutritional management. In *Handbook of Critical Care*, eds. J.L. Berk, J.E. Sampliner, J.S. Artz, and B. Vinocur. Boston: Little, Brown, 1976.
11. HOLMAN, R.T., W.O. CASTOR, AND H.F. WIESE. The essential fatty acid requirement of infants and the assessment of their dietary intake of linoleate by serum fatty acid analysis. *Am. J. Clin. Nutr.* 14:(1964)70–75.
12. WIESE, H.F., A.E. HANSEN, AND D.J.D. ADAM. Essential fatty acids in infant nutrition. *J. Nutr.* 66:(1958)345–360.
13. *Composition of Foods, Fats and Oils.* Agriculture Handbook No. 8-4. Washington, D.C.: United States Department of Agriculture, 1979.
14. GORMICAN A. AND E. LIDDY. Nasogastric tube feedings: Practical consideration in prescription and evaluation. *Postgrad Med.* 53:(1973)71–76.
15. WEINSIER, R.L. AND C.D. BUTTERWORTH, JR. *Handbook of Clinical Nutrition.* St. Louis: C.V. Mosby, 1981, p. 77.
16. KAGAWA-BUSBY, K.S., M.M. HEITKEMPER, B.C. HANSEN, R.L. HANSON, AND V.V. VANDERBURG. Effects of diet temperature on tolerance of enteral feedings. *Nurs. Res.* 29:(1980)276–280.
17. ROMBEAU, J.L. AND R.A. MILLER. *Nasoenteric Tube Feeding: Practical Aspects.* Mountain View, Calif.: Health Development Corp. (no date).

ADDITIONAL SOURCES OF INFORMATION

SMITH, J.L. AND S.B. HEYMSFIELD. Enteral nutrition support: Formula preparation from modular ingredients. *JPEN* 7:(1983)280–288.

13

PARENTERAL NUTRITION

Parenteral feeding includes any method of feeding which bypasses the digestive tract. The term *parenteral nutrition* (PN) includes the provision of partial or total nutritional requirements by the intravenous route. Parenteral nutrition can be used in addition to enteral feedings or as a sole source of nutrients. When it fills all the nutrient requirements, it is commonly referred to as *total parenteral nutrition,* or TPN. Dudrick and his colleagues (1) first developed the technique of TPN in the mid 1960s, and it is now a widely used, often life-saving, technique for the provision of nutritional support. Numerous patients have been maintained for years on home TPN.

Many institutions have *nutrition support teams* which assist in the management of the nutritional care of critically ill patients who require specialized enteral-parenteral feeding systems. The nutrition support team comprises a physician, who is often a surgeon, a pharmacist, a nurse, and a nutritional care specialist.

The nutritional care specialist working in the area of parenteral nutrition must be skilled in the assessment of nutrient needs for critically ill individuals with a variety of conditions. The conditions that most often require TPN are burns, multiple trauma, and gastrointestinal diseases that interfere with food intake, digestion, or absorption.

To care for TPN patients, you must have knowledge of the composition and availability of the components of a parenteral solution feeding system and of protocols for administering the solutions. After you assess the nutrient needs of individual patients, you must also be able to design an appropriate parenteral solution in order to make recommendations to the physician (2). You will need to record nutrient intake and parameters reflecting the nutritional status of the parenterally fed patient. These serve as the basis for

decisions concerning the discontinuation of parenteral feedings. Your work will also be essential in monitoring the transition to enteral feeding once parenteral feeding is stopped.

This chapter will draw on many concepts presented in previous chapters, especially Chapters 4 and 12. In addition, a review of the relevant chapters in your text may provide useful background information. It is especially important to complete the "To Test Your Understanding" exercises as you read this chapter. After you have completed this chapter, you should be able to assess an individual's nutrient needs and design an appropriate parenteral-feeding regimen. (The role of parenteral therapy for fluid and electrolyte disturbances is discussed briefly in *Clinical Nutrition and Dietetics* (3).

TERMINOLOGY

Parenteral feedings can be administered peripherally, usually into the veins of the arm, or centrally. *Central parenteral feeding* (CPN) usually involves infusion into the superior vena cava, which is reached via the internal jugular or subclavian vein (Fig. 13-1). *Peripheral parenteral nutrition* (PPN) involves infusion into small veins, usually in the arm (Fig. 13-2). Parenteral feeding, either PPN or CPN, may be given concurrently with enteral feeding. Another commonly used term for parenteral nutrition is "intravenous hyperalimentation," or IVH. This is misleading terminology, however, because parenteral feedings do not have to contain excessive, or "hyper," amounts of nutrients. In this chapter we will use CPN to denote central administration and PPN to denote peripheral administration of parenteral nutrition whether or not enteral feeding is also used.

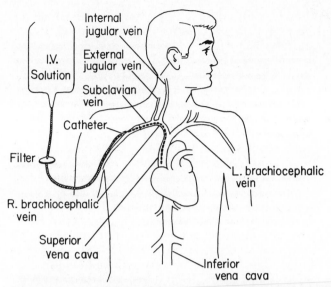

Figure 13-1 Central parenteral nutrition (CPN) is administered into large veins, such as the superior vena cava, which is reached via the internal jugular or subclavian vein.

INDICATIONS AND CONTRAINDICATIONS

The primary indication for the use of parenteral feeding is that sufficient calories cannot be ingested or absorbed enterally.

Clinical presentations that may indicate the need for parenteral feeding include

1. Nonfunctioning gastrointestinal tract
2. NPO for more than five days
3. Fistula in the gastrointestinal tract
4. Severe acute pancreatitis
5. Short bowel syndrome
6. Severe malnutrition or a 10 to 15 percent loss of body weight
7. Excessive nutritional needs which cannot be met by en-

teral feeding, and accompanying hypermetabolic states, such as burns or multiple trauma

8. Severe malnutrition or refusal to eat, as in anorexia nervosa.

There are two major contraindications to TPN support. The first is the presence of a functioning gastrointestinal tract. A useful guideline is the adage "If the gut works, use it!" The second contraindication is the existence of a terminal condition for which aggressive therapy is not provided. Advanced inoperable cancer is an example.

Hypertonic solutions containing concentrated carbohydrate calories cannot be infused into peripheral veins. The low blood flow in these veins can lead to inflammation followed by thrombosis when hypertonic solutions are infused. In practice, PN solutions from 250 to 600 mOsm/L can be administered peripherally. However, these limitations do not allow enough protein and energy to be given to meet the needs of some patients. If the solution is more hypertonic, it must be given centrally. The high blood flow in central veins results in quick dilution of hypertonic solutions, allowing for the administration of increased quantities of protein and calories from carbohydrate.

The decision to recommend CPN rather than PPN is based on the number of calories needed, the expected duration of parenteral feeding, the need to restrict total fluids, and other metabolic and financial considerations. CPN is usually indicated when calorie needs are greater than 2,000 kcal per day and parenteral feeding will be required for more than 10 days. Other individual medical factors (discussed in later chapters) must also be evaluated for each patient.

COMPONENTS OF PARENTERAL NUTRITION SOLUTIONS

The nutrient needs of a patient fed parenterally are similar to the requirements of a patient fed enterally. As always, the six major categories of nutrients—car-

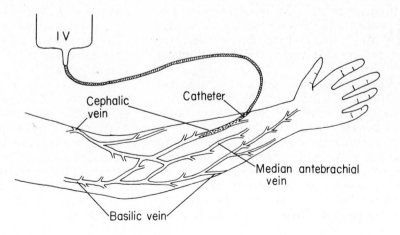

Figure 13-2 Peripheral parenteral nutrition is administered into small veins, usually in the arm.

bohydrate, protein, fat, vitamins, minerals, and fluid—must be considered, as must adequate calorie intake. However, the form of many nutrients must be specialized for direct infusion into the blood without prior digestion. Standardized concentrations and volumes of the components must also be manipulated.

Carbohydrate is given as dextrose or glucose monohydrate. This yields 3.4 kcal per g, rather than the general 4 kcal per g, because of the attached noncaloric water molecule. Dextrose is available in 5, 10, 20, 30, 40, 50, 60, and 70 percent solutions. Fifty percent dextrose in water ($D_{50}W$) is the most widely used carbohydrate solution in TPN.

Protein is supplied as amino acids which are available in 3.0, 3.5, 5.0, 7.0, 8.5, and 10.0 percent solutions. Several formulations of amino acid solutions are available. These include not only conventional amino acid solutions for adults, but also some special-purpose formulations. such as those containing a high proportion of branched-chain amino acids for trauma and liver failure, or essential amino acid formulas for renal failure. The amino acid compositions of several different types of intravenous solutions are summarized in Table 13-1. Special amino acid formulations more appropriate to the needs of growing infants have also become available. The amino acid profile of standard adult solutions differs in a number of ways from the amino acid profile of enteral formulas. These differences include the absence of glutamic and aspartic acid, low levels of cysteine and tyrosine, which are relatively insoluble, and higher levels of arginine, alanine, and glycine. Amino acid solutions provide an equivalent amount of protein, on a gram-of-amino-acid-per-gram-of-protein basis, and are calculated to provide 4.3 kcal/g when used for energy metabolism.

Fat must be provided in a parenteral-feeding regimen lasting more than 7 to 10 days in order to supply essential fatty acid (EFA) requirements. At present, 10 percent and 20 percent emulsions of soybean or safflower oil are available in 100, 200, 250, and 500 ml bottles. The basic ingredients in the fat emulsions include 10 or 20% fat from soy or a blend of safflower plus soy oil, 1.2 percent egg yolk phospholipid for use as an emulsifying agent, and 2.2 to 2.5 percent glycerin to make the emulsions isotonic. The 10 percent fat emulsions provide 1.1 kcal per ml, while 20

TABLE 13-1. Intravenous Crystalline Amino Acid Solutions

	Freamine HBC* (American McGaw)	Conventional Aminosyn 7% (Abbott)	Veinamine 8% (Cutter)	Hepatamine† (American McGaw)	Renamin‡ (Travenol)
Amino acid concentration (%)	6.9	7.0	8	8	6.5
Nitrogen (g/dl)	0.973	1.1	1.33	1.2	1
Essential amino acids (mg/dl)					
Isoleucine§	760	510	493	900	500
Leucine§	1370	660	347	1100	600
Lysine	410	510	667	610	450
Methionine	250	280	427	100	500
Phenylalanine	320	310	400	100	490
Threonine	200	370	160	450	380
Tryptophan	90	120	80	66	160
Valine§	880	560	253	840	820
Nonessential amino acids (mg/dl)					
Alanine	400	900	—	770	560
Arginine	580	690	749	600	630
Histidine	160	210	237	240	420
Proline	630	610	107	800	350
Serine	330	300	—	500	300
Tyrosine		44	—		40
Glycine	330	900	3387	900	300
Cysteine	<20		—	<20	
Glutamic acid			426		
Aspartic acid			400		
Electrolytes (mEq/L)					
Sodium	10		40	10	
Potassium	—	—	30		—
Chloride	<3	5.4	50	3	31
Magnesium	—		6		—
Acetate	57	105	—	62	60
Osmolarity (mOsm/L)	620	700	950	785	600

*Branched-chain amino acid–enriched stress formulation

†Hepatic failure formula

‡Renal failure formula

§Branched-chain amino acids

TABLE 13-2. Composition of Intravenous Fat Emulsions

Product*·†·‡	Osmolarity (mOsm/L)	Glycerin (%)	Fatty Acid Content (%)			
			Linoleic	Linolenic	Oleic	Palmitic
Soybean Oil Based						
Intralipid 10%	260	2.25	50	9	26	10
Intralipid 20%	268	2.25	50	9	26	10
Soyacal 10%	280	2.21	49–60	6–9	21–26	9–13
Soyacal 20%	315	2.21	49–60	6–9	21–26	9–13
Travamulsion 10%	270	2.25	56	6	23	11
Travamulsion 20%	300	2.25	56	6	23	11
Safflower and Soybean Oil Based (50%/50%)						
Liposyn II 10%	320	2.5	65.8	4.2	17.7	8.8
Liposyn II 20%	340	2.5	65.8	4.2	17.7	8.8

*Intralipid is manufactured by Kabi-Vitrum, Soyacal by Greencross, Travamulsion by Travenol, and Liposyn by Abbott.

†All products with 10% lipid provide 1.1 kcal/ml. All products with 20% lipid provide 2.0 kcal/ml.

‡All products contain 1.2% egg yolk phospholipid emulsifier.

percent fat emulsions provide 2.0 kcal per ml. The emulsions composed of a blend of safflower and soybean oil supply approximately 66 percent of fatty acid content as the EFA linoleate, while the emulsions containing only soy oil supply approximately 50 percent of fatty acids as linoleate. The composition of representative fat emulsions is summarized in Table 13-2. In practice, one to two 500 ml bottles of 10 percent fat may be given weekly to meet essential fatty acid (EFA) requirements.

OSMOLARITY

The osmolarity of a PN solution is an important factor in determining whether the solution will be administered via the peripheral or central route.

The osmolarity of a solution of known dextrose concentration can be readily calculated. For example, a 5 percent dextrose solution has 50 g dextrose per L divided by the atomic weight of dextrose monohydrate, 198.2 g per mole, (50g/L ÷ 198.2 g/mole), which gives 252.3 mOsm per L. A short method for calculating the osmolarity of a dextrose solution is to multiply the percentage of solution by 50. For example. the osmolarity of $D_{20}W$ would be 1,000 mOsm per L. The osmolarity of amino acid solutions can also be

calculated by a quick method which multiplies the percent amino acid concentration by 100. Using this method, a 2.5 percent amino acid solution would have an osmolarity of approximately 250 mOsm per L. Intravenous fat is isotonic to blood, with an osmolarity of approximately 300 mOsm per L. The addition of electrolytes, vitamins, and minerals also increases the osmolarity of PN solutions by approximately 300 to 400 mOsm per L.

In calculating the osmolarity of a PN solution, the component osmolarities are added together. Here is an example:

If 500 ml $D_{50}W$ (50% × 50 = 2,500 mOsm/L × 0.5 L = 1,250 mOsm) and 500 ml 8.5% amino acids (8.5% × 100 = 850 mOsm/L × 0.5 L = 425 mOsm) are mixed to make 1 L of solution, the final osmolarity would equal 1,250 + 425 = 1,675

Note that, in these examples, we are calculating osmolarity, not osmolality. Osmolarity is used because parenteral solutions are prepared using a defined number of grams of solute diluted to a final solution volume. Thus, percent concentration of a parenteral solution indicates the number of g of solute present in 100 ml of solution.

TO TEST YOUR UNDERSTANDING

1. Calculate osmolarity and calorie content for the following dextrose solutions. Show your calculations.

% dextrose/L	mOsm/L	kcal/L
5		
10		
20		
50		

2. Complete the following table for solutions with varying amino acid concentration. Show your calculations.

% amino acid/L	mOsm/L	kcal/L	g N/L
3.5			
7.0			
8.5			
10.0			

3. a. What is the calorie content (kcal/ml) and osmolarity (mOsm/L) of a solution composed of 225 ml of 10% amino acids and 350 ml of $D_{50}W$? Show your calculations.

_____ kcal/ml
_____ mOsm/L

   b. If the solution just described were infused at 20 ml/hr and a 10% fat emulsion was simultaneously infused at 10 ml/hr, what would the hourly caloric infusion rate (kcal/hr) be? _____ kcal/hr

4. a. What concentration (% or g/100 ml) of a 1 L dextrose solution would it take to equal the kcals in 500 ml of a 20% fat emulsion? _____ %

   b. What is the approximate osmolarity of the dextrose solution calculated in part a of this question? Could this solution be infused into a peripheral vein? Explain.

ASSESSING NUTRIENT NEEDS IN PARENTERAL FEEDING

CALORIES

An assessment of energy needs is the first step in planning a parenteral-feeding regimen. Measurement of gas exchange through indirect calorimetry is the preferred method for determining caloric needs, but it is not available in all hospitals. Instead, energy needs may be estimated by any of a variety of calculated methods. It is important to remember that numerous anthropometric and clinical factors affect individual energy needs, and any calculated method of establishing a caloric level is merely an estimate.

Frequent reevaluations of body weight, nitrogen excretion, and other parameters of nutritional assessment are necessary to monitor the adequacy of parenteral calorie dosage. For example, patients with cancer have an increase in basal energy expenditure (BEE), but this effect is not uniform and depends on the stage, type, and rate of growth of the cancer. Another example relates to the critically ill patient undergoing several stressful periods in sequence, such as major surgery, possible septic complications, and eventual resolution. The energy requirements of such a patient change throughout the course of an illness and need to be periodically reassessed.

One of the most widely used methods for establishing calorie needs involves calculation of BEE by the method of Harris and Benedict, followed by multiplication by an activity and injury factor (Equation 4-27).

Another approach to the estimation of calorie needs is based on requirements expressed on the basis of kcal per kg body weight per day, as shown in Table 13-3 (4). These recommendations also consider the

severity of injury and a direct relationship between nitrogen excretion and caloric expenditure (5). *As a general rule, a range of calories from 30 to 35 kcal per kg body weight per day or 1.5 times BEE is sufficient for maintenance in most patients with mild to moderate stress.* For the obese patient, calculation of BEE using actual weight may yield excessive calories, and BEE may have to be decreased by 20 to 30 percent based on actual weight. An alternative is to calculate calorie needs for the obese patient using ideal body weight.

Parenteral infusion of calories in excess of 40 kcal per kg body weight should be avoided unless clearly indicated for maintenance of body weight in conditions such as burns or severe trauma. The provision of excessive calories by the parenteral route may lead to such complications as hepatomegaly, liver dysfunction, pulmonary distress, increased energy expenditure, and hyperglycemia-induced osmotic diuresis. In providing nutritional support to the catabolic patient, the initial goal is usually to *preserve* lean body mass and then later, when the patient is more stable, to actually *replenish* nutrient reserves (6).

The nutritional support of depleted patients must

TABLE 13-3. Calorie Requirements of Hospitalized Patients

Patient Condition	Energy Requirements (kcal/kg/day)	Nitrogen Excretion (g/day)
Normal	25–30	5–10
Elective surgery	28–30	8–10
Severe injury	28–35	10–15
Sepsis		15–20
Severe trauma/burns	45–55	20–30
Severe trauma with steroids		40

Reprinted with permission from *Nutritional Support Services* Vol. 4, No. 9, Sept. 1984.

be carried out gradually. Depleted patients incorporate nitrogen more efficiently and at lower caloric levels than do normal patients, so it is easy to overestimate their calorie needs. Overzealous nutritional support of the depleted patient can lead to a "refeeding syndrome," which is characterized by hypophosphatemia, hyperglycemia, fluid retention, and cardiac arrest (7).

PROTEIN

The determination of protein needs is the next step in planning a parenteral-feeding regimen. According to the Recommended Dietary Allowance (RDA), a healthy adult needs 0.7 to 0.8 g pro/kg ideal body weight. *For the majority of patients with mild to moderate stress, 1.2 to 1.5 g pro per kg ideal body weight is indicated to promote anabolism.* Needs may increase up to 2.5 g per kg with conditions accompanied by increased nitrogen excretion, such as burns or severe trauma or stress.

The nonprotein-calorie-to-nitrogen ratio (nonpro kcal:N) must be considered in determining protein needs, as an adequate energy intake is necessary to support use of protein for anabolism. A nonpro kcal:N ratio of 250 to 300 kcal:1 g N is adequate for normal body maintenance. In stressful conditions, a nonpro kcal:N ratio of 100 to 150 kcal:1 g N is indicated to promote anabolism. Calories from protein are usually not counted in determining an individual's daily calorie needs.

CARBOHYDRATE

There is a limit to the quantity of parenteral dextrose that can be oxidized for energy without serving as a substrate for lipogenesis. Many of the earlier problems noted with TPN, such as fatty liver and liver dysfunction, are thought to have been the result of infusion of excess dextrose calories. Postoperative surgical patients have been shown to oxidize a maximum of 4 to 6 mg per kg per min, or 0.24 to 0.36 g per kg per hr, of intravenous dextrose (8, 9). In designing a parenteral-feeding regimen, the quantity of dextrose calories will be determined in large part by deciding the percentage of calories to provide as fat. *However, dextrose should not be given at a rate greater than 0.36 g per kg body weight per hr.*

LIPID

The provision of 2 to 4 percent of calories as EFA is recommended for the prevention of EFA deficiency. The provision of fat in PN reduces the calories required from dextrose and more closely approximates an enteral diet; however, impaired lipid clearance and various metabolic problems have been associated with the parenteral infusion of excess lipid calories (10). An upper limit of 60 percent of calories as fat or no greater than 2.5 g fat per kg in adults is usually set. Besides providing a source of EFAs, fat has the advantage of providing a high caloric density in an isotonic solution. This isotonicity allows parenteral-feeding solutions composed of higher proportions of intravenous fat emulsions to be administered peripherally.

A summary of various considerations affecting the provision of parenteral carbohydrate, protein, and fat is shown in Table 13-4.

FLUID

The fluid requirements of a patient will determine the percent of dextrose needed in designing a parenteral-feeding regimen. Various methods for estimating fluid requirements are outlined in Table 12-2. Patients generally need a range of 30 to 50 ml fluid per kg body

TABLE 13-4. Considerations in Parenteral Carbohydrate, Protein, and Fat Infusion for Adults

Caloric Density	Osmolarity	Availability	Requirements/Tolerance
Carbohydrate: Dextrose monohydrate 3.4 kcal/g	Estimate by multiplying solution % by 50.	5%, 10%, 20%, 30%, 40%, 50%, 60%, and 70% in a wide range of volumes. Partially filled 1 L bottles available for amino acid and electrolyte addition.	Maximum tolerance of 0.36 g dextrose/kg/hr (range of 4–6 mg/kg/min)
Protein: Crystalline Amino Acid 4.3 kcal/g amino acid or protein	Estimate by multiplying solution % by 100.	3%, 3.5%, 5%, 7%, 8.5%, and 10%. Varying amino acid formulations available.	1.2–1.5 g pro/kg for mild–moderate stress. Non-pro kcal:N ratio of 100–150:1 for anabolism.
Fat: Emulsion of soybean or safflower oil 1.1 kcal/cc (10%), 2.0 kcal/cc (20%)	Isotonic. Decreases osmolarity of dextrose–amino acid solution by approximately one-half when coinfused via a Y connector.	10% and 20% solutions in 100, 200, 250, and 500 ml units.	2%–4% kcal as fat to prevent EFA deficiency. Maximum level of 60% kcal as fat or 1.0–2.5 g fat/kg/day. Should not be mixed with electrolytes, other nutrients, or other additive solutions or used with an in-line filter.

weight to maintain hydration. Abnormal fluid losses due to fever, renal disease, or stomal losses must be added.

ELECTROLYTES

A recommendation for standard electrolyte content of parenteral-nutrition solutions is usually made in the absence of any fluid or electrolyte abnormalities. Table 13-5 summarizes standard amounts of electrolytes usually included in 1 L of PN solution. However, individual adjustment of electrolyte dosage is often required, depending on the patient's diagnosis, serum electrolyte concentration, renal function, and other modifying factors.

Electrical neutrality in plasma is maintained by equivalent amounts of cationic and anionic charges. The principal cations in plasma include Na^+ (mainly extracellular), K^+ (mainly intracellular), and lesser amounts of Ca^+ and Mg^+. The principal anions in plasma include Cl^-, HCO_3^-, and lesser amounts of SO_4^{2-}, PO_4^{3-} (major intracellular anion), organic acids, and proteins. Isotonic intravenous solutions for fluid therapy routinely include Na and K salts of acetate or chloride. Chloride and acetate are often ordered as a ratio of 2 chloride to 1 acetate, but this may vary with metabolic acid-base status. Acetate salts metabolize to yield a net HCO_3^- and are often used in greater proportion in metabolic acidosis. Additional electrolytes required for TPN solutions include calcium, usually as calcium gluconate, magnesium provided as magnesium sulfate, and phosphate supplied as a sodium or potassium salt. Magnesium and phosphate supplementation in PN solutions is needed to accompany nutrient oxidation, and potassium is important for electrolyte balance and transport of glucose and amino acids across cell membranes.

Electrolyte solutions come in various concentrations. When mixing a PN solution, electrolytes are added to the dextrose–amino acid solution usually in a total volume of approximately 80 to 100 ml per day. Some brands of amino acid solutions come premixed with standard electrolyte doses. The fat emulsions contain a small amount of phospholipid, which provides approximately 1.3 to 1.5 mmol phosphorus per 100 ml fat emulsion.

VITAMINS

Multivitamin formulations containing both fat-soluble and water-soluble vitamins are available for incorporation into intravenous infusions. The most widely used intravenous multivitamin preparation (MVI-12, Armour Pharmaceutical, Kankakee, Ill. or MVC 9+3, Lypho-Med, Inc., Chicago, Ill.) consists of two 5-ml vials which are given daily to meet maintenance requirements for adults and children age 11 years and over (11). Vial 1 provides 3,300 IU vitamin A, 200 IU vitamin D, 10 IU vitamin E, 3.0 mg thiamin. 3.6 mg riboflavin, 40.0 mg niacin, 4.0 mg pyridoxine, 15.0 mg pantothenic acid, and 100 mg ascorbic acid. Vial 2 provides 400 μg folacin, 60 μg biotin, and 5 μg vitamin B_{12}. For optimal retention. the 10-ml dose should be diluted with the entire daily volume of PN solution. Vitamin K is administered separately, usually intramuscularly (5 mg weekly), as it is not compatible with the other infusion compounds. For patients with increased vitamin requirements, multiples of the daily dosage may be given.

TRACE ELEMENTS

Recommendations for parenteral supplementation of specific trace elements are given in Table 13-6 (12). Deficiency symptoms resulting from omission of zinc,

TABLE 13-6.   Suggested Daily Intravenous Delivery of Certain Essential Trace Elements to Adults

Element	Stable adult	Stable Adult with Intestinal Losses
Chromium	10–15 μg	20 μg
Copper	0.5–1.5 mg	—
Manganese	0.15–0.8 mg	—
Zinc*	2.5–4.0 mg	Add 12.2 mg/L of small bowel fluid loss; 17.1 mg/kg of stool or ileostomy output

*An additional 2.0 mg Zn/day is suggested for the adult in an acute catabolic state.

Adapted from *J.A.M.A.* 241: (1979) 2051–2054.

TABLE 13-5.   Standard Electrolyte Levels

Electrolyte	Recommended Amount/Day	Usual Amount/L	Compatibility per L of solution
Sodium	60–120 mEq	20–50 mEq	Wide range
Potassium	60–150 mEq	20–50 mEq	Up to 80 mEq
Chloride	60–150 mEq	20–50 mEq	Wide range
Acetate	80–120 mEq	30–50 mEq	Wide range
Phosphorus*	20–40 mmol	10–15 mmol	Up to 20 mmol when combined with Ca
Calcium†	10–15 mEq	5 mEq	Up to 10 mEq when combined with P
Magnesium	8–24 mEq	8 mEq	Up to 12 mEq

*Potassium phosphate provides 0.68 mmol P/mEq K; sodium phosphate provides 0.75 mmol P/mEq Na.

†Calcium gluconate provides approximately 5 mEq Ca/g

chromium, and copper have been reported with long-term TPN (13), although short courses of PN probably do not require trace-element supplementation. Sever-

al solutions for parenteral trace-element supplementation are available (14).

TO TEST YOUR UNDERSTANDING

5. Calculate the calorie and protein needs of Mr. C.W., a 45-year-old who is 6 feet tall and weighs 80 kg. He is confined to bed while recovering from elective gastrointestinal surgery. Use an allowance of 1.5 g pro/kg, and calculate calorie needs by both BEE × activity × injury and 35 kcal/kg. How do these two calorie levels differ? Use the higher calorie level to calculate the nonpro kcal:N ratio.

    a. _____ g protein

    _____ kcal (BEE method)

    _____ kcal (35 kcal/kg)

    _____ nonpro kcal:N

    b. Using a factor of 35 ml/kg body weight to estimate Mr. C.W.'s initial fluid requirements, what would be his daily total fluid needs? _____ ml

    Rounding this to the nearest 500 ml gives _____ L/day.

6. To calculate Mr. C.W.'s EFA requirement, use a figure of 4% of total calories as EFA and the higher determination of calorie needs in part 5a. How many kcals from EFA would this include?

    a. _____ kcal EFA

    b. How many kcal/ml are provided from linoleic acid in a 10% soybean or safflower/soybean oil emulsion? Use a value of 66% of fat calories from linoleic acid in safflower/soybean emulsion oil and 50% of fat calories from linoleic acid in soybean oil emulsion. Show your calculations.

    _____ kcal/ml soybean oil emulsion

    _____ kcal/ml safflower/soybean oil emulsion

    c. How many ml of a 10% soybean or safflower/soybean oil emulsion would be needed to meet Mr. C.W.'s daily EFA requirement? Show your calculations.

    _____ ml 10% soybean oil emulsion

    _____ ml 10% safflower/soybean oil emulsion

7. Mr. C.W. receives the 10% safflower/soybean oil emulsion to meet his EFA requirement.

    a. Calculate the number of kcals from dextrose that Mr. C.W. will need in his parenteral-feeding solution in order to meet the goal of 3,060 kcal/day. How many g of dextrose would this be per day? Show your calculations.

    _____ dextrose kcal/day

    _____ g dextrose/day

    b. Would this level of dextrose be optimally utilized by Mr. C.W.? Explain your answer.

    c. What level of dextrose would you suggest supplying per day?

    d. You will provide Mr. C.W. with 3 L/day of fluid. What final concentration of dextrose and amino acids would you need in each L of TPN solution? Show your calculations.

    _____ % dextrose

    _____ % amino acids

    e. If Mr. C.W. receives 3 L/day of the dextrose–amino acid solution shown in part d and the safflower/soybean oil emulsion as outlined in part c, how many nonprotein calories will this provide per day? Show your calculations.

    f. In order to meet the goal of 3,060 kcal/day, how many *additional* ml/day of fat emulsion would have to be provided?

SOLUTION PREPARATION

You are unlikely to be responsible for the actual mixing of a parenteral feeding solution since the formula usually is prepared in the pharmacy. However, a familiarity with available solution concentrations and preparation techniques is necessary to design a parenteral-feeding regimen.

Pharmacies may vary in their methods of mixing parenteral-feeding solutions, but several generalizations apply. All component solutions must be sterile. Solutions are mixed aseptically in a laminar flow hood. Random samples of TPN solutions are routinely cultured to monitor for bacterial contamination. Assay of electrolyte content is also routinely done.

In mixing parenteral-feeding solutions, amino acid

and dextrose solutions are usually combined. This is facilitated by the use of 1-L sterile infusion bottles partially filled with a dextrose solution. Electrolyte, vitamin, and trace element solutions are also added to the amino acid–dextrose mixture.

As an example, let's consider the assembly of 1 L of a 30 percent dextrose, 3 percent amino acid solution, including additives.

We would start with a 1-L sterile IV bottle partially filled with 500 ml $D_{60}W$. Additions from other sterile solutions would include 300 ml of 10 percent standard amino acid solution, 10 ml multivitamin concentrate, 5 ml trace element solution, 45 ml elecrolyte additives as outlined in Table 13-5, and approximately 140 ml sterile water. This would give a final concentration of 30 percent dextrose and 3 percent amino acids in a 1-L volume.

In general, 100-ml portions of PN solutions are the smallest prepared. Many institutions use a standard dextrose–amino acid formulation and vary the composition for special needs. Many institutions also utilize a flexible polyvinyl chloride bag delivery system instead of the bottle system.

Intravenous fat emulsions are usually not mixed with the dextrose–amino acid base, but are instead infused from a separate sterile bottle. The fat is administered "piggyback" via a Y connector into the same line through which the dextrose–amino acid base is infused. An in-line filter (0.22 micron) is usually placed in the dextrose–amino acid line to ensure sterility of the solution being delivered. Fat is infused into the line past the filter, as the fat particles are too large

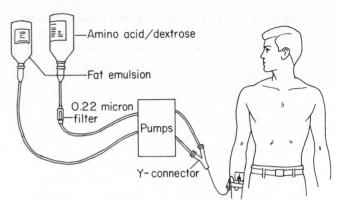

Figure 13-3 Co-infusion of fat emulsion in peripheral parenteral nutrition.

(0.45 micron) and would be impeded by the filter. A diagram of this infusion setup is shown in Figure 13-3.

An order for central line parenteral feeding of a supplemental fat infusion might read as follows:

> Daily infusion of 2 L/day TPN solution composed of 25% dextrose, 4% amino acids with standard electrolytes, vitamins, and minerals supplemented with 500 ml 10% fat emulsion. Run dextrose–amino acid solution at 83 ml/hr, and piggy-back fat emulsion over 8 hrs at 62 ml/hr.

Newer formulations of amino acids that are compatible with the lipid emulsions are now available so that all three components can be mixed and administered in a single infusion.

TO TEST YOUR UNDERSTANDING

8. We will continue with the calculation of Mr. C.W.'s TPN feeding regimen from question 5. Given your previous estimates of daily nutrient needs (summarized below), how would you assemble each L of dextrose–amino acid TPN solution for Mr. C.W.?

   120 g protein
   750 g dextrose
   3 L total volume
   Assume 100 ml/L for additives (electrolytes, vitamins, and trace elements).

   You have available 10%, 20%, 30%, 40%, 50%, 60%, and 70% solutions of dextrose in 500-ml and 1,000-ml units. You also have 3%, 3.5%, 5%, 7%, 8.5%, and 10% amino acid solutions in 500- and 1000-ml units. You have sterile, empty 1-L intravenous infusion bottles, partially filled 1-L bottles with 500 ml $D_{50}W$, and sterile water. Show your calculations.

DESIGNING A PARENTERAL-FEEDING REGIMEN

Many clinical factors affect the decision to administer parenteral feeding via the peripheral or central route. This decision is made by the attending physician, often in conjunction with a surgeon. A central line is clearly indicated for long-term feeding. Sepsis is a major problem with a central feeding line, and strict aseptic catheter care must be maintained. While solution costs are generally lower with central PN because lipid content is lower, nursing care is more extensive compared with that necessary to maintain a peripheral feeding line. The risk to the patient with the surgical placement of a central line is also greater compared with a peripheral line.

The high osmolarity of dextrose–amino acid solutions dictates that a greater percentage of calories be provided as fat in PPN. The simultaneous coinfusion via a Y connector of a lipid emulsion with the dextrose–amino acid solution decreases the final osmolarity of the mixture infused into the vein by approximately one-half, and thus decreases the incidence of phlebitis. The final concentration of dextrose usually does not exceed 10 percent in PPN, which means that a greater fluid load must be given to achieve the same calorie intake compared with CPN. Cortisol and heparin are sometimes added to peripheral dextrose–amino acid solutions to increase the tolerance of peripheral veins to hyperosmolar solutions. The addition of 5 mg per L cortisol and 500 to 1,000 U per L of heparin allows peripheral veins to tolerate solutions of up to 900 mOsm per L (15), but this practice is somewhat controversial.

We will now demonstrate how the formulation of a parenteral-feeding solution varies depending on whether it is administered centrally or peripherally. As an example, we will design both a peripheral and central PN solution for a 60-kg woman who has suffered severe trauma due to a motor vehicle accident. First, we establish her nutrient needs as follows:

$$35 \text{ kcal/kg} \times 60 \text{ kg} = 2,100 \text{ kcal}$$

$$1.5 \text{ g pro/kg} \times 60 \text{ kg} = 90 \text{ g pro or } 14.4 \text{ g N}$$

$$100–150 \text{ nonpro kcal:g N} = 1,440 \text{ to } 2,160 \text{ nonpro kcal:}14.4 \text{ g N}$$

$$2,100 \times 0.04 = 84 \text{ kcal as EFA/day, or } 588 \text{ kcal as EFA/week.}$$

(Soybean oil emulsion has approximately 0.45 kcal/ml and safflower/soybean oil emulsion has approximately 0.59 kcal/ml from linoleic acid. 1.5 L of soybean oil emulsion or 1 L of safflower/soybean oil emulsion per week would be required.)

$$35–40 \text{ ml fluid/kg} \times 60 \text{ kg} = 2,100–2,400 \text{ ml}$$

CENTRAL PARENTERAL NUTRITION SOLUTIONS

The provision of a minimal level of EFA via a central line could be handled in at least two ways. Using a 10 percent emulsion, 200 to 250 ml of emulsion could be infused via a Y connector daily. Alternatively, 500 ml of a 10 percent fat emulsion could be infused every other day. We will assume that the latter approach is used at our institution. We calculate the dextrose–amino acid solution as follows:

$$2,100 \text{ kcal/3.4 kcal/g dextrose} = 617.6 \text{ g dextrose}$$
$$\text{Maximum tolerance to dextrose} = 0.36 \text{ kcal} \times 60 \text{ kg} \times 24 \text{ hr} = 518 \text{ g dextrose}$$

Use 2 L fluid/day to make up the dextrose–amino acid solution, since we will provide 500 ml lipid emulsion every other day to average 2.25 L per day.

To allow for tolerance to dextrose, provide only 500 g dextrose per day or 500 g per 2 L, which equals 250 g dextrose per L. 90 g protein per 2 L is equal to 45 g amino acids per L.

The final concentration of nutrients would be 25 percent dextrose and 4.5 percent amino acids, and the mixture of ingredients per L would include the following:

500 ml D$_{50}$W
450 ml 10% amino acid
45 ml additives
5 ml sterile water
_____
1,000 ml total volume

Several measures can be taken to adjust the composition of the PN solution on days that lipid is also infused:

1. Reformulate the dextrose–amino acid solution to keep fluid and calorie intake constant.
2. Run the usual dextrose–amino acid solution, but decrease the rate of infusion to keep volume constant.
3. Maintain the same dextrose–amino acid composition and rate of infusion as on nonlipid days.

In addition, any of the steps just listed can be combined. The choice depends on individual clinical parameters and institutional policies. In general, reformulation of the dextrose–amino acid solution requires extra effort on the part of pharmacists and nurses, as well as a greater margin for error. Thus, the third measure listed is usually the preferred choice unless the patient's condition warrants a constant daily intake.

We will assume that the decision is to maintain a constant dextrose–amino acid composition and infuse an additional 500 ml 10 percent safflower oil emulsion every other day.

A sample TPN order for administration of the previously described CPN regimen might read as follows:

2 L/day of 25% dextrose, 4.5% amino acid solution with standard additives to run at 83 ml/hr. Every other day, infuse 500 ml 10% fat emulsion at 62 ml/hr.

The above TPN prescription would provide 90 g amino acids, 500 g dextrose, 295 kcal from linoleic acid every other day (500 ml × 0.59 kcal/ml from linoleic acid), an average fluid intake of 2.25 L per day, an average nonprotein kcal intake of 1,975 kcal per day (500 × 3.4 kcal/g dextrose + 500 ml/2 × 1.1 kcal/ml 10% fat emulsion = 1,975 kcal), and a nonpro kcal:N ratio of 137:1 (1,975 kcal/14.4 g N).

PERIPHERAL PARENTERAL NUTRITION SOLUTION

We will now formulate a parenteral feeding for delivery into a peripheral vein for our 60-kg patient. If 40 percent of calories are provided as fat, then approximately 100 g fat per day will be needed.

$$2,100 \times 0.40 = 840 \text{ kcal}/9 \text{ kcal/g} = 93.3 \text{ g fat/day}$$

We would need two 500-ml bottles of 10 percent fat emulsion or 500 ml of a 20 percent fat emulsion to supply this level of fat. The rest of the PPN solution would be formulated as follows:

500 ml 20% fat emulsion $\times$ 2.0 kcal/ml = 1,000 kcal

90 g protein $\times$ 4.3 kcal/g = 387 kcal

2,100 kcal $-$ 1,000 = 1,100 kcal

1,100 kcal/3.4 kcal/g dextrose = 323.5 g dextrose

Because a 10 percent dextrose solution is the most concentrated given in PPN, 3 L per day of a 10 percent dextrose solution would be used.

The amino acid concentration would be 90 g per 3 L, which equals 30 g amino acids per L, or 3 percent amino acid.

One liter of the PPN dextrose–amino acid solution would include the following:

500 ml $D_{20}W$
300 ml 10% amino acid
 45 ml additives
155 ml sterile water
_____
1,000 ml total volume

FORM O

```
            Physician's Orders Adult Parenteral Nutrition Orders
Date _____ Hour _____
CPN[  ]    PPN[  ]³   (Check one)
Standard Solution            Changes per
(1,000 ml)                   Bottle      Instructions

Amino acids¹        40 g                 ¹Use of nonstandard amino acids
Dextrose            250 g                   must be approved by the Clinical
Na                  60 mEq                   Nutrition Service.
K                   32 mEq               ²If patients are on 1 L of CPN for
Phos                15 mmol                  3 days or more, 10 ml of
Cl:Ac               2:1                      vitamins will be added daily.
Mg                  6 mEq                ³If PPN* is ordered, the
Ca                  5 mEq                    composition per L will be 3%
Multivitamin²       5 ml                     amino acids, 10% dextrose.
Trace element       2.5 ml                   Order in L per day. Electrolytes,
  Zn 2.0 mg                                  vitamins, minerals, and trace
  Cu 0.5 mg                                  elements will be the same as for
  Mn 0.4 mg                                  CPN†
  Cr 5.0 mcg

Daily Volume and Rate             Fat Emulsion
_____ 1 L at 42 ml/hr         10%/20% (circle one)
_____ 1.5 L at 63 ml/hr       250 ml/500 ml (circle one)
_____ 2 L at 83 ml/hr         Infuse at _____ ml/hr × _____ hrs.
_____ 2.5 L at 104 ml/hr      _____ q.d.
_____ 3 L at 125 ml/hr        _____ q.o.d.
                                    _____ Other _____
                                    Note: Each bottle of fat emulsion should not
                                    hang longer than 12 hrs.

Remarks:




Physician's Signature _____
```

*Peripheral parenteral nutrition
†Central parenteral nutrition
From: University of California—Davis, Medical Center, Sacramento.

A sample order for administration of the PPN regimen just described might read as follows:

> 3 L/day of 10% dextrose, 3% amino acid solution to run at 125 ml/hr. Infuse 500 ml 20% fat emulsion at 50 ml/hr via Y connector daily.

This TPN prescription would provide 90 g amino acids, 300 g dextrose, 1,000 kcal from fat emulsion (50% kcal), a fluid intake of 3.5 L per day, 2,020 nonprotein kcal per day (300 × 3.4 kcal/g + 1,000 kcal from fat emulsion = 2,020 kcal), and a nonpro kcal:N ratio of 140:1 (2,020/14.4 g N). The osmolarity of the dextrose–amino acid solution would be approximately 1,000 mOsm per L [(10 × 50) + (3 × 100) + (200)] = 1,000 mOsm/L, which is still too high for a peripheral infusion. However, the simultaneous coinfusion of fat emulsion would reduce the osmolarity by approximately 50 percent. This PPN regimen would be more expensive than the CPN regimen just outlined and would require infusion of 3.5 L per day compared to 2.25 L per day with CPN.

This procedure for calculating an individualized parenteral feeding is quite involved and is usually done within the pharmacy department when indicated. The dietitian needs to be aware of the limitations in calculating a parenteral feeding in order both to appreciate what is feasible for the patient to receive in terms of nutritional support and to calculate a patient's nutrient intake when receiving varying parenteral feeding. Form O is a sample routine order sheet similar to those used in many institutions. Examples are included for standard CPN and PPN solutions.

TO TEST YOUR UNDERSTANDING

9. How do CPN and PPN differ in regard to the following factors?

   Duration of PN support needed
   Calorie needs
   Septic risk
   Fluid status

PROTOCOLS FOR PARENTERAL NUTRITION

INITIATION AND DISCONTINUATION OF PARENTERAL FEEDING

Parenteral-feeding infusions are started slowly, and the total daily fluid load is gradually increased. This helps ensure patient tolerance to the lipid emulsion, concentrated dextrose solution, and total volume of infusion. Initiation methods differ, but 1 L of standard solution is usually given in the first 24 hours. If that is well tolerated, the amount is increased by 1 L per day until the desired daily amount is being delivered. Specific orders pertaining to the initiation of parenteral feeding are usually written for the nursing staff and include the following (16):

1. Check vital signs, including temperature, q 4 to 6 hr.
2. Record body weight daily.
3. Record volume of fluid intake and output daily on PN flow sheet.
4. Perform urine spot checks for glucose and ketones q shift.
5. Change IV tubing daily according to TPN protocol.
6. Change central catheter dressing q 48 hr according to TPN protocol.
7. Notify MD of temperature ≥38°C or 2+ urine glucose.

Discontinuation of parenteral feeding should be gradual to avoid hypoglycemia. This is often accomplished by decreasing the administration rate by half (for example, 83 ml/hr to 42 ml/hr, for 1 to 2 hrs, then decreasing the rate to 20 ml/hr for 1 to 2 hrs). If TPN is to be discontinued, standard IV solution may be utilized at this point. Insulin levels will usually drop within 1 to 2 hours after the cessation of concentrated carbohydrate infusion. Patients should be monitored for clinical symptoms of hypoglycemia during the weaning period.

COMPLICATIONS ASSOCIATED WITH PARENTERAL FEEDING

In general, complications associated with PPN have tended to be fewer and less serious than those resulting from CPN. A common complication with PPN is infiltration at the catheter site, necessitating placement in a new peripheral venous site.

Complications arising from CPN fall into two major categories: catheter-related problems and metabolic abnormalities (16). One of the most common catheter-related problems is *catheter sepsis*, a bloodstream infection that originates from a contaminated catheter or catheter site, contaminated PN solution, or both. Other catheter-related problems that may arise during central vein cannulation include pneumothorax, air embolus, catheter malposition, and arterial puncture or subclavian vein laceration, which may lead to hemothorax or hematoma.

Metabolic problems associated with parenteral

TABLE 13-7. Possible Metabolic Complications of TPN and Their Management

Complication	Characterized By	Usual Cause	Treatment
Hyperammonemia	Elevated blood ammonia levels Somnolence Lethargy Seizures Coma	Hepatic dysfunction Deficiency in urea cycle amino acids	Slow infusion rate Discontinue infusion
Hyperchloremic metabolic acidosis	Decrease in blood pH Decrease in serum $[HCO_3{}^-]$ Decrease in blood [base excess] Increase in serum $[Cl^-]$ Increase in serum $[Na^+]$	Excessive renal or gastrointestinal losses of base Infusion of preformed hydrogen ion Cationic amino acids greater than the concentration of anionic amino acids in TPN solution excessive chloride TPN solution	Decrease chloride excess in TPN solution by exchanging chloride ion with acetate ion
Hyperglycemia	Elevated blood glucose Glycosuria	Carbohydrate intolerance, too rapid an initiation of TPN Infection Diabetes mellitus	Decrease rate of administration Search for infection Consider insulin
Hyperosmolar nonketotic dehydration	Hyperglycemia Dehydration Increase in serum osmolality and serum sodium Somnolence Seizures Coma	Failure to recognize initial hyperglycemia and increased glucose in urine	Give insulin to correct hyperglycemia Give 5% dextrose and hypotonic saline (¼ to ½ strength), rather than TPN solution, to correct free water deficit Continue to monitor serum glucose osmolality, and sodium and potassium, and urine glucose
Hypoglycemia	Hypothermia Somnolence or lethargy Peripheral vasoconstriction	Usually due to interruption of TPN solution infusion and can be avoided by gradual withdrawal	Immediately begin appropriate dextrose infusion Monitor serum glucose and potassium
Hypokalemia	Muscular weakness Cardiac arrhythmias Altered digitalis sensitivity	Excessive gastrointestinal or urinary potassium losses deficit of potassium in TPN solution	Increase potassium concentration in TPN solution based on patient's requirements
Hypomagnesemia	Vertigo Weakness Positive Chvostek sign Convulsive seizures with or without tetany	Insufficient magnesium in TPN solution Excessive gastrointestinal or renal losses	Increase magnesium in TPN solution In an emergency, give $MgSO_4$ solution intramuscularly
Hyponatremia	Lethargy Confusion	Excessive gastrointestinal or urinary sodium losses; water intoxication Adequate sodium TPN Solution	Increase sodium concentration in TPN solution based on patient's requirements; limit free water intake to treat water intoxication
Hypophosphatemia	Paresthesia Mental confusion Hyperventilation Lethargy Decreased RBC function	Usually due to inadequate inorganic phosphate in TPN solution (concentrated glucose infusion may precipitate syndrome)	Add phosphate to TPN solution In an emergency give potassium phosphate slowly, mixed well with peripheral 5% dextrose solutions (Note: Rapid correction of hypophosphatemia may cause hypocalcemic tetany)
Prerenal azotemia	Lassitude Accumulation of nonprotein nitrogen in blood	Dehydration (possible hyperosmolar type) Calorie nitrogen imbalance	Correct free water deficit Give insulin if patient is hyperglycemic Increase nonprotein calories to achieve calorie: nitrogen ratio of about 185:1

feeding include both hyper- and hypoglycemia, glycosuria, compromised respiratory function, mineral and electrolyte abnormalities, elevation of hepatic enzymes, and trace element deficiency syndromes. Table 13-7 outlines specific metabolic complications of PN and their management.

Aseptic catheter placement, regular catheter care performed by trained personnel, aseptic preparation and delivery of parenteral feedings, and careful patient monitoring are all important if the complications of parenteral nutrition are to be minimized.

MONITORING FOR METABOLIC FUNCTION DURING PARENTERAL FEEDING

Results of a series of laboratory tests should be obtained regularly in order to detect the metabolic complications of PN (16):

1. Measure electrolytes and blood urea nitrogen (BUN) daily for the first week of parenteral feeding to monitor adequacy of hydration, renal function, and electrolyte balance. Serum calcium, phosphorus, and magnesium should be measured until blood levels stabilize.
2. Measure blood glucose levels daily and spot check urine for glucose and acetone. The detection of 2+ or 3+ glycosuria should prompt blood glucose determination and possible insulin supplementation of the parenteral-feeding solution.
3. Monitor liver enzymes—serum glutamic oxaloacetic transaminase (SGOT) or serum glutamic pyruvic transaminase (SGPT), lactic hydrogenase (LDH), and alkaline phosphatase—and serum bilirubin every 3 to 4 days to detect hepatic dysfunction related to the TPN.
4. Monitor weight daily for fluid overload. Weight gain of 1.5 kg per week or less is expected from intensive PN therapy. Weight gain above this amount probably indicates fluid and sodium retention.
5. Monitor plasma triglyceride levels to assess capacity to clear fat emulsion.

Once the course of parenteral nutrition is stable, a biweekly or weekly venipuncture schedule can be followed to monitor these parameters. Blood should not be drawn directly from the TPN catheter line for routine laboratory studies unless a Hickman catheter is used.

THE HICKMAN CATHETER

The use of long-term CPN has been facilitated by the development, in 1975 by Hickman, of a 1.6-mm silicone rubber catheter. The Hickman catheter is designed for prolonged central venous cannulation and is widely used for long-term TPN, especially home TPN, in both adults and children. Other uses of the catheter for both inpatients and outpatients include infusion of chemotherapy, antibiotic therapy, and blood products, and repeated blood sampling.

The Hickman catheter is normally inserted into the cephalic vein and threaded into the superior vena cava. The other end of the catheter is threaded through a subcutaneous tunnel and exits the skin between the sternum and the nipple. This subcutaneous tunneling of the Hickman catheter has reduced the incidence of both catheter-related sepsis and catheter displacement. The dressing-change procedure for the catheter exit site is a simple (sterile) technique that patients can perform at home.

One of the biggest advantages of the Hickman catheter is that blood sampling, medication, and CPN infusion can be done in the same line, provided that careful technique is observed. This greatly increases the comfort of the patient, who does not have to undergo repeated venipuncture. The Hickman catheter is commonly used in pediatrics, especially for cases of cancer, such as childhood leukemia, for which long-term chemotherapy and TPN support may be indicated (17).

ROLE OF THE NUTRITIONAL CARE SPECIALIST IN PARENTERAL FEEDING

The nutritional care specialist's contribution to the management of the parenterally nourished patient will vary with the institution and the existence and composition of a nutrition support team. The responsibility for assessing nutrient needs and designing the parenteral-feeding solution is often divided between the pharmacist and the dietitian. One common function is for the dietitian to evaluate whether a parenteral-feeding regimen is nutritionally adequate for a given patient.

The nutritionist must document information in the medical record relevant to the nutritional management of the parenterally fed patient. This includes an assessment of nutrient needs, actual nutrient intake, and parameters reflecting the nutritional response of the patient to the parenteral-feeding regimen. Flow sheets are often utilized to record nutrient intake and nutritional response data so that patterns can be recognized quickly and acted on promptly.

One area in which the nutritionist's input is essential is the transition of a patient from parenteral to enteral feeding. Depending on whether the patient has been consuming oral feedings during parenteral feeding, this may or may not be a big change. Patients are generally not hungry when receiving adequate parenteral support, although they miss the act of eating. Parenteral feedings are usually gradually decreased to stimulate the appetite, and enteral feedings are increased. A tube feeding or specialized nutrient composition, or both, may be indicated by the patient's condition once parenteral feeding is discontinued (see Chapter 22). It is essential that the ability to tolerate enteral feeding be established before parenteral feeding is discontinued. The dietitian is key in establishing the capacity of the patient to consume a target nutrient intake and also in recommending an appropriate transitional oral-feeding program.

TO TEST YOUR UNDERSTANDING

10. A young male patient is admitted to an intensive care unit suffering from trauma as a result of gang-related violence. The patient is 5 feet, 6 inches tall, weighs 155 pounds, and was otherwise healthy PTA. The patient is placed on the following CPN order on day 5 of admission: 2 L per day composed of 500 ml $D_{25}W$, 500 ml 7 percent amino acids and standard additives per L, plus 200 ml 10 percent Liposyn. You are asked to evaluate the nutritional adequacy of the prescribed parenteral-feeding regimen.

    a. You make an assessment of the patient's nutrient needs as follows. (Use ranges of values where appropriate.)

kcal: _____ kcal/kg, _____ kcal/day
fluid: _____ ml/kg, _____ L fluid/day
pro: _____ gm/kg, _____ g pro/day
fat: _____ minimum kcal from EFA, corresponding to
_____ ml 10% soybean oil emulsion, or _____ ml
10% safflower/soybean oil emulsion.

The maximum number of kcal from fat which would be tolerated: _____ kcal
The maximum number of g of dextrose per day which would be tolerated _____ kcal

    b. Compare your calculation of the patient's needs with the prescribed TPN regimen as follows:

	Calculated Needs	Prescribed Intake (from part a)	Adequacy
Nonpro kcal/day			
L fluid/day			
g pro/day			
Nonpro kcal:g of N			
Nonpro kcal as fat (4% to 60% minimum-maximum range)			
g dextrose/day (maximum tolerated)			

    c. How would you recommend that the parenteral-feeding regimen be changed: Give specific values for reformulating the TPN regimen.

    d. Write a SOAP note summarizing your assessment and recommendations.

PEDIATRIC PARENTERAL NUTRITION

Parenteral feeding is widely used in pediatrics, particularly in neonatology. Different standards are used to assess parenteral nutrient needs in children weighing less than 30 kg (18). The indications, complications, and monitoring parameters for parenteral nutrition are generally similar for pediatric and adult patients. For children, jugular or subclavian central venous catheters are usually used. In low-birth-weight infants, especially those weighing less than 1,500 g, catheters are sometimes placed in an umbilical blood vessel.

ASSESSING NUTRIENT NEEDS FOR PEDIATRIC PARENTERAL FEEDING

Calorie needs can be established for children over 10 years of age by using the Harris-Benedict equations to determine BEE, and then applying appropriate factors as discussed for adults. In infants (0 to 12 months), a different equation (19) should be used to determine BEE to allow for calories needed for growth:

$$\text{kcal/24 hr} = 22.10 - (31.05 \times W) - (1.16 \times H)$$

where W = weight in kg, and H = height in cm.   **(13-1)**

Another approach is to express a range of BEE requirements in kcal/kg as shown in Table 13-8. BEE is then multiplied by a stress factor (1.25 = mild stress,

TABLE 13-8. Basal Energy Expenditure for the Pediatric Population

Age	BEE (kcal/kg)*
VLBW† (<1,500 g)	85–120
0–1 year	90–120
1–8 years	70–100
8–12 years	60–75
12–18 years	45–60

*Daily energy needs = BEE × stress factor (SF). SF = 1.25 (mild), 1.50 (nutritional depletion) and 2.00 (high stress)

†Very low birth weight

TABLE 13.9. Fluid Requirements for Infants and Children

Age	Requirement
LBW* (<2,500 g)	1. Initiate 80 ml/kg; progress to 100–110 ml/kg 2. By end of first week of life 120–150 ml/kg 3. By end of second week of life 150 ml/kg
0–12 months	100–125 ml/kg/day
Older children Weight	
1–10 kg	100 ml/kg/day
11–20 kg	an additional 50 ml/each kg over 10
21 kg or more	an additional 25 ml/each kg over 20

*Low birth weight

1.50 = nutritional depletion, and 2.0 = high stress) to determine total calorie needs. BEE includes an allowance for growth in young children.

Protein requirements range from 1.5 to 3.5 g per kg, with approximately 3.0 g per kg per day required in the very-low-birth-weight (VLBW) infant (<1,500 g), 2.0 to 2.5 g per kg per day from 0 to 12 months in the normal-weight infant, 1.5 to 2.0 g per kg per day from 1 to 8 years and 1.0 to 1.5 g per kg per day from 8 to 15 years. Nonpro kcal:N ratios should be similar to adult levels.

Fluid requirements for infants and children can be calculated using the guidelines in Table 13-9.

Carbohydrate in the form of dextrose is the principal calorie source, as it is for adults. A maximum infusion rate of 6 mg dextrose per kg per min or 8.6 g per kg per day is recommended.

Fat should not exceed 60 percent of daily calories, with a range of 2.0 to 4.0 g per kg per day depending on age and tolerance. Infants, including those of VLBW, should not receive greater than 2 g of fat per kg per day, while older children may tolerate higher doses. Fat emulsion is contraindicated in infants with hyperbilirubinemia, thrombocytopenia, and cases of hyperlipidemia, and should be used with caution in VLBW babies and patients with liver disease.

Electrolyte supplementation can be determined using average recommendations (17).

Vitamin and *trace element* requirements are not well established for premature infants but are generally similar to those of term infants. Recommendations for daily vitamin and trace element supplementation for infants weighing over 3 kg and for children up to 11 years of age are presented in Table 13-10.

Several approaches can be taken to parenteral vitamin supplementation. Methods of supplementation include 10 ml per day of MVI Pediatric, 10 ml per day of MVI-12, or 1 ml per day of MVI concentrate. The composition of these multivitamin preparations is outlined in Table 13-10. Folate and vitamin B_{12} are added separately to the parenteral solutions if MVI concentrate is used. Vitamin K and iron are usually given intramuscularly if supplementation is indicated. Trace elements are also added separately to the infusion mixture.

REFERENCES

1. DUDRICK, S.J., D.W. WILMORE, H.M. VARS, AND J.E. RHOADS. Long-term total parenteral nutrition with growth, development and positive nitrogen balance. *Surgery* 64:(1960)134–142.

2. MAILLET, J.O. Calculating parenteral feedings: A programmed instruction. *J.A.D.A.* 84:(1984)1312–1323.

3. ZEMAN, F.J. *Clinical Nutrition and Dietetics.* New York: Macmillan, 1983.

TABLE 13-10. Daily Vitamin and Trace Element Requirements for Infants Weighing at Least 3 kg and Children to 11 Years

Nutrient	Requirement	MVI Concentrate (1 ml)	MVI-12 (10 ml)
Thiamin (B_1)	1.2 mg	10.0 mg	3.0 mg
Riboflavin (B_2)	1.4 mg	2.0 mg	3.6 mg
Niacinamide	17.0 mg	20.0 mg	40.0 mg
Pyridoxine (B_6)	1.0 mg	3.0 mg	4.0 mg
Ascorbic Acid (C)	80.0 mg	100.0 mg	100.0 mg
Vitamin A	2,300.0 IU	2,000.0 IU	3,300.0 IU
Vitamin D	400.0 IU	200.0 IU	200.0 IU
Vitamin E	7.0 IU	1.0 IU	10.0 IU
Pantothenic acid	5.0 mg	0	15.0 mg
Folic acid	140.0 μg	0	400.0 μg
Vitamin B_{12}	1.0 μg	0	5.0 μg
Vitamin K	0.2 μg	0	0
Biotin	20.0 μg	0	60.0 μg
Trace elements:			
Zinc	100.0 μg/kg	—	—
Copper	20.0 μg/kg	—	—
Chromium	0.14–0.2 μg/kg	—	—
Manganese	2.0–10.0 μg/kg	—	—

4. LONG, C.L. AND W.S. BLAKEMORE. Energy and protein requirements in the hospitalized patient. *JPEN* 3:(1979)69–71.

5. LONG, C.L., N. SCHAFFEL, AND J.W. GEIGER. Metabolic response to injury and illness: Estimation of energy and protein needs from indirect calorimetry and nitrogen balance. *JPEN* 3:(1979)452–456.

6. GOSS, J.C., P. EGGING, AND K. DOBYNS. Nutritional support of the stressed surgical patient. *Nutritional Support Services* 4:(1984)28–30.

7. WEINSIER. R.L. AND C.L. KRUMDIECK. Death resulting from overzealous total parenteral nutrition: The refeeding syndrome revisited. *Am. J. Clin. Nutr.* 34:(1980)393–399.

8. WOLFE, R.R., T.F. O'DONNELL, M.D. STONE, D.A. RICHMOND, AND J.F. BURKE. Investigation of factors determining the optimal glucose infusion rate in total parenteral nutrition. *Metabolism* 29:(1980)892–900.

9. GOODENOUGH, R.O. AND R.R. WOLFE. Effect of total parenteral nutrition on free fatty acid metabolism in burned patients. *JPEN* 8:(1984)357–360.

10. WOLFE, B.M. AND D.M. NEY. Lipid metabolism in parenteral nutrition. In *Parenteral Nutrition*, eds. J.L. Rombeau and M.D. Caldwell. Philadelphia: Saunders, 1986, pp. 72–99.

11. AMERICAN MEDICAL ASSOCIATION DEPARTMENT OF FOODS AND NUTRITION. Multivitamin preparations for parenteral use. *JPEN* 3:(1979)258–262.

12. AMERICAN MEDICAL ASSOCIATION DEPARTMENT OF FOODS AND NUTRITION. Guidelines for essential trace element preparations for parenteral use. *JPEN* 2:(1979)263–267.

13. McCLAIN, C.J. Trace metal abnormalities in adults during hyperalimentation. *JPEN* 5:(1981)424–429.

14. Parenteral Nutrition Therapy. In *Manual of Nutritional Therapeutics*, eds. D.H. Alpers, R.E. Clouse, and W.F. Stenson. Boston: Little, Brown, 1983, pp. 233–267.

15. ISAACS, J.W., W.J. MILLIKAN, AND J. STACKHOUSE. Parenteral nutrition of adults with a 900 milliosmolar solution via peripheral veins. *Am. J. Clin. Nutr.* 30:(1977)552–559.

16. HOOLEY, R.A. Parenteral Nutrition—General Concepts, Part 1. *Nutritional Support Services* 1:(1981)36–37.

17. WHEELER, N. Parenteral Nutrition. In *Manual of Pediatric Nutrition*, eds. D.G. Kelts and E.G. Jones. Boston: Little, Brown 1984, pp. 151–165.

18. KHALIDI, N., A.G. CORAN, AND J.R. WESLEY. Guidelines for parenteral nutrition in children. *Nutritional Support Services* 4:27–28, 1984.

19. CALDWELL, M.D. AND C.C. KENNEDY. Normal nutritional requirements. *Surg. Clin. North. Am.* 61:(1981)491–498.

14

Nutritional Care of Allergic Patients

Food allergies are usually diagnosed and treated on an outpatient basis. The function of the nutritional care specialist is to interview and counsel the patient. This counseling often includes a considerable amount of instruction on food composition and preparation, so the nutritionist must be knowledgeable about these matters. Skills in patient interviewing and counseling, which are covered in Chapters 3 and 6, are extremely important.

Occasionally, an allergy patient is hospitalized. Those with respiratory manifestations are particularly sensitive to infections. In addition, any hospital patient with any diagnosis may also have food allergies. It is the nutritional care specialist's responsibility to ensure that all patients who have food allergies are served an appropriate diet in which needs for all conditions are considered.

Nutritional care of allergic conditions may be directed toward prevention of sensitization, toward diagnosis, including identification of specific antigens, or toward management. Prior to proceeding with this chapter, you should review the anatomy and physiology of the immune system and the discussion of hypersensitivity in your text.

PREVENTION OF SENSITIZATION

Preventive actions are primarily directed toward genetically vulnerable infants—that is, those whose parents or siblings have a history of allergy. There is some evidence that infants can be sensitized in utero (1). As a precaution, patients at risk can be advised to avoid a preponderance of any particular food during pregnancy. Instead, a mixed diet without emphasis on a limited number of foods is recommended. This advice should apply particularly to those foods which are known to be especially allergenic. These are listed in Table 14-1.

After birth, breast feeding *exclusively* is the pro-

cedure most recommended for prevention of hypersensitivity in the infant. The length of time that the infant's diet should consist solely of breast milk is unknown. Commonly, a minimum of 4 to 6 months is recommended. The infant may be given added water to satisfy thirst (2) but no other food or fluid. Partial breast feeding is sometimes continued up to or after 1 year of age.

At the age of 4 to 6 months, the baby may be given cereal, fruit, vegetables, and meat in the amounts and consistency described in Chapter 8. The introduction of the foods within these groups that are common allergens may be delayed further. For example, the introduction of cereal may begin with rice since it is less often allergenic than are the other cereals commonly fed to infants. Following the introduction of rice, other cereals are added at intervals, with wheat, a common allergen, added last. Cereals should also be added one at a time so that the offending allergen may

TABLE 14-1. Common Food Allergens

Infants	Children 2 Years +	Older Children and Adults
Cow's milk	Cow's milk	Cow's milk
	Chocolate/cola	Chocolate/cola
	Wheat	Corn
	Corn	Legumes
		Egg (whites)
		Citrus
		Tomato
		Wheat
		Pork
		Cinnamon
		Fish
		Nuts

Compiled from: Breneman, J.C. *Basics of Food Allergy.* Springfield, Ill.: Charles C. Thomas, 1978; Lawlor, G.J., Jr., and T.J. Fisher. *Manual of Allergy and Immunology.* Boston: Little, Brown, 1981; Speer, F. *Food Allergy* (2d ed.). Boston: John Wright, PSG Inc., 1984.

be identified if allergic symptoms arise. Consequently, the use of mixed cereals for infants at risk should be discouraged. Similarly, when fruits and vegetables are given, applesauce, pears, carrots, and squash may be given early, with others added later. Mixtures should not be used until it is established that the infant is not sensitive to any of the individual components. Lamb is commonly used as the first meat. Vitamins for infants at risk should be uncolored (2); the reason for this will become clear later in this chapter. Eggs and citrus juices are often avoided until the infant is a year old.

Several problems can arise in connection with the protocol just described. There is evidence that infants may be sensitized to allergens in breast milk (3). Some allergic reactions have been reported to occur after the mother ate oranges, eggs, chocolate, cow's milk, strawberries, tomatoes, chocolate, apples, bananas, coffee, or tea (4). When such reactions occur, the lactating mother must be counseled on avoiding the allergen. If many foods are restricted, she must also be given advice on planning a diet for herself which is adequate for lactation. (See Chapter 7.)

A special formula is required if the infant is allergic to cow's milk, and if the mother is unable to breast feed or if the infant has a condition, such as lactose intolerance, which precludes breast feeding (4). An artificial formula that is tolerated by the infant must be used. There are several types of these (5):

1. *Casein hydrolysate–based formulas* have low allergenicity. Some are also lactose-free. Specific examples are given in Table 8-4.

2. *Soy protein–based formulas* may be useful, but must be chosen from those that are calcium- and vitamin-supplemented. (See Table 8-4.) In addition, some infants develop a sensitivity to soy (6).

3. *Goat's milk* is sometimes useful, but it has several limitations. It has an excessively high solute load for infants and must be supplemented with vitamins A, D, C, B_{12}, and folate. If it is purchased fresh, it must be boiled for 2 minutes to render it bacteriologically safe and to reduce allergenicity. However, it is also available canned or dried in some areas. In any form, goat's milk contains lactose, a problem for some infants with gastrointestinal allergy or other accompanying disorder.

TO TEST YOUR UNDERSTANDING

1. You are counseling a pregnant patient who has been sent to you by an obstetrician for information on a normal, adequate diet. The patient, Mrs. H., is 25 years old, 5 feet, 4 inches tall, and weighs 110 pounds. She is 2½ months pregnant.

    Mrs. H. is a teacher in a nursery school with 50 children and must be quite active. She also tells you that she has suffered from hay fever for 10 years. Her husband develops hives when he eats shellfish and strawberries. Neither has any other abnormal condition.

    A 24-hour recall gives you the following meal pattern, which the patient states is typical of her week days. On the weekends and holidays, she does not eat the snacks.

    Breakfast:
    4 oz orange juice
    Scrambled eggs (2)
    Sweet roll
    8 oz milk
    Coffee/sugar

    Snack (with children at school):
    8 oz carton of milk
    2 graham crackers

    Lunch (eaten with children at school):
    ¾ c cream of tomato soup
    1½ egg salad sandwich on whole-wheat bread
    Baked custard
    8 oz milk

    Snack (with children at school):
    8 oz carton of milk
    2 oatmeal cookies

Dinner:

4 oz meat loaf
½ c broccoli with ¼ c Hollandaise sauce
Sliced tomato salad/Thousand Island dressing
⅙ lemon meringue pie
Tea/lemon/sugar

a. State the basic principle(s) on which your nutritional counseling will be based.

b. The patient is required fo eat lunch with the children at the nursery school. She cannot change the menu, but it is posted a week in advance so that she knows what the meals will consist of. Indicate at the right of the menu in part a how you would suggest she modify her breakfast and dinner. Suggest two alternative box lunches for days that the school menu does not offer appropriate choices.

c. Mrs. H. is later referred to you by a pediatrician. She now has a baby boy who is 6 weeks old. Although she has been breast feeding him, she says this is too limiting on her freedom and wants to stop. What would you suggest to her and why?

DIAGNOSIS

The signs and symptoms of food allergy include many that are nonspecific, including vomiting and diarrhea as well as rashes, itching, coughing, irritability, and anemia. It is therefore necessary for the physician to differentiate food allergy from a number of other conditions. Once the condition is diagnosed as an allergy, it is necessary to determine whether the patient is sensitive to food or to pollens, drugs, or other materials. Last, the specific food antigen must be identified. The nutritional care specialist can have an important role first in confirming or disproving the existence of suspected food allergy and then in identifying the food allergen.

Diagnostic approaches include a thorough physical examination, some laboratory tests, and a detailed clinical history, of which the diet history is an important component (7). If these methods are inconclusive, diagnostic diets may be used.

PHYSICAL EXAMINATION

The physical examination includes careful observation for signs characteristic of allergy. It may be helpful in differential diagnosis to rule out other conditions, but is not generally useful in identifying specific food antigens. The physical examination also identifies malnutrition and other effects secondary to allergy.

LABORATORY TESTS

The *radioallergosorbent test* (RAST) measures the level of IgE or other immunoglobulins. The test is expensive, measures free (but not cell-bound) IgE, and cannot measure the extent of release of mediators (8). A positive test must be confirmed by dietary challenge tests, which will be described later. A variety of other tests of immune function are even less useful (7,9).

CLINICAL HISTORY

The clinical history is often the most useful diagnostic procedure. Information is obtained, usually by the physician, about the following:

nature and severity of symptoms
age of onset
possible precipitating factors
time relationship between exposure to any suspected antigen and onset of symptoms
other allergic phenomena

DIET HISTORY

The diet history may be useful both in ruling out or confirming food allergy and in identifying the allergen. To accomplish these objectives, it is necessary for the nutritional care specialist to interview the patient thoroughly and to have a detailed knowledge of foods.

The diet history interview must include a number of questions requiring detailed answers. In allergy clinics, a questionnaire form is used as a guide. Table 14-2 lists information often needed and can give you an idea of the amount of detail required.

The Food Diary

If the identity of the food allergen is not obvious to the patient and cannot be established by analysis of the diet history, the patient may be asked to keep a food diary. The number of days for which the diary should be kept will depend on the frequency of the symptoms. There must be enough days on which symptoms occur to make it possible to establish the relationship to intake of specific foods.

Unless the nutritional care specialist provides detailed directions to the patient, the procedure will be useless. The information required is similar to that

TABLE 14-2. Areas of Inquiry in the Diet History for Suspected Food Allergy

Food-Related Questions
1. List foods eaten, with frequency and amount.
2. For each food, was it home prepared? If so, describe ingredients.
3. If foods were eaten away from home, where were they obtained? Give brands and specific ingredients.
4. Was each food eaten cooked or raw?
5. Were artificial colors or flavors used in food preparation?
6. Describe the meal pattern; include the time, amount, and frequency of food intake.
7. Are any foods eaten in especially large quantities?
8. Do other family members have allergies? To foods? Which foods? Does the patient eat these foods?
9. Do symptoms develop from smelling or handling certain foods?

Other Related Questions
1. List symptoms and time of onset.
2. Do symptoms develop only in certain locations or during certain activities?
3. Does the patient chew gum? When? How often? Brand?
4. What cleaning compounds are used, including soaps, detergents, and scouring powders for dishwashing?
5. List all drugs, cosmetics, and personal hygiene products and give brand names, and time and frequency of use. Include information on toothpaste, mouthwash, lipstick, throat lozenges, prescription drugs, laxatives, and other over-the-counter drugs.
6. Is the patient under constant or recurrent emotional stress?

listed in Table 14-2. The time of intake of each food or other ingestant must also be noted, along with the time of onset and a description of symptoms. This procedure should be undertaken only if the diet history is not helpful since interpretation is time-consuming and difficult.

DIAGNOSTIC DIETS

A number of diets have been used for diagnosis of food hypersensitivity. In general, they can be classified as *food challenges* or *elimination diets*. These may be necessary if other methods are uninformative or inconclusive.

Food Challenge Tests

When an allergy to a specific food is suspected based on a diet history or food diary, the diagnosis may be tested by a food challenge. It is helpful if a diet free of all suspect foods can be followed first with the objective of having all symptoms subside. Preferably, the challenge test is a "double blind" test, in which neither the patient nor the physician knows what has been given. In an ideal situation, used when the patient is an older child or an adult, a third person places either dextrose or a dehydrated form of the suspected allergen in nonallergenic capsules. The patient is then given one or the other type of capsule and is observed for signs of allergic reaction. Since neither the patient nor the physician knows if the patient has received the allergen, the observation can be quite objective. If this

method is not possible, a "single blind" test can be conducted, in which the patient, but not the physician, is unaware of the material given. For small children, the suspected offending food can be hidden in another nonoffending food. In any case, all medications, especially antihistamines and corticosteroids, should be discontinued 1 week before the test. Patients with anaphylactic responses should not be challenged.

The challenge test may be repeated with gradually increasing doses up to 8 g. If this is tolerated, the food is given openly in large amounts conventionally prepared to evaluate the effects of preparation procedures. It may also be repeated at intervals to see if the child has "outgrown" the allergy.

Elimination Diets

Elimination diets may eliminate a few or many foods from the diet. The simplest type is *elimination of a single suspected food*. This is a useful procedure when only one food is suspected. In a child, for example, the parents may suspect a sensitivity to milk, wheat, or eggs, all common antigens in children. Since these foods are often hidden within processed foods, you will need to counsel the patient or the patient's parents on procedures for total elimination of the foods from the diet. Further information on specific foods to eliminate is given later in this chapter in the section on treatment.

When a single food has not been identified as the culprit and the antigens have not been identified, a diet might be formulated to eliminate those foods which, by previous experience, are known to have a high probability of allergenicity. The diet, sometimes called a *probability multiple-elimination diet*, eliminates common offenders for 2 to 3 weeks. If there is improvement in the symptoms, the foods eliminated are reintroduced one at a time as a challenge to identify the antigenic foods.

A difficulty may arise in deciding which foods to eliminate. Opinions differ about which foods are common offenders. There is general agreement, however, that milk is an important one, particularly in children. The list of common offenders (Table 14-1) should be coupled with the clinical and diet histories and the food diary in deciding which foods to eliminate.

If this procedure does not identify the allergen, a more stringent elimination diet may be required. A number of variations of this type of diet have been published. The principle common to all is that each consists of a limited number of foods chosen primarily from those which have been shown by past experience to be allergenic only rarely. At the same time, a sufficient number of foods must be included to make possible a diet adequate in protein and calories and to provide a little variety for acceptability. Since the number of foods allowed are quite limited, however, compliance is improved if you provide some guidance on methods of preparation and meal planning. The pa-

TABLE 14-3. Examples of Foods Allowed with Typical Elimination Diets

Rowe elimination diet #1	*Rowe elimination diet #2*	*Rowe elimination diet #3*	*Rowe elimination diet #4*
Cereals			
Rice	Corn	Tapioca	
Puffed Rice	Rye	Breads of any combination of	
Rice Flakes	Corn pone	soy, lima bean, potato starch	
Rice Krispies	Corn-rye muffin	and tapioca flours	
Tapioca	Ry-Krisp		
Rice biscuit			
Rice bread			
Vegetables			
Lettuce	Beets	White potato	
Chard	Squash	Tomato	
Spinach	Asparagus	Carrot	
Carrot	Artichoke	Lima beans	
Sweet Potato		String beans	
Yam		Peas	
Fruit or Juice			
Lemon	Pineapple	Apricot	
Grapefruit	Peach	Grapefruit	
Pear	Apricot	Peace	
	Prune		
Meat			
Lamb	Capon (no hens)	Beef	
	Bacon	Bacon	
Other			
Cane sugar	Cane or beet sugar	Cane sugar	Cane sugar
Maple sugar	Karo corn syrup	Maple sugar	Milk
Cane sugar syrup flavored with	Sesame oil	Cane sugar syrup flavored with	Cream
maple	Mazola oil	maple	Plain cottage cheese
Sesame oil	Gelatin, plain or flavored with	Sesame oil	Tapioca
Olive oil	pineapple	Soybean oil	
Gelatin, plain or flavored with	Salt	Gelatin, plain or flavored with	
lime or lemon	Baking powder	lime or lemon	
Salt	Baking soda	Salt	
Baking powder	Cream of tartar	Baking powder	
Baking soda	Vanilla extract	Baking soda	
Cream of tartar	White vinegar	Cream of tartar	
Vanilla extract		Vanilla extract	
Required Supplements			
1) multivitamin supplement	multivitamin supplement	multivitamin supplement	multivitamin supplement
2) 1 tbsp bid Calcium-Sandoz	1 tbsp bid Calcium-Sandoz	1 tbsp bid Calcium-Sandoz	
Syrup	Syrup	Syrup	

tient is also likely to need supplementation of vitamins and minerals in a hypoallergenic form.

Some suggested combinations of allowable foods that have been used as elimination diets are shown in Table 14-3. Those given are well known as *Rowe elimination diets*, named after their originator. Since all foods are potentially allergenic, there is no guarantee that all symptoms will subside in all patients. If symptoms do not subside with one diet, another composed of a different combination of foods may be tried. For infants, elimination diets may consist of the following foods:

Less than 3 months—milk substitute

3–6 months—milk substitute & rice cereal

6–24 months—milk substitute, rice cereal, applesauce, pears, carrots, squash, and lamb.

If the diet results in improvement of symptoms, foods can be added one at a time at intervals of 4 to 5 days, regardless of the patient's age. Any food that causes the patient's previous symptoms to reappear should be eliminated from the diet. The response might be tested again in 6 to 12 months.

OTHER CONSIDERATIONS IN IDENTIFYING ALLERGENS

Biological Classification

A patient who is hypersensitive to a food may also be hypersensitive to other foods in the same *biological classification*. Allergic patients should be tested for sensitivity to biologically related foods, which are shown in Table 14-4.

Intolerances to Food Additives and Other Foods

It has been suggested that patients may have an allergy or other form of intolerance to additives used in food processing. Some of these additives include monosodium glutamate, metabisulfites, and sodium nitrate, but attention has tended to focus particularly on the artificial coloring agent tartrazine, or FD&C yellow No. 5, which is used in many processed foods and on salicylate, a structurally related compound which occurs naturally in some foods and in aspirin. Although the subject is controversial, some allergists use tartrazine-free and "salicylate-free" diets for diagnosis and treatment.

TABLE 14-4. Biological Classification of Foods

Family	Members
Plants	
Apple	Apple (cider, vinegar, apple pectin), pear, quince, loquat
Arrowroot	Arrowroot
Arum	Poi, taro
Banana	Banana, plantain
Beech	Chestnut, beechnut
Birch	Filbert, hazelnut, oil of birch (wintergreen)
Buckwheat	Buckwheat, rhubarb
Cactus	Tequila
Carob	Gum acacia
Cashew	Cashew, mango, pistachio
Citrus Fruits	Angostura, citron, grapefruit, kumquat, lemon, lime, orange, tangelo, tangerine
Cola nut, cacao	Coffee, chocolate, cola, cola drinks, tea
Cocheospurnum	Guiac gum, guar gum
Composite	Artichoke, chicory, dandelion, endive, escarole, head lettuce, leaf lettuce, oyster plant, sunflower, sesame, safflower, vermouth
Ebony	Persimmon
Fungi	Mushroom, yeast, antibiotics
Ginger	Cardamom, ginger, turmeric
Gooseberry	Currant, gooseberry
Goosefoot	Beet, beet sugar, spinach, Swiss chard
Gourd	Cantaloupe, casaba, cucumber honeydew, muskmelon, Persian melon, pumpkin, squash, watermelon, citron, vegetable marrow
Grains (Grass)	Barley, malt, cane (cane sugar, molasses, corn oil, glucose), corn (cornstarch), oats, rice, rye, sorghum, wheat (bran, gluten flour, graham flour, wheat germ), wild rice
Grape	Grape, cream of tartar, raisin
Heath	Blueberry, cranberry, huckleberry, loganberry
Honeysuckle	Elderberry
Iris	Saffron
Laurel	Avocado, bay leaves, cinnamon
Lycethis	Brazil nut
Legumes	Acacia, black-eyed peas, kidney bean, lentil, licorice, lima bean, navy bean, pea, peanut, peanut oil, senna, soybean, soybean oil, stringbean, gum tragacanth
Lily	Aloes, asparagus, chive, garlic, leek, onion, sarsaparilla
Mallow	Cottonseed, okra (gumbo)
Maple	Maple syrup (maple sugar)
Mint	Basil, marjoram, mint, oregano, peppermit, sage, savory, spearmint, thyme
Morning glory	Sweet potato, yam
Mulberry	Breadfruit, fig, hop, mulberry
Mustard	Broccoli, brussels sprouts, cabbage, cauliflower, celery cabbage, collard, cress, horseradish, kale, kohlrabi, mustard, radish, rutabaga, turnip, watercress
Myrtle	Allspice, bay, cloves, guava, paprika, pimento
Nutmeg	Nutmeg, mace
Olive	Green olive, ripe olive, olive oil
Orchid	Vanilla
Palm	Coconut, date, sago, palm oil
Papaw	Papaya, papain, papaw
Parsley	Angelica, anise, caraway, carrot, celeriac, celery, coriander, cumin, dill, fennel, parsley, parship
Pea	Bean, lentil, pea, peanut, soy, alfalfa, clover, licorice, tamarind
Pedalium	Sesame, sesame oil
Pepper	Black pepper, white pepper
Pineapple	Pineapple
Plum	Almond, apricot, cherry, nectarine, peach, persimmon, plum (prune), sloe (gin)
Pomegranate	Pomegranate
Poppy	Poppy seed
Potato (nightshade)	Chili, eggplant, green pepper, paprika, pimiento, potato, cayenne papper, red pepper, tomato
Rose	Apple, blackberry, dewberry, loganberry, loquat, quince, raspberry, strawberry, youngberry
Seaweed	Agar, longan
Spurge	Tapioca, cassava
Sterculia	Cacao (chocolate), kola bean, gum karaya
Sunflower	Jerusalem artichoke, sunflower seed oil, cardoon, chicory, endive, tarragon
Walnut	Black walnut, butternut, English walnut, hickory nut, pecan
Miscellaneous	Honey
Animals	
Crustaceans	Crab, crayfish, lobster, prawn, shrimp, squid
Fish (with fins)	Anchovy, barracuda, bass, bluefish, buffalo, bullhead, butterfish, carp, catfish, caviar, chub, codfish, croaker, cusk, corvina, drum, eel, flounder, haddock, hake, halibut, harvestfish, herring, mackerel, mullet, muskellunge, perch, pickerel, pike, pollack, pompano, porgy, rosefish, salmon, sardine, scrod, scup, shad, smelt, snapper, sole, sturgeon, sucker, sunfish, swordfish, trout, tuna, weakfish, whitefish
Fowl	Chicken (chicken eggs), duck (duck eggs), goose (goose eggs), grouse, guinea hen, partridge, pheasant, squab, turkey
Mammals	Beef (butter, cheese, cow's milk, gelatin, veal), goat (cheese, goat's milk), horsemeat, mutton (lamb), pork (bacon, ham), rabbit, sheep (lamb), squirrel, venison
Mollusks	Abalone, clam, cockle, mussel, oyster, scallop
Reptiles	Turtle

Compiled from Collins-Williams, C. and L.D. Levy, "Allergy to foods other than milk," in *Food Intolerance*, ed. R.K. Chandra (New York: Elsevier, 1983); Farrell, M.K., "Food Allergy" in *Manual of Allergy and Immunology*, eds. G.J. Lawlor Jr. and T.J. Fischer (Boston: Little, Brown, 1981). Sheldon, J.M., R.G. Louell, and K.P. Matthews, "Food and gastrointestinal allergy," in *A Manual of Clinical Allergy* (Philadelphia: Saunders, 1967). Monro, J. "Food allergy and migrane," *Clin. Immun. Allergy*, 2:(1982)137–164.

This chapter considers allergies to foods. However, other patients may have *intolerances* to some of these same foods. Lactose intolerance, for example, is discussed in Chapter 16.

TO TEST YOUR UNDERSTANDING

2. Use the menu for _____ (day to be assigned by your instructor). Indicate how you would modify this diet so that it conforms to a Rowe Elimination diet #1. Circle items used and write in others as needed.
3. A patient tells you he carries his lunch, but he needs a Rowe elimination diet #2. Write a list of foods that he could pack for lunch.

TREATMENT

Once the offending foods have been identified, the diet is modified to avoid the foods in question. This type of diet is called by the general term *avoidance diet*. It is thus distinguished from an elimination diet used for diagnosis.

AVOIDANCE DIETS

Planning a diet to avoid only one or a few foods is not difficult, provided the foods to be avoided are usually eaten singly. If a person is allergic to shrimp and strawberries, for example, avoiding these foods is easily arranged. On the other hand, if the patient is allergic to many foods or if the offending foods are those in common use within many mixtures, there may be great difficulty. In particular, management of sensitivities to wheat, milk, eggs, soy, or corn is difficult.

Before we describe techniques for specific avoidances, some general principles may be established:

1. The diet should be planned initially for total avoidance of all forms of the offending food. For some individuals, the diet can be modified later to include certain tolerated forms of offending foods. Some milk-sensitive patients, for example, can tolerate milk if it is boiled. Some patients can tolerate a food if it is eaten in small quantities or at intervals at least 4 days apart, or both.
2. Nutritional adequacy must be carefully planned. When foods are omitted from the diet, alternative sources of nutrients may need to be included. If a milk-free diet is used, adequate dietary protein, energy, calcium, riboflavin, and vitamin D must be planned for. Foods or supplements suggested for replacements must be nonallergenic.
3. Specific guidance must be given to the patient on diet management. Patients must be helped to identify sources of the allergens. This is particularly true when there are many hidden forms of the allergen. Instructions on reading labels and identifying forms of the offending foods are important. Many patients also need helpful food preparation suggestions in the form of recipes.
4. It may be necessary for the patient to inquire of the manufacturer concerning the ingredients in a product. If you counsel allergy patients frequently, you will need to keep up-to-date lists of manufactured food products free of wheat, corn, milk, egg, soy, and, possibly, tartrazine and salicylates.

TABLE 14-5. Alternative Ingredients in Cooking for the Allergy Patient

Milk	Fruit juice (in cooking)
Corn	
Cornstarch	Equal amounts arrowroot starch or potato starch
	Double the amount of whole wheat, soy, or barley flour
Baking Powder containing cornstarch (1 t)	¼ t baking soda + ½ t cream of tartar
Egg	Egg substitutes (some brands contain egg white)
as emulsifier	2 T whole-wheat flour, ½ t oil, ½ t baking powder & 2 T milk, fruit juice, or water
Cocoa	Equal amounts of carob powder
Chocolate (1 sq)	3 T carob powder + 2 T milk, butter, margarine, or water
Butter	Willow Run Margarine and Parv are kosher, milk-free butter substitutes
Wheat 1 c*	1⅓ c ground rolled oats
	1¼ c rye flour
	1 c corn flour, fine cornmeal, rye meal
	⅜ c rice flour
	¾ c coarse cornmeal or coarse oatmeal
	⅝ c potato flour
	½ c barley flour
	½ c rye flour + ½ c potato flour
	⅔ c rye flour + ⅓ c potato flour
	⅝ c (10 T) rice flour and ⅓ c rye flour
	1 c soy flour + ¾ c potato starch
Wheat flour as thickener, 1 T	½ T cornstarch, potato starch, arrowroot starch, rice flour

Compiled from Ohlson, M.A. *Experimental and Therapeutic Dietetics.* (2d ed.) Minneapolis: Burgess, 1972, pp. 142–3; and *Manual of Allergy and Immunology*, eds. G.J. Lawlor and T.J. Fischer. Boston: Little, Brown, 1981, p. 467.

*To improve product quality in baking,
1. Always use soy flour in combination with another flour.
2. For smoother texture, mix rice flour or cornmeal with the liquid in the recipe, bring to boil, and cool.
3. In baking, use lower temperature and longer time. Increase in leavening to 2½ t baking powder/c of any coarse meals or flour.
4. Bake muffins and biscuits in small sizes. Yeast breads are not satisfactory without wheat flour.
5. Apply frosting or store in closed containers to preserve moisture.

In addition to these general principles, each food sensitivity has its unique aspects. Consult your diet manual for some general guidelines for diets free of cow's milk, egg, corn, soy, and wheat. Each of these foods are present in many foods, often in hidden form, and present problems in avoidance. The avoidance of wheat is particularly troublesome since there is no completely adequate substitute for wheat flour in baked goods. Table 14-5 lists substitutes for use in recipes and gives suggestions for their use. In addition, many wheat-flour products contain yeast, which is also known to be an allergen in its own right.

As previously mentioned, there is a growing belief that allergies may be developed to chemicals in foods, certain food additives, and food contaminants such as molds and yeasts. Many believe that hypersensitivity to salicylates and tartrazine causes hyperactivity and other abnormal responses, especially in children. The salicylate-free, tartrazine-free diet, often called the Feingold diet, is frequently used despite weak evidence of its effectiveness. This diet and the mold-free and yeast-free diets are found in more detailed diet manuals (10).

INDIVIDUAL FOODS AND FOOD INGREDIENTS

Nutritional care specialists must be knowledgeable about sources of foods and manufacturing procedures. This section will provide you with information useful both in identifying allergens and in counseling patients with allergies and some other types of food intolerances (11, 12).

Food Additives

Sugar, salt, smoke, vinegar, and wine have been used for centuries as additives to preserve foods and improve color and flavor. A wide variety of other substances are now used in food processing as acids, antioxidants, colors, emulsifiers, flavoring agents, mold inhibitors, preservatives, sequestrants, stabilizers, and thickeners. Many additives are listed as "generally recognized as safe" (GRAS) by the FDA. Items are sometimes removed from the GRAS list, however, when new information casts doubt on their safety. An item is more commonly removed from the list because it has become a suspected carcinogen than because it causes allergies. Nevertheless, many patients believe that additives in foods are the source of their allergies and will ask you about them. It is important for you to be able to answer their questions.

Acid Additives.   The organic *acids—acetic, benzoic, citric, fumaric, malic, oxalic, quinic, succinic,* and *tartaric—* are found in many fruits and some vegetables. They are often used in food processing and may be listed on labels as "fruit acids." *Phosphoric acid,* an inorganic acid, is also sometimes used. Acids are usually added to give tartness and flavor, to prevent discoloration of vegetables during processing, and to provide sufficient acid in making jams and jellies.

Antioxidants.   Agents used to prevent oxidation or unwanted browning of fruits and vegetables and rancidity of fats and oils are ascorbic acid, vitamin E, erythorbic acid, sodium sulfite, sulfur dioxide, butylated hydroxyanisole (BHA), butylated hydroxytoluene (BHT), and propyl gallate. BHA and BHT have been reported to cause rhinitis, wheezing, headache, and somnolence.

Coloring Agents.   Coloring agents, which may be natural or synthetic, are added to foods to improve consumer acceptance. The naturally occurring colors include beet juice, fruit juice, grape skin extract, paprika, saffron, turmeric, and caramel, all of which are plant products. Products that require an oil-soluble coloring agent, such as butter, oil, cheese, and salad dressings, are colored with carotenoids or annatto. Annatto, from the seeds of the annatto tree, is used infrequently. Of these substances, only turmeric has been reported to act as an allergen.

The question of safety of synthetic dyes has led to a great deal of confusion. Decisions about approval for use have been based on political pressure generated by those who fear that they are "poisons" or "cause cancer." The following colors are currently certified by the FDA of the United States:

> Tartrazine (FD&C Yellow #5)
> Allura (FD&C Red #40)
> lake FD&C Blue #1
> Orange B (to color sausage casing)
> Citrus Red #3 (to color orange skins)
> Erythrosine (FD&C Red #3)

These colors are included in a provisional listing:

> FD&C Red #4 (to color maraschino cherries)
> Sunset Yellow (FD&C Yellow #6)
> FD&C Blue #2
> FD&C Green #3
> Lakes of FD&C color, except FD&C red #40

The *lakes* are insoluble coloring agents made by adsorbing the dye on aluminum hydroxide. They are not believed to be allergenic.

As an example of the confusion, amaranth (formerly FD&C Red #2) has been banned in the United States while allura red is approved. In Canada, on the other hand, allura red is banned and amaranth is approved. At present, 90 percent of the manufacture of colorants consists of allura red, tartrazine, and sunset yellow.

There is some evidence of sensitivity to synthetic coloring agents. Although interest has focused on tartrazine, intolerance to other dyes may be more common. Because of the attention given to tartrazine, manufacturers must list it on labels. For others, consumers must judge for themselves whether a particular dye is present, based on the color of the product.

Common FD&C dyes used in carbonated beverages, for example, are the following:

Orange	Yellow #6, or 96% Yellow #6 + 4% Red #40
Cherry	99.5% Red #40 + 0.5% Blue #1
Grape	80% Red #40 + 20% Blue #1
Strawberry	Red #40
Lime	95% Yellow + 5% Blue #1
Lemon	Yellow #5

Emulsifying Agents. Emulsifiers serve to disperse one liquid in another. Oil-in-water emulsions are prepared in shortenings, margarine, salad dressings, ice creams, ices, sherbets, some soft drinks and baked goods. The agents used are generally mono- and diglycerides. Soy lecithin and sorbitan monostearate are used in many foods.

Flavoring Agents. Synthetic flavoring agents are used in a wide variety of foods. Common artificial flavors include the following:

Allyl caproate (pineapple)
Allyl disulfide (onion or garlic)
Anisic alcohol (peach)
Benzaldehyde (cherry)
Ethyl acetate (strawberry)
Ethyl vanillin (vanilla)
Methyl anthranilate (orange)
Methyl salicylate (wintergreen)

Mold Inhibitors. Mold inhibitors, mostly sodium diacetate and calcium or sodium propionate, are widely used in baked products. These products are presumed to be helpful to those with allergy to molds.

Preservatives. Many have questioned the safety of nitrites used in prepared fish and meat products. Nitrites also occur naturally in some vegetables, including spinach and beets. They react with amino acids to form nitrosamines, which have been suspected of being carcinogens. Allergic reactions have not been reported.

Sequestrants. Sequestrants are chelating agents used to deactivate undesirable metals in foods which otherwise catalyze lipid oxidation and cause clouding of soft drinks, and off-tastes and deterioration of foods such as canned shrimp and beans, potato salad, sandwich spreads, and other mayonnaise-containing foods.

Stabilizers and Thickeners. These materials are used to prevent separation of the contents of peanut butter, ice creams, cheese spreads, pie fillings, and salad dressings. The most common items in this category are gelatin, carboxymethyl cellulose, various vegetable gums, and cornstarch.

Useful Facts About Some Specific Foods

In order to advise the allergic patient, the counselor must be very familiar with foods, including their use in a menu and their appearance, preparation, availability, and nutritional value. This section contains information on specific food items that may be of use in identifying offending foods and in planning avoidance diets.

Baking powder: Ingredients are sodium bicarbonate (baking soda), cream of tartar (potassium acid tartrate), tartaric acid, and either monocalcium phosphate or sodium aluminum sulfate. These are not allergenic; however, some contain wheat flour, cornstarch, or powdered egg white, which may cause an allergic response.

Beef: Beef does not cross-react with cow's milk allergy. Rare beef may be more allergenic than well-done beef in some sensitive individuals.

Beer: Ingredients are yeast, hops, corn, malt, usually made from barley, and sometimes other grains. The yeast may cause difficulty for the mold-sensitive patient, and some patients are sensitive to one or more of the grains.

Buckwheat: Buckwheat is in a different botanical family from wheat, and can thus be used as a substitute for other grains, but it can be an allergen itself. Buckwheat is available as a flour and as a groat, called *kasha*.

Chewing gum: Chicle and a variety of other materials, including natural or artificial rubber and various waxes, preservatives, flavors, and colors, are used in gum manufacture. Allergies to one or more ingredients have been reported (11).

Chicken: Chicken and chicken-egg allergies do not cross-react.

Chocolate: Chocolate is prepared from the cacao nut. The defatted product is cocoa. Milk chocolate contains 20 percent milk. Chocolate is a common allergen. It cross-reacts closely with cola, and patients allergic to one are often sensitive to the other. Both contain caffeine.

Cinnamon: Cinnamon may be prepared from "true cinnamon" (*Cinnamomum zeylanicum*) or from cassia (*Cinnamomum cassia*). Either may be an antigen.

Cola (Kola): This nut is a native African plant material closely related to the South American chocolate. It is contained in cola soft drinks.

Flaxseed (Linseed): Flaxseed is contained in some whole-grain cereal. Otherwise, patients are not usually exposed to this material, and sensitivities are rare.

Honey: The hexoses (glucose and fructose) in honey are nonallergenic, but honey contains about 2 percent protein specific to the flower from which the honey is made. Some patients who are allergic to honey may also be sensitive to legumes and licorice if the source of the honey was a leguminous plant such as alfalfa. Honey allergy does not cross-react with bee venom allergy.

Licorice: Licorice is prepared from the rootstock of a legume. There is sometimes cross-reactivity between licorice and other legumes.

Milk: Allergy to milk can be a hypersensitivity to lactalbumin or casein. Albumin is species-specific and heat sensitive. A patient who is allergic to cow's milk lactalbumin may be able to tolerate goat's milk or boiled milk. The film that forms on the top of boiled milk should be removed. Casein is neither species-specific nor heat sensitive.

Nuts: English walnuts, black walnuts, pecans, and butternuts frequently cross-react. Useful substitutes are Brazil nuts, hazel nuts, almonds, and macadamia nuts. The oil in peanut butter may be corn oil.

Onion: Onion or related vegetables may be contained in items with "flavoring agents" listed on the label.

Sulfites: Sulfiting agents include sulfur dioxide and potassium and sodium salts of bisulfite or metabisulfite. They have been used to prevent darkening of processed foods and, in restaurants, in potatoes, salads, avocado dishes, and wines so that the foods do not darken on standing before they are served. Sulfites can no longer be used to prevent darkening of fresh fruits and vegetables due to asthmatic reactions in individuals allergic to sulfite compounds.

Surimi: Surimi is a fish paste prepared by mincing fish flesh and adding natural or artificial flavors. Sorbitol, sugar, and salt are also usually added. Surimi is used to prepare various foods which simulate shellfish, such as crab-, scallop-, shrimp-, and lobster-like products. It may be in the form of flakes, chunks, prebreaded portions or morsels, tails, sticks, or legs. It is often prepared from Alaskan pollock and may have a percentage of meat from the shellfish being simulated.

DRUGS

Drugs are sometimes used in management of allergies. Cromolyn sodium is thought to block mast cell degranulation in the digestive tract and thereby reduce symptoms, allowing the patient to eat restricted amounts of the offending food. Because it is poorly absorbed from the digestive tract, it is usually administered as an inhalant. Oral cromolyn sodium has been used in the treatment of food allergies, but is not FDA-approved for this purpose (7). The major justification for its use is for the patient whose nutritional status could not be adequately maintained otherwise. Antihistamines and theophylline are given for symp-

tomatic treatment, as are corticosteroids if reactions are severe. Table 14-6 lists the side effects of drugs used in the management of allergic symptoms.

TABLE 14-6. Nutrition-Related Side Effects of Drugs Used in Management of Allergies

Generic Name	Nutrition-Related Effects
Antihistamines	
Ethylenediamines	
Pyrilamine maleate	Gastrointestinal complaints common; take with meals
Tripelennamine hydrochloride or citrate	As above
Piperazines	
Hydroxyzine hydrochloride or pamoate	Dry mouth is common
Piperidines	
Cyproheptadine hydrochloride	Weight gain; do not use in newborn or premature infants
Corticosteroids	Weight gain, gastrointestinal disturbances, emotional disturbances, growth retardation in children, negative nitrogen balance, hyperglycemia, hyperlipidemia, negative calcium balance, interference with vitamin D metabolism, gastrointestinal bleeding, pancreatitis, fatty liver, peptic ulceration
Theophylline	Nausea; plasma clearance is decreased by high-carbohydrate diet or dietary methylxanthines; decreased in low-carbohydrate, high-protein diet, charcoal-broiled meats.

Compiled from Lawlor, G.J., Jr., and T.J. Fischer. *Manual of Allergy and Immunology.* Boston: Little, Brown, 1981; and Ogilvie, R.I. Clinical pharmokinetics of theophylline. *Clin. Pharmocokin.* 3:267, 1978.

TO TEST YOUR UNDERSTANDING

4. When a commonly used food or a food category is removed from a diet, the intake of certain nutrients may become inadequate. Name the nutrients that might be deficient in the diet of a patient who is allergic to the following foods, and suggest alternative sources.
   a. Milk, wheat, and egg (adult patient)
   b. Citrus fruits and tomatoes (adult patient)
   c. Chocolate, cola, and nuts (teenage patient)

5. A patient's food diary indicates that she developed hives after eating the following items: Sunday—Roast lamb; Monday—Pepperoni pizza; Thursday—Roast turkey and bread stuffing.
   What allergy would you suspect?
   What questions would you ask the patient?

6. A patient asks you if the mold inhibitor put into bread can cause cancer or asthma. What would you reply?

TOPICS FOR FURTHER DISCUSSION

1. Do you think a child's hypersensitivity could have been inherited from his atopic parents if the child is allergic to different foods and shows different allergic manifestations?

2. Do any members of the class have food allergies? Describe problems and management.

3. Groups of students may visit a nearby supermarket and examine the items in the frozen food case, canned food sections, dairy case, or baked good sections. What items would be usable by a person with an allergy to wheat? corn? soy? cow's milk? egg? all five? Evaluate these products in terms of nutrient composition, indications for use, cost, and palatability. Discuss some techniques for counseling these patients about the use of convenience foods.

4. Compile a bibliography of recipe books for allergy patients.

REFERENCES

1. Shacks, S.J. and D.C. Heiner. Allergy to breast milk. *Clin. Immun. Allergy* 2:(1982)243–255.

2. Soothill, J.F. Prevention of food allergy. *Clin. Immun. Allergy* 2:(1982)243–255.

3. Gerrard, J.W. Allergy in breast-fed babies to ingredients in breast milk. *Ann. Allergy* 42:(1979)69–72.

4. Harrison, M., A. Kilby, J.A. Walker-Smith, N.E. France and C.B.S. Wood. Cow's milk protein intolerance: Possible association with gastroenteritis, lactose intolerance and IgA deficiency. *Brit. Med. J.* 6:(1976)1501–1504.

5. Hutchins, P. and J.A. Walker-Smith. The gastro-intestinal system. *Clin. Immun. Allergy* 2:(1982)43–76.

6. Kibort, P.M. and M.E. Ament. Cow's milk and soy protein intolerance in childhood. *Ped. Ann.* 11:(1982)1, 119–123.

7. Farrell, M.K. Food allergy. In *Manual of Allergy and Immunology*, eds. G.J. Lawlor Jr., and T.J. Fischer. Boston: Little, Brown, 1981.

8. Schellenberg, R.R. and N.F. Adkinson, Jr. Assessment of the influence of irrelevant IgE on allergic sensitivity to two independent antigens. *J. Allergy Clin. Immunol.* 63:(1979)15–22.

9. Chandra, R.K. and S. Jeevanandam. Diagnostic approach. In *Food Intolerance*, ed. R.K. Chandra. New York: Elsevier, 1983.

10. *Mayo Clinic Diet Manual* (5th ed.), eds. C.M. Pemberton and C.F. Gastineau. Philadelphia: Saunders, 1981.

11. Speer, F. *Food Allergy* (2d ed). Boston: John Wright, PSG Inc., 1983.

12. Breneman, J.C. *Basics of Food Allergy* (2d ed.). Springfield, Ill.: Charles C. Thomas, 1984.

ADDITIONAL SOURCES OF INFORMATION

Dong, F.M. *All About Food Allergy.* Philadelphia: Stickley, 1984.

Dwyer, J. Commercial additives. In *Adverse Effects of Foods*, eds. E.F.P. Jelliffe and D.B. Jelliffe. New York: Plenum, 1982.

Allergy, ed. A.P. Kaplan. New York: Churchill Livingstone, 1985.

National Advisory Committee on Hyperkinesis and Food Additives. *Final Report to the Nutrition Foundation.* New York: Nutrition Foundation, 1980.

Stevenson, D.D. and R.A. Simon. Sensitivity to ingestion of metabisulfites in asthmatic subjects. *J. Allergy Clin. Immunol.* 68:(1981)26–32.

CASE STUDY III NUTRITIONAL CARE IN FOOD ALLERGY

Part I: Presentation

Present Illness: Barbara R. is a 22 y.o. commercial artist referred to Allergy Clinic by her family-practice physician. The patient C/O sporadic abdominal distention, cramping, and diarrhea 1–2 hr following some meals, with a 13 # weight loss in 2 mos. She denies other symptoms. Referral states tests had ruled out infection, chronic inflammation, abnormality of anatomy or motility of intestinal mucosa, pancreatic insufficiency, abnormality of enterohepatic circulation, and endocrine disease or malignancy; treatment for irritable bowel syndrome was not successful.

Past Medical History: Rubella and chickenpox in childhood, milk allergy as an infant, hayfever in spring for past 10 yrs.

Family History: Father has sensitivity to insect venom. Mother has asthma. No history of GI disease in immediate family.

Social History: Single, recent college graduate in first job. Shares apartment with female friends. Pt describes her employment as "very stressful."

Review of Systems: Patient has no complaints except those related to abdomen and recent weight loss.

Physical Exam:

General: White female. Ht 5 ft, 5 in, wt 112#, medium frame. *Abdomen* distended, diffusely but minimally tender. No rebound. Bowel sounds normal. No hepatosplenomegaly. Remainder of exam WNL.

Laboratory: RBC $4.0 \times 10^6/mm^3$, Hct 42%, Hgb 12.2, plasma glucose 100 mg/dl, serum albumin 3.8 g/dl, WBC $5,000/mm^3$, lymphs 35%, eos 6%.

Impression: Moderate GI distress 2° to possible hypersensitivity to unknown antigens in 22-y.-o. slightly underweight female with positive family history of allergy.

Plan: Nutrition Clinic referral for detailed diet history for identification of possible antigen and nutritional counseling. Primary physician to continue symptomatic treatment of GI symptoms.

QUESTIONS

1. Discuss the significance of the family history and employment history.

2. Compare this patient's laboratory values with normal values:

		Normal	Patient	Interpretation
A.	Hct			
B.	Hgb			
C.	Blood glucose			
D.	Plasma albumin			
E.	Leukocytes			
F.	Lymphocytes			

Part II: Nutrition Consult

Barbara R. is first evaluated in the Nutrition Clinic by a Dietetic Technician (DT), who obtains a preliminary diet history and nutritional assessment. The DT reports a TSF of 14.0 mm and a MAC of 25.7 cm, and a 24-hr. recall:

Breakfast
4 oz orange juice
¾ c ready-to-eat corn cereal/4 oz whole milk
3 Ry-Krisp wafers
Coffee/1 t sugar

Lunch
Cold plate
4 oz sliced ham
3 oz potato chips (1 oz = P-1.5; F-11; C-14 g)
½ c sliced tomato/lettuce
"A few" celery sticks

Watermelon slice, 1 sv.
Iced tea/sugar, 1 tsp.

Snack
12 oz cola drink (C-37 g)

Dinner
4 oz baked salmon/lemon
½ c buttered peas
½ c fresh fruit salad
2 chocolate brownies (P-2; F-8: C-26 g)
Coffee/1 t sugar

QUESTIONS

3. Complete Forms P and Q on the following pages for this patient. On the lower part of Form P, indicate with an **X** the major vitamins and minerals found in individual foods from the 24-hr recall. Does the diet appear to be deficient in any of the vitamins and minerals listed?

FORM P

University Medical Center
Summary of Daily Nutrient Intake

Food Group	No. of Exchanges	PRO g	FAT g	CHO g
Starch/Bread exchanges				
Milk exchanges (Circle non-fat, low-fat, or whole)				
Fruit exchanges				
Vegetable exchanges				
Meat exchanges (Circle low, medium, high fat)				
Fat exchanges				
Other				

Total g _____ _____ _____

Kcal = _____ g protein × 4 = _____
　　　 _____ g fat × 9 = _____
　　　 _____ g carbohydrate × 4 = _____

_____ Total kcal

Food	Serving Size	Vit. A	Vit. C	Thiamin	Riboflavin	Niacin	Calcium	Iron

FORM G

University Medical Center Nutritional Assessment

Patient's Name _____

Sex (Circle one)   M   F   Date of Admission _____

Age: _____ Years   Date of Assessment _____

Height and Weight:

Height: _____ ft. _____ in. _____ cm

Body weight: On admission: _____ # _____ kg

              Current _____ # _____ kg

              Usual _____ # _____ kg

              Ideal _____ # _____ kg

              Recent loss _____ # in _____ mos _____ kg

              % weight change _____ gain   or   _____ loss

Interpretation: Severely underweight   (20% < ideal) _____

(Mark X where   Severely overweight (+20% > ideal) _____

 appropriate)   Unplanned weight change, > 10% _____

              Stable and within normal limits _____

Somatic Protein:

Mark X for interpretation

Value Measured	Standard Value	Patient's Value	50th %ile	50–15th %ile	15–5th %ile	<5th %ile
TSF, mm						
MAC, cm						
MAMC, cm						

Visceral Protein:

Mark X for interpretation

Value Measured	Standard Value	Patient's Value	*Deficit* None	Mild	Moderate	Severe
Albumin, g/dl						
TIBC, μg/dl						
Total lymphocytes mm³						

Hematological:

Mark X for interpretation

Value Measured	Standard Value	Patient's Value	Acceptable	Marginal	Deficient
RBC, × 10⁶/mm³					
Htc, %					
Hgb, g/dl					
MCV, FL					
MCH, pg					
MCHC, g/dl (%)					

Nutritional Status: (Mark X where appropriate)

_____ Normal

_____ Marasmus

_____ Kwashiorkor-like syndrome

_____ Combined Marasmus-kwashiorkor

Diet Evaluation

Intake _____ kcal/24 hrs

      _____ g protein/24 hrs

BEE _____ kcal

Maintenance expenditure _____ kcal

Recommended Intake

Energy: Oral anabolic requirement

BEE × _____ = _____ kcal

Protein: Oral anabolic requirement

kg actual body weight × _____ to _____ = _____ to _____

g protein.

kcal; g N = _____; N required = _____ g;

g N × 6.25 = _____ g.

4. List additional questions *related to the 24-hr recall* that you would ask this patient when you interview her after studying the available data.

5. Your questioning reveals that her symptoms worsen when she eats chocolate. Summarize your observations, assessment, and plan in a SOAP note.

Part III: Diagnostic Diet

Three weeks after your initial consultation, the patient returns to the Nutrition Clinic. She states that she has followed your advice, but that her symptoms have not totally subsided, although they occur less frequently. Her physician has requested that she be instructed on the use of a Rowe elimination diet #3, which she is to follow for 2 weeks.

QUESTIONS

6. Explain the rationale for the diet.

7. Modify the diet for _____ (day to be assigned by your instructor) to conform to the prescribed diet.

8. If the patient refuses to eat the meats specified on the Rowe #3 diet, what would you do?

9. List the essential points of your diet instruction. (Review Chapter 6 if necessary.)

QUESTIONS

10. Two weeks later, the patient reports that all her symptoms have disappeared. The physician now authorizes additions to the basic diet. Describe how you would advise the patient to proceed.
    a. At what intervals would you recommend each new addition?

    b. How often should the newly added food be eaten during that interval?

11. If your first addition is wheat, what wheat-containing food would you recommend the patient use? Why?

Part IV: Avoidance Diet

The above procedure suggested that Barbara R. was also sensitive to wheat, milk, and eggs. You instruct her on a diet that is free of these foods and her previous avoidances.

QUESTIONS

12. For each of the following items, decide whether you would advise the patient to avoid the food. If you advise avoidance, state your reason.
    a. Sliced bologna

    b. Rye bread

    c. French bread

d. French toast

e. Buckwheat pancake and waffle mix

f. Consomme (canned)

g. Chicken-noodle soup

h. Kosher frozen dinner with beef

i. Root beer

j. Cola drink

13.   Name the nutrients that are likely to be marginal in supply in this patient's diet. Name two acceptable food sources of each for use in her diet.

                    Nutrients   Sources

14.   Using the sample menu for _____ (day to be assigned by your instructor), indicate the modifications necessary to make a diet allergen-free for Barbara R.

Part V: Drugs in the Treatment of Allergy

    Two years later, Barbara R. tells you she is engaged to John H., who is also a patient at the clinic. John was seen first in the ER a year ago. He was wheezing and pale. Closer physical examination revealed urticaria across the abdomen.

    John stated at that time that he was allergic to peas, beans, and soy, and the symptoms were similar to previous reactions to these foods. He was not aware of having eaten any of these items, but had been to a potluck supper held by his athletic club.

    John was given epinephrine 0.4 ml sc to relieve the respiratory symptoms, and oxygen was administered. Since he responded rapidly to these measures, it was felt he did not need theophylline or corticosteroids. He was released from the ER on an antihistamine, diphenhydramine·HCl (Benadryl), 50 mg t.i.d.

QUESTIONS

15.   What is the purpose of each of the drugs just mentioned?
    a. Antihistamine?

    b. Theophylline (Aminophyllin)?

c. Corticosteroids?

16. Would you expect any of these drugs to have nutrition-related side effects? Which drugs? Describe the effects and the nutritional care indicated.

17. Describe some "hidden" sources of soy John might have eaten at the potluck supper that caused his condition.

18. Since John is allergic to peas, beans, and soy, what other foods should be investigated for allergenic effects in this patient?

19. List the main points you would make in your nutritional counseling with John. Assume he has been shown to be allergic to all the items listed in question 18.

20. Using the menu for _____ (day to be assigned by your instructor), modify the menu as you would instruct John to do.

Part VI: Prevention of Allergy

After Barbara and John had been married for a year, Barbara reappears at the Nutrition Clinic. She tells you she is two months pregnant and asks if there is any advice you can give her about diet during pregnancy to prevent allergies in her baby.

QUESTIONS

21. Summarize briefly the main points of your advice.

Part VII: The Allergic Infant

After the baby is born, Barbara breast feeds him for the first 6 months. Barbara then returns to the Nutrition Clinic for advice on infant feeding for prevention of allergies. She is carrying with her a referral from the pediatrician requesting nutritional consultation. The pediatrician has given Barbara a feeding schedule which begins weaning to an iron-fortified cow's milk formula and states that solid foods should be introduced. Specific foods are to be recommended by the nutritionist at appropriate ages. Despite all efforts, the baby develops an allergy to cow's milk and corn. If these are given, the child develops a severe eczema.

QUESTIONS

22. Name some products that might be used to replace cow's milk formula for this child, and discuss their allergic potential.

23. Indicate whether you expect the infant to tolerate each of the following items. State your reasons if you expect intolerance. Then suggest a replacement in the diet.
    a. Graham crackers

    b. Gelatin dessert

    c. Margarine

    d. Sweetened chopped peaches

    e. Homemade sugar cookies

15

Nutritional Care of Patients with Diseases of the Esophagus and Stomach

Digestive system discomfort is a common experience often arising from unwise eating and drinking. Most such disorders are mild, brief in duration, and do not require professional nutritional care. However, a few conditions become sufficiently severe or chronic that nutritional care is indicated. Before proceeding, you should review, if necessary, the material in your text on diseases of the upper digestive tract.

In some circumstances, interference with food intake may be an integral part of a disorder of the gastrointestinal (GI) tract. The nutritional care specialist will thus have use for the various procedures that help improve nutrient intake. These procedures, described in Chapters 11 through 13, will not be described again here. However, they may need to be integrated with the nutritional care procedures described in this and subsequent chapters. In addition most patients will have preconceived ideas that certain foods cause distressing symptoms or, alternatively, provide unusual benefits. These beliefs, whether or not they are justified, must be considered in planning nutritional care.

In this chapter, we will emphasize nutritional care in selected diseases of the esophagus and stomach. In particular, the approaches to nutritional care of excessive contraction of the lower esophageal sphincter (achalasia), lower esophageal sphincter (LES) incompetence (gastroesophageal reflux), peptic ulcer, and dumping syndrome will be considered.

NUTRITIONAL ASSESSMENT

Many disorders of the mouth and pharynx, in addition to the esophagus and stomach, can severely affect nutritional status by altering intake; therefore, detailed nutritional assessment is important in the care of patients with disease in these tissues. These patients should be routinely considered at nutritional risk and should receive an in-depth nutritional assessment (see Chapter 4). Depending upon the specific problem, you may need to inquire about the following:

Mouth

Are teeth carious, missing, absent?

Are dentures well fitted? ill fitted?

Is there periodontal disease? ulceration of mouth or gums?

Are teeth or mouth sensitive to heat? cold?

Is mouth abnormally dry?

Esophagus

If the patient complains of dysphagia, inquire about: frequency? related to liquids? solids? both? greater with cold liquids or warm?

If the patient complains of pain on swallowing (odynophagia), ask,

Is pain precipitated by cold liquids? spicy foods? acid foods? fatty foods?

Does pain occur immediately on swallowing? after meals?

Stomach

Is distress caused by food intake? Which foods or groups of food?

Is pain relieved by food intake?

General

Life-style: smoking? alcohol intake? rest? stress? activity, including in relation to meals? medications?

Diet history: Does the diet include fiber?

What is the average meal size and frequency?

Obtain information about specific offenders.

Ask about caffeine intake and liquid intake.

ESOPHAGEAL DISORDERS

DIAGNOSIS

A variety of tests may be used to diagnose disorders of the esophagus. The *Bernstein test* consists of a normal saline drip, alternating with a 0.1 percent HCl drip, into the esophagus. Esophagitis is indicated by onset of symptoms within a half hour of the acid administration. Other common tests for esophagitis, which is the most common esophageal disorder, are *endoscopy, radiological studies* using a contrast material, and *determination of acidity* in the esophagus.

Diffuse esophageal spasm (DES) may result from reflux esophagitis (back-up of acidic gastric contents into esophagus) or various other etiologies. It is considered to be an early stage of achalasia in some patients. Diagnosis is made by *cine-esophagogram* showing disordered segmental contractions and absence of a peristaltic wave in the lower esophagus. *Manometric* studies of motility and lumenal pressure are also used.

Achalasia may be diagnosed with *radiological contrast studies* (barium swallow) which show abnormal motor function with a narrowed distal segment. *Esophagoscopy* is used for direct visualization and tissue biopsy.

NUTRITIONAL CARE

Nutritional care of esophageal disorders frequently requires measures to ensure adequate nutrient intake in general. (See Chapters 11 through 13.) In addition, there are considerations specific to certain disorders. Nutritional care procedures are given in Table 15-1 for achalasia and Table 15-2 for esophageal reflux.

OTHER TREATMENT

Medical management of reflux esophagitis is usually effective. It may consist of antacid therapy given 1 hour and 3 hours after food intake, and 300 mg of cimetidine at bedtime and with onset of symptoms for 2 to 4 weeks. Mechanical measures to reduce reflux include elevating the head of the bed on blocks (*not* propping the head on pillows), avoiding heavy exercise that increases intraabdominal pressure, not smok-

TABLE 15-1. Nutritional Care in Achalasia

Give semisolid or liquid foods as tolerated.
Provide small, frequent meals as tolerated.
Reduce protein and carbohydrate and increase fat in the diet to promote reduced gastric secretion and a decrease in lower esophageal sphincter pressure.
Avoid temperature extremes in foods.
Avoid foods such as citrus juices and highly spiced foods, which can injure the esophageal mucosa if retained.
Use a low-fiber diet if the patient finds it easier to swallow.
Encourage the patient to eat slowly.

From *Clinical Nutrition and Dietetics* by Frances J. Zeman. New York: Macmillan, 1983, p. 129. Used by permission of the publisher.

TABLE 15-2. Nutritional Care in Gastroesophageal Reflux

Increase lower esophageal sphincter pressure
Increase protein in diet
Decrease fat in diet to < 45 g/day
Avoid alcohol, peppermint, spearmint
Avoid coffee, strong tea, and chocolate if not well tolerated
Use *skim* milk

Decrease irritation in the esophagus
Avoid irritants: citrus juices, tomato, coffee, spicy foods, carbonated beverages
Avoid any other foods that regularly cause heartburn (*may* include rich pastry and frosted cakes)

Improve clearing of the esophagus
Do not recline for > 2 hr after eating
Elevate head of bed

Decrease frequency and volume of reflux
Elevate head of bed
Do not recline for > 2 hr after eating
Eat small meals, more frequent meals if necessary
Reduce weight if overweight
Sip only small amounts of fluids with meals
Drink most fluids between meals
Include enough fiber to avoid constipation (straining increases intraabdominal pressure)

Nutritional and other considerations
Monitor effect of citrus and tomato avoidance on ascorbic acid status; supplement as necessary
Monitor effect of antacids on iron status; supplement if necessary
Avoid chewing gum (causes air swallowing)
Avoid smoking immediately following meals

From *Clinical Nutrition and Dietetics* by Frances J. Zeman. New York: Macmillan, 1983, p. 131. Used by permission of the publisher.

ing, and wearing loose clothing. The patient should be advised not to lie down within 2 hours after eating and to avoid stooping over.

When these measures are insufficient, other medication can be added. These include bethanechol chloride, 25 mg q.i.d., to increase LES tone or metoclopramide hydrochloride, 10 mg q.i.d., to increase esophageal clearance and LES tone (1). If weight loss continues, a stricture forms, or there is intractable pain, surgery may be used.

In mild cases of DES, teaching the patient to avoid precipitating foods and other factors may be sufficient. Pain may be relieved with 0.3 mg sublingual (SL) nitroglycerin or 5 mg SL isosorbide dinitrate. The LES is sometimes dilated with a pneumatic bag. Surgery (myotomy) is used to treat severe cases.

Achalasia is usually treated mechanically. Surgery is undertaken if mechanical treatment is ineffective.

TO TEST YOUR UNDERSTANDING

M.H. is an 80 y.o. white male C/O "a feeling of something sticking," as he points to the epigastric and midthorax area. The symptom has been of 2 years' duration and has been worsening.

Barium swallow shows a dilated esophagus narrowing to a "beak-like" distal end, with absence of peristalsis in the distal two-thirds. Manometry confirmed absence of peristalsis and showed elevated

LES pressure with incomplete relaxation on swallowing. Esophagoscopy with biopsy was performed to R/O stricture or carcinoma.

Height is 5 feet, 10 inches, and weight is 170 pounds. Usual weight is 195 pounds. The patient states he has not been trying to lose weight. The following values are also available for nutritional assessment:

Anthropometric measures	WNL
Serum albumin	3.5 mg/dl
CBC	WNL
DCH	WNL

Problem 1 in the POMR is *achalasia.*

1. Would you judge this patient to be at nutritional risk? Why?
2. Suggest some areas of observation or questioning indicated by this patient's condition that should be included in the nutritional assessment.
3. In the course of the diet history, it becomes clear that the patient has dysphagia for both solids and liquids. He states he had pain after drinking cold grapefruit juice yesterday.

   What modifications would you recommend in the following menu for this patient? Explain the reason for your recommendations.

¾ c	Cream of tomato soup
4 oz	Meat loaf
¾ c	Hash-brown potatoes
½ c	Buttered whole-kernel corn
½ c	Tossed salad/vinegar & oil dressing
½ c	Mint ice cream/2 T chocolate sauce
	Coffee

4. Mrs. J.G. came to the Gastroenterology Clinic C/O severe, recurrent heartburn. The symptoms became worse when she bent over or lifted, and she had also vomited a little blood.

   She responded poorly to antacid therapy for 4 weeks. Therefore, a barium swallow and esophagoscopy with biopsy were performed, which ruled out neoplasia and documented inflammatory changes. Manometry showed a depressed LES pressure of 8 mm Hg.

   Nutritional assessment showed her to have normal nutritional status.

   Antacid therapy was continued with 30 ml Maalox 30 minutes after meals, snacks, and at bedtime. Metoclopramide hydrochloride 10 mg was given at 30 minutes before meals and at bedtime.

   Given the same menu as in question 3, how would you suggest it be modified for Mrs. G?
5. What advice, in addition to the diet modifications just made, would you give this patient?

PEPTIC ULCER DISEASE

DIAGNOSIS

Radiographic and *endoscopic examinations* are especially useful in the diagnosis of peptic ulcer disease (PUD). *Gastric acid levels* may also be analyzed. Gastric contents are aspirated through a tube; *basal acid output* (BAO) measures the amount of acid secreted without any stimulus. In addition, betazol hydrochloride (Histalog) may be injected to stimulate secretion for determination of *peak acid output* (PAO). Tests of acid content and output are used to detect hypersecretion and Zollinger-Ellison syndrome (ZES), rather than for diagnosis of the ulcer. Many, but not all, ZES patients have BAO > 10 mEq/h and 60% or more of PAO.

TREATMENT

Drugs are the mainstays of treatment. Surgery may be undertaken for those patients who do not respond adequately to drugs, however. In drug treatment, *antacids* are often prescribed for use after each meal and at bedtime. Cimetidine (Tagamet A) or ranitidine (Zantac) may be used to reduce acid secretion. Cessation of smoking and alcohol intake are often recommended.

Years ago, diets for patients with peptic ulcer disease (PUD) were highly restricted. They consisted initially of large quantities of milk and cream and progressed through additions of soft, "bland," or white foods such as soft cooked eggs, baked custard, and cottage cheese. In recent years, less restrictive diets have been used since the rationale for the previously used diets could not be scientifically supported. It has, in fact, been demonstrated that milk can actually increase, rather than decrease, acid production (2).

Modern treatment of PUD, centered on the use of antacids and cimetidine, commonly makes only a few dietary restrictions. Recommendations vary somewhat, depending on whether the patient is symptomatic or asymptomatic, as follows:

1. *Reduce coffee, cocoa, and tea intake.* These substances have been shown to stimulate acid production. Decaffeinated and instant coffee are stronger stimulators of acid production than regular coffee. The stimulatory effect is not proportional to caffeine content. As a consequence, you should not instruct the patient merely to reduce caffeine intake. When patients are symptomatic, these beverages should be avoided altogether.

2. *Avoid alcohol intake.* Alcohol is believed to cause back diffusion of hydrogen ion from the lumen into intercellular or intracellular sites, resulting in injury to the gastric mucosa. There is some evidence, however, that beverages with an ethanol content below 12 percent do not have this effect. For the asymptomatic patient who does not comply with a more severe restriction, it may therefore be acceptable to suggest moderate beer or wine intake (<12 percent alcohol), with avoidance of higher-proof beverages. When the patient is symptomatic, total abstinence is recommended.

3. *Avoid ground peppers.* Peppers may be irritating to the gastrointestinal tract. The patient may thus be more comfortable when avoiding their use. There is no evidence that pepper causes an ulcer or increases gastric acid secretion.

4. *Avoid fruit juices or other very-low-pH foods* **if they are irritating to the patient.**

5. *Avoid any food the patient routinely finds irritating.* You should monitor the patient's diet to ensure that it does not become so restricted that it is nutritionally inadequate.

6. *Avoid food intake before bedtime to avoid nocturnal hypersecretion.*

Many institutions list the "bland" diet in their diet manuals, despite a lack of a scientifically based rationale for its use. It is sometimes prescribed because patients associate symptom exacerbation with diet indiscretions and expect to be given a restricted diet. You should therefore be familiar with the diet, but should be cautious in recommending its use.

FEEDING THE GASTRIC SURGERY PATIENT

For those patients in whom conservative medical treatment is insufficient, surgery may be undertaken. The problems of nutritional needs in major surgery are discussed in Chapter 22. For the present, it is important for you to understand the procedures that precede and follow surgery in which general anesthesia is used.

All foods and fluids are usually withheld for at least 8 hours prior to surgery. This procedure helps to ensure that the stomach is empty, thus avoiding regurgitation and aspiration during, or immediately following, anesthesia and recovery.

In the immediate postoperative period, there may be a lack of peristalsis, known as *ileus*, in the GI tract. Ileus usually occurs following surgery on the GI tract. The patient cannot be given fluid or food orally until peristalsis returns. In the meantime, fluid and electrolyte balance is maintained by intravenous infusion.

The return of peristalsis is detected with the use of a stethoscope. The patient is lying down, and the stethoscope is placed on the abdomen. If peristalsis has returned, bubbling or gurgling noises, called *bowel sounds*, can be heard every 5 to 15 seconds. The patient is also asked whether he has passed any gas, because flatulence is another sign of the return of bowel activity. Last, the patient's abdomen should be soft and flat. (Tenderness may be present for several days after abdominal surgery and, of itself, is not a reason to delay oral feeding.)

TABLE 15-3. Nutritional Management of Dumping Syndrome

Individualize the diet to the patient's tolerance. Consult the patient frequently concerning his or her response to individual food items and to portion sizes. The following items are general guidelines.

Reduce intake of carbohydrates to 100–200 g/day. Avoid simple sugars to prevent rapid movement of food into the jejunum with formation of a hyperosmolar solution. Use *unsweetened* fruits.

Increase fat content to 30%–40% of calories to retard stomach emptying and to provide calories for weight gain.

Increase protein to 20% of calories for tissue formation and to supply energy. Include some protein in each meal.

Meals should be low in bulk, dry, and frequent. Six or more per day is common. Increase portion sizes as the patient's tolerance increases.

Provide low-carbohydrate fluids between meals, at least ½–1 hr after a meal, to retard gastric emptying. Avoid high-carbohydrate fluids.

All food and drink should be moderate in temperature. Cold drinks, especially, cause increased gastric motility.

Encourage the patient to eat slowly and then lie down for 20–30 min.

Encourage the patient to eat a variety of foods to provide an adequate diet and achievement of ideal body weight. It may be necessary to urge him or her to try foods that were being avoided preoperatively.

The possibility of lactose intolerance exists. Milk should be avoided until it is established that the patient tolerates milk.

To progress toward a more normal intake, add moderate amounts of carbohydrate with caution if the patient shows no symptoms of dumping in the first several days. Use sugar in the form of sweetened fruits and fruit juice and desserts such as sponge cake and cookies. If these are well tolerated, add more concentrated carbohydrates and foods at temperature extremes. Fresh fruits and vegetables may be added in 2–3 wk. They should be chewed thoroughly. The diet may be progressed rapidly in some patients and may be lifelong in others.

From *Clinical Nutrition and Dietetics* by Frances J. Zeman. New York: Macmillan, 1983, p. 146. Used by permission of the publisher.

DUMPING SYNDROME

Of the various potential complications following ulcer surgery, *dumping syndrome* most clearly involves nutritional care. The treatment of dumping syndrome is largely dietary and provides an opportunity for you to perform a valuable service to the patient. General guidelines for a diet for dumping syndrome are given in most hospital diet manuals, but the condition is highly variable. It is important to recognize, first, that development of the syndrome can be prevented by judicious postoperative feeding. Second, some patients have only the early symptoms of dumping, while others have only late symptoms, and still others have both. Some patients have more severe symptoms than others. Some patients have symptoms only temporarily, while others may have permanent symptoms. Thus, you must individualize the diet.

Although your diet manual will list specific foods to be used or restricted, the characteristics of the diet can be summarized as follows:

Early dumping:

Avoid concentrated sources of carbohydrate.

Restrict amounts of carbohydrate-containing foods such as fruits, cereals, and some vegetables.

Eliminate alcohol.

Use small, frequent feedings.

Use liquids only at least ½ to 1 hour following meals. Note that some fruit juices (grape and apple, for example) and carbonated beverages are very hyperosmolar and are thus inappropriate.

Increase protein and fat intake as indicated to achieve and maintain normal weight.

Late dumping:

Avoid concentrated sources of carbohydrate.

Restrict amounts of carbohydrate-containing foods, such as fruits, cereals, and some vegetables.

In addition, patients are sometimes advised to eat in a reclining position to retard stomach emptying. Milk must be eliminated from the diets of patients who do not tolerate it. The recommended diet and related factors are summarized in Table 15-3.

In time, many patients adapt, and the diet can be liberalized. Additions to the diet should be made slowly, in small quantities, until it is established that the patient can tolerate them.

TO TEST YOUR UNDERSTANDING

6. Explain briefly the theories concerning the mechanisms by which the manifestations of dumping syndrome are produced.

7. Using the diabetic exchange lists, list the exchanges that would need to be limited in a diet for dumping syndrome.

8. Many foods are not included in the diabetic exchange lists. List categories of these foods that would need to be limited or possibly omitted from a diet for dumping syndrome.

9. You have a dumping syndrome patient who is 5 pounds below ideal weight. What nutrients and categories of foods would you increase in the diet to ensure that no more body weight will be lost?

10. What advice would you give this patient concerning the form of fruit in his diet?

11. Mrs. R. is a 47 y.o. post–partial gastrectomy patient (Billroth I) who has developed early dumping syndrome. Using a hospital menu for _____ (day to be assigned by your instructor), modify the diet for Mrs. R. Assume she is 8 days postop. Use your diet manual as a guide.

12. Using the same day, modify the menu for this patient, assuming she has developed late dumping syndrome.

REFERENCES

1. GOYAL, R.K. Diseases of the esophagus. In *Principles of Internal Medicine*, eds. R.G. Petersdouf, R.D. Adams, E. Braunwald, D.J. Isselbacher, J.B. Martin, and J.D. Wilson. New York: McGraw-Hill, 1983.

2. SLEISENGER, M.H. AND J.S. FORDTRAN. *Gastrointestinal Disease, Pathophysiology, Diagnosis, Management* (3d ed.). Philadelphia: Saunders, 1983.

CASE STUDY IV   NUTRITIONAL CARE IN PEPTIC ULCER DISEASE

J.K., a 47 y.o. computer programmer, presented 12 years ago with a history of epigastric pain recurring twice. He had had an episode of hematemesis 9 years ago, with minimal blood loss. An upper GI series showed a small duodenal ulcer. A transfusion was unnecessary.

At that time, the patient was treated with a bland diet and antacids 1 to 3 hours following meals and HS. After discharge, the patient continued taking antacids, choosing to vary the type. He failed to follow the diet after 6 weeks. A year later, the pain returned but was relieved by food.

QUESTIONS

1.   What relationship is believed to exist between ulcer recurrence and the patient's failure to follow the diet?

2.   The patient stated that he occasionally changed the type of antacid he used. What nutrition-related problem might occur with the following types of antacid?
a. Magnesium salts

b. Aluminum hydroxide

c. Aluminum-containing antacids

d. Antacids in general

In the ensuing years, the episodes of pain lasted longer and became more severe. Two years ago, the pattern of pain relief with food was lost. Antacids also gave less relief. The patient lost 5 weeks' work in the past year because of ulcer symptoms.

In the past month, J.K. has lost 10 pounds. He was hospitalized when the pain became intense and was unrelieved by antacids or food.

When you read the patient's record, you find the following information:

		Normal
Lab results:		
Hct	37%	_____
Serum albumin	2.9 g/dl	_____
BUN	11 mg/dl	_____
Residual gastric contents following NG tube suction	600 ml	_____
Upper GI series results:		
Three duodenal ulcer craters, 1–3 cm in diameter, were seen just distal to the pylorus		_____
Function tests:		
Basal acid output	BAO 5.0 mEq/hr	_____
Augmented histamine test	PAO 50 mEq/hr	_____
Fasting serum gastrin	67 pg/ml	_____

No evidence of dehydration
Weight loss: 10 pounds in 4 weeks
All anthropometric measurements: WNL

QUESTIONS

3.   In the spaces provided, write the normal values for the laboratory results given above.

4. What is the most likely reason for the following tests:
   a. Serum gastrin

   b. Augmented histamine test

5. Would you consider the patient to be at nutritional risk? Why?

The residual gastric volume persisted, indicating gastric outlet obstruction, and surgery was recommended. The patient underwent an antrectomy and truncal vagotomy with a Billroth I reconstruction. Postoperatively, the patient was NPO for 2 days, and a nasogastric tube was used to remove gastric contents. He was given IV fluid and electrolyte therapy to replace losses. Feeding was resumed when bowel sounds returned.

You are the nutritional care specialist for the gastroenterology service and are asked for your recommendations on postoperative feeding.

QUESTION

6. Postoperatively, when bowel sounds resume, what feeding *pattern* (amounts and frequency) and *general types* of foods would you recommend?

At the end of 2 weeks, the patient was discharged from the hospital. He returned in a few days complaining of unpleasant symptoms following food intake. He said he felt uncomfortably full, weak, light-headed, and had some diarrhea and sweating. These symptoms soon subsided, but were followed about 2 hours later by a second episode of severe sweating, weakness, and syncope. Blood glucose level was 65 mg/dl.

Upon patient's readmission, the physician added *dumping syndrome* to the problem list.

QUESTIONS

7. Summarize the main characteristics of the diet you would now recommend for this patient.

8. Using the menu for _____ (day to be assigned by your instructor), modify the menu to be suitable for this patient. Follow the policies given in your diet manual.

The response to the diet was good. In 3 days, the symptoms had not recurred. More carbohydrates, milk, and fresh fruits and vegetables were added to the diet. The patient was discharged with a diet containing 200 g carbohydrate in 6 feedings. Six months later, the patient returned to the clinic and reported that he now observes very few food restrictions and has not had a return of symptoms.

16

Nutritional Care of the Malabsorbing Patient

The intestine plays an essential role in digestion and nutrient absorption. Therefore, most diseases of the intestinal tract have a detrimental effect on nutritional status. The resulting nutrient deficiencies may, in turn, exacerbate the intestinal disease.

A number of disorders of the small intestine have malabsorption, diarrhea, and other symptoms in common and also have common nutritional consequences. In general, malabsorption can be the result of a deficiency of pancreatic enzymes, deficiency of bile, or impairment of intestinal absorptive capacity. These will be the primary focus of this chapter.

It is important that you understand the general nutritional care procedures indicated by malabsorption and diarrhea regardless of their origin. Since the mechanisms by which diarrhea and malabsorption are produced vary, however, you will also need a command of the nutritional care procedures mandated by some of the more commonly occurring specific disease processes. Thus, this chapter will discuss the use of lactose-restricted, fat-restricted, and gluten-restricted diets. Before proceeding, you should review the related material in your textbook.

DIAGNOSIS

The diagnostic tests for malabsorption are usually used in combination, because individual tests do not establish a specific diagnosis.

MALABSORPTION

The diagnostic tests listed below are used to confirm or rule out suspected malabsorption. Normal values for many of these tests are given in Appendix E.

Qualitative fecal fat tests consist of microscopic examination for fat content of a fresh, stained stool specimen. The presence of 10 or more fat globules is considered a positive result. The test does not detect very mild malabsorption and is not useful in infants under 3 months of age.

Quantitative fecal fat tests require a diet containing 50 to 150 g (usually 100 g) long-chain fat for 2 days prior to and during the test. Stool is collected for 72 hours. The normal stool contains 1 to 3 g fat if the patient has been NPO and 3 to 5 g of fat if the patient has been on a usual diet; a value greater than 6 g per day is abnormal. Tests for fecal fat are nonspecific. They establish the existence of fat malabsorption, but they do not determine whether the lesion causes pancreatic insufficiency, bile salt depletion, or ileal dysfunction.

The *labeled carbon breath test* is also sometimes used to evaluate fat absorption. The patient is given a dose of labeled fat (triolein). Breath samples are collected hourly 3 to 6 hours later and analyzed for labeled CO_2. Fat malabsorption is indicated if less than 3.4 percent of the labeled carbon is exhaled. This test, however, does not indicate the site of the lesion.

D-xylose absorption tests may help localize the lesion. D-xylose is a 5-carbon sugar which is absorbed without pancreatic digestion and is excreted in the urine. The patient is fasted overnight because xylose absorption is delayed by food. The patient then ingests 25 g D-xylose, and serum and urine are collected for 5 hours while the patient is on bed rest and without food. For adults, normal serum xylose in 1 to 2 hours is greater than 30 mg per 100 ml; normal urine value in 5 hours is greater than 4.5 g (3.5 if the patient is over age 65). Impaired absorption indicates disease of the intestinal mucosa.

The *Schilling test* may differentiate intrinsic-factor (IF) deficiency from decreased ileal absorption. The patient is given 1 mg of vitamin B_{12} intramuscularly and an oral dose of radioactive B_{12}. About a third of the radioactive dose should appear in the urine; ileal disease or pernicious anemia are suggested if less than 7% of the radioactive dose appears in the urine. If pernicious anemia is suspected, the test is repeated and IF is also given. If B_{12} is absorbed with simultaneous administration of IF and not absorbed without it, pernicious anemia is indicated. In the case of ileal malabsorption, IF will not correct the patient's failure to absorb B_{12}. These results are valid only in the well-hydrated patient with normal renal function and without bacterial overgrowth. If bacterial overgrowth is suspected, a course of antibiotic therapy is given and the test repeated.

A variation of the Schilling test can also be used to indicate pancreatic insufficiency. The patient is given two labeled cobalamines—one attached to a protein (R) and one attached to IF. Pancreatic protease is required to release the R-bound cobalamine. If this does not occur, the ratio of cobalamine to IF-bound cobalamine decreases in a 24-hour urine sample. The normal ratio is 0.5 to 1.0. The ratio 0.02 to 0.15 is abnormal.

The *bile acid breath test* is based on the fact that bile acids secreted into the intestine are normally reabsorbed in the ileum. A small amount reaches the colon, is metabolized to CO_2 by bacteria, and expired by the lungs. In this test, the patient is given a radioactively labeled bile salt, and expired air is collected for analysis for labeled CO_2. In ileal disease and in bacterial overgrowth with bile salt deconjugation, the bile salts are not absorbed normally, and more pass into the colon. They are metabolized by colon bacteria, resulting in the production of increased CO_2. Thus, more labeled CO_2 will be expired. The normal range is 2 to 20 parts per million (ppm). Levels may increase 20-fold in malabsorption.

The *lactose tolerance test* measures the rise in blood glucose following intake of a lactose load of 50 g in adults or 50 g per M^2 of surface area in children. An increase of less than 20 mg per dl is considered positive for lactose intolerance.

The *hydrogen breath test* measures the amount of hydrogen produced by the action of colon bacteria on carbohydrate. This test is most frequently used in the diagnosis of lactose intolerance. An adult is given 1.75 g lactose per kg of body weight. Excess hydrogen production (more than 20 ppm) 90 minutes after carbohydrate ingestion indicates malabsorption of carbohydrate. The test may also be used in the diagnosis of bacterial overgrowth.

Pancreatic function tests include those for *serum amylase, urine amylase,* and *serum lipase,* all of which may be elevated in pancreatic disease. Serum immunoreactive trypsin is decreased in pancreatic insufficiency. A *sweat test* is done on infants and children to diagnose cystic fibrosis with pancreatic insufficiency. Pilocarpine is given to induce sweating. Sweat is collected on preweighed gauze, and its chloride content is measured. Cystic fibrosis is indicated by a value of over 60 mEq Cl or Na per L of sweat (1, 2).

In the *secretin test,* the patient is given secretin and cholecystokinin (CCK), and the contents of the distal duodenum are then aspirated. The material is analyzed for pancreatic enzymes and HCO_3^-. In carcinoma of the pancreas and in pancreatitis, the levels are often reduced. Decreased enzymes with normal HCO_3^- suggests partial obstruction of the pancreatic ducts. The structure of the pancreas can be visualized by a *computerized tomography* (CT) scan or an *ultrasound.*

Roentgenograms with barium contrast are useful for diagnosing some intestinal disorders, but results tend to be nonspecific. *Biopsy* of the small intestine may be useful if the disease is continuous, rather than patchy. Other methods include examination of *intestinal fluids* and assays for *intestinal enzymes. Microscopic examination of the stool for ova and parasites* (O&P) is done to rule out the possibility that parasites are causing malnutrition by altering the intestinal mucosa or absorbing nutrients.

DIARRHEA

Malabsorption is accompanied by diarrhea, the severity of which varies widely. There are multiple causes of diarrhea, and these causes must be differentiated. Some of the procedures include *stool culture* for pathogenic bacteria and examination of the stool for ova, parasites, and leukocytes. *Direct visualization* includes gastroscopy, proctoscopy, and sigmoidoscopy. Before these are used, however, a common screening test— examination of the stool for *occult* (not grossly visible) *blood,* also known as the guaiac test or Hemoccult test—is performed. This test has many false positives and false negatives. It is generally considered to be more accurate if the patient has a meat-free, high-residue diet for 24 to 72 hours prior to the test. The elimination of meat reduces the number of false positive results, while the high residue increases the accuracy of detection of lesions, thereby reducing the number of false negatives. (High-residue diets are discussed in the next chapter.)

Some specialized tests include the *lactose tolerance test* to detect lactase deficiency, *assays for serum levels of gastrointestinal hormones,* and a test for *urinary 5-hydroxyindoleacetic acid* (5-HIAA), the metabolic breakdown product of serotonin, which is increased in carcinoid intestinal tumors. The 5-HIAA test diet requires the avoidance of bananas, tomatoes, red plums, avocado, eggplant, walnuts, papaya, and pineapple juice.

TO TEST YOUR UNDERSTANDING

1. Name some specific disorders in which steatorrhea is the result of the following. (Consult your text.)

   a. Pancreatic enzyme deficiency

   b. Bile deficiency

   c. Impaired intestinal absorptive capacity

2. List the diagnostic tests that require diet manipulation as part of the test procedures, give the diet requirements, and explain why the diet manipulations are needed.

3. A patient with fat malabsorption and steatorrhea has the following test results:

Xylose tolerance: 5-hr urine xylose, 2 g
Quantitative fecal fat: 25 g/day.

Is this patient more likely to have pancreatic insufficiency or intestinal mucosal disease? Explain your answer.

NUTRITIONAL ASSESSMENT IN GASTROINTESTINAL DISORDERS

Gastrointestinal disorders may have a profound effect on the patient's nutritional status. Nutritional assessment is therefore of great importance. In addition to the standard procedures of nutritional assessment described in Chapter 4, some additional questions that may be useful are listed below. Not all are appropriate for every patient, so you will need to choose. In addition, some questions will be answered in the patient's medical record, while others are appropriate for an interview.

In General:
Weight loss? when? how much?
Anorexia?
Nausea and vomiting? How often? When (in relation to meals)?

Specific to the Gastrointestinal Tract:
Drainage? how much? composition?
Absorption site affected by past surgeries? indicated by diagnostic procedures?
Constipation?

Diarrhea? duration? nature of onset? frequency? relationship to food intake? relationship to travel?

Social History:
Drug exposure? (antibiotics? laxatives?)
Alcohol consumption?
Food intolerances? allergies?
Prior dietary restrictions? compliance? duration?
Illnesses in self or family? (diabetes, inflammatory bowel disease)

Medications:
What drugs are being given?
Are any likely to cause problems?
Do they contain lactose? large amounts of sodium? alcohol?
Do any of the drugs cause nutrient loss? which drugs? which nutrients?

The following screening tests are often recommended in suspected malabsorption: calcium, phosphate, carotene, vitamin A, alkaline phosphatase, cholesterol, triglyceride, folate, vitamin B_{12}, magnesium, iron, TIBC, and prothrombin time. (See Table F-15.) The results of such screening tests can also be useful in the nutritional assessment.

TO TEST YOUR UNDERSTANDING

4. A patient's medical record states that the site of the malabsorption disorder lies in the areas given below. In each case, what nutrient deficits would you expect to occur if the disorder is not treated? Explain your answer.

a. Duodenum and proximal jejunum
b. Ileum

5. Assume you have a patient who is receiving each of the following drugs over a long period. In each case, list the nutrients at risk.

a. Mineral oil
b. Methotrexate
c. Tetracycline
d. Milk of Magnesia

APPROACHES TO NUTRITIONAL CARE IN MALABSORPTION SYNDROMES

Nutritional care in malabsorption can be divided into two categories: supportive and specific.

SUPPORTIVE THERAPY

Some intestinal diseases leave the patient without sufficient digestive or absorptive capacity to maintain good nutrition, and it is necessary to feed the patient parenterally. In other circumstances, the patient must be fed by tube. (The procedures used are those described in Chapters 12 and 13.) Regardless of the method of feeding, fluid and electrolyte balance are important considerations.

Electrolyte and Fluid Balance

The volume of GI secretions in the adult may total 8 to 9 L. Normally, these are reabsorbed, and only about 150 ml of water are excreted daily in the feces. When the amount of fluid in the intestine is compared to a plasma volume of about 3,500 ml, it is obvious that severe fluid imbalances may result if fluid losses from the digestive tract are abnormally high. Abnormal fluid balance can be the consequence not only of malabsorption syndromes and diarrhea, but also of conditions such as intestinal obstructions and fistulas. You may, therefore, apply this information to the care of patients with a variety of disorders.

A number of abnormal routes of fluid exchange are common in GI diseases. The patient may receive additional fluid via gastric or duodenal gavage or in an enema. Some routes of abnormal loss are shown in

Table 16-1. Loss of gastric juice may reach as much as 6,000 ml in some abnormal conditions. Gastric suction or prolonged vomiting are common routes of loss. Losses from the other tissues of the body occur when fluid in abnormal amounts moves into the intestinal tract, even if it does not leave the body. This type of loss, known as "third spacing," can occur, for example, in intestinal obstruction.

The loss of electrolytes depends not only on the volume of fluid lost, but also on its composition. The site of loss is a major determinant of composition. Gastric juice contains H^+ and Cl^- plus some Na^+ and K^+, and its loss can lead to fluid deficit, metabolic alkalosis (as a consequence of H^+ and Cl^- loss), and Na^+ and K^+ deficits.

The contribution of Cl^- loss to alkalosis may require some explanation. Cl^- combines with cations in competition with bicarbonate (HCO_3^-). When Cl^- is decreased, HCO_3^- is increased to compensate because the numbers of anions and cations must be equal. Therefore, when Cl^- is lost, HCO_3^- is retained, producing *hypochloremic metabolic alkalosis*.

When a patient's gastric contents are being suctioned, water or ice should not be given by mouth. The water increases the loss of electrolytes, which are suctioned off, leaving the patient in severe alkalosis. Instead, ice chips can be made from an electrolyte solution. Commercial oral electrolyte solutions, such as Lytren, are useful (see Table G-2).

Intestinal fluid may be lost from diarrhea, intestinal suction, or fistulas. In addition to fluid deficit, loss of intestinal juice can result in metabolic acidosis (HCO_3^- loss) and Na^+ and K^+ deficits. Bile can be

TABLE 16-1. Examples of Fluid and Electrolyte Losses by Abnormal Routes

Route	Fluid Volume ml/24 hr	Na^+	Electrolytes K^+	(mEq/L) Cl^-	HCO_3^-
Vomiting	100–6,000	140	4.5	100	24
Saliva drainage	1,500–2,000	20–80	10–20	20–40	20–60
Suction, drainage, intubation losses					
Gastric juice	2,500				
with HCl*		20–100	5–10	120–160	0
achlorhydric		8–120	1–30	100	20
Bile	700–1,000	134–156	3.9–6.3	83–110	38
Pancreatic juice	>1,000	113–153	2.6–7.4	54–95	110
Small intestine juice (Miller-Abbott suction)	3,000	72–120	3.5–6.8	69–127	30
Ileostomy, new	100–4,000	112–142	4.5–14.0	93–122	30
adapted	100–500	50	3	20	15–30
Cecostomy	100–3,000	48–116	11.1–28.3	37–70	15
Transudates	Variable	130–145	2.5–5.0	90–110	
Diarrhea, secretory	500–17,000	50–60	30–50	40–45	45

*Plus approximately 90 mEq H^+/L; K^+ losses may be higher due to increased urinary excretion of K^+ in alkalosis.

Compiled from Goldberger, E. *A Primer of Water, Electrolyte and Acid-Base Syndromes* (6th ed.). Philadelphia: Lea & Febiger, 1980; Stroot, V.R., C.A.B. Lee, and C.A. Barrett. *Fluids and Electrolytes: A Practical Approach* (3d ed.). Philadelphia: Davis, 1984; Weisberg, H. *Water, Electrolytes and Acid-Base Balance* (2d ed.). Baltimore: Williams and Wilkins, 1962.

lost from fistulas or from drainage following gallbladder surgery and results in Na^+ deficit and acidosis (HCO_3^- loss). Pancreatic juice loss depletes Na^+, HCO_3^-, and Cl^-, resulting in metabolic acidosis and deficits of fluid, sodium, and calcium.

The losses from osmotic and secretory diarrhea are dissimilar, and these differences must be taken into account when fluid and electrolyte balances are calculated. A comparison is given in Table 16-2. In secretory diarrheas, such as bile salt enteropathy, diarrhea from islet cell tumors, and Escherichia coli enteritis, sodium and potassium and their cations provide a stool osmolality about equal to serum osmolality. In osmotic diarrhea, such as that found in the use of magnesium-containing cathartics and in lactase deficiency or other carbohydrate malabsorptive states, less sodium and potassium are lost. The solute gap represents contributions of osmotically active solutes other than sodium, potassium, and their anions, including magnesium and organic ions. As Table 16-2 shows, loss of these materials is particularly severe in osmotic diarrhea. The patient tends to become hypernatremic because the intestine conserves sodium and chloride more effectively than it conserves water.

Minor fluid and electrolyte deficits can be corrected by dietary alterations only. Intravenous feedings are usually ordered to correct more substantial deficits. In either case, you must be aware of the effects of fluid and electrolyte deficiencies on indicators of nutritional status. Serum albumin and hematocrit values, for example, will be elevated in the dehydrated patient.

Continuing fluid and electrolyte losses must also be considered when making recommendations for the volume and composition of tube-feeding and parenteral-feeding formulas. You will also be asked to cooperate in measuring fluid intake.

TABLE 16-2. Comparison of Clinical Features of Osmotic and Secretory Diarrhea

Clinical Feature	Osmotic Diarrhea	Secretory Diarrhea
Daily stool volume, L	< 1	>1
Stool osmolality, mOsm/kg	400	290
Stool electrolytes, mEq/L		
Na^+	50	100
K^+	35	40
Solute gap, mOsm*	280	10
Response to fasting	subsides	continues

*Solute gap = Total mOsm − [(Na^+ + K^+) × 2]
(Na^+ + K^+) is multiplied by 2 to account for the anions.

Compiled from Gardner, J.D. Pathogenesis of secretory diarrhea. In *Secretory Diarrhea*, ed. M. Field. American Physiological Society, 1980, p. 154; Krejs, G.J. Diagnostic and pathophysiologic studies in patients with chronic diarrhea. In *Secretory Diarrhea*, ed. M. Field. American Physiological Society, 1980, p. 142.

TO TEST YOUR UNDERSTANDING

6. Explain how a patient can become dehydrated as a consequence of intestinal obstruction.

7. For each of the following factors, circle the aberration you would expect to see in a patient with a prolonged, uncorrected loss of 3 L of gastric juice per day, and explain the mechanism briefly.

   a. Fluid volume (deficit or excess?)
   b. Potassium balance (deficit or excess?)
   c. Sodium balance (deficit or excess?)
   d. Acid-base balance (acidosis or alkalosis?)

8. Explain the mechanisms by which metabolic acidosis may be produced when intestinal secretions are lost in diarrhea, suction, or following ileostomy.

General Nutritional Support

Vitamins and Minerals. Patients with malabsorption disorders usually need vitamin and mineral supplements. The recommended dosages for long-term oral supplementation are given in Table 16-3. In some cases, parenteral administration may be necessary. These supplements are usually administered as drugs. As the specialist in nutritional care, however, you should be alert to evidence of existing or potential nutrient deficiency and recommend supplementation when it is appropriate.

The nutrients at risk will vary with the location of intestinal involvement. Here is a general summary:

1. Proximal bowel (duodenum and upper jejunum) involvement, seen in Billroth II reconstruction, jejunal resection, nontropical sprue, and afferent loop syndrome:
   Iron, calcium, fat-soluble vitamins
   Fat, carbohydrates, amino acids
2. Midbowel (middle and lower jejunum) involvement, seen in extensive intestinal resection:
   Magnesium
   Amino acids, carbohydrates

3. Distal bowel (ileum) involvement, seen in ileal disease, ileal resection, regional enteritis, nontropical sprue, and lymphoma:
Vitamin B_{12}, bile salts

Protein and Energy. Many patients need replacement of calories and protein, with consideration of needs for essential fatty acids and amino acids. (Procedures for increasing oral intake are discussed in Chapter 11.) If the diet assessment indicates insufficient protein and energy intake, some patients may be

TABLE 16-3. Typical Micronutrient Doses for Nutritional Care of Patients with Malabsorption Syndromes

1. **Calcium**
   Calcium carbonate (500 mg/tab), 500 mg b.i.d. to q.i.d, po.
2. **Magnesium**
   Oral: Magnesium sulfate 1.0 to 4.0 g q.i.d.
   Intramuscular: Magnesium gluconate (20% sol.) 10 ml b.i.d. or t.i.d.
3. **Iron**
   Oral: $FeSO_4 \cdot 7H_2O$, 325 mg q.d. at HS.
   Intramuscular: Imferon. Must be calculated according to severity of anemia. Detailed instructions accompany preparation.
4. **Fat-Soluble Vitamins**
   a. Vitamin A
      Oleovitamin A capsules, USP (25,000 units per capsule), 100,000 to 200,000 units daily in severe deficiencies; 25,000 to 50,000 units daily for maintenance.
   b. Vitamin D
      Synthetic oleovitamin D, USP (10,000 USP units vitamin D/gram), 30,000 units daily; increase dosage as necessary to raise serum calcium to normal. Dosage varies considerably depending on response as determined by level of serum calcium and urinary calcium.
   c. Combination A and D Vitamins
      Concentrated oleovitamins A and D, USP (50,000 to 65,000 USP A units and 10,000 to 13,000 USP D units/g) may be used rather than separate preparations.
   d. Vitamin K
      Menadione, USP, 4 to 12 mg daily, po. Vitamin K_1 tablets (Mephyton), 5 to 10 mg daily, po.
5. **Folic Acid,** USP (1 mg tablets)
   Initial: 10 to 20 mg daily
   Maintenance: 5 to 10 mg daily
6. **Vitamin B_{12} Injection, USP** (15 μg/ml)
   Initial: 1000 μg loading dose, IM
   Maintenance: 100 to 200 μg sc q 1–2 months
   If combined-system disease is present, a more intensive program is indicated.
7. **Vitamin B Complex**
   Any multivitamin preparation that contains daily requirements (thiamine 1.6 mg, riboflavin 1.8 mg, and niacin 20 mg). Use two or three tablets daily. Intramuscular preparations are available for severe deficiencies.

Compiled from Sleisinger, M.H. and J.S. Fordtran. Diseases of malabsorption. In *Textbook of Medicine* (14th ed.), eds. P.B. Beeson and W. McDermott. Philadelphia: Saunders, 1975; Stenson, W.F. Malabsorption. In *Manual of Medical Therapeutics* (23d ed.), eds. J.J. Freitage and L.W. Miller. Boston: Little, Brown, 1980.

assisted with the use of a high-protein, high-calorie liquid supplement. The patient unable to ingest enough food by these means may be given supplemental tube feedings. (Procedures are described in Chapter 12.) The feeding formula chosen must be appropriate to the patient's disorder, as discussed in the next section. If GI function is inadequate to maintain normal nutritional status by these methods, TPN may be used (see Chapter 13).

SPECIFIC NUTRITIONAL THERAPY

Three diet modifications are most often useful in nutritional care of specific types of malabsorption: *fat restriction, lactose restriction,* and *gluten restriction.* They may be used separately or in combination, depending upon the patient's needs.

The Fat-Restricted Diet

Malabsorption can affect many nutrients, but malabsorption of fat is the most common. The resulting steatorrhea may occur in the presence of bile salt deficiency, pancreatic insufficiency, or defects in the absorptive capability of the intestinal mucosa itself.

Most of these conditions require a low fat intake as part of their treatment. In these diets, the term *fat* refers to *triglycerides* and does not consider other lipids, such as cholesterol. The diet does not reverse the abnormal physiology; instead, it helps control the symptoms. As a consequence, the level of restriction must vary with the degree of malabsorption.

The diet manuals of many institutions list several levels of fat restriction from which to choose as a baseline for planning. These diet levels may be based on a percentage of total energy, such as a mild (35 to 40 percent of total kcal), moderate (25 percent) or severe (10 to 15 percent) restriction. Alternatively, diets may be planned for a specified number of g of fat, such as 30, 50, 70, or 40, 60, 75 (3–5). In any case, the diet should be adjusted to the needs of the individual patient.

For patients with minimal impairment, avoidance of high-fat meats and fried foods may be a sufficient modification. The exchange lists shown in Tables C-1 to C-8 may be used to calculate the basic diet plan and to estimate fat content for more restricted diets. Fat exchanges should be planned so that the fat intake is evenly distributed among meals.

Examples from a more detailed list of foods and their fat content, given as "fat portion exchanges," are listed in Table B-5 (6). These values are based on the same concept as the exchange lists in Tables C-1 to C-9. Each item and quantity listed provides one "fat exchange" containing 5 g fat. Using this system, a patient who requires a 50-g-fat diet could be advised to make up the day's diet to include 10 fat portion exchanges.

Although exchange lists are useful while you are learning to plan these diets, they are seldom used for this purpose by experienced nutritional care specialists in clinical situations. Some guidelines for planning specific menus are given in Table 16-4.

When fat is restricted, the diet becomes high in carbohydrate and in osmolality. If the carbohydrate is in small molecules, a carbohydrate-induced diarrhea may develop. (See Chapter 12.)

When fat is severely restricted, protein intake may be limited, since most protein foods also contain fat. If the diet does not then meet the patient's needs, it may be necessary to add a supplement to provide additional protein. At the same time, the supplement must be low in fat.

A fat-restricted diet may not meet the patient's energy needs, because many calorie-dense foods are removed. *Medium-chain triglycerides* are useful to increase the energy intake of the patient who cannot digest and absorb sufficient sources of energy.

Medium-chain triglycerides are derived from coconut oil. The oil is fractionated to separate the fatty acids that are 8 (octanoic) and 10 (decanoic) carbon atoms in length, as compared with most dietary fats, which have 16 and 18 carbon atoms in the fatty acids. When the isolated medium-chain fatty acids are re-

TABLE 16-4. General Guidelines for Planning Fat-Restricted Diets

1. Use skim milk in severe restriction; for higher fat levels, 2% milk may be useful.
2. Avoid cream cheese, hard cheeses; choose low-fat (1%) cottage cheese, sapsago cheese, other skim milk cheeses.
3. Avoid high-fat meats. Use low-fat or medium-fat meats as calculated into the diet. Meat exchanges should be broiled, baked, or boiled, not fried. Remove skin from chicken and turkey. Use skim-milk cheese with less than 5% fat.
4. Avoid most baked desserts, such as cakes, cookies, pies, and pastries. Exception: angel food cake.
5. Avoid cream sauces and gravies.
6. Avoid bread and cereal products made with fat. Examples: doughnuts, fritters, muffins.
7. Avoid candies made with chocolate, nuts, or any fat.
8. Use plainly prepared vegetables, not creamed, fried, or with sauces containing fat. Avoid olives.
9. Use fruit as desired. Exception: avocado.
10. Use fat exchanges only as calculated into the diet plan.
11. Use fat-free desserts; avoid dessert containing fat, chocolate, or nuts unless included in fat allowance.
12. Use spices and herbs as desired.
13. Limit alcohol.
14. Plan for nutritional adequacy.

TABLE 16-5. Procedures for the Use of Medium-Chain Triglycerides in the Diet

1. Combine MCT Oil with beverages:
   a. Combine 1–2 T MCT Oil with fruit juice, tomato juice, or carbonated beverages.
   b. Combine 1–2 T MCT Oil with ½ c skim milk.
   c. Combine 2–4 t MCT Oil with ⅓ c nonfat dry milk powder and ⅔ c water. Mix in a blender. Sugar and nonfat flavorings may be added.
2. Substitute MCT Oil for vegetable oils in mayonnaise, salad dressings, and sauces.
3. Use MCT Oil to stir-fry vegetables.
4. Use MCT Oil in grilling meats; use low heat because MCT Oil has a low smoke point.
5. Use MCT Oil in baking in place of regular oil, such as pancakes, waffles, muffins, and chiffon cakes. Use egg whites in place of whole eggs and skim milk in place of whole milk in such recipes.

Compiled from *Mayo Clinic Diet Manual* (5th ed.), eds. C.M. Pemberton and C.F. Gastineau. Philadelphia: Saunders, 1981.

esterified, a thin, clear oil is produced. It is available as MCT Oil (Mead Johnson, Evansville, Ind.) and in selected tube-feeding and infant formulas.

The caloric yield of MCT Oil is described in Chapter 12, and should be reviewed if necessary. It is important to note that MCT Oil contains no essential fatty acids (7).

MCT Oil should be added to the diet gradually. Most patients can tolerate 20 to 60 g, but side effects may develop if larger amounts are fed or if intake is suddenly increased. The limit on caloric yield is thus about 400 kcal. Side effects include nausea, vomiting, diarrhea, and abdominal pain and distention. MCT Oil is sometimes given as a medication; if it is used as a food, information must be provided to the patients on its use in foods and food preparation. Some suggestions are contained in Table 16-5. Recipes are available from the manufacturer (8) and elsewhere (9, 10).

MCT Oil is also available as Portagen Powder. Its fat content is 86 percent MCT, with the remainder as corn oil, and it is supplemented with vitamins and minerals (see Table G-2). The powder is reconstituted with water to make a milk-like drink. Since Portagen provides a high osmotic load, it should be given cautiously, 1 to 2 glasses per day, sipped slowly, to start. Because of the high osmotic load, it is also important to maintain adequate fluid intake.

TO TEST YOUR UNDERSTANDING

9. Your institution lists three levels of fat-restricted diets in its diet manual. The moderate restriction is set at 25% of total calories. You estimate that your patient needs 2,400 kcal per day.
   a. How many g of fat would you give a patient requiring a moderate fat restriction?
   b. How many "fat portion exchanges" would you give?
   c. How many g of fat would you give at each of three meals?

10. You have a patient who requires a diet containing 45 g of fat. Make a list of the exchanges from Tables C-1 through C-8 and note the numbers of servings of each that should be included in the diet to provide this amount of fat.

11. You have a patient who requires a severe fat restriction, and who is somewhat anorectic and cannot meet her needs for the nutrients listed below. Name supplementary sources that could be added to her food, and suggest some foods to which they could be added. (You may wish to review Chapter 12.)

12. List high-calorie, high-protein oral *liquid supplements* that might be useful for a patient on a severe fat-restricted diet who is having difficulty maintaining normal weight. Give the fat and energy content of two 8 oz servings.

13. List the tube feedings that would be useful for this patient, and note the fat and energy content of each.

14. Why is a patient on MCT always given some sources of long-chain triglycerides?

15. List oral or supplemental formulas containing medium-chain triglycerides in the following categories:

   a. Hydrolyzed protein
   b. Non-milk-based feeding
   c. Milk-based with intact protein
   d. Blenderized feeding

16. How many kcals can be obtained from ¼ c of MCT oil? Show your calculations.

17. What formula would be most useful for a 3-month-old infant with severe fat malabsorption?

18. What vitamin deficiencies would you watch for in a patient with fat malabsorption? Are these pathognomonic?

19. You have a patient who needs a 1,600-kcal diet with 30 g fat. Using the menu for _____ (day to be assigned by your instructor), plan one day's diet for this patient.

The Lactose-Restricted Diet

Lactose intolerance may be present as the patient's sole complaint or may be secondary to other conditions. It may occur with, and aggravate, the symptoms of gluten-sensitive enteropathy and regional enteritis, for example, or it may become aggravated by these conditions. Patients who are deficient in lactase will benefit from a reduction in the lactose content of their diets, but "lactose-intolerant" individuals vary widely in their ability to digest lactose. Many patients can tolerate 12 g lactose per day, the amount in 8 oz of milk, while some patients may tolerate as little as 3 g. Total lactose avoidance is not usually necessary except in galactosemia.

The goals of the diet for the lactose-intolerant patient are (1) to reduce lactose intake to a level that will not cause intestinal symptoms, and (2) to provide for adequate nutrient intake.

Diet Planning. Institutional diet manuals may contain a "lactose-free" diet for those who need complete lactose restriction, or they may present diets varying in lactose levels. In either case, the diet should be adjusted to the individual patient's tolerance. Making such adjustments is difficult, however, since information on the lactose content of foods is limited. As a result, a trial-and-error process may be required. Table 16-6 lists some values that may be helpful in initial planning. Table 16-7 offers general guidelines for a completely lactose-restricted diet and for modifications for less severe restrictions.

TABLE 16-6. Lactose Content of Selected Foods

Food	Amount	Lactose (g)
Milk, whole or skim	1 c	11
2% fat	1 c	9–13
buttermilk	1 c	10.3–12.0
skim	1 c	11–14
powdered skim	30 g	15.5
chocolate	1 c	10–12
condensed sweetened	1 c	35
goats'	1 c	8.1
Cream, light	1 T	0.6
half and half	1 T	0.6
whipped topping	1 T	0.4
Ice cream, regular	1 c	9
sherbet	1 c	4
ice milk	1 c	10
Butter	2 t	0.1
Cheese, Parmesan, Gouda, blue	1 oz	0.6–0.8
American, Cheddar	1 oz	0.5
Camembert, Limberger	1 oz	0.1–0.2
Cream	1 oz	0.8
Cottage, regular	1 c	5–6
lowfat	1 c	7–8
Yogurt	1 c	11–15
Milk chocolate	100 g	8.1

Compiled from Alpers, D.H., R.E. Clouse, and W. F. Stenson. *Manual of Nutritional Therapeutics.* Boston: Little, Brown, 1983; Gallagher, C.R., A.L. Molleson, and J.H. Caldwell. Lactose intolerance and fermented dairy products. *J. Am. Diet. Assoc.* 65:(1974) 418–419; *Handbook of Clinical Dietetics,* eds. T.T. Jensen, J.E. Staggers, and M. Johnston. Salt Lake City: Utah Dietetic Association, 1977; Hardinge, M.H. et al. Carbohydrates in foods. *J. Am. Diet. Assoc.* 46:(1965) 197–204; Walser, M., A.L. Imbembo, S. Margolis, and G.A. Elfert. *Nutritional Management.* Philadelphia: Saunders, 1984.

TABLE 16-7. General Guidelines for Planning Lactose Restricted Diets

In General:

1. Avoid or restrict as necessary milk in liquid, canned, or powdered form.
2. Labels should be read carefully for the content of milk, milk products, milk solids, skim milk, skim milk powder, skim milk solids, milk sugar, and lactose. Restrict foods containing these items as necessary to the tolerance of the patient.
3. Small amounts of cheese and butter may be tolerated.
4. Avoid use of large quantities of milk or cream in cooking.
5. Plan for nutritional adequacy. Supplementation may be necessary.

For diets with 3 g or less lactose per day:

1. Omit all milk and milk products, yogurt, ice cream, sherbet, ice milk, prepared puddings, milk drinks, malted milk products. Use soybased milks, whipped toppings, nondairy creamers.
2. Limit cheese to 1 oz/day or less.
3. Read labels carefully. Avoid products containing "lactose," "dry milk solids," or "milk sugar." "Lactic acid," "lactate," "lactalbumin," and "lactylate" are tolerated.
4. Avoid creamed or breaded meats, vegetables; avoid vegetables with lactose added in processing. (Read labels.)
5. Avoid meat products that contain lactose. (Read labels.)
6. Avoid fruits with lactose added in processing. (Read labels.)
7. Avoid prepared mixes, dry cereals with added lactose (Total, Special K, Fortified Oat Flakes, Cocoa Krispies, Instant Cream of Wheat), bread and rolls containing milk products, commercial cakes, cookies, pastries with cream fillings, or lactose-sweetened fillings.
8. Avoid any products containing chocolate.
9. Avoid instant coffee, powdered soft drinks with lactose, Kool-Aid, many candies, monosodium glutamate, soy sauce.

For patients with a greater tolerance:

1. Some patients who tolerate 10–25 g lactose may have 1–2 c milk or ice cream/day; ½ c milk or ice cream will provide 5–6 g lactose.
2. Patients tolerate lactose better if milk is taken with other foods and in small amounts throughout the day.
3. Some patients have a greater tolerance for warmed milk, buttermilk, or yogurt.
4. Consider the use of Lact-Aid to increase milk intake. Advise patients on procedures for its use.

Lactose tolerance may be improved if milk is taken along with other food to delay gastric emptying. Milk tolerance may also be improved if milk intake is divided into small, more frequent servings.

You may want to offer your nutritional-counseling patients some references for milk-free recipes. You can also give directions for use of acidophilus milk and Lact-Aid, which will be described in the next section. These may help the patient maintain an adequate calorie intake when other nutrients, such as fat or gluten, are also restricted.

Special Products. Special products are available for the lactose-intolerant patient and may be helpful in menu planning. Some have the nutrient content of milk and are useful in providing for nutritionally adequate diets.

Sweet acidophilus milk is a low-fat (2 percent) milk to which a *Lactobacillus acidophilus* culture has been added. The culture causes the hydrolysis of lactose to glucose and galactose, resulting in increased sweetness. The taste is otherwise similar to that of low-fat milk. Since the product contains reduced lactose (80 to 90 percent less), it is often tolerated by lactose-intolerant patients.

Lact-Aid (Sugar Lo Company, Atlantic City, N.J.) consists of packets of lactase enzyme, each of which is sufficient to treat 1 quart of milk. If the contents are added to 1 quart of fresh milk, mixed well, and allowed to stand in the refrigerator for 24 hours, at least 70 percent of the lactose present will be converted to simple sugars. There is 90 percent conversion in 2 to 3 days. Severely lactose-intolerant patients can convert the milk sugar to a greater degree by adding more packets to the fresh milk. Three packets per quart, for example, will convert 98 percent of the lactose present in 24 hours. The single-packet treatment is balanced to provide lactose conversion sufficient to permit an estimated 80 percent of lactase-deficient patients to enjoy treated milk.

The milk used for treatment can be fresh fluid, skim, or reconstituted from dried milk; cultured milks and dairy products other than milk cannot be treated this way. Once treated, lactase-modified milk can also be used in cooking, for preparing yogurt or buttermilk, or in any other application for which milk would be used.

Lact-Aid incorporates lactase derived from *Kluveromyces lactis*, a common food yeast, diluted with dextrose. The application of heat must be carefully controlled because the enzyme is inactivated at temperatures above 105° F. The enzyme is also pH sensitive in the acid ranges, so use of poor-quality milk interferes with the lactase action.

Products such as Mocha Mix, Coffee Rich, and Vita-Rich may also be useful in the lactose-restricted diet. These are milk-free, cholesterol-free dairy supplements which can be used as milk substitutes. Sugar content and osmolarity are high, and the taste may not be entirely acceptable. Various soy-based and lactose-free supplementary feedings, infant formulas, and tube feedings are listed in Appendix G.

TO TEST YOUR UNDERSTANDING

20. a. List the nutrients that are most likely to be deficient if a patient's diet must be milk-free. For each, give alternative food sources and commonly used supplements.
    b. Discuss the ease or difficulty of obtaining sufficient amounts of these nutrients in a milk-free diet.

21. Your patient says that she can manage 12 oz of milk per day if she does not drink more than 4 oz in 4 hours. In order to provide her with greater flexibility in menu planning, you give her a list of alternative foods that have about the same amount of lactose as 4 oz of milk. What serving sizes would you suggest for each item?

    a. Ice cream _____ c

    b. Yogurt _____ c

    c. Cottage cheese _____ c

    d. Cream soup _____ c

22. You have a patient who requires a lactose-free diet. Using the menu for _____ (day to be assigned by your instructor), write a day's diet for your patient.

The Gluten-Restricted Diet

The gluten-restricted diet eliminates glutens contained in wheat, rye, and barley protein or any derivatives from these cereals. The gluten-intolerant patient may also be sensitive to oat gluten. Rice and corn contain different glutens which are not toxic and need not be eliminated.

TABLE 16-8. General Guidelines for Nutritional Care in Gluten Intolerance

1. Omit toxic gluten from the diet.
   a. Omit wheat, rye, barley, and oats.
   b. Substitute corn, rice, potato flour, soy bean flour, tapioca, sago, arrowroot.
   c. Avoid foods containing flours of unspecified origin, graham flour, bran, bulgur, groats, starches of unspecified origin, emulsifiers, stabilizers, hydrolyzed vegetable protein, hydrolyzed plant protein, malt, malt flavoring, malt syrup, malt vinegar, malted milk, millet, modified food starch, oat germ, oatmeal, vegetable gum, wheat germ, wheat gluten, wheat starch.
   d. Read labels carefully.
   e. Use fresh meats, fish, eggs, milk, fruits, and vegetables.
   f. Unless certain that specific brands are gluten-free, be cautious about
      cereal-based beverages (Ovaltine, Postum, beer, ale, instant coffee, root beer)
      commercial ice cream, cakes, cookies and similar baked goods
      salad dressings
      canned or processed meats
      canned soups, cream soups
      candy bars
      mustard, catsup
      breaded, creamed, or scalloped products
      chocolate milk
      frozen foods with sauces
      processed cheese
2. Plan the diet to ensure adequate intake of all nutrients, since the diet is long-term. Supplement with vitamins and minerals if necessary.
3. Instruct patient carefully on
   foods to use
   foods to avoid
   hidden sources of gluten
   label reading
   diet planning for nutritional adequacy
   preparation of gluten-free products
4. Instruct patient on the following, if appropriate:
   choosing a diet in a restaurant
   additional restrictions of other nutrients (e.g. lactose, fat) if indicated.

TABLE 16-9. Substitutes for Wheat Flour

Substitutes for 1 c wheat flour
In baking:

1 c	cornflour
¾ c	coarse cornmeal
1 c (scant)	fine cornmeal
⅝ c	potato flour
⅞ c	rice flour
1¼ c	rye flour
1 c	rye meal

As a thickener:
1 T wheat flour = ½ T cornstarch, potato starch, arrowroot starch, rice flour, or 2 t quick-cooking tapioca

Cooking and baking tips
Bake more slowly and for a longer period.
Use soy flour in combination with other flours.
When cooking with rice flour or cornmeal, mix with the liquid in the recipe, bring to boil, cool before adding to the other ingredients.
Increase leavening to 2½ t/c when using coarse forms of wheat substitutes.
Bake items in small sizes.
Cakes made with wheat-flour substitutes tend to be dry. Store in closed containers. Add frosting.

Compiled from *Manual of Allergy and Immunology*. Lawler, G.J., Jr., and T.J. Fischer (eds.). Boston: Little, Brown, 1981, p. 467; Ohlson, M.A. *Experimental and Therapeutic Dietetics* (2d ed.). Minneapolis: Burgess, 1972, pp. 142–143.

General guidelines for nutritional care of the gluten-intolerant patient are listed in Table 16-8. Lists of foods allowed and not allowed, stated in general terms, are contained in most diet manuals. Such lists give information on avoiding obvious forms of wheat, rye, barley, and oats, but they often provide less information on hidden forms of gluten. These hidden forms or derivatives have been called "nebulous ingredients" (11). In order to provide adequate care, the nutritional care specialist must know these sources and instruct the patient on label reading to detect their presence. A list of food materials of which the patient must beware is also contained in Table 16-8.

It is also helpful to the patient to have a list of commercially prepared foods that are usable on a gluten-restricted diet. You should prepare a list of those that are available in your area and update it when ingredients and manufacturing procedures change. Exacerbations of the disease are often the consequence of diet errors.

The primary foods eliminated are cereals and cereal products. This obviously limits the use of many foods of which the patient may be fond, such as baked desserts. Therefore, you may want to provide suggestions and directions for substitutes. These ready-made products are expensive, however.

As an alternative to ready-made products, patients can be given directions on food preparation with ac-ceptable alternative cereal products. Some general directions are given in Table 16-9. These are useful for the patient or caregiver who can use initiative and imagination in food preparation. Most patients will also find recipes helpful. Such information is likely to increase diet compliance, encourage greater variety in food intake, and improve the likelihood that the diet will be nutritionally adequate.

TO TEST YOUR UNDERSTANDING

23. What nutrients must be considered if cereals are removed from the diet?

24. Mr. R. is suffering from an exacerbation of his gluten intolerance. He gives you the following 24-hour recall. Circle those items which might account for his current symptoms and about which you should inquire in further detail.

Breakfast:
Orange juice
Cornmeal/milk/sugar
Poached eggs
Rice crackers (no wheat)
Instant coffee

Lunch:
Ham sandwich with gluten-free bread/lettuce/catsup
Malted milk

Snack:
Chocolate-nut bar

Dinner:
Roast beef
Baked potato
Creamed peas
Head lettuce/Thousand Island dressing
Fresh fruit cup

25. Using the menu for _____ (day to be assigned by your instructor), write one day's diet for Mr. R.

26. Using the menu for _____ (day to be assigned by your instructor), write one day's diet for a gluten-intolerant patient who has also developed fat malabsorption and a lactase deficiency. He can tolerate 40 g fat and 8 oz milk per day.

TOPICS FOR FURTHER DISCUSSION

1. What conditions of organs other than the GI tract indicate a need for a low-fat diet?

2. What conditions other than lactose intolerance indicate a need to reduce milk intake? Compare the degree of restriction required for each.

3. Taste-test some of the special products described in this chapter.

4. Discuss modification of fat-, lactose-, and gluten-restricted diets for patients with ethnic origins common in your area.

5. Discuss nutritional support in inflammatory bowel disease.

REFERENCES

1. *Manual of Pediatric Nutrition,* eds. D.G. Kelts and E.G. Jones. Boston: Little, Brown, 1984.
2. *The Laboratory in Clinical Medicine* (2d ed.), eds. J.A. Halsted and C.H. Halsted. Philadelphia: Saunders, 1981.
3. AMERICAN DIETETIC ASSOCIATION. *Handbook of Clinical Dietetics.* New Haven: Yale University Press, 1981.
4. *Mayo Clinic Diet Manual* (5th ed.), eds. C.M. Pemberton and C.F. Gastineau. Philadelphia: Saunders, 1981.
5. ALPERS, D.H., R.E. CLOUSE, AND W.F. STENSON. *Manual of Nutritional Therapeutics.* Boston: Little, Brown, 1983.
6. BOYAR, A.P. AND J.R. LOUGHRIDGE. The fat portion exchange list: A tool for teaching and evaluating low-fat diets, *J. Am. Diet. Assoc.* 85:(1985)589–594.
7. PAGE, D.M. *Manual of Clinical Nutrition.* Pleasantville, N.J.: Nutrition Publications, Inc., 1983.

8. *Recipes Using MCT Oil and Portagen.* Evansville, Ind.: Mead Johnson and Company.
9. SCHIZAS, A.A., J.A. CREMEN, E. LARSON, AND R. O'BRIEN. Medium-chain triglycerides: Use in food preparation. *J. Am. Diet. Assoc.* 51:(1967)228–232.
10. *Medium-Chain Triglycerides,* ed. J.R. Senior. Philadelphia: University of Pennsylvania Press, 1968.

ADDITIONAL SOURCES OF INFORMATION

Disorders of the Small Intestine, eds. C.C. Booth and G. Neale. Boston: Blackwell, 1985.

SLEISENGER, M.H. AND J.S. FORDTRAN. *Gastrointestinal Disease: Pathophysiology, Diagnosis, Management* (3d ed.). Philadelphia: Saunders, 1983.

CASE STUDY V MALABSORPTION

 88

Part I: Presentation

Present Illness: Jocelyn W. is a 20 y.o. nursing student referred for evaluation of chronic diarrhea. She denies presence of blood or mucus in her stools. She C/O weight loss, fatigue, weakness, and diarrhea of 1 month's duration with production of 4–5 bulky, semiformed, foul-smelling stools per day. The symptoms had occurred previously but were more severe and prolonged this time. She denies recent travel to a foreign country. No one else in her residence has similar Sx, and she has no fever or joint pains. She has had no contact with any patient with diarrhea in her work as a student nurse.

Past Medical History: She had measles in childhood and a broken leg about 10 years ago. There is a history of exac-erbations and remissions of diarrhea since childhood.

Family History: An older sister died in infancy of undiagnosed diarrhea.

Social History: Single. Lives in dormitory for students and eats in student cafeteria. Very active—runs, swims.

Review of Systems: Patient has no complaints except for excess flatulence and diarrhea.

Physical Exam: Black female, 5 ft 6 in, 113 #, medium frame. Abdomen is proruberant, with a doughy consistency on palpation. No tenderness. Oral mucosa slightly dry. There is slight tachycardia with mild postural changes. Stool is heme-negative. Remainder of exam is WNL.

Laboratory:

		Normal
Serum albumin, g/dl	↓ 3.0	3.5–4.5
Total lymphocytes/mm³	↓ 1,200	↓1500 def 2000 (N)
RBC/mm³	↓ 4.0 × 10⁶	4.2-5.4
Hgb, g/dl	12.0	12-14 10-16?
Hct, %	38	37-47
Serum Na, mEq/L	↓ 135	136-145
Serum K, mEq/L	3.5	3.5-5.0
Serum Cl, mEq/L	↓ 95	100-106?
Serum HCO₃, mEq/L	20	22-26
Serum P, inorganic, mEq/L	↓ 1.9	2.5-4.5
BUN, mg/dl	↑ 30	8-25
Serum creatinine, mg/dl	1.2	0.7-1.5
Urine specific gravity	↑ 1.040	1.003-1.030
TSF, mm	↓ 12.2	16.5
MAMC, cm	↓ 18.1	23.2

(handwritten right margin:) dehyd= ↑BUN, ↑creat, ↑ sp gr or ↑BUN↓electro

(handwritten:) celiac disease

Impression: Chronic diarrhea and dehydration in a 20 y.o., slightly underweight black female with a positive history of sporadic, chronic diarrhea.

Plan: R/O gluten-sensitive enteropathy, diffuse intestinal lymphoma, Zollinger-Ellison syndrome, early collagenous sprue.

(handwritten:) celiac ↓ 2° to celiac

QUESTIONS

1. Fill in the normal values in the spaces provided above.
2. Briefly evaluate the patient's nutritional and hydration status. Indicate the data that support your evaluation.

(handwritten answer:)

① ↓13% under IBW = BEE to ↑ IBW (130) 2826
        "   " keep @ 113 = 2677

↑dehydr. ↑BUN, ↑creat ↑ sp gr, ↓elect

↑PMN – ↓TSF, ↓MAMC, ↓albumen

Part II: Diagnosis
Further laboratory studies produced the following:

		Normal
Fecal fat, g/day	↑ 20	6 1-3 *eg w/o*
Serum cholesterol, mg/dl	↓ 125	122-216 *x̄ = 124* 150-250
D-xylose absorption/5-hr urine	↓ 2.5	4.5/5 hr
Schilling test, radioactivity/24-hr urine	20%	8-40%
Serum amylase, Somogyi units/dl	100	80-160
Serum lipase, Cherry-Crandall units/ml	1.2	0-1.5
Plasma carotene, µg/dl	20	40+ 20-39 *marg*
Plasma vitamin A, µg/dl	10	20+
Bile acid breath test, ppm	15	0-20
Fecal occult blood	Negative	(-)
Prothrombin time, sec	14.8	11-12.5
Stool O&P	None seen	(-) (+) = parasites

Roentgenogram of the small intestine following a barium meal showed dilation of the small intestine with obliteration of the mucosal folds. The barium meal was fragmented and flocculent in the upper and middle portions of the jejunum. Ileal mucosa appeared normal. Endoscopic biopsy, following treatment with vitamin K given IM, revealed a flat mucosal surface with no intestinal villi. Intestinal crypts were elongated. The cells on the epithelial surface were cuboidal, with a markedly reduced brush border. Crypt cells were markedly increased, with an increased number of mitoses.

QUESTIONS

3. In the spaces provided above, give the normal values for each lab test.

4. a. Which laboratory tests are indicators of pancreatic function?

b. Based on these results, what would you conclude about this patient's pancreatic function?

D-xylose - ↓ absorption indicates disease of intestinal mucosa -- intestinal malabsorption
Schilling = not valid because she is not well hydrated
Bile acid = WNL, no malnuts.
amylase + lipase = WNL, would be ↑ if panc. disease

5. List the signs, symptoms, and laboratory results in the case study that indicate or are compatible with the following:

schilling --

a. Acidosis *- acid breath test (WNL), HCO₃ ↓*

low serum HCO₃⁻ → acidosis

b. Electrolyte depletion *Na⁺, K⁺ boarderline, Cl low*

c. Malabsorption *- fat due to fecal fat + foul smelling, stools*

6. Why is a prothrombin time value obtained prior to intestinal biopsy?

√ vit K status + eval clotting time
clotting prothime or so adm K imprior to biopsy

7. From the laboratory results, is there evidence of ileal involvement? Explain your answer.

ileum = bile salts, lab show chol no
↓ -evidence of fat malab.
and ↑ fecal fat because not abs, is passed

8. List evidence from the case study that suggests that the patient might be malabsorbing the following nutrients:

a. Protein ↓albumin↑, ↓MAMC, ↓TSF
↑BUN = nit excretion is ↑, so not absorbed

b. Fat — fecal fat, chol↓

c. Carbohydrate xylose absorp↓

d. Vitamins (Specify which) fat sol vitamins, B6, B12, folate
fat sol because of problems absorb. fat
vit A + carotene ↓, chol ↓, proteine ↑,

e. Minerals (Specify which) iron, R/T folate, B12
Hgb (borderline), Calcium (R/T D, K)   K⁺, Na⁺ = lab values
⊕ zinc R/T A + night blindness   Cl = ↓

Part III: Continued Treatment

The patient's fluid and electrolyte balances were corrected with IV feeding, after which the following laboratory results were obtained:

Hgb, g/dl	11.2
Hct, %	36
RBC/mm^3	3.8×10^6
BUN, g/dl	15
Creatinine, mg/dl	1.0

The medical record now lists the following problems:

1. Gluten-sensitive enteropathy. — sibling died as infant / diag in adults 20-30 yrs, under "stress"
2. Fat malabsorption
3. Anemia, 2° to Problem 1
4. Malnutrition, 2° to Problem 1

Plan: R/O lactose intolerance

QUESTIONS

9. List the basis on which anemia was included as a problem. ↓intake folate, B12
malabsorption of folate, B12, R/T IF?
pernicious or iron def. or megaloblastic
Iron, ↓, Hgb, Hct lower end

10. Explain why this evidence of anemia did not appear when the pt was first admitted.
because Hgb, Hct were WNL (↓ borderline) and dropped after adm, 2° problem to fat mal. dehydration set off values

Part IV: Nutritional Care

Interview of the patient elicited the following information:

Intake of large quantities of milk recently made symptoms worse. Patient had restricted milk intake to no more than 8 oz/day. Patient stated she "might be allergic" to milk, but denied other allergies.

An attempt to obtain a 24-hr recall revealed that the patient had eaten little for 3 days PTA. Her intake the previous day totaled 800 kcal and 20 g protein. Further interview elicited the following as a sample typical menu when she was feeling well: DO last.

gluten - causes damaged enterocytes + ↓ disaccharases

Breakfast:
¼ cantaloupe
¾ c Rice Krispies, ¼ c milk
1 egg
1 Danish pastry
Coffee, 1 t sugar

Lunch:
3 oz hamburger (high fat) on sesame seed roll, catsup
3 oz potato chips
½ c ice cream
12 oz soft drink

Dinner:
5 oz roast pork
½ c sweet potato
½ c buttered frozen peas
Tossed salad with Thousand Island dressing
Apple pie with ½ oz sliced cheese garnish
Tea, lemon

QUESTIONS

11. The attending gastroenterologist has corrected the fluid and electrolyte imbalances and has ordered a "gluten-free, low-fat diet; low-lactose diet as tolerated." Write the SOAP note you would place in this patient's medical record at this point.

    [handwritten notes:]
    * Recommend daily multivitamin + mineral *Fe*
      supplement (@ 100% RDA), not megadoses
    * Explain rationale of gluten free + ↓ fat, lactose
      as tol diet +
    * Handouts: * ↑ Ca foods; * gluten-free foods;
      * lactose - cont. foods; * ↑ fat foods, info
      on label reading
    * Recommend "lactaid"-type medication
    * Instructed patient how to ↑ lactose-cont.
      foods as tol
    * Eval on outpatient 3 months

    [margin notes:] Do LAST

12. Describe the mechanisms by which the fat malabsorption and lactose intolerance were produced.

    [handwritten notes:]
    fat malabsorption | lactose intol
    ↑amt fecal fat | self diagnosis=
    foul smelling stools | symptoms ↑ w/
    | ↑ intake

    [margin notes:] *patient given sample menu *patient ushed to select menu

13. Using the menu for _____ (day to be assigned by your instructor), plan a diet for one day for this patient.

§along w/ menu

²consume only in mixed meal

14. a. What changes would you make in the diet recommended in Question 11 for this patient to use when discharged from the hospital?

① limit milk to 1 c daily, eat other foods ↑ ca (give list)
give ideas for gluten replacement products and
recipe exchanges

↑ cal/protein w/ nutri dense foods

b. Prior to the present illness (PI), the patient had maintained normal weight. What difficulties would you expect her to have on the presently prescribed diet? What suggestions would you give her?

sub for wheat flour

↑ P.206!!

adherence to diet, esp ↓ fat + gluten
use of marg products, skim milk,
yogurt, ice milk
use lactaid tabs
Contact celiac asso, give info

Problem : ~~Malabsorption~~ *Gluten sen. entero;*

Contact celiac sprue asso. for
dietary support

~~#1~~
↓ intake folate, B₁₂
↑ cal to BEE level (2826 for IBW)
instruct patient for cal needs
perform c- tol test

17

Nutritional Care in Diseases of the Large Intestine

Disorders of the intestine vary from simple discomfort, such as benign flatulence, at one extreme, to life-threatening conditions, such as toxic megacolon, at the other. Nutritional care may be provided for any of these disorders; however, the procedures used are generally not specific to individual conditions. Like the fat-restricted diet, they are of use in a variety of circumstances. In this chapter, you will be introduced to the use of fiber-modified diets and to nutritional care of the ostomy patient. Before proceeding, you should review, if necessary, the relevant chapter in your text.

MODIFICATIONS OF FIBER

Although fiber is not classified as a nutrient, it has been recognized as having important health-promoting effects. Diets with *increased* fiber are reported to be protective against constipation, diverticulosis, hemorrhoids, and colon cancer. They are also sometimes recommended for patients with diabetes and with atherosclerosis. Diets with *decreased* fiber content are useful in preparation for barium enema or surgery of the intestine, and in acute diarrheal diseases, intestinal fistulas, short bowel syndrome, diverticulitis, and bleeding lesions.

TERMINOLOGY

"Fibrous" Materials

The term *fiber* refers to relatively indigestible materials associated with the cell walls of plant products. The term includes lignin, cellulose, hemicellulose, and other materials such as pectins, gums, mucilages, and algal polysaccharides. Obviously, some of these substances are not actually fibrous in nature; rather, they are somewhat gelatinous.

Information on the fiber content of foods is very limited, so modifying the fiber content of the diet can be difficult. Many tables give values for *crude fiber*—the residue remaining after the sample has been treated with solvent and hot acids and alkali. In contrast, the fiber that cannot be digested and absorbed, a much milder process, is known as *dietary fiber*. It is much more useful for diet planning. It usually measures 2 to 6 times the volume of crude fiber and is mostly from plant materials. Methods for determination of dietary fiber have become available only recently, and information is less complete. This information is necessary, however, because dietary fiber cannot be calculated from crude fiber: The relationship between the two values is too variable.

Fiber-Modified Diets

Diets with altered fiber content may bear a variety of titles. The alternative terms *roughage* and *bulk* have sometimes been used to refer to fiber. These terms are not synonymous, although they are often used as if they were. The term *fiber* has become the more commonly used and is the term we will use in this book.

Residue refers to the material left in the large intestine after digestion and absorption have been completed. It includes indigestible fibers plus some fat, the residue of intestinal bacteria, sloughed cells, and mucus. Because of the last three items, there will be residue in the intestine even if nothing has been eaten. In addition, it is important to note that all food will leave some residue. Therefore, no diet is "residue-free."

Diets which have increased and reduced fiber content are often called *high-fiber* and *low-fiber* diets, respectively. The terms *minimal fiber* and *minimal residue* are used in some institutions to indicate the lowest level that can be achieved. Because accurate information is not readily available, fiber-modified diets are not usually precisely defined. It has been estimated that the Western-type diet contains 3 to 12 g per day of crude fiber or about 20 g of dietary fiber (1). In general, low-fiber diets will contain up to 3 or 4 g per day, and minimal fiber or minimal residue diets contain 1 g or less of fiber per day.

For patients who are tube fed and need fiber restrictions, chemically defined formulas and those based on milk or hydrolyzed protein (see Table G-3) are classified as "low residue" or "low fiber." In contrast, blenderized formulas contain moderate amounts of fiber.

High-fiber diets, on the other hand, are often de-

TABLE 17-1. General Guidelines for Estimating Relative Fiber Content of Foods

1. Fiber is contained in fruits, vegetables, legumes, whole-grain cereals, and nuts.
2. Fruits
   a. Ripe fruits that are canned or well cooked may have relatively less fiber, and raw fruits, in general, may be higher in fiber. The effect of cooking is unclear.
   b. Fruits containing skin and seeds (such as grapes, berries, dates, figs, and prunes) are higher in fiber than peeled and pitted fruits.
   c. Pineapple and rhubarb are higher in fiber.
   d. Fruit juices are low in fiber.
3. Vegetables and legumes
   a. In general, raw vegetables may be higher in fiber than cooked vegetables.
   b. Vegetables, such as potatoes, are higher in fiber if unpeeled.
   c. "Cabbage-family" vegetables, peas, and beans are relatively high in fiber.
   d. Legumes have a significant gum content.
4. Cereal products
   a. Cereals and baked cereal products prepared from refined cereals, such as white wheat flour, are low in fiber.
   b. Coarse, whole-grain breads and cereals are higher in fiber.
   c. In general, "instant" products are more highly refined than the corresponding product that requires longer cooking.
   d. Oatmeal has a signficant gum content.
5. Animal foods
   a. Some meats contain indigestible connective tissue, but not fiber.
   b. Tough, fibrous meats with gristle are high in indigestible material, while tender meats, ground or well cooked, contain less.
   c. Poultry, fish, organ meats, eggs, and cheese are devoid of indigestible material.
6. Others
   Gelatin, sucrose, dextrose, corn syrup, and broth contain little or no fiber *or* residue.

fined relative to the patient's previous intake. In a patient whose usual daily fiber intake is 3 to 4 g, an increase to a level of 12 to 14 g might be considered as high (or higher) in fiber. A high-fiber diet is more often defined as containing 20 to 30 g of fiber per day, or even 50 g. In some underdeveloped countries, fiber intake may be 60 g per day. Thus, a diet history is essential in defining increased fiber for a specific patient. For patients needing formula feeding, a high-fiber formula such as Enrich (Ross Laboratories) can still be administered through a small-lumen tube.

FIBER CONTENT OF FOODS

Many tables give information on crude fiber (2) rather than dietary fiber. They do not give information on the content of individual types of fiber, such as cellulose and pectin, even though there is evidence that these various substances act in different ways. For example, pectin and guar lower serum cholesterol and modulate postprandial blood sugar levels, while bran benefits patients with diverticular disease but has little effect on elevated serum cholesterol levels. Some general guidelines for estimating the relative fiber content of foods are given in Table 17-1. A table of dietary fiber content of specific foods is given in Table B-2.

An approximation of dietary fiber intake can be obtained by using the values for dietary fiber listed in Table 17-2 in conjunction with the diabetic exchange lists in Tables C-1 through C-9. The fiber values reflect the use of whole-grain products and raw fruits and vegetables. This rough guideline for the fiber content of foods can be used to help patients monitor their daily fiber intake.

TABLE 17-2. Fiber Exchanges

Exchange	Fiber, g
Milk	0
Meat	0
Fat	0
Vegetable—raw	2–3
Beans (½ c)	6
Cereal—whole grains	3
Bread—whole wheat, 1 slice	2
Fruit—raw	2

Adapted from Anderson, J.W., Chen, W.L., and Sieling, B. *Plant Fiber in Foods.* Lexington, Ky.: HCF Diabetes Research Foundation, Inc., 1980.

TO TEST YOUR UNDERSTANDING

1. a. For each of the following cold breakfast cereals, give the dietary fiber content (g/100g) of each and rank them as sources of fiber on a weight basis, with the most fiber rated as *1*.

   All-Bran
   Puffed Wheat
   Shredded Wheat
   Corn Flakes
   Grape Nuts

b. Portion sizes for each cereal are listed below. Calculate the fiber content per serving and rank the cereals again as sources of fiber, with the cereal containing the most fiber as *1*.

All-Bran	(¾ c, 42 g)
Puffed Wheat	(¾ c, 9 g)
Shredded Wheat	(1 biscuit, 22 g)
Corn Flakes	(¾ c, 19 g)
Grape Nuts	(¾ c, 84 g)

c. How much of each of the products listed below would be required to provide the same amount of fiber (13.2 g) as 30 g of wheat bran?

Product	Fiber Content	Amount Required
Wheat Bran	44 g/100 g	30 g
All-Bran		
Corn Flakes		
Puffed Wheat		
Psyllium Seed		

THE HIGH-FIBER DIET

Diet Planning

A normal diet can be modified to increase fiber by increasing the intake of whole-grain cereal, fruits, and vegetables. A diet plan might contain, for example, 4 servings of whole grain cereals, 1 serving of beans, 4 servings of fruit, and 4 servings of vegetables. Depending upon specific choices, these foods could provide 25 to 35 g of fiber.

High-fiber diets often recommend raw fruits and vegetables. The subject is controversial, however. Cooked foods may have reduced fiber content because

1. Cooked and canned fruits, and some vegetables, are often peeled, removing much of the fiber.
2. Dietary fiber can be degraded to some degree by prolonged cooking; however, the fiber reduction produced by cooking is less than commonly believed.
3. Soluble and loosely bound components may be removed in food processing.

Some types of fiber effectively increase stool bulk and reduce constipation by absorbing water. Patients with high fiber intake should be encouraged to increase their fluid intake.

Some patients find high-fiber diet compliance difficult or impossible. Fiber may be increased for these

TABLE 17-3. Fiber Supplements

Specific Supplements	Dose	Fiber Content
Psyllium seed (Metamucil, Effersylium, Syllact, etc.)	2 t	6–7 g
Fibermed	wafer	5 g
Miller's bran	1 T	6 g

patients without changing the diet by giving fiber as a dietary supplement. Products that may be used for this purpose are listed in Table 17-3. The addition of ¼ to ½ c (½ to 1 oz) 100 percent bran cereal per day is sometimes recommended.

Table 17-4 offers some general guidelines for planning the high-fiber diet and for patient counseling.

TABLE 17-4. Planning a High-Fiber Diet

1. Increase the amount of vegetables, fruits, legumes, and nuts in the diet.
2. Emphasize raw, unpeeled fruits and vegetables when possible.
3. Use whole-grain bread and cereal in place of refined products.
4. Reduce the use of low-fiber, high-energy foods as necessary to maintain normal body weight.
5. Bran (¼–1 c) may be added to cereal, breads, and casseroles.
6. The addition of bran and other high-fiber foods should be made gradually and in divided doses throughout the day.
7. Increase fluid intake.

TO TEST YOUR UNDERSTANDING

2. A patient's diet history reveals intake of the following foods:

2 c milk	3 raw fruits
8 oz meat	3 slices whole-grain bread
1 c raw vegetable salad	2 servings whole-grain cereals
½ c cooked legumes	6 servings fat

How many g of fiber are contained in this menu? (Use exchange lists for calculation.)

Side Effects

Large amounts of fiber in the diet may bind minerals. It has been reported that small children and malnourished adults may develop mineral deficiencies if given a high-fiber diet (> 30 g) (3). Zinc is mostly likely to be bound to fiber and excreted in the stool, as are iron, copper, and calcium. As a consequence, high-fiber diets are not often recommended for these two categories of patients. Alternatively, mineral supplements may be given.

Some components of fiber, particularly soluble polysaccharides such as pectin and guar gum, can be fermented by colonic bacteria, producing excess gases such as hydrogen, carbon dioxide, and methane. Although this is not a threat to health, it can cause some discomfort and reduce compliance with a high-fiber diet.

The action of colonic bacteria on large amounts of fiber can result in the production of volatile fatty acids (VFA) such as acetate, propionate, and butyrate, which may be absorbed or metabolized by bacteria. It is estimated that 20 g of dietary fiber will result in 100 mEq of VFA, about 20 percent of which is excreted. VFA production may result in osmotic diarrhea and contribute to flatulence.

The development of flatulence and diarrhea can be minimized by increasing the fiber content of the diet gradually and giving the fiber in divided doses. An increased fluid intake is also helpful.

TO TEST YOUR UNDERSTANDING

3. Ms. S. is being tube fed over a long period with a low-residue formula. She complains of constipation. Assuming the patient is capable of digesting any formula, list the commercial formulas you might suggest as an alternative to the one presently in use.

4. A high-fiber diet has been recommended for Mr. R., who has diverticulosis. A 24-hr recall gives you the following diet, which he states is typical.

Breakfast:
4 oz orange juice
1 egg
1 slice white bread, toasted
1 t margarine
8 oz low-fat milk
Coffee

Lunch:
3 oz sliced meat
2 slices white bread
1 t mayonnaise
Chopped lettuce salad, French dressing
2 canned peach halves
8 oz low-fat milk

Dinner:
4 oz sliced beef
½ c mashed potatoes
1 serving (about 100 g) cooked asparagus
1 white roll
½ c butterscotch ice cream
Tea

a. What is the approximate fiber content of this diet?
b. Next to the menu above, write in some alterations you could suggest to this patient to increase his fiber intake to 25 to 30 g.
c. What side effects could occur in this patient as a consequence of this diet?
d. What advice would you give this patient to avoid these side effects and improve compliance?
e. If the patient was 10 percent above OBW and his fiber needed to be increased to 50 g per day, what additional suggestions could you make? Be specific as to quantity.
f. If the patient develops diverticulitis, what diet would be appropriate during the acute phase?

5. a. A patient who has a meal pattern similar to that given in question 4 needs a short-term diet that is more restricted in residue. What alterations in this menu would you suggest?

b. Evaluate the vitamin and mineral adequacy of the resulting diet and suggest care procedures if the patient will have this diet for a month. His milk intake is restricted to 8 oz per day because he has developed lactose intolerance.

c. The patient's condition deteriorates and he must be fed by tube. He is capable of digesting intact proteins, fats, and polysaccharides. Circle the tube-feeding formulas that would be appropriate for this patient, and explain your reasons for rejecting the others.

1.	Criticare	6.	Compleat B
2.	Ensure	7.	Magnacal
3.	Isocal	8.	Osmolite
4.	Enrich	9.	Precision Isotonic
5.	Meritene Liquid		

PROCEDURES FOR DECREASING DIETARY FIBER

Diet Planning

Reduced-fiber diets may be restricted to varying extents. For some patients, the removal of only the most indigestible fiber, such as bran, corn, and nuts, is sufficient. For other patients, the fiber restriction inherent in the whole soft or pureed diet is sufficient (see Table 11-1). Still other patients may require greater restriction.

In general, fiber-restricted or low-fiber diets avoid fresh or dried fruits and vegetables, whole-grain breads and cereals, and nuts, seeds, and legumes. They consist of the following food groups:

1. Refined breads, cereals, and cereal products
2. Fruits and vegetables, cooked whole, pureed, or as juice, depending on degree of restriction
3. Meat, milk, eggs
4. Any fat
5. Desserts without fruits, nuts, or seeds

Details of foods allowed and not allowed are found in the diet manuals of most institutions.

The minimal-residue or strict low-fiber diet restricts foods with even a moderate fiber content. General guidelines for planning this diet are as follows:

1. Use fruit juices and vegetable juices. Prune juice is often eliminated since it contains dihydroxyphenylisatin, a stimulant to peristalsis, which may be an intestinal irritant in these patients.
2. Avoid whole fruits and vegetables.
3. Use refined breads and cereals; avoid whole-grain breads and cereals.

Milk and connective tissue of meat are low in fiber but are believed by some to increase stool volume.

There is little scientific evidence to support this, however, and the topic is therefore controversial. In some institutions, the following guidelines are also observed.

4. Limit milk and milk products (ice cream, milk pudding, and cheese) to the equivalent of 2 c of milk per day. Milk is believed to leave a substantial residue, but does not contain fiber.
5. Eliminate meat, poultry, or shellfish with tough connective tissue.

For patients requiring a diet free of fiber, a clear-liquid diet (see Chapter 11) is sometimes used, but only for a brief period. If a fiber-free diet is needed over a long period, chemically defined formulas should be added (see Chapter 12).

Some diet manuals contain a "minimal fiber," "minimal residue," or "strict low fiber" diet. If an absolute minimum of fiber is required, fruits and vegetables are excluded, as is any meat or poultry with tough connective tissue. This diet sometimes excludes milk, which is reputed to be high in *residue, not* fiber.

Side Effects

A strict low-fiber diet will be adequate in most nutrients only if it includes 3 c of milk per day and an adequate amount of meat. It may be inadequate in vitamin A, unless liver is included in the meats, and inadequate in iron for female patients. It may be inadequate in energy content for patients with high energy requirements. Patients may thus need supplements of vitamin A and iron if the diet is used for an extended period. High-calorie fiber-free liquid supplements provide additional energy.

Patients eating a restricted-fiber diet are prone to constipation. Generally, however, the diet is used for only a limited period.

TO TEST YOUR UNDERSTANDING

6. A patient undergoing colon surgery requires a fiber-free diet. He is given a clear liquid diet. After four days he is not yet ready for a more varied diet.

   a. Evaluate the nutritional adequacy of the diet.

   b. If the restriction were needed for two more weeks, and the patient rejects tube feeding, what would you suggest? Be specific about items to be used.

7. Mr. R.R. is a white male, age 68, who has diverticulosis. He is of normal weight. You calculate his protein requirement as 60 g per day and his energy requirement at about 1,900 kcal per day. Using the menu for _____ (day to be assigned by your instructor), modify this menu for a high-fiber diet for this patient.

8. Mr. R.R. later develops diverticulitis. Modify the menu for _____ (day to be assigned by your instructor) to provide a low-fiber diet for this patient.

DIETS FOR OSTOMY PATIENTS

Ostomies may be created for feeding and for purposes of excretion. *Gastrostomies* and *jejunostomies,* used for feeding, are discussed in Chapter 12. An *ileostomy* is formed when the ileum is brought out as an opening in the abdominal wall. The colon is removed or bypassed. A *colostomy* consists of an opening of some portion of the colon through the abdominal wall. Both are used for excretion.

Many patients find that their diet can be less restricted following creation of the ostomy than it was prior to the surgery. Nevertheless, patients often benefit from nutritional counseling.

NUTRITIONAL CARE OF THE ILEOSTOMY PATIENT

In the early postoperative period, the patient is usually kept NPO. When the bowels begin to function again, the patient is given a clear liquid diet. Additions are made to bring the patient gradually to a low-fiber diet and eventually to an unrestricted diet. During this period, it may be wise to add foods one at a time so that the source of any problems can be identified. Four general problems, which will be discussed next, can develop.

Disorders of Water and Electrolyte Balance

When the colon is missing, the water, sodium, and potassium normally reabsorbed by the colon are lost in the effluent from the ileostomy. These must be replaced. Adequate fluid must be provided, with special precautions in hot weather and with heavy exercise. Since many patients will restrict their fluid intake in an attempt to decrease the amount of effluent, they should be reminded that excess fluid will not add to the effluent; it is excreted by the kidneys. In addition, foods high in sodium and potassium should be eaten daily. (Dietary sodium and potassium modifications are discussed in detail in Chapter 19.)

Danger of Mechanical Blockage

The stoma is smaller in diameter than is the colon. This is not usually a problem since the ileal content is liquid. However, blockage by large pieces of food can occur when food which has been insufficiently chewed passes intact through the intestine. Therefore, the patient should be instructed to *chew food thoroughly.* In addition, some high-fiber foods pass through the intestine unchanged; it may therefore be necessary to omit or reduce the intake of the following foods:

Corn on the cob	Raw pineapple and other raw fruits
Coleslaw	
Mushrooms	Popcorn
Nuts	Raw celery, carrots, and relishes
Tough meats	
Chinese vegetables such as pea pods, bean sprouts, bamboo shoots	Spinach
	Coconut
Orange pulp	Skins and seeds of fruits and vegetables

Odor and Flatulence

Some patients are concerned that an unpleasant odor will be noticeable. Others have problems with flatulence and pain. If odor is a problem, it may be helpful to avoid foods that form gas or particularly strong odors. The following are sometimes found to be troublesome:

Gas Forming	Odor Forming
Cabbage	Baked beans and other legumes
Broccoli	Onions

Onions	Cabbage-family vegetables
Corn	Mustard
Beans	Eggs
Nuts	Fish
Carbonated beverages	Some cheeses
Whips and meringues	Alcohol (especially beer)

It is also helpful to advise the patient to avoid habits, such as chewing gum and using a straw, that result in the swallowing of air. Yogurt and cranberry juice have been reported to reduce odor.

Excessive Effluent Volume

A large volume of effluent is often an inconvenience to the patient, even if fluid and electrolyte balances are maintained. Some foods are reputed to cause an increase in ileal output, while others cause a decrease:

Increasing Output	Decreasing Output
Beans	Applesauce
Broccoli	Bananas
Spinach	Boiled milk
Prune juice	Rice
Raw fruits, juices	Peanut butter
Licorice	
Red wine	
Beer	
Highly spiced foods	

It is important for patients to realize that they will not reduce effluent volume by limiting fluid intake: They will simply become dehydrated. If moderate adjustment of intake of the foods just listed is not successful, a low-fiber diet may be helpful. The patient may be advised to keep a diary of food intake and side effects so that troublesome foods may be detected.

NUTRITIONAL CARE OF THE COLOSTOMY PATIENT

The needs of the patient with a colostomy are determined by its location. If the colostomy is in the first part of the colon, it will behave much like an ileostomy. When the colostomy is further down, fecal matter is less liquid.

The early postoperative period is handled similarly to that for an ileostomy, as just described. Problems of fluid and electrolyte loss, odor, and excess effluent may also be handled similarly. There is less tendency to obstruction in a colostomy than in an ileostomy. High-fiber foods may increase fecal volume, however, and the patient may wish to restrict their use. The patient may learn to control volume and thickness of the stool by manipulating intake of foods that cause loose stools and increase effluent volume (raw fruits and vegetables, fruit juices, coffee) and foods that thicken and reduce the volume of effluent.

Ostomy patients are sometimes fearful of abandoning their previous diets even though the diet may no longer be necessary. Patients may need careful counseling in order to liberalize their diets. In counseling these patients, it is important to ensure that a sufficient variety of foods is available to provide an adequate diet. If a food is omitted because it causes a problem in ostomy management, it should be tried again later because some adaptation does occur.

After correction of their digestive disease, some patients tend to become obese. They may need to be counseled on weight control. It is sometimes helpful to refer patients to support groups, which may be found in many cities.

TO TEST YOUR UNDERSTANDING

9. Ms. V. has had a colon resection, and an ileostomy was created. Following discharge from the hospital, she had difficulty controlling the volume of the effluent.

   She returns to the clinic for help. Using the menu for _____ (day to be assigned by your instructor), modify the diet as to demonstrate recommended changes for this patient.

10. If Ms. V. had a sigmoid colostomy and problems with constipation, list some general advice you might give her.

TOPICS FOR FURTHER DISCUSSION

1. What suggestions could be made to a person who complains of chronic constipation?

2. Discuss the nutritional care of a patient with acute pancreatitis.

REFERENCES

1. SLAVIN, J.A. Dietary fiber. *Dietetic Currents* 10:(1983)27–32.

2. *Composition of Foods: Raw, Processed, Prepared.* Agricultural Handbook No. 8. Washington, D.C.: Agricultural Research Series, U.S. Department of Agriculture, 1976–1982.

3. HAMBRIDGE, K.M., C. HAMBRIDGE, M. JACOBS, AND J.B. BAUM.

Low levels of zinc in hair, anorexia, poor growth and hypogeusia in children. *Pediat. Res.* 6:(1972)868–874.

ADDITIONAL SOURCES OF INFORMATION

ANDERSON, J.W., W.-J.L. CHEN, AND B. SIELING. *Plant Fiber in Foods.* Lexington, Ky.: HCF Diabetes Research Foundation, Inc., 1980.

Fiber in Human Nutrition, eds. G. Spiller and R. Amen. New York: Plenum, 1976.

VAHOUNY, G.V. AND D. KRITCHEVSKY. *Dietary Fiber in Health and Disease.* New York: Plenum, 1982.

18

Nutritional Care in Diabetes Mellitus

Diabetes mellitus is a common diagnosis, and entry-level nutritional care specialists often spend a large proportion of their time counseling diabetic patients. Dietary counseling can significantly contribute to the well-being of patients with diabetes.

Our understanding of diabetes and its care has advanced significantly, but there have been only minor changes in our approaches to the diet. With the development of tissue transplant techniques and new insulin-delivery systems, as well as greater understanding of the treatment of complications, advances in nutritional care are certain to come.

This chapter provides an introduction to the currently used techniques for nutritional care of diabetic patients at various ages, with consideration of procedures to increase dietary compliance. Before proceeding, you should review the material on diabetes in your textbook.

CLASSIFICATION OF DIABETES

For purposes of this chapter, we will consider diabetic patients in the following four categories (1):

Type I, or insulin-dependent, diabetes mellitus (IDDM): These patients are usually, but not always, less than 25 years old at onset, and are insulin-deficient and ketosis-prone.

Type II, or non-insulin-dependent, diabetes mellitus (NIDDM): These patients are usually middle-aged or elderly at onset and are not ketosis-prone. They may be subdivided further into obese and nonobese groups.

Impaired glucose tolerance (IGT): These patients have some impairment of glucose tolerance. About 20 percent progress to IDDM or NIDDM.

Gestational diabetes: This condition occurs when abnormal glucose tolerance begins during pregnancy and subsides postpartum.

Thus, diabetes consists of a spectrum of disorders. All are characterized by an elevation in blood glucose concentration, and diagnostic procedures focus on this elevation.

DIAGNOSIS

There is a great deal of uncertainty about the diagnostic criteria for diabetes mellitus. This uncertainty is further complicated by the fact that different criteria are used to define the various classifications of the disease.

Patients who have signs and symptoms secondary to hyperglycemia (excessive thirst, frequent urination, increased appetite, ketonuria, glycosuria, a blood glucose over 300 mg per dl, and rapid weight loss) are relatively easily diagnosed. For many other patients, however, signs and symptoms are less marked and diagnosis is less certain.

FASTING BLOOD (OR PLASMA OR SERUM) GLUCOSE CONCENTRATION

Glucose concentrations in whole blood, plasma, or serum are determined following an 8- to 12-hour overnight fast. A fasting blood glucose (FBG) concentration over 140 mg per dl on at least two occasions in an adult or child is diagnostic of diabetes. Those with FBG levels of 110 to 140 mg per dl are classified in the IGT category and are considered at risk of developing clinical diabetes; about 20 percent do so. Normal levels for adults over 50 years of age are given in various reports as 60 to 100, 65 to 120, or 70 to 110 mg per dl. For patients over 50 years of age, FBG is reported to rise 1 to 2 mg per dl for each decade.

You will occasionally see FBG recorded in international units (mmol/L). To convert one form to the other in order to be able to interpret results, use the following equation:

$$\text{mmol/L} = 0.5551 \times \text{mg/dl} \qquad \textbf{(18-1)}$$

In tables of reference values, such as those in Appendix E, values for adults are given. The following are additional useful reference values:

Newborn, premature	20–80 mg/dl serum
Full-term infant	20–90 mg/dl serum
Children	60–115 mg/dl serum

In interpreting results, it is important to remember that FBG can also be increased in acute pancreatitis, in hyperfunction of the pituitary, adrenal, or hypothalamus, and in patients taking anabolic hormones, epinephrine, norepinephrine, benzothiadiazine diuretics, or diphenylhydantoin (phenytoin or Dilantin). FBG may be increased also if the patient is nonfasting, under stress, or receiving IV glucose.

TWO-HOUR POSTPRANDIAL BLOOD SUGAR

The *2-hour postprandial* (2hPP) *blood sugar* is elevated in the diabetic individual. In the normal person, postprandial glucose is usually less than 145 mg per dl, but may be 160 mg per dl in persons over 60 years of age. Values over 160 mg per dl are considered diagnostic of diabetes mellitus in the absence of the following: some pituitary, adrenal, or thyroid diseases; advanced liver diseases or pancreatitis, and intake of drugs such as oral contraceptives, thiazides, or phenytoin.

GLUCOSE TOLERANCE TESTS

The *glucose tolerance test* (GTT) is not used alone to diagnose diabetes because it is impaired by increasing age, obesity, inactivity, infection, and drugs such as steroids, thiazides, and phenytoin. It is useful, however, in diagnosing two types of patients:

adults under 50 years of age who are healthy and active and have FBG levels under 138 mg per dl, but who are suspected to have diabetes because of family history or current symptoms

pregnant women, to screen for gestational diabetes

Test procedures vary. A screening test on a nonfasting patient is often done first. A 50-g glucose load is given. If blood glucose exceeds 140 g per dl, the GTT is then done. For that test, it is sometimes recommended that the patient have a normal- to high-carbohydrate diet (300 g or more per day) for 3 to 7 days prior to the test in order to ensure that liver glycogen is at maximum and increased glycogen storage does not mask a diabetic response.

On the day of the GTT, a fasting blood sample is taken, and the patient is then given a glucose dose. The usual dose is 1.75 g per kg IBW, to a maximum of 75 g; it is given in an aqueous solution (25 mg per dl, often with lemon juice or in a cola drink), to be taken within 5 minutes. Blood samples are then collected by venipuncture at intervals—usually at 30, 60, 90, and 120 minutes, and sometimes also at 180 minutes (1, 2)—and then assayed for glucose.

The following criteria are examples of those commonly used for interpretation of results (1–3):

Adults: IGT—138–205 mg per dl in 120 min
Diabetes in nonpregnant adults—>205 mg per dl at 120 minutes *and* at either 60 or 90 minutes

Children: Diabetes—>200 mg per dl at 60 and/or 120 min, or
any *two* of > 175 mg per dl at 60 min
> 140 mg per dl at 120 min
> 125 mg per dl at 180 min

ACID-BASE BALANCE

When diabetes mellitus is first being diagnosed or when it is uncontrolled for any reason, it is important to determine the patient's acid-base status. For this purpose, arterial blood gases (ABGs) are measured in blood obtained from the radial, brachial, or femoral arteries. Blood bicarbonate concentration is measured at the same time. These values are used to assess the degree of acidosis caused by the lack of insulin.

The values for blood gases are given for oxygen and carbon dioxide as partial pressure, indicated as pO_2 and pCO_2. The mean and normal ranges of blood pH and ABG values are as follows:

pH	7.4 (7.35–7.45)
pO_2	90 (80–100) mm Hg
pCO_2	40 (35–45) mm Hg
HCO_3	24 (22–26) mEq/L

The first three of these are reported in the medical record in the following form:

$$ABG = 7.40/90/40$$

where pH, pO_2, and pCO_2 are given in sequence.

These values and serum bicarbonate are used not only to determine the patient's acid-base status, but also to differentiate among the four types of disturbances in acid-base balance: metabolic acidosis, respiratory acidosis, metabolic alkalosis, or respiratory alkalosis. Such disturbances are found in a variety of disorders. The patient with uncontrolled diabetes mellitus may develop metabolic acidosis.

Some general guidelines may be used for interpretation of these laboratory values. To simplify the examples, we will use the mean values just given and ignore the ranges.

First, determine the direction of the change from normal by examining the pH: It is increased in alkalosis and decreased in acidosis. Thus, a pH of 7.2 indicates acidosis; 7.5 indicates alkalosis.

Then, determine the type of acidosis or alkalosis by identifying the parameter that is predominantly abnormal. The value for pCO_2 represents the respiratory effect on pH. An increase contributes to acidosis and indicates hypoventilation. A decrease contributes to alkalosis and indicates hyperventilation. The pO_2 is not used in assessment of acid-base balance, but is an indicator of oxygenation.

The bicarbonate represents the metabolic (non-respiratory) effect on acid-base balance. A high value indicates alkalosis, while a low value is associated with acidosis.

Interpretation can be confirmed and quantified as follows: Determine the difference between the patient's pCO_2 and the normal value. Let us assume, for example, that the medical record gives the values 7.32/90/50. Then, 50–40 = 10. Next, calculate the theoretical pH, assuming that *each change of 10 mm Hg in pCO_2 causes a change in pH of 0.08 units in the opposite direction.* If pCO_2 increases, pH will decrease (become more acid); if pCO_2 decreases, pH will increase (become more alkaline). Note carefully that the carbon dioxide represents the acid and the bicarbonate represents the base in acid-base balance calculations. Thus, continuing the calculation,

$$7.4 - 0.08 = 7.32$$

If calculated and measured pH are very similar, the changes are caused by alterations in pCO_2; thus the changes are respiratory. In this example, the results indicate *respiratory* acidosis.

Another useful distinction is the differentiation between acute and chronic respiratory conditions. As a general rule of thumb, if the *change* in pH is of the order of 0.8 units, the respiratory acidosis or alkalosis is acute, while if the change is 0.2 to 0.3 units, the condition is chronic. The patient in the example, then, has acute respiratory acidosis.

In *metabolic* acidosis or alkalosis, a change in serum pH results from a change in serum bicarbonate. Bicarbonate values and pH vary from normal in the same direction, while the patient's pCO_2 changes from normal in a direction to compensate for the change in bicarbonate.

A patient who presents with an elevated pH resulting from increased bicarbonate (a base) will have a compensatory increase in pCO_2 (an acid). This patient is in metabolic alkalosis, a condition often referred to as *base excess.* For example, if values are ABG = 7.62/90/50, and serum bicarbonate is 50 mEq per L, the patient is in metabolic alkalosis. Since the base (bicarbonate) has increased more—from 24 to 50, or 100 percent—than the pCO_2 (acid)—from 40 to 50, or 20 percent—the patient is considered to have a base excess.

On the other hand, a patient who presents with a depressed pH resulting from bicarbonate loss will have a compensatory decrease in pCO_2. This patient is in metabolic acidosis, often referred to as *base deficit.* For example, if the record states that ABG = 7.20/90/25 and blood bicarbonate is 10 mEq per L, the patient has metabolic acidosis. Since the base (bicarbonate) has decreased more than pCO_2 (acid), the patient is considered to have a base deficit. (It is also possible to have a mixed respiratory and metabolic acidosis or alkalosis, but these conditions are beyond the scope of this text.)

Metabolic acidosis can be caused by the addition of a strong acid or by the loss of base (via the GI tract or kidney). In order to distinguish between these two causes, the *anion gap* (AG) is calculated from concentrations of Na^+, K^+, Cl^-, and HCO_3^-:

$$AG = (Na^+ + K^+) - (Cl^- + HCO_3^-) \quad \text{(18-2)}$$

where all values are stated in mEq per L. Normal anion gap is 12 to 16 mEq per L.

If the anion gap is greater than 16, there is a decrease in bicarbonate balanced by an increase in unmeasured H^+, instead of an increase in Cl^-. The patient has *normochloremic acidosis*, also called *anion gap acidosis.* This may occur in *diabetic ketoacidosis* (DKA), in other conditions causing increased acid production or decreased acid excretion, or when certain poisons have been ingested.

If the patient loses bicarbonate, balanced by an increase in chloride, the result is *non–anion gap (hyperchloremic) acidosis.* This condition may result from GI or renal loss of bicarbonate.

TO TEST YOUR UNDERSTANDING

1. Assume that in your institution, normal fasting plasma glucose levels are considered to be 70 to 110 mg/dl. You have a patient whose fasting plasma glucose level is 40 mmol/L. By your institution's standard, is this value considered to be within normal limits, high, or low? Show your calculations.

2. In each of the following situations, write in the space to the right the diagnosis you would expect to see. Use the following code: DM—Diabetes mellitus; IGT—Impaired glucose tolerance; WNL—Within normal limits

   a. 8 y.o. girl with FBG 145 mg/dl. GTT showed 210 mg/dl at 60 min, 190 mg/dl at 120 min. _____

   b. Nonpregnant 23 y.o. woman with FBG 100 mg/dl. GTT showed 160 mg at 60 min, 135 mg/dl at 120 min, and 110 mg/dl at 180 min. _____

   c. 60 y.o. man with FBG 120 mg/dl. GTT showed 190 mg/dl at 120 min. _____

3. The following values are given for a patient:

	Patient	Normal
Blood glucose, mg/dl	504	_____
Urine glucose (by test strip)	+++	_____
ABG: pH	7.21	_____
pCO$_2$, mm Hg	27	_____
HCO$_3$, mEq/L	11.2	_____
Electrolytes: Na$^+$, mEq/L	133	_____
K$^+$, mEq/L	5.3	_____
Cl$^-$, mEq/L	100	_____
BUN	35	_____

a. Fill in normal values in the spaces provided above.
b. Calculate the anion gap. Show your calculations.
c. Calculate the patient's serum osmolality. Show your calculations.
d. Circle the conditions indicated by these results and give the values that indicate the conditions you circle.

Respiratory acidosis	Dehydration
Metabolic acidosis	Normal hydration
Respiratory alkalosis	Normochloremic acidosis
Metabolic alkalosis	Hyperchloremic acidosis

NUTRITIONAL ASSESSMENT

The nutritional assessment procedures described in Chapter 4 are used for diabetic patients, with emphasis on some specific points. Achieving and maintaining normal weight is emphasized for overweight patients. On the other hand, the pregnant woman or child who is diabetic must be assessed for normal growth and development, as described in Chapters 7 and 8.

For patients who have other conditions, such as renal disease, in addition to diabetes, nutritional assessment procedures may have to be combined. For example, if the patient has renal or cardiovascular disease, assessment of nutritional status might include the additional procedures described in Chapter 19 or 20. Laboratory values for blood cholesterol and triglycerides, BUN, urine protein, and serum creatinine should be routinely monitored.

In general, patients are more likely to follow a diet if it is designed to fit into their current life-style. In order to plan such a diet, you must have detailed information about the patient. You must consider income and food budget, as well as cultural, social, religious, and ethnic factors. The home and family should be evaluated. What are the physical facilities for food storage and preparation? Who plans and prepares the food? The diet should accommodate the patient's work and activity schedule, particularly in IDDM, in which diet, insulin, and activity must be integrated; therefore, the patient's occupation, work hours, and scheduled meal hours and coffee or milk breaks must be known. It is also important to assess the patient's attitude toward the disease. Is the reaction one of acceptance and compliance or of denial, depression, anxiety, or fear? Also, what is the patient's motivational level? What are the learning capabilities and limitations? What is the patient's reading level? What is the level of current knowledge? When you have all this information, you and the patient *together* should plan a meal pattern with which the patient is willing to comply.

TO TEST YOUR UNDERSTANDING

4. List some general information that you would need to have in order to plan good nutritional care for each of the following patients. List items other than those that apply to all.
   a. 16 y.o. girl, IDDM patient, newly diagnosed.
   b. 47 y.o. man, IDDM of 30 years' duration; retinopathy.
   c. 82 y.o. woman, NIDDM of 20 years' duration.

MONITORING CONTROL

Because of the chronic nature of diabetes mellitus, control of the disease is assessed at more frequent intervals than is nutritional status. However, both processes are necessary for appropriate nutritional counseling.

Maintenance of blood glucose level within normal limits is usually used as the criterion for good control. As part of the health care team, you will need to interpret the results of monitoring procedures. Therefore, it is important that you be familiar with these monitoring methods.

BLOOD TESTS

Blood tests include both the measure of blood glucose that has been used for many years and the more recently developed test for glycosylated hemoglobin.

Blood Glucose

Monitoring of glucose levels is considered to be a very effective procedure for monitoring short-term diabetic control. A small drop of blood is placed on the reactive pad of a test strip. The test procedure causes a color change in the pad proportional to the blood glucose level; the change is interpreted visually or in a meter. Meters vary in price and some are expensive, but most third-party payers (medical insurance) are now willing to cover the cost. *Self-blood-glucose monitoring,* or SBGM (also called *home blood glucose monitoring,* or HBGM) is especially valuable in patients who have wide fluctuations in blood glucose, patients with renal thresholds which vary markedly from normal, and pregnant diabetic women and gestational diabetics.

Results obtained from properly used meters can then be used as the information base for decisions on altering diet or insulin dose in order to maintain blood glucose within normal limits. An SBGM program often begins with premeal, 2-hour postmeal, and bedtime determinations, seven times a day for at least a week. It then progresses, as control is achieved, to biweekly determinations at fasting, 2-hour postprandial, and at bedtime. The achievement of control is confirmed by determination of glycosylated hemoglobin at intervals of 4 to 12 weeks.

Glycosylated Hemoglobin

The determination of glycosylated hemoglobin, particularly HgbA$_{1c}$, is very useful. Its use is based on the fact that an irreversible C-N bond can form between the terminal amino group of hemoglobin and the number-2 carbon of glucose. This type of reaction occurs in browning of cooked meat, baking or toasting of baked goods, and browning of sliced fruits. It is known as the *browning reaction* in these situations. When the same reaction occurs in human tissue, it is called the *glycosylation reaction.*

The glycosylation reaction between the red cell hemoglobin and glucose increases when the blood glucose level rises. The reaction is irreversible, but the life span of the red cell averages 120 days. As a result, the amount of glycosylated hemoglobin reflects the average blood glucose level for the previous 120 days, and HgbA$_{1c}$ indicates the degree of control of diabetes. Patients cannot then mislead you by being careful about their diets or by taking more insulin only immediately prior to clinic appointments.

Normal glycosylated hemoglobin values range from 3.5 to 8.5 percent. Levels above 8.5 percent indicate lesser control of diabetes, as follows (4):

<8.5%	Excellent control
8.5–9.5%	Good control
9.5–10.5%	Fair control
10.5–12%	Fair to poor control
>12%	Poor control

A common protocol consists of determining HgbA$_{1c}$ during the initial visit. The patient is then evaluated sequentially during succeeding visits. If the diabetes is in good control, as reflected by glycosylated hemoglobin levels, and if the patient keeps good SBGM records, HgbA$_{1c}$ need be monitored only once or twice a year. If, however, self-monitoring records are inadequate, control is poor, or if the HgbA$_{1c}$ levels do not agree with and confirm the self-monitoring records, glycosylated hemoglobin testing will be repeated in alternate months, with an accompanying effort to improve control (5).

URINE TESTS

Urine testing is less accurate than blood testing, but it is still used by some patients.

Limitations of Urine Testing

An important limitation of urine testing is the lack of information on specific blood glucose values at levels below renal threshold. Additional sources of error are increased renal thresholds in advancing age or in renal or heart failure and decreased renal threshold in the young, in pregnancy, with severe exercise, and in fever. In addition, the patient needs to provide a "double-voided" urine sample. Urine is voided first, and the urine is discarded. Another sample is then collected after a known interval and used for the testing. Some patients have difficulty with this procedure.

Urine Glucose

If blood glucose rises above the renal threshold (usually 150 to 180 mg glucose per dl blood), glucose will appear in the urine. This may be used as a rough indicator of a blood glucose concentration *above renal threshold.*

Four products are commonly used for urine glucose testing: Chemstrip uG, Clinitest, Diastix, and Tes-Tape. Clinitest may be used with the "5-drop" method (5 drops urine and 10 drops water) or the "2-

TABLE 18-1. Summary of Results of Urine Sugar Tests Comparing Plus
and Percent System

Plus System:	0	0.1	0.25	0.5	0.75	1.0	2.0	3.0	5.0
Chemstrip uG	neg*	0.1	0.25	0.5	–	1%	2%	3%	5%
Clinitest, 5 drop	neg	neg	tr	+	++	+++	++++	–	–
2 drop	neg	neg	tr	½	–	1	2	3	5
Diastix	neg	tr*	+	++	–	+++	++++	–	–
Tes-Tape	neg	+	++	+++	–	–	++++	–	–

*Neg. = negative; tr. = trace.

drop" method (2 drops urine and 10 drops water). Color charts are provided for interpretation of results. Results used to be expressed on the "plus system"— 1+, 2+, 3+, and 4+—and some long-term patients will use this terminology. Test results are now given in percentages. Table 18-1 provides a translation from the plus system to the percentage system.

A number of factors affect the accuracy of tests performed with these products. Diastix and Tes-Tape are less accurate in the presence of ketonuria. False positive Clinitest results may occur in patients receiving barbiturates, L-dopa, or high doses of some antibiotics. The reaction of Diastix is inhibited by L-dopa and high doses of salicylates, such as aspirin. Large quantities of ascorbic acid cause false positive Clinitest results and false negatives with the other three products in Table 18-1. Diabetic patients using urine testing should therefore be strongly urged to avoid megadoses of ascorbic acid.

Patients with stable NIDDM need to test their urine twice a day—before breakfast and before the evening meal. IDDM patients should test their urine before each meal and at bedtime. Results of urine tests may then be used to adjust the insulin dosage. Alert, competent patients can be taught to make such adjustments for themselves. As an example, let us assume that a patient has 2 percent glycosuria in the morning, with good control the rest of the day. The patient might then cautiously increase the evening insulin dose until morning glycosuria is in the "trace" category or less. Instruction on this procedure is given by the physician.

Urine Ketones

Urine ketones can be monitored with Acetest tablets, Ketostix, or Chemstrip uK. Ketodiastix and Chemstrip uGK are combinations of Ketostix and Diastix or Chemstrip uG and uK, respectively. The patient should test for the presence of ketones during infections or other illness, when under emotional stress, or when there is an increase in glycosuria for any reason. Directions for use of these materials are given on the packages. Phenylketones and sulfobromophthalein can cause false positives. Acetest and Ketostix show false positives in patients taking L-dopa.

TO TEST YOUR UNDERSTANDING

5. You are advising a highly motivated IDDM patient who feels it is important to maintain her blood glucose concentration within normal limits. The patient monitors her condition before each meal and at bedtime. Evaluate the following methods for their ability to provide the most accurate information to achieve the closest possible control on a daily basis.

    a. Urine glucose
    b. Urine ketones
    c. Blood glucose
    d. Glycosylated hemoglobin

6. Your instructor will demonstrate the use of the urine- and blood-monitoring systems, using aqueous glucose and acetoacetic acid solutions.

    In the space below, indicate the color you see for a negative reading for each of the following and the color and dimensions of change. Indicate the highest measurable level. Your instructor may provide other samples.

    Clinitest, 5 drop
    Tes-Tape
    Dextrostix
    Acetest

TREATMENT

The four main aspects of treatment of diabetes mellitus are a blood glucose–lowering agent (not invariably used), diet, exercise, and education. Because they are interrelated, you need to understand all aspects.

BLOOD GLUCOSE–LOWERING AGENTS

There are two types of glucose-lowering agents: insulin and oral hypoglycemic agents (OHAs).

Insulin

Insulins are available in the following forms, listed in the order of decreasing tendency to cause insulin resistance or allergy:

> improved single-peak with less than 20 ppm of impurities
> single monocomponent ("purified") with less than 10 ppm of impurities
> "human" insulin (sold as "Humulin" by Eli Lilly or "Novolin" by Squibb-Novo) prepared by "genetic engineering" methods

Types of Insulin. Insulin dose and time of administration are integrated with food intake on the basis of their speed of onset, time to peak action, and duration of action. The insulins available in the United States and their properties are shown in Table 18-2. For patient use, most are available in concentrations of 100

units per ml (U-100), with hypodermic syringe sizes to match. Some are also sold as U-40.

Administration of Insulin. Patients routinely give themselves insulin by subcutaneous injections at rotating sites, but insulin may be given to them IM or IV in acute situations. Some patients receive insulin through a pump, which delivers a constant baseline dose with an increased amount in a bolus prior to meals. The pump is expensive ($1,000 to $3,500) and requires much patient participation, but it is useful for patients who cannot otherwise achieve control.

Beginning Insulin Therapy. Patients first diagnosed as having IDDM may be treated in a hospital or on an outpatient basis. Brief hospitalization may be recommended for initial stabilization of IDDM and for pregnant patients; it is more strongly indicated for patients with acute complications such as diabetic ketoacidosis or infection, and for evaluation of patients suspected of having chronic complications. The dosage of insulin varies with the patient's age, severity of symptoms, and the existence of other illnesses. Insulin, prescribed by the attending physician, is sometimes given 3 to 4 times a day, but once or twice is more usual. Patients are sometimes given regular insulin for initial control and later changed to a longer-acting type. A number of protocols have been found to be effective.

In an example of one procedure, the starting dose is one AM injection of intermediate insulin (NPH or

TABLE 18-2. Types of Insulin

Insulin	Onset (hrs)	Peak Action (hrs)	Peak Duration (hrs)	Types Available/Source*·†·‡ Purified		Improved	
				Name	Species§	Name	Species
Rapid-acting	½–1	2–4	5–7	Regular*	b,p,h	Regular*	b+p
				Regular†	p,h	Regular†	p
				Regular‡	p	Semilente*	b+p
				Semilente*	b+p	Semilente†	b
				Semilente†	p		
Intermediate-acting	2–4	6–12	18–24	Lente*	b+p	Lente*	b+p
				Lente†	p,h	Lente†	b
				NPH*	b,p,h	NPH*	b+p
				NPH†	b,h	NPH†	b
				NPH‡	p	Globin†	b+p
				Mixtard‡ (30% RI, 70% NPH)	p		
Long-acting	2–6	18–24	36+	Ultralente*	b+p	Ultralente*	b+p
				Ultralente†	b	Ultralente†	b+p
				PZI*	b+p	Lente*	b+p
						PZI†	b

*Eli Lilly
†Squibb-Novo
‡Nordisk-USA
§b = beef; p = pork; h = human; b+p = beef and pork

Lente). Dosage size (U/kg/24 hr) may be estimated from the following (6):

Normal-weight adult	0.2–0.5
Moderately active adult	0.6
Luteal phase of menstrual cycle	0.7
Child	0.5–1.0
Puberty	1.0–2.0

Dose increases may be necessary in growth, pregnancy, adrenal steroid treatment, stress, illness, or increased food intake. Insulin need may decrease with exercise, decreased food intake, and illnesses such as renal failure. The following are some commonly used dosages (6):

Athlete in training	0.4–0.5
Infection, trauma, stress	1.0
Diabetic ketoacidosis	2.0–4.0
Pregnancy, first trimester	0.7
Pregnancy, second trimester	0.8
Pregnancy, third trimester	0.9–1.0
Lactation	0.4–0.6

Generally, the dose is increased in obese patients. Note that these guidelines do not apply in hyperosmolar nonketotic coma.

Once the total per day is determined, the number and size of doses are scheduled. Doses must be carefully integrated with food intake. The blood glucose is monitored and the insulin titrated to produce (1) a blood glucose concentration of less than 180 mg per dl, or (2) "tighter" control and normal blood glucose levels. The most desirable degree of control is controversial, and medical opinion varies. Some sample schedules are given in Table 18-3.

TABLE 18-3. Suggested Schedules for Insulin Administration

1. Combined insulins: NPH (or Lente) and regular
   AM dose: NPH (or Lente) and regular, two-thirds total dose
   PM dose: NPH (or Lente) and/or regular, one-third total dose
2. Regular insulin at each meal, Semilente at bedtime
3. Triple AM mixture: Regular, Lente, and Ultralente
4. Ultralente and regular in AM; regular at lunch and supper
5. Ultralente and regular in AM; regular at lunch; Ultralente and regular before supper
6. Regular insulin at each meal and Ultralente at supper
7. AM: NPH (or Lente) and regular; regular insulin before lunch if necessary
   PM: Regular insulin before supper; NPH (or Lente) at bedtime

Reprinted by permission of Elsevier Science Publishing Co., Inc., from The clinical use of insulin and the complications of insulin therapy, by J.A. Galloway and R.D. de Shazo. In *Diabetes Mellitus: Theory and Practice* (3d ed.), eds. Ellenberg and Rifkin, p. 522. Copyright 1983 by Medical Examination Publishing Company, Inc.

For the patient using a pump and receiving constant subcutaneous insulin infusion (CSII), the basal dose is frequently 0.3 U per kg per 24 hours. Boluses of additional insulin are then given as necessary. One recommended procedure (5) is to provide 1 U insulin per 100 kcal carbohydrate 30 to 45 minutes before the start of the meal. These values are approximate and may need to be higher at breakfast. The amount is determined with blood or urine testing for glucose. In all cases, the insulin regimen must be individualized.

Continuing Insulin Therapy. Once the baseline dose is established by the physician, it may be altered as necessary to achieve glycemic control for the individual patient. Examples of procedures are given in Table 18-4. Alternatively, the diet may be altered by redistribution of food intake.

TABLE 18-4. A Suggested Algorithm for Insulin Dosage Adjustment Based on Blood Glucose Determination (Blood, Plasma, or Serum)*

1. Initial doses: Use NPH or Lente insulin, start with 0.2–0.5 U/kg.
2. On subsequent days increase AM (prebreakfast) NPH or Lente according to fasting blood glucose as follows:
   a. Give 1 U for every 20 mg/dl the fasting blood glucose (FBG) exceeds 140/mg/dl. Example: If FBG is 260 mg/dl give 6 additional U.
   b. When AM dose reaches 50 U, or if presupper hypoglycemia occurs, then reduce the AM dose by 20% giving that 20% before supper. Example: Patient is taking 40 U of NPH and complains of nervousness and hunger at 5:00 PM, FBG is 210 mg/dl, reduce AM dose of NPH to 30 U and give 10 U before supper. Use presupper insulin dose to control FBG, increasing this dose by 1 U/10 mg/dl if the FBG exceeds 140.
3. An occasional patient will exhibit persistent fasting hyperglycemia in spite of a marked increase in the presupper NPH or Lente (where the presupper dose is equal to or greater than the prebreakfast dose). Two procedures are indicated in such patients:
   a. Rule out rebound hypoglycemia (the Somogyi effect). This is done by checking the blood glucose one or two times between 2:00 and 6:00 AM.
   b. If hypoglycemia is not occurring, then move the presupper dose of NPH or Lente to before bedtime.
4. When the FBG has been optimized using the above techniques, then prelunch and prebedtime hyperglycemia is treated using regular insulin mixed with the prebreakfast or presupper NPH or Lente. Dosage change is 1 U/30 mg/dl over 140.
5. For hypoglycemia, decrease dose by 2–4 U of NPH or regular (except for 2b above) and inquire of patient about changes in dietary intake and physical activity.

*This schedule assumes that patient is receiving an optimum diabetic diet and that reliable plasma glucose data are available from hospital or home glucose monitoring.

Reprinted by permission of Elsevier Science Publishing Co., Inc., from The clinical use of insulin and the complications of insulin therapy, by J.A. Galloway and R.D. de Shazo. In *Diabetes Mellitus: Theory and Practice* (3d ed.), eds. Ellenberg and Rifkin, p. 522. Copyright 1983 by Medical Examination Publishing Company, Inc.

TABLE 18-5. Oral Hypoglycemia Agents

Product	Dosage (mg/day)	Duration of Action (hrs)	Half-life (hrs)	Doses/Day
Tolbutamide (Orinase)	500–3,000 b.i.d. or t.i.d.	6–12	4–5	2–3
Acetohexamide (Dymelor)	250–1,500 q.d. or b.i.d.	12–24	1–2	1–2
Tolazamide (Tolinase)	100–1,000 q.d.	12–24	7	1–2
Chlorpropamide (Diabinase)	100–500 q.d.	36–60	36	1
Glipizide (Glucotrol)	2.5–40	24	8	1–2
Glyburide (Micronase) (DiaBeta)	1.25–2.0	24	10	1–2

Oral Hypoglycemic Agents

Oral hypoglycemic agents are controversial and are not prescribed by all physicians. When used, they are given to NIDDM patients. They are most effective for patients who are not obese and have no concurrent disease. The available products, dosage, and duration of action are given in Table 18-5. They should not be used in IDDM or pregnancy, or for patients with kidney or liver dysfunction. Their action is increased by anticoagulants, salicylates. alcohol, and propranolol and decreased with the use of thyroid drugs, corticosteroids, and thiazide diuretics.

DIET MANAGEMENT

Diet is important in the treatment of all diabetic patients. The overall objectives of nutritional care can be summarized as follows (7):

1. Provide for optimal nutrition throughout the life cycle.
2. Restore normal blood glucose and lipid concentrations.
3. Maintain consistent timing of meals and snacks to prevent large swings in blood glucose levels for people with IDDM.
4. Control weight for obese people with NIDDM.
5. Individualize a meal plan according to a person's lifestyle and based on a diet history.

The Diet Prescription

Although the original diet prescription has traditionally been determined by the attending physician, there is a trend toward delegating this procedure to the nutritional care specialist. When nutritional needs are met, and the diet is a constant, the physician adjusts the insulin dosage as necessary. If this is the case, you might proceed as follows:

Step 1: Establish the Total Energy Content. The energy needs of diabetic patients who are not losing energy via glycosuria do not differ from those of nondiabetics. As in nondiabetics, energy intake must be adjusted for age, activity, physiologic state, and sex. The true test of proper calorie intake is the attainment and maintenance of desirable weight. However, this takes a long time to evaluate. Meanwhile, you have to start somewhere.

Some common rules of thumb are as follows:

Estimate ideal body weight (IBW). (See Chapter 4.)
Calculate energy requirements based on IBW (8):

For adults: Basal energy (kcal) = IBW (in pounds) × 10
Then add the following for activity:
Sedentary: IBW × 3
Moderate: IBW × 5
Strenuous: IBW × 10

For women *over* 50 years of age, subtract 200 kcal from the total. For men *under* 50, add 200 kcal. If appropriate, add calories for needed weight gain (500 kcal per day for 1 pound of weight gain per week) or for pregnancy or lactation. (See Chapter 7.)

If appropriate, subtract calories for desired weight loss. (A 500 kcal deficit per day will provide a *mean* weight loss of 1 pound per week.)

In an alternative system, energy needs may be calculated from the following values, which consider weight and activity:

	Kcal/kg actual body weight		
	Sedentary	Moderate	Very active
If above IBW	20–25	25–30	30–35
If at IBW	25–30	30–35	35–40
If below IBW	30–35	35–40	40–45

For children, estimate energy requirements using the NRC Table of Recommended Dietary Allowances. Some additional guidelines are as follows:

Age 4–6 yrs: 90 kcal/kg
7–10 yrs: 80 kcal/kg

Growth is traced on a growth chart (see Chapter 8) and adjusted as necessary to achieve normal growth.

Step 2: Establish the Protein Content. Commonly, 15 to 20 percent of the total energy in the diet is devoted to protein. A 1,600-kcal diet with 20 percent protein would contain the following:

$$1,600 \times 0.20 = 320 \div 4 = 80 \text{ g protein}$$

This is, of course, above the minimum requirement, unless the patient has complications requiring an increased protein intake. If the patient is satisfied, this amount can be planned into the diet, but patient food preferences and ability to afford the diet should be considered, as should ethnic and religious factors and vegetarianism when indicated.

Step 3: Distribute Remaining Energy Between Carbohydrate and Fat. The optimum distribution of energy between carbohydrate and fat is unknown and is controversial. Recognizing the tendency of diabetics to develop cardiovascular disease, a larger proportion of carbohydrate is now being recommended than was formerly the case. This also makes a more typical diet possible, does not appreciably increase the insulin requirement, and may be less costly. Therefore, diets often consist of 50 to 60 percent carbohydrate and 20 to 30 percent fat (7). The content of a 1,600-kcal diet might then be, for example

Carbohydrate:	$1,600 \times 0.5 = 800 \div 4 = 200$ g
Fat:	$1,600 \times 0.3 = 480 \div 9 = 53.3$ (usually rounded to 55)

For patients with NIDDM, total calories are more important than the amount of carbohydrate.

Another controversial matter is the form of carbohydrate to be included. The effects of mono- or disaccharides on blood sugar depend on the amount consumed and the nature of other foods consumed at the same time. In order to control blood sugar level, the consensus is that disaccharides should not provide more than 10 percent of the *total* energy (8). The remainder is in the form of polysaccharides.

There is some evidence that polysaccharides vary in their potential to raise the blood glucose level—that is, in their "glycemic index" (9–11). At present, however, the potential clinical usefulness of the glycemic index is unknown. There is also some evidence of improved glucose tolerance when diets are fiber-enriched. The mechanism of these effects is unknown; nevertheless, there is a trend toward recommending increased fiber in diets for diabetics.

Because diabetics tend to develop earlier and more severe cardiovascular disease, it is also considered advisable to restrict the diet to 300 mg or less of cholesterol and to restrict saturated fat. Guidelines to accomplish this are given in your diet manual.

Step 4: Distribute Nutrients Among Meals and Snacks. The nutrients must now be distributed among meals and other feedings, with the primary objective of maintaining blood glucose levels within normal range. The procedure varies somewhat, depending on the category of patient. Also, in some institutions, the policy is to divide the carbohydrate, while in others, the total kcals are divided. We will use the division of carbohydrate (not kcals) in our examples and problems.

For NIDDM patients, the primary objective is to avoid wide variations in blood sugar level. Therefore, the restricted amount of carbohydrate is relatively evenly divided among three meals. For example, depending on patient preferences, one-third of the carbohydrate might be eaten at each of three meals, or one-quarter at each meal plus a snack. Patients preferring a smaller breakfast could have a one-fifth, two-fifths, two-fifths division.

For IDDM patients, meals are planned so that carbohydrate is coordinated with the insulin doses to avoid wide fluctuations in blood sugar and to provide for consistent intake from day to day. The procedure to accomplish this must be determined by trial and error. Most diabetics take insulin in the morning before breakfast. This dose is often a combination of a rapid-acting and an intermediate- or slow-acting insulin. The net effect is not entirely predictable, because the insulins interact to some extent and the rate of absorption varies. Results from SBGM are very useful in determining the optimal division. There are two general guidelines:

Patients taking an intermediate-acting insulin will probably need an afternoon snack.
Patients taking a long-acting insulin in the morning will probably need an evening snack.

It may be desirable to distribute the carbohydrate into even more divisions in order to reduce the amount taken at one time. Adults and children aged 10 and over may be given four or five meals or snacks a day with carbohydrate or calories distributed, for example, 20 percent at breakfast, 30 percent at lunch and dinner, and 10 percent midafternoon and at bedtime. For children up to age 9, six feedings a day may be recommended with, for example, 20 percent of the carbohydrate at breakfast and lunch, 20 percent at dinner, and 10 percent each at midmorning, midafternoon, and at bedtime, with some protein food at each meal. The diet must also fit the patient's activity pattern and the family's meal pattern.

In summary, the initial diet prescription gives the number of g of protein, fat, and carbohydrate, and the distribution of calories or carbohydrate among meals and snacks. Here are some examples:

2,000 kcal; 100 g protein; 65 g fat; 250 g
    carbohydrate
    Divide: 20%, 25%, 10%, 35%, 10% (for IDDM)

or

1,200 kcal; 60 g protein; 40 g fat; 150 g
    carbohydrate
    Divide: ⅕, ⅖, ⅖ (for NIDDM)

The Patient's Diet Plan

The nutritional care specialist must translate the diet prescription into a meal plan of familiar foods for the patient. The exchange-list system, developed by the American Diabetes Association, the American Dietetic Association, and the U.S. Public Health Service, is most often used for this purpose. It allows for variety in meals from day to day while still providing for consistency of intake by the conscientious patient.

Exchange Lists. The six exchanges, along with the average protein, fat, carbohydrate, and calorie content of each, are listed in Table C-1 (12). *Before proceeding, you should stop now and memorize these values.* It will save you a great deal of time as you continue with this chapter.

Now, let us look at the individual lists which follow in Tables C-2 through C-9. You will see that some items in each list are set in italic type. These are the foods that should be chosen preferentially to reduce the saturated fat in the diet. You will also see that the milk, fruit, and vegetable exchanges each consist of similar products that have similar uses in meal planning. The meat list consists of meat, poultry, fish, and also cheese and eggs, used similarly in meals. However, the bread/starch exchange list contains not only a variety of breads, but also cereals and cereal products, such as breakfast cereals, pastas, crackers, and biscuits. It also contains legumes and starchy vegetables. The fat exchange list consists not only of butter, margarine, solid shortenings, and oils, but also of nuts, bacon, salt pork, cream, and salad dressings.

You will also see that there is a "free" list (Table C-8). These foods contain under 20 calories per serving and can be used freely in addition to the calculated meal plan if no serving size is specified. No more than 2–3 servings per day of a free food with a specified serving size should be eaten. The "free" food list is quite popular with patients, as it provides a relief from the feeling of regimentation.

Calculation of the total exchange lists in the diet: Armed with the exchange lists, we will now calculate a meal plan for a patient. For illustrative purposes, we will assume that the diet prescription is as follows:

2,000 Kcal; 100 g Protein; 70 g Fat; 250 g Carbohydrate
Divide carbohydrate: B, 1/6; L, 2/6; PM 1/6; D 2/6

First, we need to establish the number of each of the exchanges to be included in the diet for the day. Let us see how we could arrive at the calculations given in Form R.

Step 1: List the exchanges in the order given—that is, milk, fruit, and vegetables in any order first, followed by the bread exchanges, then the meat exchanges, then the fat exchanges.

Step 2: Estimate the number of milk exchanges that will fit into the diet. For an adult, a minimum of two exchanges to a maximum of one exchange for each meal and snack are usually used. The amounts for adolescents and children are adjusted for age. In all cases, the amounts should be adjusted for patients' preferences.

For purposes of our calculation. we'll assume that our patient wants an 8 oz glass of milk at breakfast, lunch and supper, for a total of three milk exchanges. Note that we use *skim* milk in the calculation. The three milk exchanges contain 24 g protein and 36 g carbohydrate. If 2-percent or whole milk is used instead of skim milk, the exchanges contain 5 g and 8 g of fat, respectively.

Step 3: Estimate the number of vegetable exchanges that will fit into the meal plan. Two exchanges, one at midday and one at the evening meal, are customary. Again, however, some patients prefer more or less. If a patient is a vegetarian, for example, the number of vegetable exchanges would almost certainly be increased.

For our patient, we will calculate three vegetable exchanges into the meal plan. These contribute 6 g protein and 15 g carbohydrate to the diet.

Step 4: Estimate the number of fruit exchanges that will fit into the meal plan. It is customary to include a minimum of one for breakfast, and one at each of the other two main meals to serve as a dessert. The maximum is usually one for each meal or snack; however, if the patient prefers more fruit, for example, double servings could be included.

We'll assume that the patient in our example says he prefers one serving of fruit at each meal and snack. These four servings will then contribute 60 g carbohydrate to the total intake.

Step 5: Total the carbohydrate you have calculated into the diet thus far and subtract from the prescribed amount: 36 + 15 + 60 = 111; 250 − 111 = 139.

Step 6: To find the number of bread exchanges needed to provide the total carbohydrate, divide the amount still needed by the amount in one bread exchange: 139 ÷ 15 = 9 (rounded to the nearest whole number).

Note that nine bread exchanges add 27 g protein and 135 g carbohydrate to the diet plan in Form R.

Step 7: Find the total protein included thus far and substract from the total needed: 24 + 6 + 27 = 57. Then, 100 − 57 = 43.

Step 8: To find the number of meat exchanges needed to fill the prescription, divide the amount needed by the amount in one meat exchange: 43 ÷ 7 = 6 (rounded to the nearest whole number).

Note that six medium-fat meat exchanges add 42 g protein and 30 g fat to the diet. It is recommended that meal plans be calculated with medium-fat meats. However, clients should be encouraged to use lean meats whenever possible, and high-fat meats should be limited to not more than three servings per week (13).

Step 9: Total the fat included thus far and subtract from the amount prescribed: 70 − 30 = 40.

Step 10: To find the number of fat exchanges needed to provide the total fat, divide the amount still needed by the amount in one fat exchange: 40 ÷ 5 = 8.

Step 11: Add the total amounts of protein, fat, and carbohydrate. The protein and carbohydrate totals should agree with the prescription within an acceptable range of ±5. If the diet does not meet these restrictions, go back and adjust as necessary.

FORM R

Calculating a Meal Pattern

Total Calories 2000
Carbohydrate (% calories) ______ (g) 250
Protein (% calories) ______ (g) 100
Fat (% calories) ______ (g) 70
Division of carbohydrate: 1/6, 2/6, 1/6, 2/6 ______

Daily Meal Pattern

Exchange	# of Exchanges	Protein (g)	Fat (g)	Carbohydrate (g)
*Milk—(NF) LF, whole	3	24		36
Fruit	4			60
Vegetable	3	6		15
Subtotal		(30)		(111)
*Bread/Starch	9	27		135
Subtotal		(57)		
*Meat—lean, (medium,) high fat	6	42	30	
Fat	8		40	
TOTAL		99	70	246

*Circle the one used in calculating the meal pattern

Distribution of Exchanges at Meals and Snacks

Exchanges	Total # of Exchanges	Breakfast	AM Snack	Lunch	PM Snack	Dinner	HS Snack
Milk, NF	3	1 (12)	( )	1 (12)	( )	1 (12)	( )
Fruit	4	1 (15)	( )	1 (15)	1 (15)	1 (15)	( )
Vegetable	3	( )	( )	1 (5)	( )	2 (10)	( )
Bread	9	1 (15)	( )	3 (45)	2 (30)	3 (45)	( )
Meat, med.	6	( )	( )	2 ( )	1 ( )	3 ( )	( )
Fat	8	1 ( )	( )	4 ( )	( )	3 ( )	( )
Total		(42)	( )	(77)	(45)	(82)	( )

The meal plan: The exchanges just calculated must now be distributed among the meals and snacks. The distribution is influenced by the type of insulin the patient is receiving in IDDM. In NIDDM, the food, or the carbohydrate at least, is divided relatively evenly into three meals in order to keep variations in blood glucose to a minimum.

We'll assume our example patient is taking NPH insulin and needs an afternoon snack. This is reflected in the prescription for one-sixth of his carbohydrate at that time. (An example of the procedure is shown in Table 18-6). The diet contains 246 g carbohydrate. Therefore, 41 g (246 ÷ 6 = 41) should be included in the breakfast and afternoon snack and twice that, or about 82 g at lunch and dinner. You can see that the milk exchanges are distributed one to each meal and the fruit exchanges are distributed one to each meal and snack as requested by the patient, and the vegetable exchanges are scheduled for lunch and dinner. The bread exchanges are then distributed to meet the prescribed distribution of carbohydrate.

Meat and fat exchanges are distributed according to patient preference if only carbohydrate is distributed. In those institutions where calorie distribution is prescribed, meat and fat would be distributed to meet that requirement.

Planning daily menus: Using the meal plan, a series of daily menus can be planned for or by the patient. For each exchange on the meal plan, a choice is made from the corresponding exchange list. Choices are made *within* the list, not *between* lists. A sample menu is shown in Table 18-6.

Some foods are almost free of protein, fat, and carbohydrate. These foods, listed in Table C-8 may be added to the planned diet in reasonable amounts as desired to vary the menu. You will see that coffee, tea, broth, vinegar, dill pickles, and lettuce have been added to the menu in Table 18-6 as "free" foods not calculated into the meal plan.

Expanding the exchange lists: A variety of information sources on food values can be used to expand the exchange lists. Table C-9 gives exchange values for various combination foods. A number of fast-food restaurant chains publish the composition of their products in terms of the diabetic exchange lists.

Sample dietary plans and exchange lists that are useful in feeding diabetic infants are also available (14). Some of these may be useful in feeding diabetic patients with complicating illnesses requiring pureed foods.

Special foods for diabetic diets: A number of special foods are available for use by diabetic patients. Although most are unnecessary, there are a few that are useful. *Unsweetened canned fruits* are helpful, especially during seasons when the variety of fresh fruits is limited.

Some persons prefer to use *artificial sweeteners*. Aspartame is a current favorite, used in a variety of prepared products and as a sweetener to be added to beverages or other foods. Saccharine is also available, but some complain that it leaves a bitter aftertaste.

There are also "diabetic" or "dietetic" candies, frozen desserts, gelatin desserts, and salad dressings. In general, these are not necessary and are usually expensive. They are sometimes lower, but are rarely higher, in energy content than are the corresponding conventional items.

Patients should be acquainted with the specific meanings of labeling terminology. Government regulations give the following definitions:

Low calorie—a food that contains no more than 40 kcal per specified serving.
Reduced calorie—a food that contains at least one-third fewer kcals than a similar food for which it can be substituted.

TABLE 18-6.   Sample Diabetic Diet Menu

Exchange	Food	Exchange	Food
Breakfast		*Lunch*	
1 Fruit	½ Grapefruit	—	1 c Broth (no fat)
1 Bread	1 Slice whole-wheat toast	1 Bread	6 Saltines
1 Fat	1 t Margarine	2 Meat	2 oz Hamburger patty
1 Milk, skim	1 c Milk, skim	4 Fat	4 t Mayonnaise
—	Coffee, black	2 Bread	1 Hamburger bun
		—	Dill pickles; Leaf lettuce
		½ Vegetable	¼ c Sliced tomato
		½ Vegetable	¼ c Carrot and celery sticks
		1 Fruit	4 Fresh apricots
		1 Milk, skim	1 c Milk, skim
		—	Coffee black
PM *Snack*		*Dinner*	
1 Fruit	1 Small pear	3 Meat	3 oz Roast pork loin
2 Bread	12 Saltine crackers	1 Vegetable	½ c Tomato juice
1 Meat	1 oz Mozzarella cheese	1 Vegetable	½ c Broccoli
		2 Bread	⅔ c Sweet potato
		1 Bread	1 Plain roll
		1 Fruit	⅛ Honeydew melon
		3 Fat	3 t Margarine
		1 Milk, skim	1 c Milk, skim
		—	Tea, black

Foods not recommended: There are few foods that are absolutely forbidden for inclusion in a diabetic diet, but some categories of foods are generally considered to be poor choices. One of these categories includes foods that are *concentrated sources of simple carbohydrates.* Sweetened baked goods, other very sweet desserts, candies, sugars, jams, jellies, and syrups are the primary components of this group. Even so, exceptions can be made if substitutions are skillfully handled and infrequently used for special occasions.

Another less-commonly used category comprises foods that are *mixtures of unknown composition.* These foods may be difficult to fit into the diet when composition is unknown, but several procedures are available to accommodate a patient who has a special desire for such foods:

1. If the food is a commercially prepared convenience food, obtain the protein, fat, and carbohydrate content. This information may be on the label or in tables of food values issued by the manufacturer. (It is wise for you to collect these as they become available.)

If all else fails, you can write to the manufacturer on your institution's letterhead stationery and request the information.

Foods not recommended or foods that are mixtures of unknown composition can be assigned values in terms of exchange lists. A food which contains 6 g protein, 30 g carbohydrate, and 10 g fat would be considered, for example, to be equivalent to two bread exchanges and two fat exchanges. The food can then be included in the diet in place of other foods providing these exchanges.

2. Alternatively, you can suggest to patients that they prepare their own mixed dishes using the exchanges on the meal plan. For example, a patient could make spaghetti and meat balls with 1 c cooked spaghetti equal to two bread exchanges, 3 oz medium-fat ground beef equal to three medium-fat meat exchanges, ½ c tomatoes equal to one vegetable exchange, plus desired "free" seasonings. Many recipes of this kind are available in cookbooks for diabetic diets.

TO TEST YOUR UNDERSTANDING

7. You have an adult NIDDM patient who weighs 220 pounds. His DBW is 180 pounds. The attending physician asks you to recommend a diet for the patient that will eventually bring him to DBW. Based on an interview, you determine that the patient has a sedentary life-style. The patient is receiving an oral hypoglycemic agent, but the physician hopes to discontinue this medication when DBW is achieved. You know that a safe rate of weight loss is 1 to 2 pounds per week. Write your answers in the blanks provided.
   _____ g protein; _____ g fat; _____ g carbohydrate; _____ division of carbohydrate

8. You have another patient whose diet prescription is P-100; F-65; C-190; divide Carbohydrate- 2/7, 2/7, 1/7, 2/7, with a 4:00 P.M. snack. The patient has the following preferences:

   No more than 1 pt milk per day
   Carries her lunch, usually one or more sandwiches
   Wants at least one egg for breakfast
   Dislikes breakfast cereals

   a. Calculate on Form S the number and types of exchanges that could be included in her diet.
   b. Write a daily meal plan for the patient, also on Form S.
   c. Using the menu for _____ (day to be assigned by your instructor), plan a day's menu for this patient.

9. Your IDDM patient's diet contains the following exchanges for lunch and dinner:

   4 lean meat, 1 vegetable, 1 fruit, 3 bread, 4 fat, and 1 skim milk.

   He tells you that he has a favorite food, a frozen entree, that he would like to include in his diet occasionally. Your information from the manufacturer says that a one-serving package contains 36 g carbohydrate, 14 g protein, and 15 g fat. What would you tell the patient to remove from his exchange lists when he includes this entree in his meal?

10. A patient tells you that she would like to make a "chili" containing beans, ground beef, onions, and tomatoes, plus desired "free" seasoning. Using the meal plan given in question 8, how much of these ingredients could she use to make a mixture that fits into her meal plan?

FORM S

Calculating a Meal Pattern

Total kcal _____
Carbohydrate (% kcal) _____ (g) _____
Protein   (% kcal) _____ (g) _____
Fat   (% kcal) _____ (g) _____
Division of carbohydrate: _____

Daily Meal Pattern

Exchange	# of Exchanges	Protein (g)	Fat (g)	Carbohydrate (g)
*Milk—NF, LF, whole				
Fruit				
Vegetable				
Subtotal				
*Bread/Starch				
Subtotal				
*Meat—lean, medium, high fat				
Fat				
TOTAL				

*Circle the one used in calculating the meal pattern

Distribution of Exchanges at Meals and Snacks

Exchanges	Total # of Exchanges	Breakfast	AM Snack	Lunch	PM Snack	Dinner	HS Snack
Milk		( )	( )	( )	( )	( )	( )
Fruit		( )	( )	( )	( )	( )	( )
Vegetable		( )	( )	( )	( )	( )	( )
Bread		( )	( )	( )	( )	( )	( )
Meat		( )	( )	( )	( )	( )	( )
Fat		( )	( )	( )	( )	( )	( )
Total		( )	( )	( )	( )	( )	( )

11. Plan a noon Thanksgiving-day meal for the patient described in question 9.

12. A list of products prepared for use in diabetic diets is listed here. For each product, define a serving and give the protein, fat, and carbohydrate content. If the product is available, evaluate its taste. Your instructor may add additional items in the space provided:

Product (Brands)	Servings	Pro (g)	Fat (g)	CHO (g)	Taste	Other comments
Water-pack canned fruit						
Juice-pack canned fruit						
Aspartame (NutraSweet)						
Saccharine						
Unsweetened gelatin dessert						

13. Visit a nearby supermarket and list below the products available (other than those in question 12) that are labeled "diabetic," "low calorie," "dietetic," or that otherwise imply they are useful for diabetic diets or are reduced in calorie content. Evaluate each as indicated in the table:

Product (Brand)	Label	Food Value (g) Protein	Fat	CHO	Comments (Usefulness, desirability, truth in labeling, etc.)

Compensatory Changes. There are a number of circumstances in which it is appropriate to change a diabetic diet once control has been established. These include special occasions involving food, changes in activity routines, eating in restaurants, travel, and illness. In order to control blood sugar levels with *food*, *insulin*, and *activity*, if there is a change in one of these three components of control, at least one other component must be altered to compensate. The nutritional care specialist is often called upon to suggest compensatory modifications in the diet or procedures to avoid changes in diet. In this discussion, we will describe some useful procedures.

General approach to diet modification for glycemic control: We will assume that the patient has been regulated as well as possible based on the information available concerning his usual activity and eating habits. The original plan must then be tailored to the individual, since each patient's response to treatment is unique, and the patient must be taught to make necessary temporary changes.

Ideally, the patient is on SBGM and brings records of the results to the clinic for you to review. Results of urine tests are less informative, but still useful.

If results show periods of hyperglycemia at certain times each day, you can sometimes move foods from the immediately preceding meal to another meal, preferably at a time when blood glucose is lower than

desirable. Alternatively, you can explore with the patient the possibility of rescheduling some activity. If periods of hyperglycemia or hypoglycemia are sporadic, it is appropriate to question the patient about the reasons for these changes, such as variation in diet, exercise, insulin dosage, and emotional upsets.

You may see circumstances in which diet change alone will not correct the lack of control. Patients may need to have their insulin dosage increased or decreased. These patients should be referred to their physician.

Precautions in hypoglycemia: IDDM patients are advised to carry some form of simple carbohydrate, such as sugar cubes or hard candy, with them at all times. These are used to compensate for low blood sugar. A patient who reports frequent hypoglycemic episodes should be referred to his physician. If the patient is compensating for excess insulin by taking additional food, the result will be undesirable weight gain.

Alcohol use: The use of alcoholic beverages by diabetic patients is not usually recommended. The energy content of alcohol (7 kcal/g) may be responsible for unwanted weight gain. It may be responsible for hypoglycemia in the IDDM patient, especially if meals are missed or delayed. The hypoglycemia may be difficult to distinguish from alcohol intoxication and may result in a delay in needed treatment. The oral hypoglycemic agents given to NIDDM patients may interact with even very small amounts of alcohol to produce a reaction resembling alcohol intoxication.

Despite these contraindications, it must be recognized that alcohol consumption is an important part of the social life of many patients and is likely to continue. Some patients find alcohol consumption a necessary part of their occupations. The patient who has decided to consume alcoholic beverages must be taught about its effects and about setting reasonable limits.

There is some evidence that the moderate intake of alcohol is relatively harmless in the well-controlled diabetic. Moderate intake has been defined as less than 6 percent of the total kcals per day from alcohol, not more than once or twice a week (15).

Because alcohol is metabolized in two-carbon fragments similar to fat, it is usually incorporated into diabetic diets in place of the fat exchanges. In fact, it has been suggested that an "alcohol equivalent" be considered to be equal to two fat exchanges. Some alcoholic beverages also contain carbohydrate, and some bread exchanges are removed to compensate for this.

The substitutions are recommended only for NIDDM patients. No food is removed from the diet of the IDDM patient because of the risk of alcohol-induced hypoglycemia (16). Insulin is not required for alcohol metabolism. In either case, the need for *moderate* intake or less should be emphasized to the patient.

The patient may be given a list of exchange values for alcoholic beverages. A typical list is given in Table C-10.

Eating out and travel tips: If diabetic patients are to lead normal lives, they need to know how to order meals in restaurants and how to take care of themselves while traveling.

In restaurants, simple foods that follow the prescribed diet should be ordered. The diabetic should ask that gravies and sauces not be added to food and that salad dressings be served "on the side" so that the amount used can be controlled. Most restaurants serve more food in a meal than a diabetic diet allows, and most are happy to provide a container so that the excess can be taken home.

Travel generally does not present a problem for NIDDM patients. For the patient with IDDM, however, certain precautions may be necessary.

All IDDM patients should be instructed to carry with them at all times some foods that can be used to avoid hypoglycemic reactions. Procedures vary with the means of transportation and length of trip. The following guidelines may be given to the patient:

Car travel—If driving, especially for more than a half hour and if the time is during peak insulin action, have some food, such as a half sandwich (one meat, one bread, one fat), taken from your next meal. Do *not* have any alcohol before driving; it tends to cause hypoglycemia, which may not be distinguished from intoxication. Always carry some sugar or candy with you—even if you are just a passenger.

Air travel—Carry an emergency supply of sugar. Find out whether meals will be served. Airlines will serve special diets if ordered well in advance. Carry sandwiches in case there is a mix-up about meals.

Ship travel—Food is usually available. The main problem may be seasickness. A liquid diet or the diet for "morning sickness" (see Chapter 7) may be helpful.

Rail travel—Long-distance trains usually have food available. It is a good idea to carry some sandwiches and fruit as a precaution in case of problems with the dining car. Commuter-train travel is likely to require only an emergency sugar supply.

Bus travel—Commuter-bus travel is similar to travel by commuter train. Long-distance bus travel is difficult because there is no food on buses and schedules are often erratic. Patients should carry enough food to provide all meals in transit.

TO TEST YOUR UNDERSTANDING

14. Your NIDDM patient who is controlling his diabetes with diet alone has a diet which contains, for the evening meal, four low-fat meat, one vegetable, one fruit, three bread, one skim milk, and four fat exchanges. He tells you that he occasionally entertains with afternoon cocktails and occasionally likes to "have a beer while watching the football game." He asks how he can continue to do this and still stay within the limits of his diet.

    Given the following possible combinations, indicate the adjustment he should make to his evening meal to allow for the intake specified:

	Food & Drink Items	Amount	Exchange Value	Total Removed from Next Meal
a.	Whiskey	1.5 oz		
	Calorie-free mixer			
	Potato chips	15		
b.	Scotch	1.5 oz		
	Soda			
	Corn chips	15		

Food & Drink Items	Amount	Exchange Value	Total Removed from Next Meal
c. Sherry, dry	2 oz		
Almonds	10 whole		
d. Vodka in calorie-free mixer	1.5 oz		
Peanuts, Spanish	20 whole		
e. Champagne, dry	4 oz		
Olives	5 small		
f. Chablis	4 oz		
Cheese, Cheddar	1 oz		
Crackers, Saltine	6		
g. Cabernet Sauvignon	4 oz		
Cream cheese	2 T		
Crackers, butter-type	5		
h. Beer	12 oz		
Pretzel sticks	25		

15. A patient tells you his favorite restaurant is a "steak house," where the menu consists of:

   Steaks (broiled) or roast beef
   Baked or French-fried potatoes
   Sliced tomato salad with choice of dressings
   Assorted rolls, butter
   Ice cream
   Coffee, tea

   The restaurant has a full bar.
      Describe how you would counsel this patient.
   (*Hint:* See Chapter 6.)

Adjusting for illness: Concurrent illnesses sometimes interfere with control of diabetes. Some illnesses, such as infections, increase the demand for insulin, causing hyperglycemia; decreased activity may further increase blood glucose. Ill patients should check their blood glucose frequently and be guided primarily by those results.

The ill diabetic may be unwilling or unable to eat part of the food in a meal. If the patient is not receiving a hypoglycemic drug, particularly if obese, no substitution needs to be made. If the patient has received the prescribed insulin, however, failure to eat food can lead to a hypoglycemic reaction. A patient who is taking an OHA may also need a substitute for uneaten food for a short period since some products have a half life of 1 to 2 days.

All institutions have procedures to deal with such situations. Common procedures are as follows:

1. No substitutions are needed if the uneaten food contains only protein and fat (that is, meat or fat exchanges).

2. No substitution is offered if the uneaten food contains less than a specified amount of carbohydrate. In many institutions, the specified amount is 5 g or less. Thus, ¼ c milk or a serving of vegetable would not require substitution.

3. Substitutions are offered for foods containing more than 5 g of carbohydrate. Usually, the food offered is in a form easier to eat (or drink) and in a smaller volume than the rejected food.

In institutions, it is common practice to use *unsweetened* fruit juice as the substituted food, using a graduated cylinder to measure. For these purposes, the fruit juices are considered to contain the concentrations of carbohydrate given in Table C-4. For larger amounts, which would require great volumes of juice, foods may be given in combinations—for example, 45 g of carbohydrate can be provided in 240 ml pineapple juice plus 3 graham crackers. Sugar is sometimes added to grapefruit or orange juice to reduce the volume needed. Hard candy provides carbohydrate without the liquid volume, which can aggravate vomiting.

Alternatives to Diet Planning with Exchange Lists

The use of the exchange-list system in diet planning is not suitable for all patients. Some patients need a simpler system. For this purpose, there is a system with fewer exchanges:

		Pro	Fat	CHO
1.	Milk (1 c) or	8	10	12
	Meat (2 oz)	14	10	
2.	Fruits/Vegetables	2		15
3.	Starches	2		15

The vegetables in the fruits/vegetables exchange are those in the bread/cereal exchange of the standard exchange list. Fats are listed for the patient as the total per day, to be used as desired. The vegetable list from the standard exchange list is considered "free" food in this system.

A diet might thus be planned as follows:

Breakfast	Lunch	Dinner	HS
1 Fruit/Veg	2 Meat	2 Meat	1 Milk

1 Meat	1 Free Veg	2 Fruit/Veg	1 Starch
1 Starch	2 Starch	1 Starch	
	1 Fruit/Veg		
	1 Milk		

+ 3 fat as desired

+ free vegetables as desired

Another approach is particularly useful for NIDDM patients who are not obese. It may also be useful for IDDM and obese NIDDM patients if the patient is unwilling to follow a more structured program. In this diet, the following instructions are emphasized:

Avoid concentrated carbohydrates.

Eat three regular meals of approximately equal size per day, plus HS snack if indicated.

Each meal should contain both protein and carbohydrate. Patients are also given instruction on

Treatment for insulin reaction

Modification of the diet during illness and for exercise

TO TEST YOUR UNDERSTANDING

23. Mr. S. is a 89 y.o. IDDM patient who lives alone in a small apartment. His diabetes has become less well controlled over the past two years, and he tells you, "I can't seem to remember all those numbers any more." You decide to try the "three-exchange" system for him.

    a. His current lunch consists of 1 milk (skim), 1 fruit, 1 vegetable, 2 bread, 2 meat (medium-fat), and 2 fat. You note also that he has 2 fat exchanges at each meal.

    Translate this meal plan into the "three-exchange" system.

    b. Besides a new list of exchanges, what additional information would you give him?

    c. Assuming the patient has a hamburger, green beans, fresh peaches, baked potato, bread, and milk available, write a lunch menu from your meal plan in part *a* above.

24. Ms. K is a 37 y.o. obese IDDM patient who has been diabetic for 15 years. She understands her diet and other aspects of treatment, but refuses to follow a diet. She has stated that, "It isn't worth it to go through all that, and I'm *not* going to bother." She has signs of advanced vascular disease for her age but has never been hospitalized for diabetic ketoacidosis (DKA).

    You take a 24-hr recall, which reveals the following:

Breakfast:	½ grapefruit
	1 Danish pastry
Coffee break:	1 doughnut
	Coffee with cream and sugar substitute
Lunch:	Vegetable-beef soup (canned)
	12 Saltines
	Vegetable salad/French dressing
	Soft drink (artificially sweetened)
Dinner:	3–4 oz serving meat or poultry (no skin)
	Potato, rice, or noodles with butter, occasionally gravy
	Buttered vegetable or salad with dressing
	Tea
Snack:	Fruit, unsweetened, canned or fresh
	or
	½ c "dietetic" ice cream

You have referred the matter to Social Services, and they are working with the patient. In the meantime, the patient continues to refuse to follow a more structured diet with exchange lists.

a. List some appropriate objectives for counseling at this time.

b. Choose one of your objectives in part *a*. What changes in her meals, indicated by her 24-hr, recall would be necessary to accomplish this?

EDUCATION OF THE PERSON WITH DIABETES

The greatest portion of the care of diabetic patients must be provided by the patients themselves. In order to provide adequate self-care, the patient must be willing to accept that responsibility and must also be capable of carrying out the necessary procedures. As a consequence, patient education is of great importance.

The education of the diabetic patient requires a team effort if it is to succeed. The team must comprise, at least, the physician, the nurse, the nutritional care specialist, and most important, the patient. A podiatrist, a social worker, members of the patient's family, a public health nurse, teachers of a diabetic child, employers, and others may be included as necessary.

Unfortunately, many, if not most, patients in the past have not received sufficient education to enable them to take adequate care of themselves. Proper education is essential if diabetic patients are to live active and productive lives. In addition, it is essential that patient education, as well as evidence that the patient has been effectively informed, be documented in the medical record.

In order to be effective, patient teaching must be conducted over a prolonged period, with concepts reviewed at intervals. It is suggested that the education

TABLE 18-7. Sample Lesson Plans for Education of the Newly Diagnosed Diabetic

Day 1	*Day 2*
Objectives 1. Pt or significant other is able to give one reason that diet is important. 2. Pt or significant other is able to list foods to avoid that are high in concentrated CHO and foods that are free. 3. Pt will read assigned pages in instruction booklet before next lesson.	*Objectives* 1. Pt and/or significant other answers review questions correctly. 2. Pt or significant other will read remainder of instruction booklet. 3. Pt or significant other will complete sample menu using exchange plan by next lesson. 4. Pt or significant other verbalizes appropriate treatment for hypoglycemic reaction.

Content:
1. Rationale of diabetic diet in terms of
  a. definition of diabetes
  b. need for diet to avoid concentrated CHO and provide regular meals of approximately equal amts each day.
2. What foods high in CHO must be avoided.
3. Free foods and when to use.
4. Give pt ADA exchange booklet to review before next lesson.
	Content:
	1. Assessment of pt's understanding of previous session.
	2. Exchange system:
	  a. Foods of similar composition grouped with average CHO, protein, fat.
	  b. Review content of exchange lists and portion sizes.
	  c. Concept of exchanging within lists, not between.
	3. Give pt meal pattern for writing sample menu.
	4. Ask pt to read remainder of booklet.
	5. Symptoms and treatment of hyper- and hypoglycemia; importance of having concentrated CHO available.
	6. Answer questions.

Documentation: **S:** Pt comments about usual diet habits, especially sugar comsumption; pt ability to list foods to avoid, free foods; pt response to question, "Why do you need to avoid sugar?" **O:** Diet Rx, Ht, Wt, ideal weight, insulin, blood glucose, % meal consumption; pertinent medical info, lab data **A:** Assessment of difficulty with adherence; adequacy of present food intake and weight, reason for contacting MD for diet change **P:** Exchange meal pattern adjusted per preferences. Discussed rationale for diet. Pt given instruction booklet to read before next session. Contact MD for diet order revision.	*Documentation:* **S:** Pt comments on diet, statements about diet procedures. **O:** Diet Rx, blood glucose, meds, % meal consumption, etc. **A:** Accuracy of pt answers to review questions; has pt read booklet?; grasp of principles of exchange system. **P:** Pt to complete sample menu for 1,500-kcal diet with HS snack and finish instruction booklet by (date).
Example: **S:** "I eat a sweet dessert every day"; pt listed foods with sugar to be avoided to control BS; pt likes diet drinks for free food. **O:** Diet Rx—1,500 kcal, 4 fdg, Ht 5 ft, 6 in; Wt 140#; DBW 130–140#, Start 20 U NPH + 10 U RI: FBG—140 mg/dl; 2h PP: B—170, L—180. 100% meal intake. **A:** WM 35 y.o. at DBW with adequate diet. Diet will involve many changes for pt but receptive to info; 1,500 kcal appropriate for wt maintenance at present activity level. **P:** Pt selected 1,500 kcal menu with HS snack, modified per preferences. Discuss rationale for diet; given instruction booklet to review for next lesson.	*Example* **S:** "When I feel shaky and sweaty, I need to eat a sugar cube." **O:** Diet Rx—1,500 kcal with HS; FBG—105; 2h PP: B—100; L—110, Incr. NPH to 27 U. 100% food intake. **A:** Pt answering review questions correctly; has read instruction booklet; seems to grasp principles of exchange system. **P:** Pt to use prescribed diet for completing sample menu and finish reading instruction booklet.

of the patient is divided into 3 phases (21). The first phase provides the IDDM patient with introductory information about the disease, how to test for glucose, insulin administration, how to plan meals, and how to deal with acute complications. These are the essentials for survival and are usually also provided in written form.

Next, the patient is given information to make the regimen easier to "live with," such as how to order in restaurants, exercise and diabetes, use of alcohol, meal planning during illness, and chronic complications. Previous information is also reviewed in greater depth.

The third phase, which has been termed "continuing education," reviews and expands basic concepts at intervals. During all phases, keep in mind the principles of patient education that you learned in Chapter 6. The first two phases proceed over lengths of time that vary with the interest and aptitude of the patient. The third phase should continue as a permanent part of nutritional care. An example of a plan for part of the education of a diabetic patient, and documenta-

tion of that education, is given in Table 18-7. When the early stages of the program are finished and the patient is discharged from the hospital, the name and telephone number of a nutritional consultant should be provided, and the patient should be scheduled to attend outpatient classes for diabetics.

In all groups of patients, there are those for whom exceptions must be made. Diabetic patients who have some mental dysfunction, or who are being transferred to a nursing care facility where meals are provided, are among such patients. If a diet instruction is ordered less than 24 hours prior to discharge, a comprehensive diet instruction is also not possible. In some cases, patient aptitude or interest makes proper diet instruction on the exchange-list system unfeasible. In such circumstances, one of the previously described alternatives can be used.

The main thrust of education for obese NIDDM patients is weight control. In addition, food is distributed throughout the day, with avoidance of simple carbohydrates to prevent wide variations in blood sugar levels.

TO TEST YOUR UNDERSTANDING

25. Mr. B. is a 40 y.o. patient who has been admitted to your hosptial for the first time. His surgery for hernia repair was done two days ago. The patient is an insulin-dependent diabetic of 25-years' standing.

    During your interview, Mr. B. is alert and cooperative, and says he understands his diet. However, you pick up two pertinent comments:

    "My diet has 4 ounces of meat at noon and night, but I can never figure out how much 4 ounces of meat is, especially if the meat has a bone in it, like a pork chop."

    "My diet has three bread exchanges at dinner and two graham crackers in the afternoon snack. I get awfully tired of graham crackers every afternoon. Two slices of bread and a potato every night gets tiresome, too, so I sometimes have baked desserts for more variety."

    a. Write a note in the patient's medical record in which you evaluate his understanding of his diet.

    b. The patient is being discharged shortly, but will return to the Diabetic Clinic in two weeks. You can only deal with one of his problems today. Which would you choose? Why?

    c. Outline a short lesson plan to educate the patient on the subject you have chosen as having first priority.

26. You have a patient who has had the instruction described in Table 18-7. It is now the patient's third hospital day, and she will be discharged the next morning, but will return to the Diabetic Clinic for further instruction.

    a. List the items you would teach today and those that would be deferred until a later clinic visit.

    b. List your objectives for this day's instruction.

    c. List the items you might write as a SOAP note in the patient's record.

DIABETES AND PREGNANCY

Pregnant diabetics may be classified into two groups— the diabetic woman who becomes pregnant (pregestational diabetes) and the patient with gestational diabetes mellitus. In both cases, the pregnancy is considered high risk; rigid control of the diabetes is therefore required in both cases and requires great effort. Without adequate control, there is increased risk of congenital anomalies. preterm delivery, macrosomia,

intrauterine growth retardation, newborn hypoglycemia, and newborn hyperbilirubinemia.

THE PREGNANT WOMAN WITH PREGESTATIONAL DIABETES

Patients who are diabetic when they conceive, but who are not well controlled, are often hospitalized for control of diabetes, review and correction of previous education, education on aspects of pregnancy and self-monitoring techniques as soon as pregnancy is diagnosed. The NIDDM patient who becomes pregnant will need insulin during pregnancy.

Monitoring

SBGM is considered important, even essential, for successful outcome. Desired glucose levels are 60 to 100 mg per dl for fasting levels and a maximum of 140 mg per dl 1 to 2 hours after meals. The standards for control are more rigid than are those for the nonpregnant woman. When the patient brings you her SBGM records, it is important to ensure that blood glucose has remained within normal limits.

Diet

The diet should have at least 200 g carbohydrate per day and 1.5 to 2.0 g protein per kg per day. Recommended total energy intakes are 30 kcal per kg IBW in the first trimester and 38 kcal per kg IBW in the second and third trimesters, with 50 to 60 percent carbohydrate, 20 to 37 percent fat, and 12 to 20 percent protein. An evening snack, containing a minimum of 25 g complex carbohydrate, is always included in order to avoid hypoglycemia during the night. It is a common practice to give six equal meals, or three meals and three snacks, to the IDDM pregnant diabetic.

During the first trimester of pregnancy, food intake may decline with symptoms of nausea and vomiting, and insulin doses may need to be decreased. Starvation ketosis, characterized by hypoglycemia and ketonuria, is common during the first trimester, and it is important to adjust the diet to foods that can be tolerated in order to ensure an adequate calorie intake and avoid ketonuria (see Table 7-6).

Insulin is given by multiple subcutaneous injections (MSI) or by CSII and is carefully balanced with the diet. Long-acting insulins are usually avoided. More rapid-acting insulin in multiple doses or CSII gives better control.

The NIDDM patient is often obese. It must be kept in mind that pregnancy is not the time for stringent weight reduction; however, excessive weight gain should be avoided. There is controversy concerning the optimal energy level to include in the diet. It has been stated that a diet of 1,500 to 1,700 kcal per day will provide for fetal growth (22). Alternatively, it has been suggested that 36 kcal per kg of current, or of ideal, body weight should be used. However, the use of current body weight as a base may result in a large overestimation of energy requirement. In the final analysis, it is necessary to monitor weight gain and adjust the diet to achieve a gain of 15 to 16 pounds over the course of gestation. For thin diabetics, 2,000 to 2,400 kcal per day (36 kcal per kg or more) are recommended.

Careful nutritional counseling and individualized treatment are essential. It is important to keep in mind that the nutritional needs for pregnancy must be met (see Chapter 7). In addition, ketonuria should be carefully avoided since there is evidence of fetal brain damage in ketosis.

GESTATIONAL DIABETES

Gestational diabetes mellitus (GDM) is, by definition, diabetes that begins during the second half of pregnancy and is reversible postpartum. Its diagnosis is important because these patients also have an above-normal risk of complications. Therefore, many physicians now screen all pregnant women for GDM.

Patients at Risk

Patients at risk of GDM include those with a previous history of GDM, those with glycosuria or other symptoms of DM, or those with fasting plasma glucose levels at or above 120 mg per dl. Patients who are obese, defined as having a body mass index of greater than or equal to 27 before pregnancy, are also at risk. Previous reproductive history may also reveal risk factors: a previous infant weighing over 4,100 g (9 pounds) at birth, previous unexplained stillbirth, previous infant with a congenital anomaly, or development of polyhydramnios (22).

Diagnosis

The diagnostic tests for GDM are listed in Table 18-8. A positive screening test is an indication to proceed to the loading test, in which the patient is given a 50-g glucose (Glucola) load. In some clinics, the loading test is used as the screening test. A 3-hour glucose tolerance test is done if the loading test is positive. HgbA$_{1c}$ is used to distinguish GDM from previously undiagnosed NIDDM.

Treatment

Some GDM patients, but not all, require insulin to control hyperglycemia. OHAs are not used because

---

TABLE 18-8   Tests for Hyperglycemia During Pregnancy

Screening:
   Abnormal if a fasting plasma glucose level ≥ 105 mg/dl or if a 2-hr or more postprandial random plasma glucose ≥ 120 mg/dl
Loading
   50-g glucose load given orally at random
   Abnormal if 1-hr postload plama glucose ≥ 150 mg/dl
Tolerance Test:
   1. Plasma glucose in fasting state
   2. 100-g glucose load given orally
   3. Plasma glucose at 1, 2, and 3 hr postload
   Results
      Abnormal if two or more values ≥ fasting, 105 mg/dl; 1 hr, 190 mg/dl; 2 hr, 165 mg/dl; 3 hr, 145 mg/dl

Reproduced with permission from Barden, T.P. and H.C. Knowles, Jr. Diagnosis of diabetes in pregnancy. *Clin. Obstet. Gynec.* 24: (1981) 3–17.

of the risk of teratogenesis. An appropriate diet is needed by all. The pattern of the diet for the non-obese patient is similar to that described for IDDM and NIDDM patients (20), except that the patient is usually given three meals and one evening snack, rather than three snacks per day. The desired weight gain for the obese GDM patient is controversial. It has been suggested that an intake of 25 kcal per kg, or not less than 1,700 to 1,800 kcal per day, is a safe level (23). All GDM patients need extensive instruction because, unlike most pregestational diabetics, they have not had previous instruction.

TO TEST YOUR UNDERSTANDING

27. Mrs. R. is a pregnant patient who has been diabetic (IDDM) for 8 years. She lost one previous child by miscarriage and is anxious that this pregnancy be successful. She has been monitoring her own blood glucose for the last two years. The following data are in her medical record:

Age 24 yrs
Ht 5 ft, 6 in
Wt 132 #; IBW 132 #
EDD (date given indicates pt is at 6 wks gestation)
FBG 90 mg/dl
HgbA$_{1c}$ 7.2%
Grav II, Para O
Previous insulin 10 U RI and 32 U NPH. Changed to RI—14 U t.i.d. prior to each main meal.

a. You receive a referral asking that you recommend a diet for Mrs. R. for the first trimester. Indicate the diet you would recommend.

Protein	_____
Fat	_____
Carbohydrate	_____
Division of carbohydrate	_____

b. How might you need to adjust the content of the diet during the first trimester to avoid ketonuria?
c. What diet would you recommend at the beginning of the second trimester? Assume Mrs. R. now weighs 61.5 kg.

Protein	_____
Fat	_____
Carbohydrate	_____
Division of carbohydrate	_____

28. Mrs. C. has been tentatively diagnosed as having gestational diabetes. Her medical record gives the following data:

Age 20 yrs
Height 5 ft, 8 in
Weight 176 # Weight at conception 166 #
EDD (date given indicates pt is at 23 wks gestation)
FBG 175 mg/dl
Loading test 200 mg/dl
GTT fasting 140 mg/dl; 1 hr—190; 2 hr—160; 3 hr—140
Para I, Grav O
No insulin has been ordered.

a. Explain why the diagnosis of gestational diabetes is tentative.
b. What is patient's IBW? What total weight gain is desirable?

OTHER USES OF EXCHANGE LISTS FOR DIET PLANNING

The diabetic exchange lists are useful for planning other than diabetic diets. *Obese* patients may find them helpful for planning weight-reduction diets. The results are similar to a diet for an obese NIDDM patient except that there can be greater flexibility in distributing food throughout the day.

A diet for patients with *functional reactive hypoglycemia* can be planned by varying the proportions of the major nutrients. A suitable diet might contain, for example, 125 g protein, 100 g carbohydrate, and sufficient fat to maintain normal weight. The protein and fat are evenly divided throughout the day. As many as six feedings may be necessary.

The *ketogenic diet* is sometimes used, though rarely, for epileptics. The same exchange lists can be used to plan a moderate-protein, low-carbohydrate, and very-high-fat diet.

The basic principles on which these exchange lists are based are also useful with other types of groupings. In the chapter on renal disease, for example, you will see exchange lists based on the protein, sodium, and potassium content of foods. Other lists are based on the amino acid content of the foods. Skill in using exchange lists is therefore useful in a number of clinical situations.

TOPICS FOR FURTHER DISCUSSION

1. What is the rationale for the increase in dietary carbohydrate prior to a glucose tolerance test?

2. The following drugs affect the results of tests used for urine glucose or blood glucose. Discuss the type of patients for whom these drugs are used and in whom you must be alert for errors in testing results: levodopa, sulfobromphthalein, thiazide diuretics, anticoagulants, propranolol.

3. Why is plasma glucose higher than whole-blood glucose?

4. Why is it recommended that patients check for urine ketones during infections or other stresses?

5. From information obtained in the literature (including advertisements), make a list of the products currently available for home blood glucose monitoring. Note the range of values they will record and compare their advantages and limitations.

6. Why are oral hypoglycemic agents not used in IDDM, pregnancy, and kidney or liver dysfunction?

7. How could one of the diets in this chapter be modified for a strict vegetarian? an Orthodox Jew?

8. Discuss procedures for reducing the cost of a diabetic diet if the patient complains of being unable to afford it.

9. What is the glycemic index and what is its significance in diet planning?

10. Discuss the relative sweetness of artificial sweeteners and the safety of their use.

11. Discuss the metabolism of fructose and its use in diabetic diets.

12. How are diabetic diets modified to increase fiber content?

13. Discuss modification of the diabetic diet for various ethnic groups in your area.

14. Discuss modification of the diabetic diet for various religious groups in your area.

REFERENCES

1. DANIELS, J.S. AND N. FISHMAN. Diabetes mellitus and hyperlipidemia. In *Manual of Medical Therapeutics* (23d ed.), eds. J.J. Freitag and L.W. Miller. Boston: Little, Brown, 1980.

2. BAKERMAN, S. *ABCs of Interpretive Laboratory Data* (2d ed.). Greenville, N.C.: Interpretive Laboratory Data, Inc., 1984.

3. NATIONAL DIABETES DATA GROUP. Classification and diagnosis of diabetes mellitus and other categories of glucose intolerance. *Diabetes* 28:(1979)1039–1957.

4. GUTHRIE, D.W. AND R.A. GUTHRIE. The disease process of diabetes mellitus. Definition, characteristics, trends and developments. *Nurs. Clin. N. Amer.* 18:(1983)617–630.

5. PETERSON, C.M., L. JOVANOVIC, AND M. BROWNLEE. Home blood glucose monitoring. In *Diabetes Mellitus: Theory and Practice* (3d ed.), eds. M. Ellenberg and H. Rifkin. New York: Medical Examination Publishing Co., Inc., 1983.

6. GALLOWAY, J.A. AND R.D. deSHAZO. The clinical use of insulin and the complications of insulin therapy. In *Diabetes Mellitus: Theory and Practice* (3d ed.), eds. M. Ellenberg and H. Rifkin. New York: Medical Examination Publishing Co., Inc., 1983.

7. AMERICAN DIABETES ASSOCIATION. Nutritional recommendations and principles for individuals with diabetes mellitus: 1986. Diabetes Care 10:(1987)126–132.

8. ARKY, R.A. Nutritional management of the diabetic. In *Diabetes Mellitus: Theory and Practice* (3d ed.), eds. M. Ellenberg and H. Rifkin. New York: Medical Examination Publishing Co., Inc., 1983.

9. CRAPO, P.A., G. REAVEN, AND J. OLEFSKY. Plasma glucose and insulin responses to orally administered simple and complex carbohydrate. *Diabetes* 25:(1976)741–747.

10. JENKINS, D.J.A., A. LEEDS, M.A. GASSULL, B. COCHET, AND K.G.M.M. ALBERTI. Decrease in postprandial insulin and glucose concentrations by guar and pectin. *Ann. Int. Med.* 86:(1977)20.

11. JENKINS, D.J.A., T.M.S. SOLEVER, R.H. TAYLOR, H. GHARARI, A.L. JENKINS, H. BARKER, AND M.J.A. JENKINS. Rate of digestion of foods and postprandial glycaemia in normal and diabetic subjects. *Brit. Med. J.* 28:(1980)14–17.

12. COMMITTEES OF THE AMERICAN DIABETES ASSOCIATION AND THE AMERICAN DIETETIC ASSOCIATION. *Exchange Lists for Meal Planning*. Chicago: American Dietetic Association and American Diabetes Association, in cooperation with the National Institute of Arthritis, Metabolism, and Digestive Disease and the National Heart, Blood, and Lung Institute. U.S. Department of Health, Education, and Welfare, 1986.

13. FRANZ, M.J., P. BARR, H. HOLLER, M.A. POWERS, M.L. WHEELER, AND J. WYLIE-ROSETT. Exchange lists: revised 1986. J. Am. Diet. Assoc. 87:(1987)28–34.

14. BENZ, M.M. AND E. KOHLER. Baby food exchanges and feeding the diabetic infant. *Diab. Care* 3:(1980)554–556.

15. FRANZ, M.J. Diabetes mellitus: Considerations in the development of guidelines for the occasional use of alcohol. *J. Am. Diet. Assoc.* 83:(1983)147–152.

16. WALSH, D.H. AND D.J. O'SULLIVAN. Effects of moderate alcohol intake on control of diabetes. *Diabetes* 23:(1974)440–442.

17. KONISHI, F. Food energy equivalents of various activities. *J. Am. Diet. Assoc.* 46:(1965):187–188.

18. ZOKMAN, L.R. *Beyond Diet: Exercise Your Way to Fitness and Heart Health.* Englewood Cliffs, N.J.: CPC International, 1974, pp. 20–21.

19. LEON, A.S. *Nutrition and Athletic Performance.* Palo Alto: Bull Publishing, 1981, p. 233.

20. RUDERMAN, N. et al. *Diet and Exercise: Synergism in Health Maintenance.* Chicago: AMA, 1982, p. 143.

21. ETZWILER, D.D. Patient education and management: A team approach. In *Diabetes Mellitus: Theory and Practice* (3d ed.), eds. M. Ellenberg and H. Rifkin. New York: Medical Examination Publishing Co., Inc., 1983.

22. HOLLINGSWORTH, D.R. *Pregnancy, Diabetes and Birth.* Baltimore: Williams & Wilkins, 1984.

23. ALGERT, S., P. SHRAGG, AND D.R. HOLLINGSWORTH. Moderate caloric restriction in obese women with gestational diabetes. *Obstet. Gynecol.* 65:(1985)487–491.

ADDITIONAL SOURCES OF INFORMATION

COHEN, S., M. MILLER, AND R.L. SHERMAN. Metabolic acid-base disorders. *Am. J. Nursing.* Part 1, October 1977; Part 2, January 1978; Part 3, March 1978.

FINER, N. Sugar substitutes in the treatment of obesity and diabetes mellitus. *Clin. Nutr.* 4(1985)207–214.

CASE STUDY VI   DIABETES MELLITUS

Part I: Presentation

Present Illness: Eileen H. is a 10 y.o. child who was brought to the clinic by her mother. Mother reported that Eileen has had excessive thirst and frequent urination of 1 week's duration, in addition to increased appetite and a weight loss of 8 pounds in 4 weeks. Pt is normally active, complains of minor malaise.

Past Medical History: Pt was the product of a normal pregnancy and delivery. She had rubella at age 6 and a broken arm 6 months ago.

Family History: Parents L&W. Maternal aunt has IDDM. Paternal grandfather died of cardiovascular disease 2° to NIDDM. Other grandparents L&W.

Social History: 10 y.o. female at usual school grade for age. Lives with parents, one older brother, and one younger sister.

Review of Systems:

GI: No history of nausea, vomiting, diarrhea.

GU: No history of any urgency, frequency, or burning except for present complaint.

CNS: No history of loss of consciousness, convulsions, or difficulty with gait or station.

Physical Exam:

   General: Slightly underweight white female; ht 138 cm (50th percentile); wt 29 kg (25th percentile)

Vital signs: T 98.2° F; P 120; R 27 with fruity odor; BP 100/50 in right arm, supine

Lungs: Clear to percussion and auscultation

Heart: Normal sinus rhythm, no murmurs

Abdomen: Flat, liver not enlarged

Genitalia: Prepubertal

Extremities: Normal

CNS: Normal gait and station; normal deep tendon reflexes

   Laboratory:
      FBG: 450 mg/dl
      Urine: 4+ sugar, large acetone
      Serum Acetone: 3.0 mg/dl

Impression: Diabetes mellitus in 10 y.o. slightly underweight female with positive family history of DM.

Plan: Admit and place on RI until stabilized, then adjust to NPH. Place on 2,000-kcal diet, P-100; F-65, C-250, divide into equal thirds.

   Nutritionist to evaluate pt and recommend changes in diet as necessary. Also recommend diet for home use.

   Begin routine diabetes education of pt and significant others.

QUESTIONS

1. Discuss the significance of the family history.

2. Compare this patient's laboratory values with normal values:

    a. FBG

    b. Urine sugar

    c. Urine acetone

    d. Serum acetone

Part II: Nutritional Consult

During the next two days, the patient is given regular insulin t.i.d. You briefly meet with Eileen and her mother to obtain a 24-hr recall, offer a general explanation of a diabetic diet, and review the selected menu.

The routine nutritional assessment provides the following information:

TSF: 7.5 mm (5th percentile)
MAC: 17.5 cm (5th percentile)
24-hr recall:

Breakfast:

8 oz orange juice
1 c cornflakes, ½ c whole milk, 1 T sugar
2 eggs, fried
2 slices toast, 4 t margarine, 4 T jelly
8 oz whole milk

AM Snack:

8 oz whole milk (at school)
4 cookies

Lunch:

Bowl cream of tomato soup
2 tunafish salad sandwiches on rye bread
Large apple
4 cookies
8 oz whole milk

PM Snack:

Soft drink, sweetened, 12 oz
4 graham crackers
1 apple
1 chocolate bar

Dinner:

6 oz meat loaf
1 lg baked potato, 2 T margarine
½ c buttered broccoli
½ c molded fruit salad
1 c chocolate ice cream, chocolate sauce
8 oz whole milk

Evening Snack:

8 oz whole milk
1 doughnut

QUESTIONS

3. Describe what you would initially say to Eileen and her mother about the diabetic diet before reviewing the selected menu.

4. Develop a meal plan to be used for hospital meals for Eileen. Use Form T.

5. Using the menu for _____ (day to be assigned by your instructor), plan one day's menu for this patient while she is hospitalized.

6. Based on the information gathered in the 24-hr recall, what points might be important to stress in the diet instruction?

7. One day, Eileen complains about the lunch menu and refuses to eat some of the food. She leaves her vegetable, 2 oz meat (medium fat) and a roll on her tray. What would you do? Show your calculations.

FORM T

Calculating a Meal Pattern

Total Calories _____
Carbohydrate (% kcal) _____ (g) _____
Protein   (% kcal) _____ (g) _____
Fat   (% kcal) _____ (g) _____
Division of carbohydrate: _____

Daily Meal Pattern

Exchange	# of Exchanges	Protein (g)	Fat (g)	Carbohydrate (g)
*Milk—NF, LF, whole				
Fruit				
Vegetable				
Subtotal				
*Bread/Starch				
Subtotal				
*Meat—lean, medium, high fat				
Fat				
TOTAL				

*Circle the one used in calculating the meal pattern

Distribution of Exchanges at Meals and Snacks

Exchanges	Total # of Exchanges	Breakfast	AM Snack	Lunch	PM Snack	Dinner	HS Snack
Milk		( )	( )	( )	( )	( )	( )
Fruit		( )	( )	( )	( )	( )	( )
Vegetable		( )	( )	( )	( )	( )	( )
Bread		( )	( )	( )	( )	( )	( )
Meat		( )	( )	( )	( )	( )	( )
Fat		( )	( )	( )	( )	( )	( )
Total		( )	( )	( )	( )	( )	( )

Part III: Calculating the Discharge Diet

Eileen is in school from 9:00 AM to 12:00 Noon and from 1:15 to 3:00 PM. Travel time on the school bus is 30 minutes. She carries her lunch. Milk is available at school at 10:30 AM and at noon. Recess is at 10:30 AM, and lunch hour is from 12:00 to 1:15 PM.

Eileen's mother works part time and returns home at 5:00 PM, 3 days a week. She prepares all meals.

Eileen takes music lessons and is normally active at play after school.

8. You estimate that Eileen's increased activity after discharge will add 250 kcals to her total daily need. The pediatric endocrinologist specifies that Eileen should receive three meals and three snacks per day and that each snack should contain half as much carbohydrate as a meal.
    a. How much protein, fat, and carbohydrate would you recommend?
    b. Plan a meal pattern at this level, assuming the same carbohydrate division. Use Form U.

FORM U

Calculating a Meal Pattern

Total Calories _____
Carbohydrate (% kcal) _____ (g) _____
Protein   (% kcal) _____ (g) _____
Fat   (% kcal) _____ (g) _____
Division of carbohydrate: _____

Daily Meal Pattern

Exchange	# of Exchanges	Protein (g)	Fat (g)	Carbohydrate (g)
*Milk—NF, LF, whole				
Fruit				
Vegetable				
Subtotal				
*Bread/Starch				
Subtotal				
*Meat—lean, medium, high fat				
Fat				
TOTAL				

*Circle the one used in calculating the meal pattern

Distribution of Exchanges at Meals and Snacks

Exchanges	Total # of Exchanges	Breakfast	AM Snack	Lunch	PM Snack	Dinner	HS Snack
Milk		( )	( )	( )	( )	( )	( )
Fruit		( )	( )	( )	( )	( )	( )
Vegetable		( )	( )	( )	( )	( )	( )
Bread		( )	( )	( )	( )	( )	( )
Meat		( )	( )	( )	( )	( )	( )
Fat		( )	( )	( )	( )	( )	( )
Total		( )	( )	( )	( )	( )	( )

9. Following this diet plan, write a menu for
a. a lunch she can carry to school

b. an afternoon snack she can get for herself after school

c. Assuming the school provides 8 oz skim milk at 10:30 AM, what should Eileen carry for her morning snack?

10. Eileen was in the hospital for 4 days and was scheduled to return on Saturday mornings 2 weeks later and for 5 succeeding Saturdays with her mother, for instruction.
a. In addition to the patient and her mother, who should receive instruction?

b. In addition to the people just listed, who else in Eileen's life should learn about diabetes?

c. List the topics related to diet that you would attempt to teach the patient and her mother prior to discharge.

d. You have 3 hours to add further information in the Saturday morning sessions. List the topics you would include.

Part IV: The Sick Diabetic

When Eileen is 13 years old, she has an episode of throat pain and requires a liquid diet. Her diet plan states that her lunch should contain 1 skim milk, 2 fruit, 1 vegetable, 2 bread, 3 lean meat, and 4 fat.

QUESTIONS

11. Plan a liquid diet compatible with her sore throat.

12. During the sore throat episode, Eileen is eating less and asks if she should reduce her insulin dose.
a. How would you answer her question? Why?

b. What additional advice would you give her?

Part V: The Adolescent Diabetic

By the time Eileen is 15 years old, she becomes somewhat resistant to the limitations of her diet. The control of her diabetes becomes poor. The physician suggests to her parents that SBGM might be helpful.

Eileen is now 5 ft, 5 in tall and weighs 105 pounds. She is active in school sports, and you estimate her energy needs to be about 2,400 kcal per day. Her prescribed diet is P-100; F-65; C-250; divide 2/7, 2/7, 2/7, 1/7, with HS feeding.

Eileen admits to you that she had not been following her diet. She says that she and her friends gather after school and she usually has "a cheeseburger and a diet Coke." The fast-food chain they patronize lists their cheeseburgers as containing 2 bread, 2 meat, and 1 fat exchange. Since she began SBGM, she has followed her diet more carefully, but she would still like to snack with her friends. She lists the following additional problems:

Both her parents are working and she has to get her own breakfast. She sometimes feels groggy in the morning and doesn't want to prepare as much breakfast as is presently listed on her diet. She has to be in school at 8:00 AM.

She gets very hungry and "a little light-headed" before lunch, which is scheduled for 12:30 in her school program.

She needs to carry her lunch.

Her mother prepares dinner. However, Eileen's brother gets home late from football practice, so the meal is not prepared until 7:00 PM.

The physician asks you to recommend a diet with which Eileen will be willing to comply and states he will change the insulin dosage as necessary.

QUESTION

13. What changes in the diet prescription would you recommend? Why? Indicate the number of meals and snacks, the reason for each, and the general direction (increase or decrease) of the change in the size of each. It is not necessary to calculate the diet in detail.

The physician accepts your recommendation and changes Eileen's insulin prescription accordingly. Eileen returns in 2 weeks with her SBGM records from the previous week. She tells you she is much happier with her diet and has been following it carefully. She reports, however, that she still feels groggy in the morning. She refuses to agree to a bigger breakfast. She has gained 2 pounds in the previous 2 weeks.

Her SBGM record lists the following blood glucose levels:

7:00 AM	FBG	60 mg/dl
1:30 PM	1 hr after lunch	140 mg/dl
8:00 PM	1 hr after dinner	120 mg/dl

Her AM snack is scheduled for 10:30 to fit in with her school schedule. The PM snack is at 4:00 PM and the HS snack is at 9:00 PM.

QUESTION

14. What alterations would you suggest in the carbohydrate distribution in the diet at this point? Why?

Part VI: The Non–Insulin Dependent Diabetic

The next time you see Eileen, she is accompanying her grandfather, Mr. M., who was found to have a high blood sugar level during a physical examination. You find the following relevant items in his medical record:

Present Illness: Mr. M. is a 66 y.o. retired businessman c/o lethargy, polyuria, and blurring of vision.

Physical Examination:

General: Overweight male; ht 5 ft, 9 in: wt 220 pounds; IBW 160 pounds.

Eye examination shows presence of arcus senilis and cataracts. Fundoscopy is unremarkable. Hands have slight tremor. Remainder of PE is unremarkable.

Laboratory:

FBG: 220 mg/dl

Cholesterol: 310 mg/dl

Urinalysis: Glucose 2+, ketones negative, protein negative

Impression: NIDDM

Plan: Refer to nutritionist in Diabetic Clinic for 1,800-kcal reduction diet instruction.

You learn that Mr. M. has been very inactive since retirement. He reads and watches television much of the day. He enjoys sports but only watches them on television, and he snacks during this period.

Mr. M. tells you that he is familiar with Eileen's diet and the use of exchange lists, and you find that this is true. He expresses a willingness to lose weight.

QUESTIONS

15. Why did the attending physician decide not to order insulin for this patient?

16. How would you evaluate the potential effectiveness of this diet? What would you suggest?

17. What division of carbohydrate would you suggest for this diet? Why?

18. The patient asks you what you suggest for a snack while he watches a football game. What would you suggest? Give an example.

Part VII: The Pregnant Diabetic

When Eileen is 24 years old, she and her husband come to talk to you about a diet during her pregnancy. The pregnancy was planned. LMP was 6 weeks ago.

Eileen's weight prior to her pregnancy was 135 pounds, and she has gained 1 pound in the past 6 weeks. Her height is 5 ft, 7 in. Her medical record and her SBGM records indicate that her diabetes is in very good control. $HgbA_{1c} = 6.8$ percent.

She is working as a secretary from 8:30 AM to 5:30 PM with an hour for lunch, noon to 1 PM. Coffee breaks are at 10:00 AM and 3:00 PM. She plans to continue to work.

The physician plans to change her insulin prescription to regular insulin t.i.d.

QUESTIONS

19. What diet would you recommend for Eileen at this point? Show your calculations.

   Calories _____
   Pro _____ g
   Fat _____ g
   CHO _____ g
   CHO Division _____

20. Eileen tells you that she and her husband usually have a dry martini before dinner every Friday night. What would you advise her concerning this practice?

21. At the end of the first trimester, Eileen has gained 4 pounds and now weighs 139 pounds. $HgbA_{1c}$ = 9.0 percent. She complains of hunger. What diet would you recommend for the next trimester?

   Calories _____
   Pro _____ g
   Fat _____ g
   CHO _____ g
   CHO Div _____

22. In the next 4 weeks, the pattern of Eileen's weight gain is as follows:
   Beginning of second trimester (June 1)   139 #
   Two weeks later (June 15)   140 #
   Four weeks later (June 30)   141 #
   a. Evaluate the desirability of this rate of gain.

   b. What diet recommendation would you make at this time?

19

Nutritional Care in Renal Disease

Nutritional care of patients with renal disease is extremely demanding. It requires an understanding of fluid and electrolyte balance, acid-base balance, and nitrogen balance. Since the patient's condition changes with time, the nutritional care specialist must be able to alter the care to meet changing needs. Nutritional care must also be adjusted to the type of treatment afforded to the patient, including drug treatment, hemodialysis, peritoneal dialysis, and renal transplant. Before proceeding, you may need to review the material on kidney disease in your text.

Chronic renal failure (CRF), the presence of irreversible nephron damage, may develop either relatively rapidly or slowly, over periods varying from months to decades. Several stages in the progression of the renal insufficiency have been arbitrarily defined as *mild* (40 to 80 percent of normal function), *moderate* (15 to 40 percent of normal function) and *severe* (2 to 20 percent of normal function) (1). The severity of the disease is often clinically defined in terms of decreases in creatinine and urea clearances and increases in serum concentrations of creatinine and urea nitrogen. Since the kidneys have a large reserve capacity, patients are often unaware of the existence of renal disease until it is quite advanced.

If managed properly, patients may remain symptom-free until glomerular filtration rate (GFR) has decreased from a normal level of 80 to 120 ml per min to less than 10 ml per min, and sometimes to less than 5 ml per min. The condition at this point is called *end-stage renal disease* (ESRD). In this advanced stage of the disease, patients have lost their ability to cope with stresses such as dehydration, overhydration, large amounts of nitrogenous waste products, limited or excessive amounts of electrolytes, hypertension, infection, or the presence of a renal toxin. Proper management then becomes even more important.

The general objectives of nutritional care are the following:

1. to maintain optimal quality of life for the patient as the disease progresses, including reduction of the severity of symptoms
2. to minimize secondary effects, such as renal osteodystrophy
3. to retard progression of renal failure if possible
4. for some patients, to delay the necessity for dialysis as long as possible

Treatment of CRF may be divided into three phases. The first phase consists of *conservative management,* primarily using diet and drugs. The diet consists of changes in intake of protein, sodium, potassium, phosphorus, and fluid. Many of the drugs interact with certain foods, as we shall see.

As renal function declines, a second phase develops, during which the patient is *dialyzed.* The diet changes somewhat, but the same nutrients are the major concerns. During the third phase, the patient receives a *transplanted* kidney. Some patients go through all phases, while others skip some phases. Each phase varies markedly in length and has some unique requirements for nutritional care.

NUTRITIONAL ASSESSMENT

MODIFICATIONS IN ROUTINE PROCEDURES

Nutritional assessment is important in renal disease because these patients have a high incidence of malnutrition. The procedures for assessment described in Chapter 4 are generally applicable to the renal disease patient; however, some differences in methods and interpretation must be taken into account. In addition, since CRF is a long-term, progressive disease, the assessment must be repeated at intervals to evaluate changes in the patient's condition, the effectiveness of the diet, and compliance with the diet. Some of the procedures therefore monitor not only the patient's nutritional status, but also the response to and adequacy of the diet as it relates to the progress of the disease. Some special considerations are:

Anthropometric Measurements

Weight and Height.   Body weights of renal patients should be obtained after the bladder has been emptied and with similar clothing at each weighing. For patients who are edematous, calculations involving body weight are usually based on *dry weight*—that is, weight at normal hydration. A patient is assumed to be at dry weight when blood pressure is normal, there is no evidence of edema, and serum sodium is within normal range. Dry weight in the dialyzed patient is the weight at the end of a dialysis treatment when normal blood pressure is reached.

The weight best used as the standard for interpretation in renal patients is not known (2). *Usual weight*—that is, the weight before the onset of illness—is often used as the standard for adults. Alternatively, the patient's weight is compared to optimal body weight (see Chapter 4) or relative weight (average body weight of normal individuals of similar age, height, frame, and size (3). Once true dry weight has been established, subsequent changes compared with previous weights will indicate the direction of changes in nutritional status.

In repeated assessments of the CRF patient, percent of usual body weight should be calculated as shown in Equation 4-7. Standards for interpretation are given in Table 19-1. Rate of weight loss is also important. Rapid weight loss is considered to be more clinically significant than a slow loss.

Height is a special concern in children; it is often severely affected by renal disease. It is therefore important to monitor height in children and compare it to standard height for age, as described in Chapter 8.

Muscle Mass and Body Fat.   Midarm muscle circumference and triceps skinfold measurements may be useful in evaluating the extent of the wasting syndrome frequently seen in CRF and in monitoring the efficacy of nutritional care. Thus, they should be repeated at intervals separated by at least 2 weeks. Useful values are given in Table 19-1, but it is important to keep in mind that standards for triceps skinfold for uremic patients are based on few data. However, serial measurements are useful in determining *direction* of change. Low body fat stores are generally seen in male hemodialysis patients.

When MAMC is measured in hemodialysis patients, the use of the "nonaccess" arm is recommended—that is, the arm that is *not* attached to the dialyzer. Some degree of error is introduced if the nonaccess arm is the dominant arm, but sequential measurements may still be useful to indicate direction of change. Arm anthropometry is not used if both arms contain access sites. Suggested values for interpretation are given in Table 19-1.

The extent to which these measurements are altered by edema is unknown. As a consequence, some treatment centers do not use them in evaluating edematous CRF patients. If possible, the interpretation of data should be based on the patient's dry weight.

Biochemical Measurements

Serum albumin is a poor early indicator of malnutrition since it has a long half-life and a large pool in the body. It also generally does not respond well to supplementary feeding. Nevertheless, serum albumin is extensively used because its determination is inexpensive and readily available, and because CRF is a long-term disease. Serum albumin is frequently decreased in the patient with CRF, but it should be maintained within normal range, if possible.

Serum transferrin, with its smaller body pool and shorter half-life, is considered a better indicator. Transferrin levels should not be calculated from total iron binding capacity, which is altered by the iron deficiency commonly seen in renal failure. Low serum transferrin levels are often found in hemodialysis patients. This may be the consequence of low protein intake, amino acid losses, and iron loads with medications such as iron dextran. (See Table 19-1 for interpretation.)

Serum transferrin and albumin are useful mainly in monitoring the effect of treatment over an extended period. It is sometimes helpful to maintain a flow sheet, recording sequential values over many months so that trends of change can be readily seen.

The usefulness of *total lymphocyte counts* (TLC) and *delayed cutaneous hypersensitivity testing* (DCH) has been questioned. The effect of uremia on TLC is unclear, and DCH is reduced in dialyzed patients. Both tests are also sensitive to immunosuppressive drugs given

TABLE 19-1.   Standards for Interpretation of Nutritional Assessment in Chronic Renal Failure

	Deficit		
Nutritional Parameter	Normal/Mild	Moderate	Severe
Dry weight as % of usual relative body weight	85–95	75–85	<75
Triceps skinfold (mm)			
Men		4–6	<4
Women		8–12	<8
Arm muscle circumference (cm)			
Men		22–24	<22
Women		18–20	<18
Serum albumin (g/dl)		2.8–3.3	<2.8
Serum transferrin (mg/dl)		150–180	<150

to transplant patients and to those whose renal disease is a consequence of autoimmune diseases such as lupus erythematosus and vasculitis.

Diet Assessment

The diet history obtained from the patient with chronic renal disease must be detailed if it is to be useful, and must consider intakes of fluid and electrolytes, as well as protein, fat, and carbohydrate. A 24-hour recall is often insufficient for this type of patient. A food intake record kept by the patient for 3 to 4 days is more appropriate, and it should be redone every few months. The patient's family, social worker, and primary care givers are often good sources of information.

Diet analysis should include the proportion of protein that is of high biological value, as well as total protein and estimates of intake of sodium, potassium, calcium, phosphorus, iron, ascorbic acid, and fluids.

You will need to inquire about the use of various types of special products. For example, it is important to know whether the patient is using salt substitutes, and if so, the brand, and the amount. In addition, you should inquire as to whether the patient is using any "special diet" products, the type, nutritional value, and amount. The use of vitamin and mineral supplements should also be determined along with the brand, content, and dose. Form V is a typical form for gathering and recording relevant data.

Other sources of both nutrients and losses must also be considered, including losses in hemodialysis and the additional calories from peritoneal dialysis.

FORM V

University Medical Center Nutritional Assessment for Renal Patients

Name	Birthdate	Recommended Diet Order	
Address	Phone	Height	Weight
Dialysis Schedule	First Dialysis	Dialysate	MD

Intradialytic wt. gain: HD _____ CAPD _____

Summary of Intake Analysis (Circle or star inadequacies)

Date	Kcal	Pro gms	HBV %	CHO gms	Fat gms	Na^+ mgs	K^+ mgs	Ca^{++} mgs	PO_4^{-3} mgs	Fe mgs	Vit C mgs	Fluids mls

BEE _____   Pro req _____   HBV_____

Describe present eating habits, patterns, likes, dislikes, use of special dietary products (e.g. low protein, low sodium)

Medical needs affecting (diagnosis, other med. disorders, allergies, or medications):

Physical needs affecting nutrition (ability to ambulate, eyesight, dental care, housing):

Social needs affecting nutrition (depression leading to noncompliance, poor appetite, economic and ethnic considerations, language barriers):

Evaluation (compliance with diet, understanding of diet, acceptance, nutritional status, compliance with medications):

Recommendation and long-term goals (care plan):

Questions for Interview

1. Is current appetite   excellent ____, good ____, fair ____, or poor ____?
2. Has there been a change of appetite recently?   Yes ____ No ____
3. Cause of change in patient's appetite?

4. Has weight changed recently?   Yes ____, no ____. Cause of change?

5. Desired weight: _____.
6. Is patient on a "special diet" now? Describe.

7. Has patient had previous diets? Describe.

8. What is the most difficult part of present diet?

9. When does patient have the most difficulty following diet?

10. What "special diet" products does patient purchase?

11. Does patient take vitamins and/or minerals. If so, what kind?

12. Does patient take phosphate binders with meals? Yes _____ No _____
    Type _____
13. Is patient allergic to any foods? List.

14. What foods does patient strongly dislike?

15. What foods does patient especially like?

16. Does patient salt food at the table? During cooking?

17. Does patient use a salt substitute? _____ Brand? __
18. Has patient experienced any taste changes? Describe.

19. Does patient eat anything not usually thought of as food? Specify.

20. Does patient do own cooking? If not, who does?

21. Does patient usually eat breakfast? _____ lunch? _____ dinner? _____
22. Does patient usually snack midmorning? _____ midafternoon? _____
    before bed? _____ during night? _____
23. Does patient eat most meals at home? _____
    Eat away from home? Times/week _____.
24. Is patient inactive? _____ moderately active? _____
    very active? _____
25. Does patient exercise regularly? _____
26. Is patient employed? Full-time _____ Part-time _____ No _____

MONITORING PROCEDURES FOR RENAL PATIENTS

In addition to the above routine procedures, the following can be especially useful in monitoring the efficacy of nutritional care in renal disease and, in some cases, adherence to the various aspects of the prescribed diet.

Monitoring Protein Homeostasis

Creatinine is produced at a fairly constant rate from metabolism of muscle creatine and is excreted by the kidneys. The amount of creatinine in the serum is thus dependent only on muscle mass and on the ability of the kidney to excrete it. It is not diet-related unless the patient has a diet with a high meat intake. *Serum creatinine* is used to measure the extent of renal failure at the time of diagnosis and to monitor the efficacy of treatment. It may be useful as an indicator of an increase or decrease in muscle mass, but only if values are obtained over a long period during which treatment has not changed markedly, and if the adequacy of renal function has not changed in the interim. *Creatinine clearance* (Cl_{CR}) is an indicator of the GFR and serves as a measure of renal damage. It is not diet-related. Creatinine clearance is depressed in renal failure; consequently, serum creatinine is elevated. Creatinine-height index is thus not useful as a measure of muscle mass.

Serum urea nitrogen (SUN) or *blood urea nitrogen* (BUN) may also be an indicator of the extent of renal failure but is affected by many other factors. If the renal disease patient is stable, SUN is closely correlated with dietary protein. While increased SUN may be associated with excessive protein intake, it can also be caused by dehydration; catabolic states, such as surgery, infections, burns, or other trauma; the intake of catabolic medications, such as steroids, in high doses; and gastrointestinal bleeding. Levels of 60 to 80, or sometimes up to 100, mg per dl are considered acceptable for the patient with CRF since uremic symptoms generally do not develop until SUN is 80 mg per dl or more. If values are less than 40 mg per dl, the patient should be checked for malnutrition.

Urea clearance (Cl_{UREA}) may also be used to indicate renal filtration ability. True GFR or inulin clearance is difficult to measure directly in clinical settings. Cl_{CR} tends to overestimate GFR, whereas Cl_{UREA} tends to underestimate it. In clinical settings, GFR may be obtained by averaging Cl_{CR} and Cl_{UREA}. The estimate obtained is most accurate in patients with severe renal disease.

The *SUN/serum creatinine ratio* is closely correlated to protein intake in CRF patients who are not receiving dialysis since, at a given level of renal function, SUN is relative to protein intake, but serum creatinine is independent of diet. The relationship is shown by the curve in Figure 19-1 or may be calculated from the formula also given in the figure. Because of this relationship, the patient's average protein intake can be

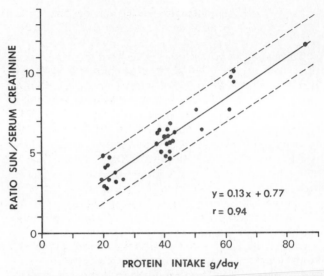

Figure 19-1 Direct relationship between the ratio of the serum urea nitrogen (SUN) to serum creatinine concentrations and the protein intake in nondialyzed men with chronic uremia. Each symbol represents a separate metabolic study. Interrupted lines are 95% confidence limits.

(From Kopple, J.D., Evaluation of chronic uremia: Importance of serum urea nitrogen, serum creatinine, and their ratio. *JAMA* 227:(1974):41–44. Used with permission of the author.)

estimated. For example, if a man has a SUN level of 100 mg per dl and serum creatinine of 10 mg per dl, his SUN-to-creatinine ratio is 10. His average protein intake per day is about 78 g (Fig. 19-1).

If a protein-restricted diet has been prescribed, estimated intake can be compared with the prescription to assess compliance. However, several sources of error must be kept in mind. First, when dietary protein is changed, it takes 2 to 3 weeks for SUN to stabilize and for the SUN-to-creatinine ratio to reflect the new regimen. Secondly, Figure 19-1 is based on values for men with normal muscle mass. For women, children, small men, and muscle-wasted men, muscle mass will be reduced, and the SUN-to-creatinine ratio will be higher. Oliguria and catabolic stress will also increase the ratio (4).

Urinary urea nitrogen (UUN) can be used to assess recent protein intake in clinically stable, chronically uremic patients, and thus to monitor adherence to the diet (5). The amount of urea in the urine per day (UUN) is obtained in the laboratory and recorded in the patient's chart. In assessing protein intake, recent nitrogen intake is first calculated from the equation

$$\text{Recent mean N intake} = 10/9 \times \text{UUN} + 1.8$$
$$\text{where all values are given in g per day.} \quad \textbf{(19-1)}$$

The value 1.8 is for fecal, respiratory, and integumental losses (4). Protein is then calculated from nitrogen. Protein intake can also be calculated directly, with the equation

$$\text{Protein intake} = (7.0 \times \text{UUN}) + 11$$
where all values are in g per day.   **(19-2)**

Urea nitrogen appearance (UNA) is the sum of urinary urea nitrogen (UUN) plus the change in SUN in g per day. When the patient is retaining, rather than excreting, nitrogen, UNA may be used to provide a more precise estimate of nitrogen balance than is obtained by the method described in Chapter 4 and can be used to estimate *recent* protein intake. UNA is also useful for other purposes, as we shall see next.

Each day, about 3 g of urea are degraded by bacterial urease in the GI tract. The difference between total urea production and the amount degraded is the UNA, usually expressed as g of urea nitrogen per day.

The change ($\triangle$) in body urea nitrogen is calculated with the following equation (4). It is based on the assumptions that (1) urea freely crosses membranes and is thus present in all body fluids at the same concentrations and (2) short-term changes in body weight are composed of fluid.

$$\triangle \text{Body urea N(g)} = (\text{SUN}_f - \text{SUN}_i) \times (0.6 \text{ L/kg} \times \text{BW}_i) + [(\text{BW}_f - \text{BW}_i) \times \text{SUN}_f] \quad \textbf{(19-3)}$$

where i and f = initial and final values for the
  period of measurement
  SUN = g serum urea nitrogen per L
  BW = kg body weight
  0.6 = fraction of body weight which is water
UNA (g N/day) may then be calculated with the equation
$$\text{UNA} = \text{urinary urea N} + \triangle \text{ body urea N} \quad \textbf{(19-4)}$$

in which urinary urea N is obtained by laboratory analysis. All values in Equation 19-4 are given in g per day.

If the patient is being dialyzed, the formula is as follows:

$$\text{UNA} = \text{urinary urea N} + \text{dialysate urea N} + \triangle \text{ body urea N}$$
where all values are given in g per day.   **(19-5)**

In the above equations, the fraction of body weight that is water may need to be decreased in women (to 0.5) and in the obese, whereas it is increased in infants, edematous patients, and very lean patients. The weight change that occurs during the 1 to 3 days during which measurements are made is assumed to consist entirely of water.

Since we now have our estimate of UNA, we can proceed to relate it to nitrogen intake and output, and thus to nitrogen balance, as follows:

If nitrogen intake has been estimated from the diet history, and UNA is known, then output in the stable, nondialyzed CRF patient can be estimated with the following equation:

$$\text{Total N output (g/day)} = 0.97 \text{ UNA (g/day)} + 1.93 \quad \textbf{(19-6)}$$

If you have an estimate of protein intake obtained from the diet history, output and intake can be compared to arrive at an estimate of nitrogen balance:

$$\text{N balance (g/day)} = N_i - N_o$$
  where N_i = g/day nitrogen intake calculated from
protein intake
  and N_o = g/day nitrogen output from Equation
19-6.   **(19-7)**

If the patient is in approximate nitrogen balance, UNA will be closely correlated with nitrogen intake. The relationship is as follows:

$$\text{Dietary N intake (g/day)} = 0.69 \text{ UNA (g/day)} + 3.3 \quad \textbf{(19-8)}$$

If intake and UNA are known, output can be estimated from Equation 19-6, and the nitrogen balance from Equation 19-7.

These equations have uses in addition to estimation of nitrogen balance. If UNA is known and intake is known from the diet history, they can be used together to estimate whether high UNA is the consequence of increased nitrogen intake, or increased protein breakdown (negative nitrogen balance), or both. On the other hand, if UNA is low, the equations can be used to indicate whether this is due to decreased nitrogen intake, or positive nitrogen balance, or both (5).

The relationship between UNA and nitrogen intake is altered in anabolic patients, for example, during nutritional repletion or pregnancy. The relationship between UNA and either nitrogen output or intake are altered in patients who are losing protein in nephrotic syndrome or peritoneal dialysis, or in acidotic patients who have sufficient renal function to excrete a quantity of ammonia.

Anemia in CRF patients may also be used to monitor protein homeostasis to some extent. It must be recognized, however, that while the anemia may be nutritional in origin, this cannot be assumed to be so. *Hematocrit* is usually low when the renal disease is advanced since the kidney may be unable to produce erythropoietin. Both *serum iron* and *ferritin* detect the presence of iron deficiency, which may be superimposed on the anemia of uremia.

Monitoring Sodium Homeostasis and Fluid Balance

Serum sodium concentration is an indicator of the balance between sodium and water. Used alone, it does not give information on deficiency or excess; it must be combined with other indicators of hydration status.

If weight is stable, *urinary sodium* is an indicator of sodium intake. In nonsteady state, when weight is changing, it may indicate sodium retention with concurrent fluid retention or sodium wasting.

Daily *urine volume* does not always change with changes in fluid intake in renal disease. It is important that daily volume be known, as well as any *change in volume*. Urine volume should be compared with *fluid intake* and changes in body weight. Intake and output (I & O) of inpatients are recorded in the patient's medical record by the nursing staff.

Blood pressure may also be a useful guide to hydration status. In the absence of hormonal or other lesions, decreased blood pressure may indicate dehydration, while an elevated blood pressure may result from overhydration. Ideally, treatments related to body weight should be based on dry weight—that is, body weight in the absence of excess fluid and the weight above which the patient becomes hypertensive.

Monitoring Potassium Homeostasis

Serum potassium concentration may not rise until the creatinine clearance falls to 20 ml per min or less. However, potassium levels may be increased if the patient takes potassium-containing medications or salt substitutes containing potassium, in severe catabolic disease, in metabolic acidosis, or following blood transfusion. It may rise with very high potassium intake, very low sodium intake, or both.

Monitoring Serum Calcium and Phosphate Homeostasis

Serum calcium is often depressed and *serum phosphate*, elevated in CRF patients. Because these changes lead to severe bone disease, normalization of these values is important. Increased *serum alkaline phosphatase* often signals early renal bone disease. Serum *parathyroid hormone* (PTH) is also monitored. The results must be interpreted in relation to serum calcium. Normal serum calcium and serum PTH of 100 to 600 pg per ml are consistent with normal parathyroid function. In chronic renal disease, secondary hyperparathyroidism is indicated by a serum calcium level less than 9.4 mg per dl and a serum PTH level over 800 pg per ml.

Monitoring Effects of Medications

Renal patients often take substantial amounts of a variety of medications. These may be prescribed or may consist of self-medication with nonprescription drugs. The intake of medications containing sodium or potassium or those affecting phosphate absorption and excretion are of particular interest in nutritional monitoring. Some patients are given phosphate binders by prescription. You should inquire about the amount and about when these are taken in relation to the time of food intake. Poor compliance with the medication regimen is a common problem and should be investigated.

The composition and function of medications taken by renal patients should be familiar. Some of the references listed at the end of the Introduction to this volume are useful sources of information.

TO TEST YOUR UNDERSTANDING

1. A renal patient's usual weight was 160 pounds prior to his current illness. Four months later, the patient weighs 128 pounds, and he is 5 ft, 10 in tall.
    a. Calculate his weight as a percent of usual weight.
    b. How would you interpret his nutritional status based on weight only?
    c. How would you alter your interpretation in the following circumstances? (Explain your reasoning for each.)
        1) The patient's weight has increased 10 pounds in 2 weeks. Blood pressure is 135/95.
        2) You obtain a 3-day diet record and find that the patient's fluid intake is 1,500 ml per day. His medical record says his maximum urine output is 1,200 ml per day.

2. A reasonably well-nourished male patient with CRF has the following laboratory values:

	Patient	Normal
SUN, mg/dl	100	_____
Serum creatinine, mg/dl	10	_____
Urinary urea nitrogen, g/24	4.1	_____

    a. In the space provided, fill in the normal values.
    b. Calculate the patient's SUN-to-creatinine ratio.
    c. Using Figure 19-1, estimate his average protein intake.
    d. You are a clinical dietitian who reads the above values in the medical record. It is not your custom to carry a copy of Figure 19-1 with you; however, you do know the formula given for the curve. Estimate the patient's protein intake using the formula.
    e. A diet containing 40 g protein per day had been prescribed for the patient. How would you evaluate the patient's compliance with the diet?
    f. Calculate the patient's intake from the UUN.
    g. Does the value obtained in part f confirm your evaluation in part e? If not, explain the discrepancy.

3. If a patient's diet contains 50 g protein, what is the nitrogen content of the diet?

4. You have the following data on Ms. L., a CRF patient who is not being dialyzed.

Initial SUN, mg/dl	60.0
SUN, 72 hrs later, mg/dl	100.0
Initial body weight, kg	70.0
Body weight, 72 hrs later, kg	75.0
Urinary urea nitrogen, g/24 hrs	3.0

   a. Calculate the change in body urea nitrogen. (*Hint:* Observe the *units* of measure carefully.)

   b. Calculate the urea nitrogen appearance for Ms. L. (*Hint:* Note that the change indicated by the data just given is for 3 days.)

   c. Your calculations from the diet history indicate that the protein intake was 40 g per day. Calculate the expected nitrogen output.

   d. Estimate the patient's nitrogen balance.

   e. Using your calculation of UNA, estimate Ms. L.'s nitrogen intake.

   f. How much protein does this intake represent?

   g. Using the calculated nitrogen intake, rather than that obtained from the diet history, what is the nitrogen balance?

   h. What would you conclude is the source of the increased SUN for this patient?

   i. Calculate the patient's protein intake from the UUN.

   j. Does the result from part i confirm your results from part f? If not, what factors might account for the discrepancy?

5. What is contained in the following nonprescription drugs that makes them of questionable value for patients with renal disease: Alka-Seltzer? Bromo-Seltzer? Sal-Hepatica?

PREDIALYSIS NUTRITIONAL CARE IN CHRONIC RENAL FAILURE

Depending on the etiology of the disease, the stage of progression of renal failure, and medications being used, CRF patients may require either increases or decreases in dietary protein, sodium, potassium, and fluid. Although energy requirements are not increased, appetite is often depressed, and a concerted effort must be made to ensure normal energy intake. For some patients, phosphorus restriction may also be necessary. You must be able to recognize the indications for the specific modifications and to manipulate the diet to meet these requirements.

PROTEIN MODIFICATIONS

As CRF progresses, the ability of the kidneys to excrete nitrogen metabolites declines and the concentration of these metabolites in the blood rises, indicating the need for *protein restriction.* On the other hand, patients whose renal disease includes nephrotic syndrome lose protein and may need to *increase* their protein intake. Nitrogen retention and proteinuria can coexist.

Protein Restriction

Recommendations for protein restriction are based on the GFR, which is given in the patient's medical record. Common recommendations are as follows (6):

GFR (ml/min)	Protein Allowance	
	g/day	g/kg usual body weight/day
>25	No restriction	No restriction
20–25	60–90	1.3
15–20	50–70	1.0
10–15	40–55	0.7
5–10	40 (males)	0.55–0.6
	35 (females, small males)	

If there is urinary protein loss, the amount lost in 24 hours is added to the calculated intake. The protein intake of children should be at least 1.0 g per kg of body weight, and may be as high as 2.0 g per kg.

Another basis for determining the need to restrict protein intake is to monitor the SUN level. A SUN level of 80 mg per dl or more is often associated with the onset of uremic symptoms; therefore, protein intake is restricted to a level sufficient to keep the SUN under 80 mg per dl and sometimes lower.

The need for protein can also be estimated by using SUN-to-creatinine ratios. For example, let us assume that a patient's serum creatinine is 10 mg per dl, and the nephrologist considers it desirable to maintain the SUN at 60 mg per dl or less. The SUN-to-creatinine ratio would then equal 6.0. Figure 19-1 or the formula for the curve shows that this SUN level can be maintained with a protein intake of 40 g. This value may also be used to evaluate adherence to the diet.

You can see that there is substantial loss of renal function, from a normal GFR of about 125 ml per min to less than 25 ml per min, before any restriction is required. Note also that the lowest level of protein suggested is 35 to 40 g. The extent to which protein should be restricted is controversial, and lower protein intakes, down to 20 g, are occasionally used. Low-protein diets tend to be quite unpalatable, however, and it is difficult for the patient to maintain a protein intake as low as 20 g and still take in enough food to meet energy needs. If energy needs are not met with carbohydrate and fat, protein will be used for energy, aggravating the wasting syndrome and increasing production of nitrogenous waste products. Thus, the 35-to-40-g-protein diet is most often used. When this restriction is no longer effective, dialysis may be considered.

In addition to the quantity of protein, its quality must be considered. Therefore, 70 to 80 percent of the protein in the diet should be high-biological-value (HBV) protein. HBV proteins are those which contain all essential amino acids in concentrations proportional to the minimum daily amino acid requirements and in which most of the nitrogen is in the form of essential amino acids. When sufficient HBV protein is provided, the patient can meet needs for essential amino acids and use the remaining nitrogen to synthesize those that are nonessential, thus reducing the amount of urea to be excreted.

Egg protein has the highest biological value—0.94 on a scale of 0 to 1.0. Milk, lean meat, poultry, and fish are also HBV proteins. Eggs and milk have less of nonessential amino acids than do meats, so 10 to 15 g of HBV protein should come from these sources. Gelatin and the plant proteins in grains and vegetables are low in biological value and make up the remaining 20 to 30 percent of the diet protein.

If a protein-restricted diet is prescribed and the SUN-to-creatinine ratio equals 10 or more, the patient may not be following the diet. On the other hand, inadequate protein intake may be detected by decreasing serum albumin, weight loss, and declining MAMC.

Once the desired level is determined, the protein content of the diet may be planned using exchange lists like those provided in Appendix K. Similar lists are found in many institutional diet manuals, although there are minor variations among them. You may recall from Chapters 5 and 18 that in an exchange list system, foods used similarly in meal planning are grouped according to their nutrient content. The exchange lists used in planning diets for diabetic patients are grouped according to their protein, fat, and carbohydrate content. Exchange lists that group foods according to other nutrients have also been developed. The exchange lists used in planning diets for renal patients are based on the protein, sodium, and potassium contents of foods; also, the protein content is stated more specifically than it is in the exchanges for

diabetic diets. If you compare the two lists, for example, you will find that fruit is listed as containing 0.5, 0.6, or 0.7 g protein per serving in exchanges for renal patients, while this small amount is ignored in the lists for diabetics. Meat and eggs are listed as containing 8 g of protein, while the diabetic diet lists 7 g protein as the value.

When planning the diet, the number and types of exchanges can be calculated to meet the prescription. For the moment, in order to clarify the procedure, we will ignore the sodium, potassium, and fluid information in the exchange lists in Appendix K, and work with the protein prescription only. As an example, let us assume that your patient requires a 60-g protein diet with 75 percent HBV. The needed 45 g of HBV protein is obtained from eggs, meat exchanges, and milk. Since egg protein has the highest biological value, at least one egg is usually included per day. The diet could then contain the following:

Exchange	Number	Protein (g)
Egg	1	8
Meat	4 (oz)	32
Milk	1 (½ c)	4
Total		44

This leaves 16 g of the total remaining to be obtained from the LBV protein in the other foods used to make up the menu. These might be provided as follows:

Exchange	Number	Protein (g)
Starch	5	10
Vegetables	2	2
Fruit	4	2
Total		14

An average value of 0.6 g protein per serving of fruit is used in these calculations. Once the number of each protein-containing exchange is established, the exchanges are distributed among the meals so that a source of HBV protein is included in each meal. In addition, some high-carbohydrate foods are served with the protein. For example, the exchanges in the example just given might be distributed as follows:

Breakfast	g Pro	Lunch	g Pro	Dinner	g Pro
2 Fruit (#3)	1.4	2 Meat	16.0	2 Meat	16.0
1 Cereal	2.0	1 Veg (#1, 2, or 3)	1.0	1 Starch	2.0
1 Egg	8.0	2 Fruit	1.2	1 Veg (#1, 2, or 3)	1.0
4 oz Milk	4.0	1 Bread	2.0	1 Fruit (#1)	1.0
2 Bread	4.0				
Total	19.4		20.2		20.0

The meals for the day may be made up by choosing items from the list for each exchange. In planning the menu for this day, the patient might have for breakfast, for example:

8 oz orange juice (two exchanges of Fruit #3)
⅔ c cornflakes
1 egg
4 oz whole milk
2 slices toast
Margarine, butter, jam, or jelly as desired
Coffee with sugar, if desired

Multivitamin and calorie supplements should be used routinely with diets restricted to 40 g protein or less. These diets are inadequate in all vitamins and minerals except Vitamin C. The 60-g protein diet is likely to be inadequate in calcium and also in iron for premenopausal women.

High Protein Diets

The patient with nephrotic syndrome loses protein, primarily albumin, in the urine. Depending on the extent of the proteinuria, nephrotic syndrome may make it necessary to increase the patient's protein intake. A common recommendation is 1.5 to 2.0 g protein per kg usual body weight per day. If urinary losses are high, that amount may be added (7); the diet frequently contains 100 to 150 g protein per day. Of this amount, 80 percent should be high biological value.

Nephrotic syndrome and renal failure may occur simultaneously. If the patient becomes azotemic, high protein intakes are contraindicated. These patients may be given 0.7 g protein per kg usual body weight *plus* the amount of protein lost in the urine.

When the nephrotic patient is edematous, diuretic medication is used to control the edema. If diuretics are ineffective, sodium is restricted. The effects of diuretics on nutritional management are discussed later in this chapter.

ENERGY INTAKE

The energy needs for CRF patients are highly variable and must be estimated on an individual basis. Sufficient energy must be provided to prevent catabolism of protein for energy in the patient on a protein-restricted diet. If possible, sufficient energy must also be provided to maintain the patient at ideal weight. Calculations of BEE (see Chapter 4) may be used as a baseline and adjusted for activity, the patient's present weight, and stress factors. In general, energy needs are 35 to 50 kcal per kg ideal body weight. Children may need 100 to 150 kcal per kg per day (8). In practice, recommended energy intakes are usually increased as GFR, and recommended protein intake, decline:

GFR (ml/min)	Recommended kcal (/kg IBW)
>20	40–45
10–20	45
<10	45–50

Fewer kcals are given if the patient is obese—defined as body weight at least 120 percent of normal weight.

Deficient energy intake is common in CRF since patients are often anorectic. Many patients have intakes under 75 percent of the RDA for energy, and maintenance of appropriate energy intake presents a major challenge. Patients frequently complain that the diet is "too sweet and too greasy."

Since most staple foods contain protein and cannot be used in larger quantities, additional calories must be derived from those sources of carbohydrate and fat which have been separated from their natural food source. These may be categorized as

1. high-carbohydrate foods lacking in protein. (Some of these are listed in the "Protein-Free" list of Appendix K.)
2. concentrated fats. (See the "Miscellaneous" list of Appendix K.)

If the patient's fluid prescription will allow, high-carbohydrate, low-protein, low-electrolyte liquid supplements can be used. (Some of these are listed in Appendix K.) You must always keep in mind, however, that as fluid is restricted, the fluid content of these formulas must be included within the prescribed amount.

Commercial formula products designed to provide energy sources without adding protein or unacceptable amounts of electrolytes are CalPower, Controlyte, Hycal, Moducal, Polycose, Sumacal, and Lipomul. Two products designed particularly for use by the renal patient are Travasorb Renal and Amin-Aid. They contain a small amount of protein. These products, including their sodium and potassium content, are described in further detail in Table G-2. In addition, a number of mixtures developed by renal dietitians are valuable for increasing patients' intakes of protein and energy. They provide various levels of sodium, phosphorus, and potassium and thus must be chosen with the patient's total needs in mind. When you counsel renal patients, you will find it useful to make a collection of these recipes.

It is particularly important to provide specific suggestions for increasing energy intake to patients who are underweight. Some examples of strategies for increasing the energy content of the diet include the following:

1. Add allowed butter or margarine to cooked cereals, vegetables, rice, potatoes, and pasta products.
2. Use butter generously on bread, toast, and rolls.
3. Use cream in place of milk on cereals and in cooking.
4. Use the higher-calorie foods from each exchange list.
5. Sweeten beverages such as tea and coffee, and use sweetened soft drinks in place of water.
6. Add "free foods."
7. Add powdered supplements like Polycose or Sumacal to cooked dishes such as casseroles, puddings, and cereals.
8. Use all the exchanges on the diet each day.

All the suggestions listed are not always useful for every patient. You will need to choose those compatible with the limitations of the individual patient's diet.

TO TEST YOUR UNDERSTANDING

6. You have an adult male patient with CRF at OBW of 70 kg whose medical record shows the following values:

		Normal
Cl_{CR}	18 mg/min	_____
Cl_{UREA}	8 mg/min	_____

   a. Give normal values in the spaces at the right.
   b. What is the patient's approximate GFR?
   c. Approximately how much protein per day would you expect to be ordered for this patient?

7. a. You have a patient for whom a 40-g-protein diet has been prescribed. Using Form W, make a list of the exchanges and the number of exchanges that would fill this prescription. Use the average serving values in Table K-1.
   b. Using Form W, plan a meal pattern for this patient.

FORM W

University Medical Center
Protein, Sodium, Potassium, and Fluid-Restricted Diet

Prescribed: Pro _____ g; Na _____ mg; K _____ mg;
             Fluid _____ ml; _____ kcal
             _____ % HBV = _____ g HBV protein

List	Amount	Pro g	Na mg	K mg	Fluid ml	Kcal
Egg						
Meat, Low Na						
High Na						
Dairy						
SUBTOTAL						
Bread, etc.						
Low Na						
Regular						
Vegetable #1						
#2						
#3						
#4						
Fruit #1						
#2						
#3						
Fats, Regular						
Unsalted						

Sweets
_____
_____
_____

Salt List _____

Miscellaneous _____

TOTAL _____

Meal Plan: _____

BREAKFAST	Serving	Pro	Na	K	Fluid	Kcal
# _____ Fruit _____						
Meat list, High Na _____						
Low Na _____						
Egg _____						
Bread, Regular _____						
Low Na _____						
Dairy _____						
Fats, Regular _____						
Unsalted _____						
Misc. _____						

SUBTOTAL _____

LUNCH
Meat list, High Na _____
        Low Na _____
Bread list, Regular _____
        Low Na _____
_____ Veg list _____
_____ Veg list _____
_____ Fruit list _____
Dairy list _____
Fats, Regular _____
        Unsalted _____
Misc. _____

SUBTOTAL _____

DINNER
Meat list, High Na _____
        Low Na _____
Bread list, Regular _____
        Low Na _____
_____ Veg list _____
_____ Veg list _____
_____ Fruit list _____
Dairy list _____
Fats, Regular _____
        Unsalted _____
Misc. _____

SUBTOTAL _____

SNACKS AND SUPPLEMENTS _____
_____
_____

GRAND TOTAL _____

8. Using the exchange lists from Appendix K or your diet manual, and the menu for _____ (day to be assigned by your instructor), plan the menu for a patient whose diet contains the following exchanges:

   1 egg
   4 oz meat
   1 c milk, whole
   2 vegetables
   2 fruit
   1 starch
   10 fat

9. A female patient weighed 110 pounds and was at her ideal weight. She had a GFR of 15 ml/min. The prescribed diet contained 50 g protein. Estimate her energy requirement.

10. Your institution stocks CalPower, Controlyte, Hycal, and Polycose. Which product would you recommend for each of the patients described?

    _____ a. Needs added carbohydrate; protein is severely restricted and is already in the calcu-lated diet; electrolyte prescription has also been filled.
    _____ b. Patient dislikes strong-flavored drinks. Needs additional energy, but fat is restricted since patient has a high serum lipid level. Electrolyte prescription is slightly in excess of amounts calculated into the diet.
    _____ c. Fluid is restricted; energy may be obtained from either carbohydrate or fat; limited added electrolytes acceptable; to be added to food exchanges calculated in diet.

11. An adult male patient weighing 72 kg has a GFR of 12 ml/min, SUN of 80 mg per dl, and serum albumin of 4.8 g/dl. He has nephrotic syndrome and is losing 20 g protein per day in his urine.
    a. What protein intake would you recommend?
    b. What protein intake would you recommend if the GFR were 40 ml/min, SUN was 18 mg/dl, and serum albumin 1.5 g/dl?

12. A diet containing 1.0 g protein/kg body weight/day with 75 percent HBV protein is prescribed for an adult male patient. The medical record gives the following values:

		Normal
Body weight, kg	70.0	
Body weight prior to illness, kg	64.0	
Urine volume/day, ml	800.0	
Creatinine clearance, ml/min	15.0	_____
Serum creatinine, mg/dl	8.0	_____
SUN, mg/dl	100.0	_____
Blood pressure	140/90	_____
Serum albumin, mg/dl	2.0	_____
Urine protein, g/day	20.0	_____

    a. List normal values in the spaces provided.
    b. List the values that are compatible with a diagnosis of CRF and indicate how they compare to normal values.
    c. List the values that are compatible with a diagnosis of nephrotic syndrome, and indicate how they compare with normal values.

MODIFICATIONS IN SODIUM INTAKE

Not all forms of renal failure affect sodium balance in the same way. Patients who retain sodium need so-dium restriction, while "salt wasters" require added salt. Nephrotic patients are given sodium-restricted diets, which may be as low as 500 mg. However, the use of diuretics usually makes it possible to allow more sodium.

Sodium-Restricted Diets

Sodium restriction is useful in the nutritional care of a wide variety of conditions. These include some dis-eases of the kidneys, liver, and cardiovascular system, as well as other conditions associated with edema or hypertension. Therefore, we will first discuss the plan-ning of low-sodium diets in some detail and follow with a discussion of their use in renal disease.

Terminology. Some institutions use the terms *low-salt* and *salt-free* or *salt-poor*. The critical substance is sodium, however, so better terminology is *sodium-restricted* or *low-sodium*.

The diet prescription should also state the amount of sodium allowed on the diet. In some institutions, it is customary to express the sodium content of the diet in milligrams (mg) while in others it is expressed in milliequivalents (mEq). You will need to be able to use both systems and convert one to the other since the sodium contents of foods in tables are usually given in mg. (Atomic weights and valences of a number of elements of interest are given in Appendix H.)

TO TEST YOUR UNDERSTANDING

13. A patient is given a diet containing 1,200 mg sodium. How many mEq of sodium are contained in the diet?
14. What percent of the total weight of NaCl is sodium?
15. A patient is told by her physician that she can use ½ t (2½ g) salt with her food each day. How many mg of sodium will the salt (NaCl) provide?

Commonly Used Diets. As you can see from your answer to the question 14, sodium chloride is approximately 40 percent sodium. This factor is sufficiently accurate for most calculations in clinical situations. Therefore, 2,500 mg NaCl can be considered to contain $2,500 \times 0.40 = 1,000$ mg Na.

The sodium content of unrestricted American diets has been estimated to be 2,500 to 8,800 mg, a quantity often much in excess of the minimum requirement. An intake of 1,000 to 3,300 mg per day is considered reasonable and safe for the normal adult.

Most institutions will offer a series of sodium-restricted diets with differing sodium contents. The most common are

250 mg	(11 mEq)	"Severe" restriction (rarely used)
500 mg	(22 mEq)	"Strict" restriction (often the lowest level in use)
1,000 mg	(44 mEq)	"Moderate" restriction
2–3 g	(87–130 mEq)	"Mild" restriction
4 g	(174 mEq)	"No added salt"

For most cardiovascular conditions, the amount specified is the maximum allowable. A range down to 10 percent lower is acceptable, but 10 percent higher is not. For most renal patients, the acceptable range is ± 10 percent.

Dietary Sources of Sodium. Sources of sodium in the diet fall into 4 categories:

1. Sodium compounds, primarily table salt (NaCl), and including baking soda ($NaHCO_3$), baking powder, monosodium glutamate, and soy sauce.
2. Foods in which sodium is naturally contained. Animal foods—meats, eggs, and dairy products—have a substantial inherent sodium content as do some vegetables. The quantities of these foods in the diet must be controlled even if no salt or other sodium-containing compounds are added.
3. Foods with added salt or additions of other sodium compounds.
4. Sodium in the water supply.

In addition, some medications contain appreciable quantities of sodium.

The water supply is naturally high in sodium in some areas. Patients requiring 20-mEq-sodium diets should use bottled, distilled water if the sodium content of their water supply exceeds 40 parts per million. This is equivalent to 3 mEq or 40 mg of sodium per L. Information on sodium in the water is usually available from the Department of Public Health or the local Heart Association.

Water softeners add appreciably to the sodium content of the drinking water. Table 19-2 indicates the sodium added by softeners to water of varying hardness. If the diet is restricted to 22 mEq of sodium or less, the softener should be attached to the hot water line only, and patients should be advised to use the cold water for drinking and cooking. Alternatively, the patient can buy bottled, distilled water, but the expense is greater.

Planning the Sodium-Restricted Diet. Exchange lists are frequently used for planning the sodium-restricted diet. For renal patients, the combined protein, sodium, and potassium exchanges are useful. For pa-

TABLE 19-2. Sodium Content of Softened Water

Initial Water Hardness (gr/gal)	*Sodium Added by Cation Exchange Softener (mg Na/qt water)*
1	7.5
5	37
10	75
15	112
20	150
30	225
40	300

tients who do not require protein or potassium restrictions, the less restrictive exchange lists found in some diet manuals are more serviceable.

Some general guidelines for planning a 500-mg-sodium diet are as follows:

1. No salt or salty seasonings (for example, garlic salt, celery salt, soy sauce) are added during food preparation or at the table.
2. Foods processed with sodium compounds are avoided unless the sodium content is less than 10 mg per serving.
3. Avoid condiments such as catsup, mustard, relishes, sauces, pickles, and olives.

4. Avoid processed, smoked, and cured meats and fish.
5. Avoid salted snack foods such as peanuts, popcorn, potato chips, and pretzels.
6. Avoid prepackaged frozen foods and packaged mixes for casseroles, sauces, and gravies, soups, flour mixes, and baking mixes unless prepared without salt by the manufacturer.
7. Avoid frozen peas and lima beans, sauerkraut, frozen fish fillets, and shellfish (except oysters) and all canned meats and vegetable products unless prepared without salt.
8. Avoid bread, butter, cheese, and peanut butter unless made without salt.

TABLE 19-3. Sodium Composition Chart

Food	Unit Size	Mg Na Unit	250-Mg Sodium	Na/Food	500-Mg Sodium	Na/Food	1-G Sodium	Na/Food	2-G Sodium	Na/Food	3-G Sodium	Na/Food	4-G* Sodium	Na/Food
Milk, LS	8 oz	12	2	24	1	12	—	—	—	—	—	—	—	—
Milk, regular	8 oz	120	—	—	2	120	2	240	2	240	2	240	2	240
Meat, LS	1 oz	25	4	100	5	125	6	150	5	125	3	75	3	75
Cottage cheese, regular	¼ c	130	—	—	—	—	1	130	2	260	2	260	2	260
Fresh shellfish	1 oz	50	—	—	—	—	—	—	1	50	1	50	1	50
Peanut butter, regular	1 T	80	—	—	—	—	—	—	2	160	2	160	2	160
Eggs	1 ea	65	—	—	1	65	1	65	1	65	1	65	1	65
Vegetables LS	½ c	10	3	30	2	20	2	20	2	20	2	20	1	10
Higher value LS	½ c	40	—	—	1	40	1	40	1	40	1	40	1	40
Vegetables, regular canned	½ c	250	—	—	—	—	—	—	—	—	—	—	1	250
Fruits	½ c	2	3	6	3	6	3	6	3	6	3	6	3	6
Bread, LS	1 sl	5	6	30	5	25	3	15	—	—	—	—	—	—
Bread, regular	1 sl	120	—	—	—	—	2	240	5	600	4	480	4	480
Quick breads	1 ser	300	—	—	—	—	—	—	—	—	1	300	1	300
Fat, LS	1 t	1	6	6	6	6	6	6	—	—	—	—	—	—
Fat, regular	1 t	50	—	—	—	—	—	—	6	300	6	300	5	250
Salad dressing, regular	1 T	350	—	—	—	—	—	—	—	—	—	—	2	700
Soup, LS	1 c	25	1	25	1	25	1	25	1	25	1	25	1	25
Desserts, LS	1 ser	15	2	30	2	30	2	30	2	30	1	15	1	15
Desserts, regular	1 ser	300	—	—	—	—	—	—	—	—	1	300	1	300
Salted vegetable juice	½ c	200	—	—	—	—	—	—	—	—	—	—	1	200
Salt	1 t	2,300	—	—	—	—	—	—	—	—	¼ t	575	¼ t	575†
Total sodium:				251		474		967		1,921		2,911		4,001

*When a "no-added-salt" diet is ordered, the 4-g-sodium diet will be served.

†In the hospital, the salt has been added to the foods during preparation. No salt will be added to the tray.

Note: The diets have been calculated with high average values and total less than the specified amount to allow flexibility for the patient, and for a small amount of sodium to be present in the water.

9. Specify amounts of foods that must be limited because of their inherent sodium content.
10. Avoid locally bottled beverages if the local water is high in sodium.

Various combinations of foods can be used to plan the 500-mg diet. An example is given in Table 19-3. It is important to plan a variety of foods for nutritional adequacy.

Some patients find that the use of salt substitutes helps to make the sodium-restricted diet more acceptable. Available products are listed in Table 19-4. Salt substitutes are not recommended to patients without a prescription from the attending physician. Most contain less than 1 mEq sodium per teaspoon but large quantities of potassium (30 to 70 mEq per teaspoon) and may be hazardous to patients with renal disease in particular. Those containing ammonium salts are not usable for hepatic-failure patients.

To adjust the sodium content of the diet for other levels, one can begin with a plan such as that for the 500-mg-sodium diet and adjust up or down, as shown in Table 19-3.

250 mg Use "low-sodium milk" (Lonalac or LSM) in place of regular milk. Reduce meat and egg to 4 oz meat. Increase low sodium breads and vegetables.

1,000 mg Use 3 servings regular (salted) bread with unsalted butter per day and all regular milk

or

2 slices regular bread (240 mg) plus 4 t regular butter or margarine (200 mg) plus 1 serving of a high-sodium vegetable (50 mg)

or

give the patient a list of favorite foods with their sodium content which he can use to "spend" the additional 500 mg.

2–4 g. Progressively more regular (salted) items are allowed on the diet as indicated in Table 19-3. On the 3-g and 4-g diet, the patient may be allowed ¼ t salt to add to food or use in food preparation. Note that in some institutions, the 4-g-salt diet is called a "no-added-salt diet." The

TABLE 19-4. Potassium Content of Salt-Substitute Products

Product	Potassium (mEq/t)
Morton's Salt Substitute	70
No Salt (Norcliff Thayer, Inc.)	68
Diamond Crystal	66
Adolph's Salt Substitute	65
Featherweight K Salt Substitute (Chicago Dietetic Supply, Inc.)	49
Nu-Salt (Sugar Foods Corporation)	55
Morton's Seasoned Salt Substitute	50
Featherweight Garlic Salt Substitute	53
Featherweight Seasoned Salt Substitute	43
Adolph's Seasoned Salt Substitute	33
Featherweight Poultry Seasoning	16
Featherweight Meat Seasoning	16
Featherweight Fish Seasoning	15

patient is given regular salted foods, eliminating those especially high in salt content, but is instructed not to salt food at the table.

Patient Counseling. Many patients need a restricted-sodium diet for extended periods. In order to comply with the diet, they need information on sources of usable products, food preparation methods, and eating out on a diet.

Patients should be encouraged to eat primarily fresh, rather than processed, foods. They also need to learn to read labels carefully. The chemicals used in processing must be recognized and avoided. In addition, the following definitions apply to labeling:

"Unsalted" or "Having no salt added": Processed without salt in food normally processed with salt. Sodium content must be stated.
"Reduced sodium": Processed to reduce usual sodium level by 75%.
"Low sodium": 140 mg or less/serving
"Very low sodium": 35 mg or less/serving
"Sodium-free" or "Salt-free": Less than 5 mg Na/serving

The sodium content of a wide variety of foods, including many brand-name processed foods, can be obtained from commercial publications (9) or by writing to the manufacturer.

Patients should be given information on alternatives to salt for seasoning and flavor; suggestions are available from many sources (10, 11). Wines can be used to add flavor in cooking. but those labeled "cooking wine" are high in salt content and should not be used. Various herb combinations, homemade or purchased already mixed, can be used in a shaker. Patients with CRF appreciate such flavorings because they have decreased taste acuity (12).

Many recipe books are available to help patients use these seasonings, to provide recipes for new dishes, and to provide reduced-sodium substitutes for familiar foods. Another useful product is sodium-free baking powder: 2 T *each* cream of tartar, potassium bitartrate, arrowroot starch, and potassium bicarbonate. (*Caution:* Sodium-free baking powder is not to be used by patients who are at risk of retaining potassium.)

Eating out presents a challenge, so guidelines based on the information in the diet manual are helpful. Recall from Chapter 6 that practice with actual menus is helpful. Travelers can ask for low-salt meals on airplanes. Sandwiches for carried lunches can be made with low-sodium bread, pita bread, or unseasoned crisp breads. Cold, sliced roast meats can be used as fillings. Fresh tomatoes, lettuce, and celery can be included, as can fresh fruit.

Increased Sodium in the Diet

Some patients have a decreased capacity to conserve sodium and a resultant need for increased intake. For these "salt losers," additional sodium can be provided with more highly salted foods, with bouillon cubes (2,500 mg Na per cube), and by generously salting their food. (A list of high-salt items is included in Appendix K as the "Salt List.") Some patients are given sodium chloride as medication. If a patient becomes severely depleted, the sodium and fluid balance must be corrected intravenously.

Dietary Sodium in Chronic Renal Failure

The healthy kidney reabsorbs about 99 percent of the sodium filtered by the glomerulus, adjusting the amount reabsorbed to the need. As renal failure progresses, however, the ability to adapt to changes in sodium intake is lost. The objective then becomes to make daily sodium intake equal to daily loss.

To establish the appropriate intake level, patients may be given a moderate-sodium diet (4 to 8 g salt; 1,600 to 3,200 mg Na). Dietary intake is then adjusted to urinary sodium excretion.

The sodium content of the diet is established at a level to avoid either a large fluid excess or volume depletion. A large fluid excess, with attendant edema, can lead to pulmonary edema and congestive heart failure (CHF). Volume depletion can reduce renal blood flow and further compromise renal function. Therefore, patients are commonly maintained in a slightly edematous state to achieve the maximum possible GFR while avoiding CHF.

A reduction in weight or a drop in blood pressure can indicate the need for a higher sodium intake, provided the patient is not fluid overloaded. Accompanying decreases in serum or urinary sodium, or both, may also indicate sodium deficit. On the other hand, a sudden increase in body weight or development of hypertension may indicate developing edema and the need to reduce sodium intake to prevent CHF. These may be accompanied by increases in serum or urinary sodium or both.

Most conservatively managed renal patients are maintained on mild sodium restrictions of 2 to 3 g per day. As renal failure progresses, however, the sodium intake may have to be further restricted. For patients who are not hospitalized, the 1,000-mg or 500-mg diets may be usable. Compliance is low at lower dietary sodium levels.

MODIFICATIONS IN FLUID INTAKE

The fluid needs of renal disease patients also vary widely. In patients who have lost renal concentrating ability and have polyuria, intake requirements may be 3,000 ml per day to excrete the solute load. If thirst does not stimulate this intake, the prescription may state "force fluids" or "encourage fluids."

If sodium balance is properly maintained, the patient's thirst mechanism may control water balance appropriately (commonly at 1,500 to 3,000 ml of fluid) until the GFR falls to 5 ml per min or less. It eventually becomes necessary to monitor fluid intake to prevent fluid overload. For the patient who is not dialyzed, the volume of urine output in 24 hours, plus 500 to 1,000 ml for replacement of insensible losses plus abnormal losses (like vomiting), is considered an appropriate fluid intake once the patient is brought to normal hydration (as indicated by approximately normal blood pressure, normal serum sodium, and absence of edema). Insensible losses may also be estimated as 10 ml per kg body weight. This intake will usually maintain a stable weight. It should be adjusted as necessary if the patient gains or loses weight in a short period. Patients should weigh themselves daily and measure urine output. Each 1,000 ml of retained fluid will add a kg of body weight.

Any intake of 2,000 ml fluid or less per day is considered a restriction. In planning for fluid content of the diet, the following sources of fluids must be counted:

1. Obvious sources of fluids such as drinking water, milk, juices, soups, gruels, coffee, tea, soft drinks, and alcoholic beverages
2. Syrup or juice served with canned fruit
3. Foods that are liquid at body temperature, even if they are relatively solid as served, such as gelatin, ice cream and other frozen desserts, and ice; the following are used as the approximate fluid contents of these products:

½ c ice cream, ice milk, or sherbet	70 ml
½ c Jello or other gelatin	100 ml
1 ice cube	30 ml

4. Foods containing the normal fluid allowance, such as milk in puddings and sauces

Another source of fluid is the water content of solid food, which can be estimated as 14 ml per 100 kcal. This is considered only if the patient's condition demands a severe fluid restriction with very careful control. This amount is ordinarily considered to counterbalance the insensible losses. Water from metabolism of protein, fat, and carbohydrate is not included in these calculations.

Careful compliance with the sodium restriction tends to limit the feeling of thirst. Some patients do complain of thirst, however, particularly at the more restricted levels. The problem may be worsened when part of the fluid ration must be used for liquid medications or to swallow medications in solid form. For hospitalized patients, the fluid ration for each patient is divided between the dietary department for use in meals and the nursing service for use in administering drugs. If increasing the energy intake is a concern, medications may be taken with the high-calorie, low-protein, low-electrolyte liquids previously described.

The following suggestions can be made to ease the discomfort of the nonhospitalized patient:

Suck on sliced lemon wedges to stimulate saliva.
Use sour hard candy or chewing gum to stimulate saliva.

Rinse the mouth with water but do not swallow it, or use a spray mouth wash.

Freeze allowed fruit juices or water in ice cube trays. Ice is more satisfying because it stays in the mouth longer.

Put lemon juice in ice cubes (a half lemon per tray).

Freeze lemonade into individual popsicles in an ice cube tray.

When thirsty, eat something allowed from the diet. This food may alleviate the dry mouth.

Try eating allowed fruits and vegetables ice cold between meals.

If possible, take medications with liquids allowed at mealtime.

Use very small cups and glasses.

Avoid very-high-sodium foods.

TO TEST YOUR UNDERSTANDING

16. A patient's normal dry weight is 145 pounds. The patient's energy intake is adequate for weight maintenance. In each of the following circumstances, all of which developed in a short period, would you consider the sodium intake too low, too high, or about right? Describe your reasoning.
    a. Body weight is 135 #; BP 115/75
    b. Body weight is 150 #; BP 122/79
    c. Body weight is 160 #; BP 130/90
    d. Weight gain of 2 kg in 2 days

17. a. Make a list of the type and number of allowed exchanges for a patient who requires a 1,000-mg-sodium diet. Base your calculations on the exchanges in Table K-1 and information in Table 19-3.
    b. Using the menu for _____ (day to be assigned by your instructor), plan the menu from the diet plan you calculated in part a.

18. Using the menu _____ (day to be assigned by your instructor), modify this menu to be a "no-added-salt" (4-g-salt) diet.

19. You have a prescription for a diet as follows:
    Protein, 40 g; Sodium, 1,000 mg; Fluid, 1,500 ml. Nursing service requires 600 ml of fluid for administration of medications.
    a. Using Form X and the exchange lists in Appendix K, plan a meal pattern for this patient.
    b. Using the menu for _____ (day to be assigned by your instructor), plan the day's diet for this patient.
    c. The patient tells you of a canned tuna product he enjoys and asks if he can use it on his diet. He says it is labelled "reduced sodium." What would you tell him?

FORM X

University Medical Center
Protein, Sodium, Potassium, and Fluid-Restricted Diet

Prescribed: Pro _____ g; Na _____ mg; K _____ mg;
            Fluid _____ ml; _____ kcal
            _____ % HBV = _____ g HBV protein

List	Amount	Pro g	Na mg	K mg	Fluid ml	Kcal
Egg						
Meat, Low Na						
High Na						
Dairy						
SUBTOTAL						

Bread, etc. _____

   Low Na _____

   Regular _____

Vegetable #1 _____

       #2 _____

       #3 _____

       #4 _____

Fruit #1 _____

    #2 _____

    #3 _____

Fats, Regular _____

   Unsalted _____

Sweets _____

_____

_____

_____

Salt List _____

Miscellaneous _____

  TOTAL _____

Meal Plan: _____

BREAKFAST	Serving	Pro	Na	K	Fluid	Kcal
# ____ Fruit						
Meat list, High Na						
Low Na						
Egg						
Bread, Regular						
Low Na						
Dairy						
Fats, Regular						
Unsalted						
Misc.						
SUBTOTAL						
LUNCH						
Meat list, High Na						
Low Na						
Bread list, Regular						
Low Na						
# ____ Veg list						
# ____ Veg list						
# ____ Fruit list						
Dairy list						
Fats, Regular						
Unsalted						

Misc. _____
_____
_____

SUBTOTAL _____

DINNER
Meat list, High Na _____
           Low Na _____
Bread list, Regular _____
           Low Na _____
_____ Veg list _____
_____ Veg list _____
_____ Fruit list _____
Dairy list _____
Fats, Regular _____
       Unsalted _____
Misc. _____
_____

SUBTOTAL _____

SNACKS AND SUPPLEMENTS _____
_____
_____

GRAND TOTAL _____

20. Calculate the fluid content of the following menu for a renal patient:

   1 c cream of tomato soup
   2 oz beef patty
   ½ c buttered green beans
   Molded vegetable salad on lettuce (⅓ c gelatin, 2 T chopped vegetables)
   ¾ c ice cream
   6 oz iced tea with 2 ice cubes and 2 t sugar

POTASSIUM INTAKE

Serum potassium levels that are abnormally low (*hypokalemia*) or abnormally high (*hyperkalemia*) can occur in patients with renal disease. Either can be life-threatening.

Hypokalemia

Hypokalemia as a consequence of inadequate intake is unlikely because potassium is present in most foods. It is more often the consequence of (1) increased losses due to vomiting and diarrhea, or (2) the use of diuretics that cause the kidney to excrete potassium.

Diuretic medications are classified into three categories:

1. the thiazides, which principally decrease sodium reabsorption in the distal tubules
2. the loop diuretics, which decrease NaCl reabsorption in the ascending limb of the loop of Henle and in the proximal tubule
3. the potassium-sparing diuretics, used to prevent the potassium-losing effects of the other two types

Diuretics are used not only in the treatment of renal disease, but also in cardiosvascular disease and liver disease. Therefore, you should be familiar with these drugs and their relationship to nutritional care.

In general, in nutritional care of the CRF patient receiving diuretics, you need to have information on baseline body weight, BUN, serum creatinine, and serum electrolytes. Fluid intake and output should be monitored, as should body weight. Some considerations are specifically related to the type of diuretic used. You can see from Table 19-5 that the thiazide and loop diuretics can result in hypokalemia. Thiazide diuretics are less frequently used in renal disease since they become ineffective in renal insufficiency at a GFR below 30 ml per min. Furosemide is more commonly used (13).

If the patient has a tendency to become hypokalemic, treatment is preferably via oral intake, and a potassium supplement is usually prescribed. The least expensive forms of these are the potassium-containing salt substitutes. Some patients on sodium-restricted diets are already using these. An appreciable amount

TABLE 19-5. Uses and Side Effects of Diuretic Drugs

Generic Name	Brands	Uses	Side Effects
Thiazides and their congeners			
Chlorothiazide, hydrochlorothiazide, bendroflumethiazide, methylclothiazide, hydroflumethiazide, benzthiazide, polythiazide, cyclothiazide, trichlormethiazide	Naturetin, Aquatag, Exna, Diuril, Anhydron, Esidrix, HydroDiuril Aretic, Saluron, Enduron, Renese, Metahydrin, Naqua, Hygroton, Zaroxolyn, Hydromox	Treatment of edema (in toxemia, nephrosis, congestive heart failure) Control of hypertension Diabetes insipidus Hypercalciuria	Hypokalemia (especially with large NaCl intake) Hyponatremia (with excess water intake) Hypercalcemia Hyperglycemia Hyperuricemia Circulatory volume contraction (can lead to renal failure) Gastrointestinal irritation Dry mouth; bad taste
Loop Diuretics			
Ethacrynic acid Furosemide	Edecrin Lasix	Treatment of edema (in nephrosis, cirrhosis, congestive heart failure) Treatment of oliguria (in acute tubular necrosis, drug intoxication, stone in ureter) Control of hypertension Hypercalcemia	Hypokalemia Alkalosis Hyperuricemia Hyperglycemia Plasma volume contraction Decreased GFR and progressive azotemia Gastritis Rash
Potassium-Sparing Diuretics			
Spironolactone Triamterene	Aldactone Dyrenium	Control of hypertension Treatment of ascites of liver disease	Hyperkalemia Spironolactone: hyponatremia, gastrointestinal irritation Triamterine: hyperglycemia, megaloblastic anemia

Compiled from Kemp, G. and Kemp, D. Diuretics. *Am. J. Nurs.* (June 1978) 1000–1010; Gifford, R.W., Jr. A guide to the practical use of diuretics. *J.A.M.A.* 235:(1976)1890–1893.

of fluid is needed for the administration of potassium-supplement medications since potassium salts are gastric irritants; this can be an important consideration if the diet is fluid-restricted.

An increase in dietary potassium alone is sometimes sufficient. High-potassium foods that are particularly useful for this purpose are listed in Appendix L. It is also helpful to ensure that patients limit their sodium intake since excess sodium excretion increases potassium loss. Precautions must also be taken to ensure that energy intake does not become excessive when foods are added to the diet for the primary purpose of supplying potassium.

Hyperkalemia

The kidney maintains its potassium-excreting ability until GFR is severely compromised. Patients who have a Cl_{CR} over 30 ml per min usually will not become hyperkalemic, especially if they maintain sufficient urine output. There are exceptions, however: patients who have a catabolic illness in which catabolized cells release intracellular potassium into the extracellular fluid, patients who are acidotic or oliguric, and, occasionally, those with a very high potassium intake. Hyperkalemia as a consequence of ex-

cess intake alone is unlikely, however. Some drugs, such as penicillin, have a high potassium content. Triamterene (Dyrenium) and spironolactone (Aldactone), the "potassium-sparing" diuretics, can cause severe hyperkalemia and are not used for patients in renal failure (7).

It is important that serum potassium be kept within normal limits. Severe hyperkalemia (serum K over 6.5 mEq per L) is life-threatening and is a medical emergency. For less marked elevation of serum potassium or for prevention of hyperkalemia in the patient who does comply with the diet, an exchange resin, sodium polystyrene sulfonate (Kayexalate), may be given by mouth. One t contains 7 to 12 g of resin, and each g exchanges approximately 1 mEq of potassium for 1.3 to 1.7 mEq sodium. Since it contributes sodium, it is used cautiously in patients who are volume overloaded. Also, Kayexalate is constipating and is therefore given with an osmotically active substance, such as sorbitol.

Potassium-restricted diets are used to prevent potassium accumulation. In severe failure, patients generally do not receive more than 70 mEq of potassium per day, and some diets are restricted to 40 mEq. Lower levels than these are not achievable over an extended period since potassium is present in most foods. Hyperkalemia which persists when the diet is at 40 mEq per day is an indication for dialysis.

The usual daily intake of potassium is estimated to vary from 2,000 to 6,000 mg per day (50 to 100 mEq). (Potassium exchanges are given in Appendix K, in combination with protein and sodium exchanges.) Since meats, milk, vegetables, and fruits are the most concentrated sources, they are the most often restricted.

The potassium content of foods can be altered in processing. In general, more highly refined foods, such as refined cereals, are lower in potassium than are whole grains. Bran and germ are even higher. Similarly, among dairy products, butter and cream products are lower than cheeses, other than cream cheese, while fluid, dried, evaporated, and condensed milk are highest.

Higher-potassium forms of fruits are whole fruits, including raw, dried, or frozen fruits. The potassium level is lowered when fruit is canned if the surrounding liquid, into which potassium is leached, is discarded. The same principle applies to vegetables. The high potassium concentrations in vegetables present a problem in menu planning since only limited amounts of vegetables can be used. This tends to limit vitamin intake from food. In addition, vegetables contribute greatly to the color and general appearance of food. In their absence, the aesthetic value of meals is reduced. To some extent, potassium can be extracted from vegetables by *leaching*. The vegetables are peeled, cut in small pieces, and soaked in distilled water for two hours or more. They are then rinsed and boiled in a fresh supply of distilled water. This process removes 50 to 75 percent of the potassium but has a deleterious effect on the color of green vegetables and on the texture of most vegetables.

The high potassium content of strong, brewed coffee can be moderated by using a weak, instant coffee. Candies can be low in potassium if they consist primarily of refined sugar and do not contain additions such as chocolate, nuts, coconut, and raisins (14).

Some other pointers in diet planning:

1. Be certain that energy intake is adequate. Cell breakdown as a consequence of energy deficit releases potassium.
2. Distribute potassium-containing foods evenly throughout the day.

Patients should also be encouraged to exercise to the extent possible in order to prevent cell breakdown and promote movement of carbohydrate into cells.

Because potassium restriction becomes necessary only late in renal failure, it is seldom the only diet modification. Instead, it is often combined with protein, sodium, and fluid restriction.

STEPS IN CALCULATING THE PROTEIN-, SODIUM-, POTASSIUM-, AND FLUID-RESTRICTED DIET PLAN

Calculation of a diet that contains restrictions of all four materials is more complex than planning the simple protein-restricted or sodium-restricted diet previously described. The following steps might be helpful if considered in the order given:

1. Calculate the amount of HBV protein.
2. Using the average values for each group in Appendix K, determine the number of servings of meat, egg, and milk from each group (meat and dairy list) to provide the HBV protein. Remember that one egg is usually included because of the high biological value of eggs.
3. Using the average values for each group, determine the number of servings of fruits, vegetables, and bread/cereal/starch to provide the LBV protein, sodium, and potassium. (Acceptable range: Na ± 10 mg, K ± 5 mg.)
4. Add to find totals of protein, sodium, potassium, fluid, and kcals. Alter Step 3 if any values are in excess of prescription or are insufficient.
5. Add sources of additional kcals from fat and carbohydrate ("Miscellaneous" list).
6. Add items from the "Salt" list if necessary to reach the prescribed sodium intake. (This is only likely to be necessary for salt losers.)
7. Add desired beverages, if possible, within prescribed fluid intake.

In calculating the menu pattern, a small amount of variation from the prescribed diet is allowable for ease of calculation. The amount varies from one center to another and also with the condition of the patient. For example, the policy at a given center might be to allow the protein intake to differ from the prescription by ±2 g for nondialyzed patients and ±5 g for hemodialysis patients. On the other hand, if a patient has a problem controlling the urea level, perhaps only the prescribed amount or 5 g less, but not more, would be acceptable. The proportion of HBV protein should vary toward the high side.

An example of a prescription and calculation of the exchanges is shown in Table 19-6.

PHOSPHORUS, CALCIUM, AND VITAMIN D INTAKE

Phosphorus is present almost entirely as phosphate and is excreted primarily in the urine. The elevated phosphate and reduced calcium levels in the serum of patients with a GFR less than 20 ml per min must be controlled in order to avoid renal osteodystrophy. It has been recommended that serum phosphate or phosphorus, which is what is actually measured, be maintained at 3 to 4 mg/dl or less (2). This is difficult to achieve, and a serum phosphorus of 5 to 6 mg/dl with normal serum PTH is more often the objective. Average adult daily phosphorus intake in the United States is 1,500 to 1,600 mg/day (15). In order to control serum phosphorus levels by diet, the intake must be 600 to 1,200 mg/day or less (4).

Low-phosphorus diets are often omitted from institutional diet manuals. Phosphorus is contained pri-

TABLE 19-6. Sample Diet

Prescribed: 60 g Pro (75% HBV), 850 mg Na, 2,000 mg K, 2050 Kcal, 1,000 ml fluid:
Calculate: HBV protein = 60 × 0.75 = 45

Exchange	Serving	Pro	Na	K	Kcal	Fluid
Meat, low Na	4	32.0	120	400	240	
Egg	1	8.0	30	100	60	
Dairy	2	8.0	140	370	400	240
SUBTOTAL		48.0	290	870	700	240
Veg, Group 1	1	1.0	10	100	15	
Group 2	1	1.0	20	170	20	
Group 4	1	2.5	20	200	50	
Fruit, Group 1	1	0.5	5	100	60	
Group 2	2	1.2	10	350	130	
Bread, low Na	3	6.0	15	90	195	
Fat, reg.	3	0.3	420	9	306	
Sweets:						
Jelly	3 T		9	42	318	
Sugar	1 T				46	
Gum drops	6 pieces		20	2	196	
Coffee, instant	6 oz		2	65	2	180
TOTAL		60.5	821	1998	2038	420

a meal pattern:

Breakfast	Serving	Lunch	Serving	Dinner	Serving	Snack	Serving
Fruit #1	1	Low-Na meat	2	Low-Na meat	2	Gum drops	6 pc
Egg	1	Low-Na bread	1	Vegetable #4	1		
Low-Na bread	1	Vegetable #1	1	Vegetable #2	1		
Dairy list	1	Reg margarine	1	Low-Na bread	1		
Reg margarine	1	Fruit #2	1	Reg margarine	1		
Jelly, T	1	Dairy list	1	Fruit #2	1		
Coffee, inst.	6 oz	Jelly, T	1	Jelly, T	1		
Sugar, T	1						

marily in protein foods; therefore, low-protein diets tend to be low in phosphorus. For purposes of estimating the phosphorus content of diets, the following values for the various exchanges are useful (15):

	mg/g protein
Milk, cream, ice cream	30
Nuts	30
Cheese (except cottage)	20
Meat, egg, fish	15
Bread (except whole grain)	15
Rice, pasta	15
Potato, vegetables	15
Cottage cheese	10
Fruit	3

The following are some general guidelines for planning a phosphorus-controlled diet:

1. Omit milk, yogurt, and ice cream. Substitute nondairy cream products, such as Mocha Mix, Poly-Perx, Coffee-Rich, Cool Whip, Dessert Whip, or Rich's Whip Topping.
2. Use meat, fish, poultry, and egg only in amounts compatible with reduced protein intake.
3. Exclude whole-grain cereals or breads and any products containing bran.
4. Exclude dried beans and peas.
5. Omit beverages made with milk, cola beverages, and powdered fruit beverage mixes.

A diet containing 50 g protein will contain 700 to 800 mg phosphorus with the above guidelines. A 40-g-protein diet contains 500 to 650 mg phosphorus (16). Efforts to restrict phosphorus intake further make the diet unpalatable since so many foods must be excluded. Therefore, phosphate-binding gels composed of aluminum carbonate or hydroxide, such as Amphalume, Basaljel, Alutabs, Dialume, and Alternagel, are often used to decrease phosphate absorption from the gastrointestinal tract. There is a current controversy regarding use of aluminum-based phosphate binding gel because of undesirable side effects associated with increased aluminum absorption from these gels. If a phosphate binder is prescribed, it must be taken with meals to be effective. Patients complain that they are hard to swallow, requiring excess fluid, are inconvenient, cause constipation, and have an unpleasant taste. Some suggestions on varying the taste of the binders may improve compliance. Alternatively, binders can be added to foods. If you work extensively with renal patients, you may wish to develop recipes incorporating the binders usually prescribed on your unit.

Patients who develop constipation from phosphate binders might profit from suggestions to increase fiber in the diet or, if not fluid-restricted, to increase fluid intake. The physician may, instead, recommend a stool softener since many foods providing fiber contain large amounts of phosphate.

Calcium intake in CRF patients is usually low because calcium-rich foods contain large amounts of protein, phosphorus, and sometimes fluid. As a result, after serum phosphorus has been reduced to normal, a calcium supplement, usually 1 to 2 g per day, is given. A common dose is 1.5 g calcium carbonate b.i.d. with meals to provide 40 percent calcium (1,200 mg per day). Alternatives are calcium citrate (24 percent Ca), calcium chloride (36 percent Ca, but not used in acidosis), calcium lactate (18.4 percent Ca), calcium gluconate (9.4 percent Ca), or calcium gluconogalactogluconate (92 mg per 4 ml of a syrup, useful for small children).

Vitamin D is also given in some form. Since the names and abbreviations for these forms vary, they are summarized here:

Vitamin D_3 as it first appears in serum is cholecalciferol or 7-dehydrocholesterol.

Hydroxylation in the liver forms 25-hydroxycholecalciferol, also known as 25-hydroxyvitamin D, $25(OH)D_3$, 25-HCC, or calcidiol.

Further hydroxylation in the kidney forms the active metabolite, 1,25-dihydroxycholecalciferol, also known as 1,25-dihydroxyvitamin D, $1,25-(OH)_2D_3$, 1,25-DHCC, or calcitriol. (In this chapter, the term 1,25-DHCC will be used.)

Treatment with the active form of the vitamin, 1,25-DHCC (Rocaltrol), is postponed until serum phosphorus is normalized. It then begins with 0.25 to 0.5 µg/day by mouth. Serum calcium levels are monitored. If they do not rise to normal within 4 to 6 weeks, the 1,25-DHCC dose is increased by similar increments until serum calcium is normal. It is also important to monitor serum phosphorus levels to be sure that the calcium-phosphorus product (mg serum Ca × mg serum P) does not exceed 77; at this point, the risk of soft tissue calcification increases.

IRON INTAKE

Iron deficiency anemia in patients with CRF may be treated with oral or parenteral iron compounds. Anabolic steroids may be given to stimulate erythropoiesis if the patient is iron deficient. Serum ferritin assay is used to monitor iron stores. Most anemia in renal patients is secondary to decreased production and survival of red cells, however, and will not respond to iron therapy.

LIPIDS

Hyperlipidemia may develop in CRF patients. Its management is described in Chapter 20.

VITAMINS

Vitamin A is not given because CRF patients have elevated serum vitamin A levels.

Water-soluble vitamins are supplemented daily as follows (17): 1.5 mg thiamin, 1.8 mg riboflavin, 20 mg niacin, 5 mg pantothenic acid, and 3 µg Vitamin B_{12} in a multivitamin preparation plus 70 to 100 mg ascorbic acid, 5 mg pyridoxine hydrochloride, and 1 mg folic acid.

ALKALINIZING AGENTS

Many CRF patients develop mild metabolic acidosis due to a decreased ability to excrete hydrogen ions, loss of bicarbonate, and retention of fixed anions, such as sulfate and phosphate. The restricted dietary protein reduces acid production. Calcium carbonate to correct calcium deficiency and to bind intestinal phosphate also contributes to correction of acidosis. Some patients require sodium bicarbonate medications (2 to 4 g or 24 to 48 mEq per day in 300 to 600 mg tablets), although the sodium may contribute to hypertension. The sodium does not usually accumulate. Others use Shohl's solution, in which 98 g sodium citrate and 140 g citric acid in 1 L of solution yields 1 mEq $NaHCO_3$ per ml.

TO TEST YOUR UNDERSTANDING

21. Show your calculations for each of the following.
    a. How many mg of potassium are contained in 40 mEq?
    b. How many mEq of potassium are contained in 1 g of KCl?

22. You have a patient who is using a potassium-losing diuretic. Using the menu for _____ (day to be assigned by your instructor), modify this menu to increase the potassium content without increasing its kcal content.

23. You have a patient whose diet prescription is as follows:

Protein	40	g
Sodium	40	mEq
Potassium	50	mEq
Fluid	1,000	ml
Kcal	2,200	

a. Using the exchange lists in Appendix K, calculate a meal plan for this patient on Form Y.

b. Using the menu for _____ (same day as question 22), plan the day's menu for this patient.

FORM Y

University Medical Center
Protein, Sodium, Potassium, and Fluid-Restricted Diet

Prescribed: Pro _____ g; Na _____ mg; K _____ mg;
Fluid _____ ml; _____ kcal
_____ % HBV = _____ g HBV protein

List	Amount	Pro g	Na mg	K mg	Fluid ml	Kcal
Egg						
Meat, Low Na						
High Na						
Dairy						
SUBTOTAL						
Bread, etc.						
Low Na						
Regular						
Vegetable #1						
#2						
#3						
#4						
Fruit #1						
#2						
#3						
Fats, Regular						
Unsalted						
Sweets						

Salt List _____

Miscellaneous _____

  TOTAL _____

Meal Plan: _____

BREAKFAST	Serving	Pro	Na	K	Fluid	Kcal
# _____ Fruit						
Meat list, High Na						
Low Na						
Egg						
Bread, Regular						
Low Na						
Dairy						
Fats, Regular						
Unsalted						
Misc.						

  SUBTOTAL

LUNCH

Meat list, High Na _____
      Low Na _____
Bread list, Regular _____
     Low Na _____
_____ Veg list _____
_____ Veg list _____
_____ Fruit list _____
Dairy list _____
Fats, Regular _____
   Unsalted _____
Misc. _____

  SUBTOTAL

DINNER

Meat list, High Na _____
      Low Na _____
Bread list, Regular _____
     Low Na _____
_____ Veg list _____
_____ Veg list _____
_____ Fruit list _____
Dairy list _____
Fats, Regular _____
   Unsalted _____
Misc. _____

  SUBTOTAL

SNACKS AND SUPPLEMENTS

  GRAND TOTAL

24. You have an adult female patient whose diet prescription reads as follows:

Protein   50 g
Sodium   3 g

Her medical record lists the following values:

	Current	Normal
Fluid intake, ml	2,000	
Fluid output, ml	1,000	
BUN, mg/dl	120.0	_____
Serum creatinine, mg/dl	5.0	_____
Serum sodium, mEq/L	140.0	_____
Serum potassium, mEq/L	6.5	_____
Creatinine clearance, ml/min	20.0	_____
Body weight change, 1 week, kg	3 ½	
BP	140/92	_____

a. Fill in normal values in the spaces provided.
b. Which values are expected to remain high? What values would be your objective for these?
c. What changes, in your opinion, should be made in the diet prescription, assuming you are satisfied that the patient is complying with the currently prescribed diet? Explain your answer.

25. Your patient is complying with a diet containing 40 g protein, 40 mEq Na, and 40 mEq K. Serum phosphate is elevated, and the attending physician asks you to ensure that phosphorus intake is under 1,000 mg per day.

a. What modification in the diet is indicated?
b. The physician prescribes Amphojel for the patient. What nutrition-related problems might you anticipate, and what action on your part do these suggest?
c. The patient complains that the diet is tasteless. She asks whether she can use a salt substitute. What is your response?

NUTRITIONAL CARE IN HEMODIALYSIS

The same nutrients are of concern in the hemodialyzed patient, but the requirements vary, as do the standards used in monitoring the patient. The same methods for planning the diet and the same exchange lists are used.

PROTEIN MODIFICATION

The hemodialyzed patient loses amino acids and peptides to the equivalent of 1 to 2 g of protein per hour of dialysis. Therefore, a patient who is dialyzed for 6 hours per day, 3 days per week, could lose 18 to 36 g of protein. As a consequence, one common recommendation for protein intake, provided body weight is within the normal range, is 0.75 to 1.25 g per kg body weight, with 50 to 65 percent of HBV. This recommendation is based on *dry* body weight—that is, body weight postdialysis. Higher levels are used for repletion. The amount to be eaten by the individual patient will depend on the blood chemistries.

In monitoring the patient, a common objective is to maintain the BUN at 60 to 80 mg per dl following the longest interdialysis interval. Some dialysis centers aim for values under 100 mg per dl. In the stable patient, BUN will correlate with protein intake, but it is not expected that BUN levels will be normal.

The following are some useful guidelines for patient monitoring:

A BUN value over 100 mg per dl and maintenance of weight suggest excess protein intake.

If BUN is unusually elevated, but other values are as expected, the patient is probably taking too much low-biological-value (LBV) protein.

If BUN and phosphate are elevated without other increases, look for excessive cheese intake.

Increased BUN, potassium, and phosphate are usually the result of too much total protein, often in the form of meat and milk.

Calculation of UNA for the interdialytic interval may also be informative.

Weight loss with high BUN indicates protein catabolism.

If BUN is relatively low for a CRF patient, and if serum albumin is also low, inadequate protein intake may be indicated. Weight should be checked, and the degree of edema should be noted.

Serum creatinine is elevated in the dialysis patient. A range of 10 to 20 mg per dl is acceptable prior to dialysis, and 5 to 10 mg per dl is acceptable immediately postdialysis. The value may increase or decrease slightly if the patient is building or losing muscle mass. However, serum creatinine is largely a measure of the effectiveness of the dialysis. Increases are not usually diet-related unless the patient is catabolic. If so, serum albumin is likely to be decreased at the same time.

Albumin levels, which should be within normal range, are useful as a check on *long-term* protein nutrition and general nutritional status.

ENERGY INTAKE

Energy requirements do not differ from those recommended during conservative management—that is, 35 to 50 kcal per kg body weight. The energy intake must be sufficient to spare protein for tissue formation and to maintain normal dry body weight. Wasting often continues in dialysis patients not only from loss of nutrients in the dialysis fluid, but also because some patients are nauseated during and for several hours after dialysis and are unable to eat. If the amount of activity changes when the patient is being dialyzed, energy intake must also be modified. The normoglycemic patient loses 20 to 50 g glucose for each hemodialysis when glucose-free dialysate is used. This amount must be replaced in the diet. To monitor the adequacy of the energy intake, the patient's dry weight should be recorded at the end of dialysis. If energy intake is inadequate, calorie supplements such as those described previously may be helpful.

GLUCOSE

Blood glucose levels are usually normal in non-diabetics, but about 25 percent of patients with end-stage renal disease (ESRD) are diabetic. When monitoring blood glucose, the following should be kept in mind:

The normal kidney degrades insulin; therefore, in ESRD, the half-life of insulin is prolonged.

Predialysis blood samples are usually not fasting samples.

Dialysis removes glucose and will therefore transiently lower blood sugar.

Increased glucose may result in fluid retention, diluting blood chemistries. For example, a normal BUN in a hyperglycemic patient may actually be elevated when the hyperglycemia is corrected. Hyperglycemia may also affect values associated with acid-base balance.

For further discussion of diabetes, see Chapter 18.

PROPORTION OF MAJOR NUTRIENTS

Hemodialysis does not improve a patient's hyperlipidemia. Therefore, recommended kcal distribution is usually 15 percent from protein; 35 percent from fat, with emphasis on polyunsaturated oils; and 50 percent from carbohydrate, primarily polysaccharides.

SODIUM AND FLUID INTAKE AND WEIGHT GAIN

Sodium and fluids are restricted to a level that will limit weight gain between dialyses to 0.5 kg per day. A patient who is dialyzed on Monday, Wednesday, and Friday could gain 1.0 kg between Monday and Wednesday, and between Wednesday and Friday, and 1.5 kg between Friday and Monday.

To maintain this limit, a common recommendation is 1 to 1.5 g sodium per day (43 to 55 mEq) and 500 to 1,500 ml of fluid, not including the fluid content of solid food if the patient is anuric (5). If the patient is not anuric, the urinary excretion of sodium and fluid are added to this allowance. The success of this regimen is determined by monitoring serum sodium, blood pressure, body weight, and, particularly, weight change between dialysis treatments.

The following are some additional guidelines:

Excess weight gain (over 0.5 kg per day) with normal serum sodium indicates excessive intake of both salt and water.

Excessive weight gain with low serum sodium suggests excess fluid but not salt.

Excess sodium intake can result in edema, hypertension, and even congestive heart failure.

Weight loss, hypotension, decreased urine output (if the patient is not anuric), and an increasing BUN suggest inadequate salt intake.

POTASSIUM

Potassium is controlled in the same manner as it is in conservative management. Patients generally should not receive over 70 mEq of potassium per day since they generally do not become hyperkalemic at this level. If the patient still tends to become hyperkalemic, potassium is restricted further in the compliant patient. The objective, as with the conservatively managed patient, is to maintain serum potassium within normal range. An elevated potassium level suggests increased potassium intake by ingestion of too many fresh fruits and vegetables or the use of salt substitutes. Acidosis may also contribute to hyperkalemia. It will be seen with reduced serum bicarbonate values.

CALCIUM, PHOSPHORUS, AND VITAMIN D

Hemodialysis does not diminish the tendency to bone disease in the CRF patient because phosphate is not removed efficiently by dialysis. In addition, the increased protein in the diet tends to increase phosphorus intake. Elevated serum phosphate may reflect excess phosphorus intake or failure to take phosphate binders. High serum alkaline phosphatase levels indicate bone demineralization. Hence, the use of phosphate binders and restriction of dietary phosphate continues. Once serum phosphate is normalized, patients are usually given a calcium supplement of 800 to 1,200 mg per day. Serum calcium levels must also be monitored, with observation of the Ca × P product. Patients often need a calcium supplement of 1 g per day. High serum calcium with normal serum phosphate may occur in patients on vitamin D therapy or oral calcium supplements. Reduced calcium with normal phosphate suggests the patient is not taking the prescribed vitamin D or calcium. Calcium and phosphate levels are also affected by acidosis and by parathyroid hormones.

IRON

Serum iron should be maintained within normal limits. Hemodialyzed patients lose some blood with each dialysis, increasing the tendency to anemia. They should be evaluated with serum ferritin determination. They are usually given an iron supplement, either orally or parenterally. High iron values may be the result of multiple transfusions. Usual values for dialysis patients include hemoglobin values of 8 to 10 g per dl and a 20 percent or higher hematocrit.

BICARBONATE

Dialysis usually corrects the acidosis in these patients. In some patients, however, an accumulation of acid accompanies the increase in protein intake. For these patients, decreased protein intake to decrease the acid from protein metabolism, or medication with bicarbonate to neutralize the excess acid, may be necessary.

VITAMINS

Water-soluble vitamins are lost in dialysis. Therefore, patients are given a multivitamin supplement containing the RDA of thiamine, riboflavin, niacin, biotin, pantothenic acid, and vitamin B_{12}. In addition, 10 mg pyridoxine, 1 mg folate, and 100 mg ascorbic acid are given. Vitamin preparations should not be taken within several hours prior to dialysis, or the vitamins may be removed. Vitamin A is not given because it is not dialyzed; serum levels thus tend to remain high. The vitamin preparation given should not contain nondialyzable substances such as magnesium and other trace elements.

OTHER MEDICATIONS

In addition to phosphate binders, calcium and vitamin D supplements, anabolic steroids, and vitamin supplements, patients with renal disease may be given other drugs of nutritional significance. Hypertension often cannot be controlled by sodium or fluid restriction or by dialysis, so the patient may be given an antihypertensive drug (examples are propranolol HCl [Inderal], minoxidil [Loniten], and hydralazine HCl [Apresoline]). Side effects include nausea, vomiting, and abdominal distress. CRF patients with CHF may be given digitalis therapy. Digoxin is not significantly removed by dialysis, and patients can be susceptible to digitalis toxicity. In addition to cardiac arrhythmias and visual disturbances, signs of digitalis toxicity include nausea and vomiting.

INDICATIONS FOR NUTRITIONAL CONSULTATION

The patient load often is such that it is impossible for you, as the provider of nutritional care, to see each patient each time he is dialyzed. Instead, many dialysis centers set criteria to indicate the need for nutritional consultation. Typical criteria consist of the following:

Serum sodium, mEq/L	<132, >148
Serum potassium, mEq/L	<3.0, >6.0
Predialysis BUN, mg/dl	<40, >100
Serum creatinine, mg/dl	>20
Serum calcium, mg/dl	<8.0, > 11.0
Serum phosphate, mg/dl	>5.0
Serum albumin, g/dl	>3.0
Dry weight, kg	Any unexplained weight change
Weight change over longest interdialytic interval, kg	>2 kg
Other	New diet order
	Patient dissatisfaction

It is important to note that many values are not expected to stay within the range of what is normal for those with normal renal function.

NUTRITIONAL CARE IN PERITONEAL DIALYSIS

The diet for the patient who is undergoing *peritoneal dialysis* (PD) is, in general, less restricted than that required in hemodialysis. It varies slightly depending on whether the dialysis is intermittent (IPD) or continuous ambulatory (CAPD).

PROTEIN

About 1.5 to 3.5 g per day free amino acids are removed by peritoneal dialysis. In addition, patients lose about 13 g protein in 10 hours of maintenance IPD or 9 g in 24 hours of CAPD. Below-normal serum albumin levels are common. The usual recommendation for protein intake is 1.2 to 1.5 g per kg IBW. Of the total, 50 percent should be of high biological value (3). The higher protein intake should be used for the patient who needs to rebuild muscle or following an episode of peritonitis. For repletion, an alternative method is to base protein intake on desired, rather than actual, body weight (3).

ENERGY

Energy intake is generally recommended to be 35 kcal per kg IBW. It is necessary to adjust the level for differences in activity. In addition, precautions must be taken to ensure that the patient does not become obese. Obesity is a particular hazard in CAPD since the glucose in the dialysate (1.5 or 4.5 g per dl) is absorbed and contributes to the patient's energy intake.

SODIUM, FLUID AND POTASSIUM

IPD patients often require the same restrictions as hemodialysis patients do. On the other hand, CAPD patients may tolerate a more liberal intake of 2 to 3 g sodium and 2,000 to 3,000 ml of fluid (3). Some are unrestricted and may need supplemental sodium. Sodium and fluid levels are based on fluid retention and blood pressure. Sodium intake may need to be decreased if peritonitis develops. Potassium intakes are based on serum potassium. In general, patients should not receive more than 70 mEq per day.

CALCIUM AND PHOSPHORUS

Serum phosphorus levels remain elevated in PD. Dietary phosphorus in excess of 1,200 mg per day is often permitted, however, to allow for the increase in dietary protein, and phosphate binders continue to be used. The increased dietary protein may provide additional calcium so that a supplement may be unnecessary. Total calcium intake should be 1.4 to 1.7 g per day (3). If a supplement is necessary, it should not be given until serum phosphate is normalized (3 to 4 mg per dl) (3).

VITAMINS

Water-soluble vitamins are lost in PD. Vitamin supplements are given in doses similar to those given to hemodialyzed patients. If patients are receiving antibiotics, they may need a vitamin K supplement.

In summary, in monitoring the dialysis patient, regardless of method, the following may be considered acceptable: Serum levels of sodium, potassium, calcium, phosphorus, total protein, albumin, and serum ferritin, as well as body weight, should be in normal range. Blood glucose should be in normal range, or may be slightly higher for diabetics. BUN is high, but should be under 100 mg per dl. Serum creatinine is high, at 10 to 15 mg per dl. Total CO_2 may be lower, indicating some acidosis. Hematocrit is usually lower than normal.

TO TEST YOUR UNDERSTANDING

26. When you are monitoring a hemodialysis patient's progress, what data would you look for to determine whether intakes of the following are at appropriate levels?

a. Protein
b. Sodium
c. Potassium
d. Fluid

27. You have a patient who is beginning hemodialysis.

Body wt = 70 kg	Ideal body wt = 84 kg
MAMC = 19.8	Urine output = 200 ml/day
TSF = 10.1	SUN = 180 mg/dl

The diet prescription reads as follows:

1 mg protein/kg, 50 percent HBV; 2,800 kcal; 1,500 ml fluid; 55 mEq Na; 70 mEq K

a. What changes would you suggest later if the patient's predialysis lab values are as follows? (Assume for this and succeeding parts of this question that the patient is complying with the diet.)

SUN	100 mg/dl
Serum Na	WNL
Serum K	WNL
Serum albumin	2.9 g/dl
MAMC	unchanged
TSF	unchanged
Body wt (estimated dry)	70 kg
Urine output	200 ml/day
Weight gain between dialyses	1.5 kg/3 days
No edema	

Explain the basis for your answer.

b. SUN	180 mg/dl
Serum NA	WNL
Serum K	WNL
Serum albumin	3.1 g/dl
MAMC	21.4 cm
TSF	11.2 mm

Body weight (estimated dry)	72 kg
Blood pressure	140/92
Urine output	200 cc/day
Weight gain between dialyses	3 kg/3 day
Edema	3+, pitting

Explain the basis for your answer.

c.

SUN (increase of 30 from previous month)	150
Serum Na	130 mEq/L
Serum albumin	3.3 mg/dl
MAMC	21.4 cm
TSF	11.2 mm
Body weight (estimated dry)	68 kg
Blood pressure	112/70
Urine output	75 ml/day
Weight gain between dialyses	0.5 kg/3 days
Edema	None

Explain the basis for your answer.

28. The following products have been used by patients with CRF. Briefly state the purpose of each product.

   a. Paygel
   b. Lonalac
   c. Hycal
   d. Controlyte
   e. Nephramine
   f. Diasal
   g. Kayexalate
   h. Dialume

NUTRITIONAL CARE FOLLOWING RENAL TRANSPLANT

Renal transplantation is a major surgical procedure. The nutritional care of the prospective transplant patient should be targeted toward maintaining the patient in the best possible condition prior to surgery. Immediate postoperative feeding will include the clear liquid and transitional diets described in Chapter 11.

Once the transplanted kidney is functioning well, the patient's dietary needs are very different. The following nutritional problems may occur:

1. Tendency to excessive weight
2. Need to rebuild muscle and other tissue
3. Need to replace calcium losses from bone
4. Need to reduce or control hyperlipoproteinemia
5. Sodium and fluid retention
6. Carbohydrate intolerance

A commonly recommended diet, therefore, consists of the following:

High protein (100 g or more)
Eliminate simple sugars and concentrated sweets; use 40 percent of energy from complex carbohydrate. The diet is moderated as the immunosuppressant (glucocorticoid) dose is decreased.
High calcium (1.2 g or more)
Low cholesterol with high polyunsaturated : to : saturated fat ratio
Kcals to maintain normal weight
Moderately low sodium (about 2,000 mg)

TOPICS FOR FURTHER DISCUSSION

1. If a growing child has CRF, how would her protein and energy needs per kg of body weight compare to those of an adult?

2. How is nutritional status assessed in a child with CRF?

3. List and price some special low-protein products and low-sodium products. Compare cost per serving with the regular, salted counterpart. If products are available for tasting, compare their acceptability.

4. What is the sodium content of your local water supply? Discuss the implications of this in planning for a 500-mg-sodium diet for someone using this water.

5. A 14 y.o. CRF patient has a height age of 9 years and a bone age of 12 years. Is this patient's final height likely

to be shorter, taller, or normal for age? Describe the physiological basis for your answer.

6. In nutritional care of the pregnant dialysis patient, what changes are made in the laboratory criteria for control? Discuss potential necessary changes in the diet?

7. Discuss adjustment of TPN procedures for renal patients.

8. Using the menu from a local restaurant, choose some meals for renal patients requiring various diet restrictions.

9. Discuss nutritional care of patients with various types of renal stones.

REFERENCES

1. COLBURN, J.W. General concepts and management of chronic renal failure. In *The Kidney: Diagnosis and Management,* eds. N.S. Bricker and M.A. Kirschenbaum. New York: John Wiley, 1984.
2. BLUMENKRANTZ, M.J., J.D. KOPPLE, R.A. GUTMAN, Y.K. CHAN, G.L. BARBOUR, C. ROBERTS, F.H. SHEN, V.C. GANDHI, C.T. TUCKER, F.K. CURTIS, AND J.W. COBURN. Methods for assessing nutritional status of patients with renal failure. *Am. J. Clin. Nutr.* 33:(1980)1567–1585.
3. HARVEY, K.B., M.J. BLUMENKRANTS, S.E. LEVINE, AND G.L. BLACKBURN. Nutritional assessment and treatment of chronic renal failure. *Am. J. Clin. Nutr.* 33:(1980)1586–1597.
4. KOPPLE, J.D. Nutrition and the kidney. In *Human Nutrition: Metabolic and Clinical Applications,* ed. R.E. Hodges. Vol. 4 of *Human Nutrition: A Comprehensive Treatise,* eds. R.B. Alfin-Slater and D. Kritschevsky. New York: Plenum, 1979.
5. KOPPLE, J.D. Significance of diet and parenteral nutrition in chronic renal failure. In *The Kidney: Diagnosis and Management,* eds. N.S. Bricker and M.A. Kirschenbaum. New York: John Wiley, 1984, pp. 333–352.
6. KOPPLE, J.D. Nutritional therapy in kidney failure. *Nutr. Rev.* 39:(1981)193–206.
7. DAROVITCH, E.M. Sodium-retaining states: The edematous patient. In *The Kidney: Diagnosis and Management,* eds. N.S. Bricker and M.A. Kirschenbaum. New York: John Wiley, 1984.
8. MARTIN, K.J. Renal disease. In *Manual of Medical Therapeutics* (23d ed.), eds. J.J. Freitag and L.W. Miller. Boston: Little, Brown, 1980.
9. KRAUS, B. *The Barbara Kraus 1985 Sodium Guide to Brand Names and Basic Foods.* New York: New American Library, 1984.
10. MAYES, K. *The Sodium-Watcher's Guide.* Santa Barbara, Calif.: Pennant Books, 1984.
11. *The Renal Family Cookbook,* ed. M. Law. Downsview, Ont.: The Renal Family Inc., 1983.
12. ANONYMOUS. Decreased taste acuity in chronic renal patients. *Nutr. Rev.* 39:(1981)207–210.
13. NORDLICHT, S.M. Congestive heart failure. In *Manual of Medical Therapeutics* (23d ed.), eds. J.J. Freitag and L.W. Miller. Boston: Little, Brown, 1980.
14. SUITOR, C.W. AND M.F. CRAWLEY. *Principles and Application in Health Promotion* (2d ed.). Philadelphia: Lippincott, 1984.
15. PAGE, L. AND B. FRIEND. The changing United States diet. *Bioscience* 28:(1978)192–198.
16. WALSER, M. AND E.C. CHANDLER. Phosphorus. In *Nutritional Management,* eds. M. Walser, A. Imbembo, S. Margolis, and G.A. Eefert. Philadelphia: Saunders, 1984.
17. ALPERS, D.H., R.E. CLOUSE, AND W.F. STENSON. *Manual of Nutritional Therapeutics.* Boston: Little, Brown, 1983.

ADDITIONAL SOURCES OF INFORMATION

CHANTLER, C. Nutritional assessment and management of children with renal insufficiency. In *End-Stage Renal Disease in Children,* eds. R.N. Fine and A.B. Gruskin. Philadelphia: Saunders, 1984.

DWYER, J., E. FOULKES, M. EVANS, AND L. AUSMAN. Acid/alkaline ash diets: Time for assessment and change. *J. Am. Dietet. Assoc.* 85:(1985)841–845.

NELSON, P. AND J. STOVER. Principles of nutritional assessment and management of the child with ESRD. In *End-Stage Renal Disease in Children,* eds. R.N. Fine and A.B. Gruskin. Philadelphia: Saunders, 1984.

CASE STUDY VII   CHRONIC RENAL FAILURE

Part I: Presentation

Present Illness: Ellen R. is a 20 y.o. university student referred to the Renal Clinic from the university's Student Health Center for evaluation of renal function. She had come to the Health Center C/O fatigue, weakness, anorexia, periorbital and pedal edema, and sudden weight gain. The Health Center reports data listed below.

Past Medical History: T&A at age 7; streptococcal infection of throat at age 11, followed by glomerulonephritis; fractured arm at age 14.

Family History: Parents are a&w. Brother age 16 a&w.

Social History: Single. Resides in university residence hall.

Review of Systems: Patient c/o mild, intermittent headache; nocturia 1–2 times/night; fatigue; anorexia; mild pruritis

Examination:

General: White female; 5 ft, 7 in; 57 kg; medium frame. BP 128/85, right arm, sitting. P 72, regular. R 15. T 37° C. Fundi normal. Lungs clear. Heart without murmur or gallop. Extremities show 2+ pedal edema. Rest of exam WNL.

Impression: Nephrotic syndrome with renal insufficiency in a 20 y.o. normal-weight female with medical history of poststreptococcal glomerulonephritis.

Plan: Nutrition Clinic referral for instruction on 4–6-g-salt diet. Rx: furosemide (Lasix) 60 mg q.d.; phosphate binder (Dialume) 3 × 500 mg tab t.i.d. with meals; docusate sodium (Colace), prn. RTC in 1 wk for BP check and serum K assay, renal biopsy.

BP	135/90
Albuminuria	3+
BUN	50 mg/dl
Serum albumin	2.8 g/dl
Current body wt	140 #
Pre-illness wt	128 #

Laboratory:	*Units*	*Normal*	*Patient*	*Interpretation*
BUN	mg/dl	____	50	____
Serum creatinine	mg/dl	____	2.2	____
Creatinine clearance	ml/min	____	40	____
Serum sodium	mEq/L	____	138	____
Serum potassium	mEq/L	____	4.0	____
Serum albumin	g/dl	____	2.0	____
Serum calcium	mg/dl	____	7.3	____
Serum phosphate	mg/dl	____	6.0	____
Urine pH		____	6.2	____
24-hr urine protein	g/24 hr	____	7.00	____
Urine specific gravity		____	1.004	____
Urine volume	ml/24 hr	____	2,000	____
Hgb	g/dl	____	9.8	____
Hct	%	____	33	____
Rheumatology W/U		NL		____
Microscopic urine exam			broad casts	____
Radiology (KUB)			kidney size	

QUESTIONS

1. The patient's complaints of anorexia and weight gain and the fact that she is at approximately normal weight seem incompatible. Explain how these conditions can coexist.

2. In the above column headed "Normal," write in the normal values.

3. In the above column headed "Interpretation," write *P* for any value that suggests the kidney disease is affecting Ellen's protein and nitrogen homeostasis.

4. In the same column, write *S* for any value that indicates that the disease is affecting the kidney's ability to conserve or excrete solutes.

5. In the same column, write *F* for any value that suggests that the disease is compromising the kidney's ability to maintain fluid balance.

6. In the same column, write *B* for any value suggesting that the patient might develop skeletal abnormalities.

7. Explain the purpose of

   a. The dietary sodium restriction

   b. Furosemide

   c. Phosphate binder

   d. Colace

8. Explain why a protein restriction was not ordered.

9. a. Would you suggest any other diet modification? If so, what? Explain your reasoning.

   b. If you answered positively to part a, describe in general terms the content of your suggestions to the patient.

10. a. Describe side effect(s) of furosemide.

    b. What nutritional care procedures do these side effects indicate?

Part II. Medical Management of Renal Insufficiency

Ellen continued on this program of conservative management for the next 3 years. During this time she graduated from college, began her career as an elementary school teacher in a rural community, and was married. She was followed by her personal physician and was not seen in the Renal Clinic for several years.

Three years later, she was again referred to the Renal Clinic. She C/O more frequent headaches, nausea and vomiting, severe itching, and an unpleasant taste in her mouth. She also C/O muscle cramps and twitching, weight loss, weakness, and drowsiness, with difficulty concentrating. The examination and interview provided the following information:

BUN	100 mg/dl
Serum creatinine	4.8 mg/dl
Creatinine clearance	30.0 ml/min
Urea clearance	16 ml/min
Serum sodium	142 mEq/L
Serum potassium	5.7 mEq/L
Serum phosphate	8.5 mg/dl
Serum calcium	7.5 mg/dl
Serum albumin	2.8 g/dl
Hgb	19.2 g/dl

Hct	28%
Serum transferrin	150 mg/dl
BP	180/120, standing, right arm
Proteinuria	Negative
Urine pH	7.31
Serum alkaline phosphatase	18 units/dl (King-Armstrong)
Blood CO_2	14.8 mEq/L
Urine volume	500 ml/24 hr
Dry weight	52 kg (estimated by urologist)

Bone roentgenogram demonstrates renal osteodystrophy.

Parathormone level is elevated.

Impression: Chronic renal failure in a 23 y.o. underweight female with history of renal insufficiency and nephrotic syndrome.

Plan: Nutrition Clinic referral for advice on diet: protein, 40 g; Na, 1,000 mg; K, 40 mEq; fluid, output + 500 ml. Rx: furosemide (Lasix), 60 mg t.i.d.; methyldopa (Aldomet), 250 mg t.i.d.; sodium bicarbonate, 1 g t.i.d.; phosphate binder (Dialume), 4 × 500 mg tab t.i.d.

QUESTIONS

11. From the laboratory values given, calculate Ellen's GFR.

12. Explain the purpose of each of the following, and list the data indicating the need for the treatment:

a. Methyldopa

b. Sodium bicarbonate

c. Protein restriction

d. Sodium restriction

e. Potassium restriction

f. Fluid restriction

g. Phosphate restriction

13. a. Since the patient showed evidence of renal osteodystrophy and serum calcium was low, why were calcium and vitamin D supplements not ordered?

b. If we assume that the calcium and vitamin D supplements were to restore serum calcium to at least normal levels (8.5 mg/dl or more), at what point would it be safe to begin prescribing them? Why? What is the common practice in this regard?

c. Why was a low-phosphorus diet not ordered?

14. When you see Ellen in the Nutrition Clinic, you note that the diet prescription does not specify a calorie content.
a. How many kcals would you try to include in her diet? Show your calculations and explain your reasoning.

b. On Form Z, calculate a diet plan for this patient.

FORM Z

University Medical Center
Protein, Sodium, Potassium, and Fluid-Restricted Diet

Prescribed: Pro _____ g; Na _____ mg; K _____ mg;
Fluid _____ ml; _____ kcal
_____ % HBV = _____ g HBV protein

List	Amount	Pro g	Na mg	K mg	Fluid ml	Kcal
Egg						
Meat, Low Na						
High Na						
Dairy						
SUBTOTAL						
Bread, etc.						
Low Na						
Regular						
Vegetable #1						
#2						
#3						
#4						
Fruit #1						
#2						
#3						

Fats, Regular _____

    Unsalted _____

Sweets _____

_____

_____

_____

Salt List _____

Miscellaneous _____

TOTAL _____

Meal Plan: _____

BREAKFAST	Serving	Pro	Na	K	Fluid	Kcal
# _____ Fruit						
Meat list, High Na						
Low Na						
Egg						
Bread, Regular						
Low Na						
Dairy						
Fats, Regular						
Unsalted						
Misc.						

SUBTOTAL

LUNCH						
Meat list, High Na						
Low Na						
Bread list, Regular						
Low Na						
# _____ Veg list						
# _____ Veg list						
# _____ Fruit list						
Dairy list						
Fats, Regular						
Unsalted						
Misc.						

SUBTOTAL

DINNER						
Meat list, High Na						
Low Na						
Bread list, Regular						
Low Na						
# _____ Veg list						
# _____ Veg list						
# _____ Fruit list						
Dairy list						
Fats, Regular						
Unsalted						
Misc.						

SUBTOTAL

SNACKS AND SUPPLEMENTS
_____
_____

GRAND TOTAL _____

c. Using the menu for _____ (day to be assigned by your instructor), plan one day's menu for this patient.

d. The patient tells you she has a salt substitute which she uses "sparingly." What action would you take at this point?

15. When Ellen comes to see you again, you find the following data in her medical record:

	March 5	March 8
SUN, mg/dl	95.0	98.0
Body wt, kg	52.0	52.0
UUN, g/24 hr	4.3	4.3

You interview Ellen at some length. She assures you she is following her diet. You take a 24-hour recall and your calculations show that her diet contained approximately 40 g protein.

a. Calculate her UNA, her nitrogen output, and her nitrogen intake as indicated by the laboratory values.

b. Do your results confirm that the patient is following her diet? Show your calculations.

c. Is the protein content of the diet sufficient to avoid tissue catabolism? Explain your answer.

d. Is her energy intake adequate for protein sparing at her current activity level? Explain your answer.

16. Ellen tells you that she feels thirsty all the time. She would like to have more fluid, but the attending physician is reluctant to allow this. She says that she needs most of her fluid allotment to take her medications. What procedures could you suggest to her?

Part III: Hemodialysis

Ellen is no longer able to keep up her work at the school. Her GFR is 16 ml/min. Her physician recommends a transplant, but a kidney is not immediately available. As a consequence, hemodialysis is recommended.

An arteriovenous fistula was surgically created in Ellen's left forearm. A month later, she is admitted to the hospital. Her serum potassium level has risen further and SUN is 110 mg/dl. Her BP has also risen. She is started on hemodialysis 5 hours, three times per week.

Her diet prescription now reads as follows: protein, 1 g/kg; Na, 55 mEq; fluid, 1,500 ml; K, 70 mEq; phosphate, 1,200 mg. She was instructed to continue her previously prescribed phosphate binder and calcium supplement and to discontinue the bicarbonate and steroid. She was also given vitamin supplements.

Her postdialysis weight was 50 kg.

QUESTIONS

17. How much protein per day would you recommend for Ellen? Explain your reasoning.

18. At one time, Ellen's laboratory values were as follows:

BUN (predialysis)	110 mg/dl
Serum sodium	140 mEq/L
Serum potassium	4.6 mEq/L
Serum albumin	3.1 g/dl
BP	145/95
Interdialytic weight gain	2 kg
MAMC	19.5
TSF	13.2

a. How would you interpret the data?

b. What action would you take?

c. Which values would you monitor to determine the *long-term* adequacy of the diet?

19. Explain the rationale for the following:
a. Phosphate binders, calcium supplement, and dietary phosphate restriction

b. Water-soluble vitamin supplements

20. Why are the following not given:
a. Vitamin A

b. Bicarbonate

Part IV: Peritoneal Dialysis

The three trips a week to the Dialysis Center from her rural community become a hardship for Ellen as months pass, and a kidney for transplant is still not available. Her physician considers home hemodialysis, but they are concerned that the power and water supplies are not sufficiently reliable. In addition, her husband's work does not allow him to be of enough help in the process.

A decision is made to have Ellen use continuous ambulatory peritoneal dialysis. She and her husband are both carefully instructed in the procedures.

The diet prescription is as follows: protein, 120 g; kcal, 2,100; Na, 3 g; fluid, 2,000 ml; phosphate, 1,200 mg.

QUESTIONS

21.   a. What nutritional problems might arise?

   b. Describe the nutritional care procedures indicated.

Part V: Renal Transplant

One day, Ellen receives a telephone call telling her that a kidney is available for her transplant. She leaves for the hospital immediately and receives her transplant late that evening.

She is given a clear liquid diet for three days and then advanced to a more adequate diet. She is given immunosuppressants and a diet is prescribed. Six months later, you see Ellen for the last time. She reports that she is teaching again and is expecting her first child.

20

Cardiovascular Diseases

Cardiovascular disease is the principal cause of death in the United States. Atherosclerosis and hypertension are the major forms of diet-related cardiovascular disease. This chapter focuses on those aspects of cardiovascular disease which have a nutritional component and are commonly seen in a clinical setting—hypertension, hyperlipidemia, myocardial infarction, and congestive heart failure. The emphasis is on integration of clinical care and nutritional management, specific aspects of nutritional assessment, and pertinent educational considerations in the approach to individuals with these cardiovascular disorders. Before you proceed, you may want to review the related chapters in your text. You will also need to refer to information contained in Chapter 19 on sodium-restricted diets.

HYPERTENSION

SCREENING AND DIAGNOSIS

The level of blood pressure (BP) at which a diagnosis of hypertension is made has been established somewhat arbitarily as a *systolic* pressure of 140 mm Hg or greater and a *diastolic* pressure of 90 mm Hg or greater. Epidemiologic studies have suggested that the risk of cardiovascular disease increases above these levels. The Hypertension Detection and Follow-Up program of the National Heart, Lung and Blood Institute (1) has shown that aggressive treatment of individuals with levels of diastolic blood pressure 90 mm Hg or more results in a significant reduction in complications. The report also suggests screening of blood pressure in childhood, with repeated measurements to determine the relationship of the child's blood pressure to age-specific percentile levels.

INTEGRATION OF CLINICAL CARE AND NUTRITIONAL MANAGEMENT

If the hypertensive patient's diastolic blood pressure is between 90 and 105 mm Hg, the patient is usually given a diet and counselled on reducing stress factors and starting an exercise program (2). The main features of the diet include the following:

1. Calorie manipulation to achieve and maintain OBW
2. Restriction of dietary sodium to 2 g or 86 mEq per day
3. A daily intake of potassium of at least 4 g or 100 mEq and intakes of calcium and magnesium which provide the RDA
4. Reduction of excess alcohol intake to one or two drinks or 10 to 20 g alcohol per day and moderation in caffeine intake

If the diet and stress-reduction therapy are unsuccessful, it is usually necessary to begin drug therapy. The 2-g-sodium diet is usually continued since drug dosage, drug-related side effects, and potassium losses can be minimized with a concomitant sodium restriction. In general, the use of drug therapy makes severe sodium restriction of 500 mg or less per day unnecessary.

KEY POINTS OF NUTRITIONAL ASSESSMENT

Three specific aspects of nutritional assessment are important in the hypertensive patient. First is the consideration of the patient's body weight compared to optimal body weight. Second are possible side effects associated with diuretic therapy, especially potassium balance, and interaction with cardiac drugs such as digitalis. (Food sources of potassium are given in Appendix L.) Third, sodium intake, including sodium present in food or added by the patient, is of concern. Approximately 50% of the average daily sodium intake from food comes from grain products, meat, poultry, fish, milk, and dairy products (3). These foods are also major sources of calcium, iron, magnesium, and pyridoxine. These nutrients should be

given particular attention when evaluating the diet of a hypertensive patient who adheres to a low-sodium diet.

TO TEST YOUR UNDERSTANDING

1. What is the mechanism of increased potassium losses seen with thiazide and loop diuretic therapy?
2. Describe the symptoms of hypokalemia.
3. Why is hypokalemia of particular concern with a combination of digitalis and thiazide or loop diuretic therapy?
4. What is the potassium content of 1 t (5 g) salt substitute? (Assume pure KCl.)
   a. _____ g K/t KCl
   b. _____ mEq K/t KCl
5. List three examples of food choices which could provide 40 mEq of K and no more than 300 kcal. (List each food's portion, mEq K, and Kcal.)

HYPERLIPIDEMIA

EVALUATION OF LIPIDS AND LIPOPROTEINS

Clinically, the measurement of total serum or plasma cholesterol is the most common, the simplest (available from most automated chemistry panels), and the best-documented index of the risk of atherosclerosis. The sum of the cholesterol carried by the very low density lipoprotein (VLDL), low density lipoprotein (LDL), and high density lipoprotein (HDL) fractions equals the total plasma cholesterol. Triglyceride measurements are also routinely available but must be done on a blood sample obtained from a fasting subject. Triglyceride level as an independent risk factor for coronary heart disease has not been established.

The relative amounts of the lipoprotein classes VLDL, LDL, and HDL are estimated by determining cholesterol content in each of these fractions. Elevated HDL-cholesterol levels, which have been shown to be associated with a reduced risk of coronary heart disease, can be measured clinically by simple methods. VLDL-cholesterol can be estimated as 20 percent of the triglyceride value for levels of triglyceride less than 300 mg per dl and LDL-cholesterol, the most atherogenic lipoprotein, can be estimated from the following equation:

$$\text{LDL Chol} = \text{Total Chol} - (\text{HDL Chol} + 0.2\,\text{TG}) \qquad (20\text{-}1)$$

A simple technique for determining the abnormal presence of chylomicrons and VLDLs involves allowing a fasting plasma sample to stand for 18 to 24 hours at 4° C, the so-called refrigerator test. If abnormal chylomicron metabolism exists, a cream layer will form on top, and elevated VLDL levels will produce turbidity throughout the tube. Thus, from measurement of serum cholesterol, triglyceride, and HDL-cholesterol, extrapolation to LDL-cholesterol, and a

refrigerator test, a preliminary assessment of the levels of chylomicrons, VLDL, LDL, and HDL can be established. An elevation in plasma cholesterol and triglyceride levels is often further characterized by electrophoresis to provide additional information on the lipoprotein profile.

Hyperlipidemia is defined as an elevation of plasma lipids including cholesterol, cholesterol esters, phospholipids, and triglycerides. When hyperlipidemia is defined in terms of class or classes of elevated plasma lipoproteins the term *hyperlipoproteinemia* is used. The simplest nomenclature for defining the type of lipoprotein(s) present in excess is the phenotyping system proposed by Fredrickson and Levy in 1980 (4). Although widely used, this system offers no information about the causes of the different forms of hyperlipoproteinemia. A summary of the lipoprotein phenotypes follows:

Phenotype	Plasma Lipoprotein Present in Excess
I	Chylomicrons
IIA	LDL
IIB	LDL + VLDL
III	Beta VLDL (cholesterol-rich VLDL remnants)
IV	VLDL
V	Chylomicrons + VLDL

The levels of blood lipid and lipoprotein patterns that require dietary modification are controversial. The risk associated with various plasma cholesterol levels was the subject of a 1984 National Institutes of Health Consensus Development Conference on Lowering Blood Cholesterol(5). The panel recommended that "safe" cholesterol levels are those below 200 mg/dl, a level exceeded by approximately one-half of the adult population of the United States. They suggested that individuals with plasma cholesterol levels above the 90th percentile are at "high risk," and those with values between the 75th–90th percentiles

TABLE 20-1. Cholesterol Values for Classifying Men, Women, and Children as Moderate or High Risk for Developing Coronary Heart Disease

	Cholesterol Level (mg/dl)	
Age (yr)	Moderate Risk	High Risk
2–19	>170	>185
20–29	>200	>220
30–39	>220	>240
40 and over	>240	>260

are at "moderate risk" as outlined in Table 20-1 (5).An average upper limit for plasma triglyceride concentrations is suggested to be 200 mg per dl. Triglyceride levels in the range of 250–500 mg/dl can be a marker for secondary disorders or for a subset of patients at increased risk due to genetic forms of hyperlipoproteinemia. Age-specific percentile values for plasma cholesterol and triglyceride and LDL- and HDL-cholesterol are listed in Tables F-17 to F-20. These values are based on a 1980 United States population survey conducted by the Lipid Research Clinic (6).

NUTRITIONAL MANAGEMENT

Current research suggests that a single basic diet may be used initially in the management of all types of hyperlipidemia (7). The main exception to this statement involves fasting chylomicronemia, which requires individualized total fat restriction and the restriction of alcohol in hypertriglyceridemia. The single-basic-diet concept is in contrast to earlier diet recommendations which suggested an increase in polyunsaturated fat intake, a decrease in carbohydrate intake for those forms of hyperlipidemia associated with hypertriglyceridemia, and inconsistent recommendations for the level of cholesterol intake (4).

The suggested single basic diet is in accordance with the United States Dietary Goals and includes three major recommendations:

1. Calories to achieve and maintain OBW, with reduction in the intake of simple sugars and alcohol
2. A reduction in intake of total fat, especially cholesterol and saturated fat
3. An increase in complex carbohydrate and fiber intake

TABLE 20-2. Variations on the Single Basic Diet for Management of Hyperlipidemia

Nutrient	Phase 1–Prudent Diet	Phase 2	Phase 3
Fat (% calories)*	30	25	20
Cholesterol (mg)	300	200–250	100–150
Carbohydrate (% calories)	55	60	65
Protein (% calories)†	15	15	15

*Equal amounts of saturated, monounsaturated and polyunsaturated fatty acids.
†3–6 oz/day of fish, poultry, lean meats (10% fat after cooking), and low-fat cheeses. Emphasize meatless dishes.

The aggressiveness with which the single-diet approach is applied depends on the degree and type of hyperlipidemia. Table 20-2 outlines three phases of the single basic diet (8).

Phase 1, or the American Heart Association Prudent Diet is a moderately low-fat, low cholesterol diet that can be used by individuals who have normal lipids and want a "preventive" eating plan. The Phase 1 diet is also used initially for individuals classified as "moderate" or "high risk" as outlined in Table 20-1. If response to the Phase 1 diet is not adequate, then Phase 2 and Phase 3 diets are used. Individuals classified as "high risk" often need drug therapy in addition to diet, to reduce blood lipid levels. Reduction of elevated LDL-cholesterol levels via reduction in dietary saturated fat and cholesterol intake is a primary objective of all three diets.

Drug Therapy

A variety of lipid-lowering drugs are used as an adjunct to diet in the treatment of hyperlipoproteinemia. None of these drugs is effective in treating all lipoprotein disorders, and most are associated with side effects. Lipid-lowering drugs can be broadly divided into four classes: agents that decrease the synthesis of VLDLs and LDLs, such as niacin; agents that enhance VLDL clearance, such as clofibrate and gemfibrozil; agents that enhance LDL catabolism, such as cholestyramine and colestipol; and agents that inhibit cholesterol synthesis, such as the experimental drugs compactin and mevinolin (9).

TO TEST YOUR UNDERSTANDING

6. a. Using the diabetic exchange lists in Appendix C and Form AA, calculate a 2,000-kcal meal *pattern* for a Phase 2 diet as described in Table 20-2.

b. Using the meal pattern you just calculated, write a menu for use at home on Form BB. Assume that you are calculating the meal plan for an individual who is generally agreeable to modifying dietary fat and carbohydrate intake and has no major food preferences other than consuming only 1 c of milk per day.

Form AA

Calculating a Meal Pattern

Total Kcal _____
Carbohydrate   (% kcal) _____ (g) _____
Protein   (% kcal) _____ (g) _____
Fat   (% kcal) _____ (g) _____
Division of Carbohydrate: _____

Daily Meal Pattern

Exchange	# of exchanges	Protein (g)	Fat (g)	Carbohydrate (g)
*Milk—nonfat, low fat, whole				
Fruit				
Vegetable				
Subtotal				
Bread/Starch				
Subtotal				
*Meat—lean, medium, high fat				
Fat				
TOTAL				

*Circle the one used in calculating the meal pattern.

Distribution of Exchanges at Meals and Snacks

Exchanges	Total # of exchanges	Breakfast	AM Snack	Lunch	PM Snack	Dinner	HS Snack
Milk		( )	( )	( )	( )	( )	( )
Fruit		( )	( )	( )	( )	( )	( )
Vegetable		( )	( )	( )	( )	( )	( )
Bread		( )	( )	( )	( )	( )	( )
Meat		( )	( )	( )	( )	( )	( )
Fat		( )	( )	( )	( )	( )	( )
Total		( )	( )	( )	( )	( )	( )

7. What advice could you offer an individual for the selection of a margarine with a high P:S ratio? (See Table B-3.)

8. Assume that you are counseling a patient who carries her lunch. Plan two menus that you could give her as examples of lunchbox meals that conform to the Phase 2 Diet. Use the 2,000-kcal meal plan you calculated in question 6.

Form BB

Nonselect Menu

Diet _____

Breakfast	Lunch	Dinner

_____ Margarine
_____ Milk—no fat, low
      fat, whole
Coffee, Tea, Sanka
Salt, Salt Substitute
Pepper
Sugar, Sugar Substitute

Snacks:

_____ Margarine
_____ Milk—no fat, low
      fat, whole
Coffee, Tea, Sanka
Salt, Salt Substitute
Pepper
Sugar, Sugar Substitute

Snacks:

_____ Margarine
_____ Milk—no fat, low
      fat, whole
Coffee, Tea, Sanka
Salt, Salt Substitute
Pepper
Sugar, Sugar Substitute

Snacks:

9. Visit a local grocery store in groups of two or three students and name at least two brands of products in each of the following categories that would be acceptable for an individual following the Prudent diet.

Flavored beverage	Margarine
Prepared bread mix	Oil
Cereal	Frozen meat dish
Crackers	Salad dressing
Cream substitute	Soup
Cheese	Sauce mix
Egg substitute	Dessert

NUTRITIONAL MANAGEMENT IN MYOCARDIAL INFARCTION

Nutrition is important in both the prevention and the acute and long-term management of *myocardial infarction* (MI).

PREVENTION

The association between high plasma cholesterol levels and an increased incidence of heart disease is well established and forms the basis of the Diet-Heart hypothesis. This hypothesis states that a reduction in plasma cholesterol levels will reduce the risk of heart disease. Studies have shown that adherence to a Prudent diet can reduce plasma cholesterol by 10 to 15 percent. A linear decrease in serum cholesterol with dietary intakes of cholesterol in the range of 0–400 mg/1000 kcal is observed. Each mg cholesterol per 1000 kcal is projected to increase serum cholesterol by approximately 0.1 mg/dl (10). Thus, with a 2500 kcal diet an increase in cholesterol intake of 100 mg is expected to increase serum cholesterol by approximately 4 mg/dl.

The 1984 National Heart, Lung and Blood Institute Coronary Primary Prevention Trial (11) provides support for the Diet-Heart hypothesis. In this study, a group of American middle-aged men with cholesterol levels in the 95th percentile (>265 mg/dl) took the drug cholestryamine, which reduced their blood cholesterol levels by an average of 8.5 percent in comparison with a placebo group. In association with lower cholesterol levels these men had a 19% reduction in the incidence of total coronary heart disease deaths and non-fatal MIs. This study demonstrates that each 1% reduction in total cholesterol results in a 2% reduction in the incidence of coronary heart disease morbidity and mortality in men with high blood cholesterol levels.

The Nutrition Committee of the American Heart Association issued an updated position statement in 1986 entitled "Dietary Guidelines for Healthy Americans" (12). The purpose of the statement is to propose an optimal preventive diet for coronary heart disease. Here is a statement of the specific dietary guidelines.

1. Saturated fat intake should be less than 10% of calories.
2. Total fat intake should be less than 30% of calories.
3. Cholesterol intake should be less than 100 mg/1,000 cal, not to exceed 300 mg/day.
4. Protein intake should be approximately 15% of calories.
5. Carbohydrate intake should constitute 50 to 55% or more of calories, with emphasis on increased complex carbohydrates.
6. Sodium intake should be reduced to approximately 1 g/1,000 cal, not to exceed 3 g/day.
7. If alcoholic beverages are consumed, the caloric intake from this source should be limited to 15% of total calories but should not exceed 50 ml of ethanol per day.
8. Total calories should be sufficient to maintain the individual's best body weight.
9. A wide variety of foods should be consumed.

IMMEDIATE POSTINFARCTION CARE

The rationale for nutritional management of an individual in the immediate postinfarction period follows a knowledge of the physiologic response to MI. The objectives of nutritional care during this period include the following:

1. Reduction of potential arrhythmias by elimination of caffeine and use of a liquid diet in the first 24 hours, when nausea and choking are common
2. Reduction of cardiac workload with small, frequent feedings of soft or liquid foods
3. Individualization of sodium restriction according to sodium and fluid status
4. Provision of consistent dietary information as a basis for later education for long-term nutritional management

LONG TERM MANAGEMENT

Patients most likely to benefit from long-term dietary intervention after an MI are those with the best prognosis—in general, younger patients without functional impairment of the heart. Cardiac rehabilitation programs—which include cessation of smoking, gradual increase in exercise, and adherence to a Prudent diet—are felt to be of value in improving the quality of life and arresting, retarding, or possibly reversing the atherosclerotic process. In general, older patients with long-standing heart disease will not benefit greatly from adherence to a Prudent diet; with the elderly patient, however, it becomes especially important to individualize the diet to customary food practices.

Patients who have had an MI and have various complications, such as hypertension or diabetes mellitus, should have appropriate nutritional management in addition to the Prudent diet. Many cardiologists feel that since congestive heart failure is a common long-term complication of MI, all MI patients should be advised to follow a moderate sodium restriction of 3 to 4 g per day during the postinfarction period.

For patients with persistent or recurrent angina, slow eating of frequent, small meals may reduce pain. Also, resting before and after a meal may be of benefit. Weight reduction may help decrease angina in the obese patient with significant chest pain.

Programs promoting a rapid weight reduction—a weight loss of greater than 2 pounds per week—should be used with caution in the postinfarction patient. The elevation in plasma free fatty acid levels which accompanies rapid weight reduction can induce cardiac arrhythmias. In addition, the fluid and electrolyte alterations which accompany rapid weight reduction can be particularly dangerous to the post-MI patient maintained on diuretic and digitalis therapy.

THE CORONARY BYPASS PATIENT

The postinfarction patient who has successful coronary bypass surgery also needs appropriate sodium restriction and adherence to a Prudent diet. Atherosclerosis may progress more rapidly in bypass graft vessels than in the native circulation. Patients often consider themselves cured because of dramatic relief of symptoms after bypass surgery and must be carefully counseled on their nutritional needs.

CONGESTIVE HEART FAILURE

The nutritional management of congestive heart failure (CHF) comprises several aspects. Sodium restriction to reduce fluid retention and cardiac workload is essential in the management of CHF. (See Chapter 19.) A patient in severe cardiac failure may require a sodium restriction of 500 mg per day, while patients with moderate failure may tolerate as much as 2 to 3 g sodium per day. It is important to control obesity with a restricted calorie intake in order to reduce cardiac workload. Diuretic and digoxin therapy are commonly used in the management of CHF, and serum potassium levels are usually followed closely to guard against hypokalemia and associated digitalis toxicity. Small, frequent feedings may be useful in the case of severe cardiac failure. Alcohol depresses myocardial contractility and should not be consumed in excess by the CHF patient. The use of caffeine is controversial, but it should not be used if there is a history of MI or cardiac arrhythmia.

TO TEST YOUR UNDERSTANDING

10. Explain the potential dangers of routinely using a sodium-restricted diet for all MI patients in the acute phase.

11. In physiological terms, what is the rationale for a sodium-restricted diet in CHF?

CONSIDERATIONS IN NUTRITIONAL COUNSELING

DIET MODIFICATIONS

Nutritional counseling of patients with cardiovascular disease involves the guiding of dietary behavior to achieve weight control and a modified intake of sodium or fat or a combination of both. The process of changing life-long eating habits is slow. It is usually best accomplished with gradual changes in eating patterns and by enlisting the support of family members to help prevent a relapse in eating patterns. Teaching about the composition of processed foods and about how to read food labels are important aspects of counseling patients to modify dietary intakes of fat and sodium. Dietary modifications currently under investigation include the effects on blood lipids of monounsaturated fats such as olive oil and intake of cold water fish which contain omega-3 fatty acids.

Modification of dietary fat intake to lower plasma cholesterol includes reducing the total dietary intake of fat, especially the intake of both cholesterol and saturated fat. In counseling patients to modify their dietary fat intake, it is useful to teach how to compare foods according to their content of cholesterol and saturated fat. The *cholesterol–saturated fat index* (CSI) is a simple formula which allows patients to make these food comparisons (13). The CSI of a food can be calculated according to the equation:

$$\text{CSI} = (1.01 \times \text{saturated fat}) + (0.05 \times \text{cholesterol}) \quad \textbf{(20-2)}$$

where saturated fat is given in g and cholesterol is given in mg. A lower CSI indicates that the food has less cholesterol and saturated fat. For example, we can compare the CSI of fish versus ground beef. A 3½ oz portion of cooked fish contains 66 mg cholesterol and 0.2 g saturated fat; this contrasts with a cholesterol content of 92 mg and a saturated fat content of 12.5 g for the same amount of 30-percent-fat beef. The CSI for the fish is 4, while that of the beef is 18. The CSI can be a useful tool for teaching modification of dietary fat intake, as it allows a comparison of foods in terms of their relative contents of cholesterol and saturated fat.

MEASURING ADHERENCE TO A FAT-MODIFIED DIET

Assessing adherence to a fat-modified diet can be difficult because a number of changes in food intake are usually involved. The nutritional counseling program of the Multiple Risk Factor Intervention Trial (MRFIT) has developed a system entitled Food Record Rating (FRR) (14). The FRR can be used to assess an individual's average daily intake of fat and cholesterol and to predict the relative effect of specific changes in eating habits on blood lipids.

FRR is based on a scoring system of classifying foods containing saturated fat, polyunsaturated fat, or cholesterol according to the food's predicted blood cholesterol-raising or cholesterol-lowering effect. This is called *blood lipid effect*, or *B-value*. A food with a positive B-value has an excess of saturated fat or cholesterol over polyunsaturated fat and will raise blood cholesterol more than a food with a lower B-value. The B-value of a food is calculated from its lipid composition using the equation

$$B = 0.475 \, (\text{SFA} - 0.5 \, \text{PFA}) + 0.02 \, \text{CHOL} \quad \textbf{(20-3)}$$

where SFA and PFA represent saturated and polyunsaturated fat as g per food portion and CHOL represents cholesterol in mg per food portion.

Complete instructions for using the FRR system can be obtained from the Department of Health and Human Services (14). The use of the system on an individual basis requires sufficient time and an intelligent, highly motivated client. Application of the system to group instruction has been reported to be useful.

Another alternative for evaluating type and amount of fat intake utilizes a food grouping system developed jointly by the National Heart, Lung, and Blood Institute and the U.S. Department of Agriculture (15). This grouping system was originally developed to identify food use patterns in various population groups but may be applied to individuals or small groups.

OTHER CHANGES IN LIFE-STYLE

In counseling patients who have, or who are at risk of developing, cardiovascular disease, it is important to be aware of other changes in life-style, in addition to dietary changes, that may be necessary. Ideally, an attempt to prevent heart disease through reduction of risk factors should be a primary objective. The three variables which have the strongest correlation with premature coronary heart disease include high blood cholesterol, high blood pressure, and cigarette smoking. Other risk factors include diabetes, obesity, a sedentary life-style, stress, and a family history of premature coronary heart disease. The initial assessment can help identify the risk factors that are pertinent to an individual and the modifications that may need to be considered in nutritional counseling. Counseling on stopping smoking, taking antihypertensive medication, or starting an exercise program is frequently integrated with nutritional counseling.

TOPICS FOR FURTHER DISCUSSION

1. Demonstrate the use of the FRR system using a sample menu of choice.
2. Describe principles of nutritional support for a cardiac transplant patient.
3. Compare and evaluate the most recent recommendations on diet for prevention of cardiovascular disease.
4. Discuss and describe procedures for establishing counseling programs on diet for prevention of cardiovascular disease.
5. Discuss principles of childhood nutrition for long-term prevention of atherosclerosis.

REFERENCES

1. HYPERTENSION DETECTION AND FOLLOW-UP PROGRAM CO-OPERATIVE GROUP. Five-year findings of the hypertension detection and follow-up program. *J.A.M.A.* 242:(1979)2562–2577.
2. McCARRON, D.A., J. STANTON, H. HENRY, AND C. MORRIS. Assessment of nutritional correlates of blood pressure. *Ann. Intern. Med.* 98:(1983)715–720.
3. WOLF, I., N. RAPER, AND J. ROSENTHAL. USDA activities in relation to the sodium issue: 1981–83. *Food Tech.* 37:(1983)59–63.
4. FREDRICKSON, D.S. AND R.I. LEVY. *Dietary Management of Hyperlipoproteinemia: A Handbook for Physicians and Dietitians.* National Heart and Lung Institute. DHEW Publication No. (NIH) 80-110, 1980.
5. CONSENSUS CONFERENCE. Lowering blood cholesterol to prevent heart disease. *J.A.M.A.* 253(1984), 2080–85.
6. U.S. DEPARTMENT OF HEALTH AND HUMAN SERVICES, PUBLIC HEALTH SERVICE, NATIONAL INSTITUTE OF HEALTH, LIPID METABOLISM BRANCH, NHLBI. *The Lipid Research Clinic: Population Studies Data Book,* Vol. 1. Bethesda: NIH Publication No. 80-1527, 1980.
7. CONNOR, W.E. AND S.L. CONNOR. The dietary treatment of hyperlipidemia: Rationale, technique and efficacy. *Med. Clin. N. Amer.* 66:(1982)485–518.
8. AMERICAN HEART ASSOCIATION. Recommendations for the treatment of hyperlipidemia in adults. *Arteriosclerosis* 4:(1984)445A–468A.
9. SCHAEFER, E.J. AND R.I. LEVY. Pathogenesis and management of lipoprotein disorders. *N. Eng. J. Med.* 312:(1985)1300–1310.
10. HEGSTED, D.M. Serum-cholesterol response to dietary cholesterol: a re-evaluation. *Am. J. Clin. Nutr.* 44:(1986)299–305.
11. LIPID RESEARCH CLINICS PROGRAM. The lipid research clinics coronary primary prevention trial results 1: Reduction in incidence of coronary heart disease. *J.A.M.A.* 251:(1984)351–374.
12. NUTRITION COMMITTEE, AMERICAN HEART ASSOCIATION. Dietary Guidelines for Healthy American Adults. American Heart Association, Dallas, 1986.
13. CONNOR, S.L., J. GUSTAFSON, S. WILD, N. BECKER, D. FLAVELL, AND W.E. CONNOR. *The Cholesterol–Saturated Fat Index of Foods: A Description of their Atherogenicity.* Abstract XIII, International Congress of Nutrition. Brighton, U.K., August 1985.
14. *Heart to Heart: A Manual on Nutrition Counseling for the Reduction of Cardiovascular Disease Risk Factors,* eds. C. Raab and J.L. Tillotson. Publ. No. 83-1528. Washington: NIH, 1983.
15. BREWER, E.R., N. KASSIM, F.J. CRONIN, B.H. DENNIS, R.J. KUCZMARSKI, S. HAYNES, AND K. GRAVES. Food group system of analysis with special attention to type and amount of fat—methodology. *J. Am. Diet. Assoc.* 87-(1987) 584–92.

ADDITIONAL SOURCES OF INFORMATION

GRUNDY, S.M., D. BILHEIMER, H. BLACKBURN, W.K. BROWN, P.O. KWITEROVICH JR., F. MATTSON, G SCHONFELD, AND W.H. WEIDMAN. Rationale of the Diet-Heart Statement of the American Heart Association: Report of the Nutrition Committee. *Circulation* 65:939A–854A, 1982.

NATIONAL INSTITUTES OF HEALTH. *Lowering Blood Cholesterol: A Consensus Report.* Washington: NIH, 1984.

NATIONAL INSTITUTES OF HEALTH. *Treatment of Hypertriglyceridemia.* NIH Consensus Development Conference Summary. *Arteriosclerosis* 4:296–301, 1984.

Nutrition and Heart Disease, ed. E.B. Feldman. New York: Churchill Livingstone, 1983.

Rehabilitation of the Coronary Patient (2d ed.), eds. N.K. Wenger and H.I. Hellerstein. New York: Wiley, 1984.

CASE STUDY VIII   CARDIOVASCULAR DISEASE

Part I: Presentation

Present Illness: Jim C. is a 42 y.o. engineering technician referred to his family physician for evaluation of arterial hypertension detected during a preemployment examination and confirmed one week later. He relates no prior history of elevated BP but had been warned to "watch his weight." He denies current symptoms of chest pain, shortness of breath (SOB), edema, or visual symptoms. He smokes one pack of cigarettes a day and plays tennis once or twice a week. His body weight has been steadily increasing by 2 to 4 pounds per year for the last ten years.

Past Medical History: He had measles, mumps, and chickenpox in childhood, and an appendectomy approximately 20 years ago. There is no history of rheumatic fever, diabetes, or kidney disease.

Family History: Father died at 48 years of age from an acute MI, and mother is being treated for essential hypertension.

Social History: Has two children; wife works as a legal secretary.

Review of Systems: Patient has no complaints except for occasional mild tension headaches.

Physical Exam: General: somewhat overweight white male; 5 ft, 10 in, 180 #, small frame. BP 155/103, right arm, sitting, without postural changes. P 76 and regular. R 15. HEENT—fundoscopic exam revealed normal A-V ratio, no A-V nicking, with flat discs and no hemorrhages or exudates. Neck without thyromegaly, venous distention, or bruits. Lungs clear to P&A. Heart—regular rhythm, without murmur or gallop. Abdomen slightly obese, soft, and without bruit. Extremities revealed no edema. Screening neurological exam, including mental status exam, is completely WNL.

Laboratory: Hct 51%, Hgb 15.8 g, glucose 118 mg/dl. BUN 18 mg/dl. Cholesterol 280 mg/dl, Triglyceride (fasting) 120 mg/dl, HDL-cholesterol 30 mg/dl. U/A negative for glucose, protein, and blood. EKG revealed normal sinus rhythm with a rate of 80, normal intervals, and no evidence of ischemia, strain, or hypertrophy. CXR was unremarkable.

Impression: Essential hypertension in a 42 y.o., slightly obese, otherwise healthy male with a positive family history of CHD.

Plan: Nutrition Clinic referral for instruction in 1,500-kcal, 2-g-sodium Prudent diet. Encourage cessation of smoking and increase in exercise. RTC in 2 weeks for BP check.

QUESTIONS

You are the dietitian for the Nutrition Outpatient Clinic associated with the local University Hospital. Mr. C. comes to you for initial dietary counseling with a physician referral which reads as follows: Instruct in 1,500-kcal, 2-g-Na Prudent diet. You have access to his medical chart as outlined in Part I.

1. List 4 major points or areas that you will need to explain to Mr. C. in order for him to follow a 2-g-Na diet.

2. List 3 major points or areas that you will need to explain to Mr. C. in order for him to follow a Prudent diet.

3. List the points you will stress when teaching Mr. C. how to use an exchange meal plan.

4. Calculate a 1,500-kcal, 2-g-Na Prudent diet meal plan for home use for Mr. C., using Form CC and the low-Na diabetic exchange lists provided in your diet manual. You may find it helpful to add a column to Form CC to summarize the Na content of the exchange lists. Consult Table 19-3 for approximate values of Na content for the exchange lists. Assume that Mr. C. has decided to stop smoking and has no major food preferences other than a distaste for nonfat milk and the need to take a lunch to work.

Form CC

Calculating a Meal Pattern

Total Kcal _____
Carbohydrate   (% kcal) _____ (g) _____
Protein   (% kcal) _____ (g) _____
Fat   (% kcal) _____ (g) _____
Division of Carbohydrate: _____

Daily Meal Pattern

Exchange	# of exchanges	Protein (g)	Fat (g)	Carbohydrate (g)
*Milk—nonfat, low fat, whole				
Fruit				
Vegetable				
Subtotal				
Bread/Starch				
Subtotal				
*Meat—lean, medium, high fat				
Fat				
TOTAL				

*Circle the one used in calculating the meal pattern.

Distribution of Exchanges at Meals and Snacks

Exchanges	Total # of exchanges	Breakfast	AM Snack	Lunch	PM Snack	Dinner	HS Snack
Milk		( )	( )	( )	( )	( )	( )
Fruit		( )	( )	( )	( )	( )	( )
Vegetable		( )	( )	( )	( )	( )	( )
Bread		( )	( )	( )	( )	( )	( )
Meat		( )	( )	( )	( )	( )	( )
Fat		( )	( )	( )	( )	( )	( )
Total		( )	( )	( )	( )	( )	( )

5.   Using Equation 20-1, calculate Mr. C.'s LDL-cholesterol level, and comment on his potential risk of cardiovascular disease.

6. Summarize your observations, assessment, and plan of action in a SOAP note.

Part II: Medical Management of Hypertension

Mr. C. keeps his F/U appointments and is evaluated several times in the next 2 months. He successfully quits smoking and reduces his sodium intake, but he gains approximately 5 #. PE reveals a weight of 185 #, and BP of 152/99; other assessment factors are unchanged. He is considered to have failed dietary and exercise management of his hypertension and is started on hydrochlorothiazide (HCTZ) 50 mg po qd, in addition to maintaining his

1,500-kcal, 2-g-Na Prudent Diet, with a suggested K intake of 125 to 275 mEq/day. He is also referred back to the Nutrition Clinic for follow-up. His medical record states:

Problem 1: Essential Hypertension
Problem 2: Excess Body Weight

QUESTIONS

You see Mr. C. in Nutrition Clinic for F/U 10 weeks after your initial consultation. He has started HCTZ, now weighs 186 #, and has a recent serum K of 4.0 mEq/L. He tells you that he has stopped using salt but is always hungry since he quit smoking. A 24-hr diet recall reveals the following intake (assume that no added salt is used in preparation):

Breakfast:
- 1 c apple juice
- 3 c puffed cereal
- 1½ c low-fat milk
- 2 c coffee

Lunch:
- 2 tuna sandwiches (4 slices bread, 1 c water-packed tuna, ¼ c mayonnaise)
- large apple
- 1 small candy bar
- Diet cola

Dinner:
- 2 broiled, skinned chicken breasts (7 oz total meat)
- Large baked potato
- 1 T margarine
- 1 c green beans
- Tossed salad
- 2 T oil for dressing
- ½ c ice cream

7. a. Compare the content of the 24-hr recall to the diet prescription (1,500-kcal, 2-g-Na Prudent diet, 125 to 175 mEq K/day). (Use Form DD, Table B-5, and a handbook on food composition to assist with your intake calculations.)
   b. List the major differences between the prescribed and reported intake.

8. What *positive* feedback can you give Mr. C. regarding his dietary intake?

Form DD

Food Intake Calculation Guide

Food	Kcal	Portion	CHO (g)	Pro (g)	Fat (g)	Na (mg)	K (mEq)	Cholesterol (mg)
Total								

% kcal as CHO _____
% kcal as Pro _____
% kcal as Fat _____

Part III: Angina

Mr. C. continues F/U with his physician. His BP is maintained with HCTZ at 130–140/86–92 during repeated visits. He starts smoking again approximately 4 years after stopping, manages to reduce his weight to 175 #, and generally adheres to a low-cholesterol, low-fat, 3–4-g-Na diet. A repeat cholesterol determination after nutritional counseling and weight loss is 210 mg/dl.

Approximately 10 years after his initial presentation, Mr. C. at age 52 begins to notice vague retrosternal discomfort during moderate physical activity, which he describes as a dull, heavy sensation that always subsides after a few minutes of rest. PE at this time is again essentially unchanged, and he has normal blood chemistries. An EKG shows mild left ventricular strain, and a treadmill stress test is considered equivocal. Nitroglycerin (NTG), 0.4 mg sublingually prn for chest pain and before exercise, is prescribed. He notices an improved exercise tolerance with NTG.

Mr. C.'s medical record now contains the following problem list:

Problem 1: Essential Hypertension
Problem 2: Excess Body Weight
Problem 3: Angina

Part IV: Myocardial Infarction

At age 55, the patient reports a 3-hr history of severe retrosternal pain associated with SOB, which occurred while he was painting a room in his house. This pain is only partially relieved with NTG and radiates to his jaw and left arm. There is also associated diaphoresis, nausea, and light headedness, but he denies palpitations.

On PE he is found to be moderately overweight and extremely anxious. BP is 115/90, P 96, and R 28 and regular. Skin is dusky, cold, and moist. Fine rales are heard in both lung bases, and there is a dyskinetic pulse at the fifth intercostal space lateral to the midclavicular line. Peripheral pulses are symmetrical but of decreased volume. There is an audible fourth heart sound. His EKG reveals ST-segment elevation and a poor R-wave progression in the anterior precordial leads.

Laboratory tests reveal a white count of 12,500, with a normal differential, cholesterol of 200 mg/dl, and triglycerides of 180 mg/dl. His CPK on admission is 125 units. (Normal is less than 150.)

Mr. C. is admitted to the CCU to R/O MI, and is given oxygen at 2 L per minute by nasal passage prongs, minidose subcutaneous heparin, parenteral morphine sulfate, and a prophylactic lidocaine drip. During his first day in the hospital, his CPK peaks at 677, with an MB isoenzyme fraction of 11 percent, confirming the diagnosis of MI. He has no recurrence of chest pain and only occasional ventricular premature contractions.

Mr. C.'s medical record now contains the following problem list:

Problem 1: Essential Hypertension
Problem 2: Excess Body Weight
Problem 3: Angina
Problem 4: Chest Pain → MI

His CCU diet orders include the following:

Day 1: 2 g Na, clear liquid, no caffeine, 6 small feedings of no more than 360 ml each.
Day 2: 2 g Na, 1,200 kcal, soft, low cholesterol, low fat (Prudent diet), no caffeine, 6 feedings, with fluids restricted to 360 ml per feeding.
Day 3 and on: 2-g-Na, 1,200-kcal Prudent diet, no caffeine.

His activities follow routine protocol with bed rest until he is transferred from the CCU to the general ward on day 3. He then begins a program of rehabilitation, with passive exercises followed by progressive ambulation. He is discharged from the hospital on the tenth day, fully ambulatory, with instructions to limit his activity to leisurely walking with a slowly progressive exercise program. He is again strongly encouraged to stop smoking and told that his prognosis is generally favorable. The patient has lost 5 # during hospitalization and now weighs 170 #. He is discharged on a 2-g-Na Prudent diet as well as NTG, propranolol, and HCTZ. He returns to work 5 weeks after his MI.

Angiography is performed 2 months after hospital discharge to evaluate the status of the coronary arteries. The angiogram reveals a 70% occlusion of the right coronary artery and distal lesions of the left circumflex artery. Since surgery (coronary artery bypass graft [CABG]) has not been shown to be superior to medical management in patients with this pattern of atherosclerosis, medical management is continued.

QUESTIONS

9. Discuss the significance of the WBC and CPK levels and the MB isozyme level.

10. Is a cholesterol determination valid in the immediate postinfarction period? Answer *yes* or *no*, and explain your answer.

11. Explain the rationale and, where appropriate, the nutritional significance of the following therapies:

a. Oxygen by nasal prongs

b. Lidocaine

c. Morphine sulfate

d. Heparin

e. Propranolol

f. Hydrochlorothiazide

g. Nitroglycerin

12. Why is caffeine eliminated from the diet?

13. Explain the rationale for a calorie restriction of 1,200 kcal and small feedings with limited fluids in the post- (5—8 days) infarction period.

Part V: Congestive Heart Failure

Over the next 15 months, Mr. C.'s angina is controlled on the above regimen, with pain occurring approximately once every 2 to 3 weeks and easily controlled with sublingual NTG. He then presents with symptoms of increasing SOB and DOE. PE at that time reveals BP of 142/85, with bilateral rales a quarter of the way up from the lung bases and 2+ bipedal edema. Cardiac exam reveals an audible third heart sound and evidence of increased CVP. He is felt to have moderate CHF, and to his problem list is added

Problem 5: Congestive Heart Failure

The propranolol is stopped, and digoxin 0.125 mg/day is started. Symptoms of SOB and DOE persist, and the HCTZ is stopped and furosemide begun. Mr. C. finally becomes stable on digoxin, with 80 mg of furosemide po every AM and continued adherence to a 2-g-Na Prudent diet. Routine evaluation, approximately 2 months after initiation of this therapy, reveals a serum K of 3.0 mEq/L. After a trial of increasing dietary K intake, Mr. C. is begun on a 10% KCl solution, 1 T po b.i.d.

QUESTION

14. What is the primary nutritional concern with combined use of the drugs digoxin and furosemide?

Part VI: Cardiac Cachexia

Mr. C. decides to retire at age 62 due to increasing weakness and SOB. He succeeds in quitting smoking and generally follows his diet, but he never increased his activity level after his first MI. His weight progressively decreases. At age 66 he weighs 145 # and is becoming increasingly weak and losing muscle mass. Medical management with adjust- ment of drug dosage is continued, as Mr. C. is not a surgical candidate. The diagnosis of early cardiac cachexia is made. His medical record states

Problem 6: Cardiac Cachexia

QUESTIONS

15. What is cardiac cachexia and what are potential mechanisms associated with its occurrence?

16. Describe an appropriate diet for Mr. C. now that he is in the early stages of cardiac cachexia.

21

Liver Disease and Alcoholism

The liver plays a key role in the digestion and intermediary metabolism of nutrients. Liver disease directly affects nutritional status and frequently necessitates dietary modifications of protein, fluid, and sodium intake. The most widespread and significant liver disease in the United States is alcohol-related. Cirrhosis is usually the end stage of liver disease. Ninety percent of all cirrhosis in the United States is secondary to alcoholic liver injury. This chapter discusses nutritional assessment, dietary management, and methods of feeding the patient with liver disease.

NUTRITIONAL IMPLICATIONS OF LIVER DISEASE

Diseases of the liver are often associated with malnutrition. Malnutrition reflects inadequate food intake and, with advancing liver disease, alterations in the digestion, absorption, and metabolism of nutrients.

Poor dietary intake is the principal cause of malnutrition in alcoholic liver disease (1). Reduced food intake in alcoholics is a result of both socioeconomic considerations and anorexia secondary to hepatic dysfunction and the high calorie content of alcohol. Individuals with alcoholic cirrhosis primarily consume carbohydrates, with inadequate amounts of protein, vitamins, and minerals. Folic acid is the vitamin most often deficient in the diet of cirrhotics (2). This deficiency is manifested by reduction in plasma and red cell folate values with or without megaloblastic anemia. Inadequate intake and altered metabolism of thiamin and pyridoxine also frequently occur. Thiamin deficiency can be associated with Wernicke-Korsakoff syndrome or cardiac beriberi in alcoholics. In addition, dietary deficiencies of zinc, vitamin A, riboflavin, and nicotinic acid are also commonly associated with alcohol abuse (3).

Individuals with liver disease due to alcoholism frequently demonstrate both maldigestion and malab-

sorption. Evidence suggests that alcohol results in reduced exocrine pancreatic secretion, damage to the intestinal mucosa, and a specific interference in thiamin and folate absorption. Steatorrhea is the most common manifestation of malabsorption in cirrhotics. Loss of fat calories and deficiency of the fat-soluble vitamins both result from steatorrhea. Possible causes of steatorrhea in patients with liver disease include lipase and bile salt insufficiency, diminished intestinal absorption of long-chain fatty acids, and drug administration.

Drugs used in the treatment of liver disease which contribute to steatorrhea include neomycin, lactulose, and cholestyramine. Neomycin and lactulose are used to treat hepatic encephalopathy by reducing ammonia production. Neomycin decreases the content of ammonia-producing organisms in the intestinal flora and may be associated with mucosal toxicity and fat malabsorption. Lactulose traps nitrogen and increases its fecal loss, but often causes an osmotic diarrhea. Cholestyramine, used to reduce itching in jaundiced patients, is a bile salt chelator, which may cause steatorrhea by limiting fat hydrolysis and absorption.

NUTRITIONAL ASSESSMENT

A careful nutritional assessment of dietary, clinical, anthropometric, and biochemical data is necessary before designing a dietary regimen for the patient with liver disease.

DIETARY

Long-standing alcohol abuse is frequently the cause of chronic pancreatitis and chronic liver disease. Whether or not these alcohol-related diseases occur depends on the pattern and duration of alcohol abuse, intake of other hepatotoxic drugs, diet, and other poorly understood factors. Alcohol-related symptoms of pancreatitis and cirrhosis can appear after 15 to 30

(±10) years of heavy alcohol consumption in excess of 150 g per day (4). To evaluate the risk of alcohol-related liver disease, it is important that the dietary assessment include an evaluation of the pattern, quantity, and duration of alcohol intake, the usual dietary intake, and the various socioeconomic factors affecting eating habits.

Determination of an individual's alcohol intake requires information on the onset of excessive drinking, the frequency and quantity of alcohol intake, which alcoholic beverages are consumed, and how and where these beverages are consumed. This information may be obtained from the patient or from a reliable friend or family member. Table 21-1 contains an Alcohol Intake Questionnaire designed to elicit this information (4).

The Alcohol Intake Questionnaire should be evaluated to determine intake of alcohol in grams and caloric value of the alcohol intake. Alcohol yields 7 kcal per g and in large quantities can supply the majority of the day's calorie intake, resulting in little intake of nutrient-rich foods. The average percent alcohol content based on weight per volume of various forms of alcohol is as follows: beer, 4 to 6 percent; wine, 9 to 12 percent; and distilled alcohol such as whiskey, rum, gin, or brandy 35 to 50 percent.

Alcohol concentration of distilled beverages is often expressed as "proof"; one proof equals 0.5 percent alcohol. For example, 80-proof whiskey contains 40 percent alcohol. Distilled alcohol is customarily measured in a "jigger," which is 1½ oz, or 45 ml. Two jiggers, or approximately 3 oz, or 90 ml, of 80-proof whiskey would provide 36 g alcohol and 252 kcal according to the following calculation:

$$3 \text{ oz} \times 30 \text{ ml/oz} \times (40 \text{ g}/100 \text{ ml}) = 36 \text{ g alcohol}$$

$$36 \text{ g alcohol} \times 7 \text{ kcal/g} = 252 \text{ kcal}$$

Beverages used for mixing with distilled alcohol also must be included to estimate daily calorie intake.

A combined alcohol-food record for a drinking day should be obtained to check information on alcohol consumption patterns and to show the relationship between eating and drinking patterns. You could obtain a 24-hour recall if the previous day had been a drinking day, or simply ask the patient to describe usual food intake on a drinking day. A daily alcohol-food record for an alcoholic with compensated liver disease is shown in Table 21-2. Based on this example, you can see why marasmus and specific vitamin and mineral deficiencies are common in this population.

Further assessment of dietary intake is best obtained using a food-frequency questionnaire (4). This will give information on foods consumed or not consumed, which, coupled with further questioning, will give a clue to potential maldigestion or malabsorption. In addition to fat malabsorption, lactose intolerance is common in individuals with excess alcohol consump-

TABLE 21-1.   Alcohol Intake Questionnaire

1. How many days a week do you drink alcoholic beverages? (Circle number of days)
    0 <1 1 2 3 4 5 6 7
2. Where do you drink?
    a. at home
    b. at a friend's home
    c. at a bar
    d. at work
    e. in the car
    f. other (specify) _____
3. Which alcoholic beverages do you consume? (Circle letters.)
    a. beer
    b. table wine
    c. fortified wine (sherry, port)
    d. gin
    e. whiskey
    f. vodka
    g. rum
    h. other (specify) _____
4. How do you determine how much you drink? (Circle letter(s) to indicate all methods that apply.)
    a. I count the number of beer cans.
    b. I count the number of wine glasses.
    c. I count the number of shots of liquor I pour.
    d. I count the number of bottles of wine.
    e. I count the number of bottles of liquor I use per day or week.
    f. I don't know exactly how much I drink.
    g. Other method of determining alcohol intake (specify)

Further information about current alcohol intake can be obtained from answers to the following questions which pertain to drinking days:

5. On any drinking day, how many drinks do you usually have? (Circle letter(s) indicating drinks consumed and number within each category consumed to indicate number of drinks in that beverage category per day.)

a.	beer	1	2	3	4 >5
b.	table wine	1	2	3	4 >5
c.	port wine	1	2	3	4 >5
d.	gin	1	2	3	4 >5
e.	whiskey	1	2	3	4 >5
f.	vodka	1	2	3	4 >5
g.	rum	1	2	3	4 >5
h.	other (specify) _____	1	2	3	4 >5

6. For how long have you been drinking this quantity?
7. Do you drink this amount regularly or sporadically?

Adapted from Roe, D.A. and A.B. Lasswell. Nutritional assessment and assessment tools. In *Nutrition for Family and Primary Care Practitioners*, eds. A.B. Lasswell, D.A. Roe, and L. Hochheiser. Philadelphia: George F. Stickley Co., 1986.

tion. It is also important to know whether the patient is taking a multivitamin-mineral supplement and specific fat-soluble vitamin supplements, such as vitamin A or protein supplements, which could worsen liver pathology. A screening for intake of drugs that are hepatotoxic or that influence nutrient absorption, such as neomycin or lactulose, should be done.

Because individuals who abuse alcohol have a tendency to deny their drinking problems, they will often give fictitious information about food and alcohol consumption. When obtaining an alcohol-food record, it is important to pose open-ended questions, and to phrase them several ways, in order to double-check

TABLE 21-2. Sample Alcohol-Food Record

Time	Place	Beverage or Food	Amount
6 AM	Home	Whiskey	3 shots*
7 AM	Home	Coffee, black	3 c
9 AM	Office	Coffee, black	1 c
11 AM	Office-restroom	Whiskey	3 shots
Noon	Restaurant	Chili	1½ c
		Saltines	6 crackers
		Coffee, black	1 c
5 PM	Bar	Wine	750 ml—10% alcohol, W/V
		Pretzels	12
7 PM	Home	TV dinner	1
10 PM	Home	Beer	3-12 oz cans

*shot = 1½ oz. 80-proof whiskey

the accuracy of information. Completing a food-frequency questionnaire after obtaining the alcohol-food record is one way of doing this; another approach is to double-check information with reliable family members or significant others. Professionals who work with alcoholics often advise that self-reported intakes of alcohol be *doubled.*

It is also important to be aware of various dietary risk factors associated with the development of alcohol-related diseases. A history of a high fat intake increases the risk of developing pancreatitis in individuals with a chronic intake of excess alcohol (5). For example, individuals who consume 150 g per day of alcohol for 10 or more years in conjunction with more than 100 g per day of fat have an increased risk of developing chronic pancreatitis.

A history of a high intake of alcohol or a high consumption of both salt and alcohol is associated with an increased incidence of hypertension. Asking the alcoholic if he salts food when eating in a restaurant can give an indication of preference for salty foods. The patient who goes on alcohol binges without eating increases the risk of acute metabolic crises, including thiamin-dependent cardiac beriberi, Wernicke's encephalopathy, hypoglycemia, porphyria, and hepatic encephalopathy.

CLINICAL

Because protein-energy malnutrition is common in individuals with excessive alcohol intake, it is not unusual to find clinical manifestations of avitaminosis and mineral and trace element deficiencies in this population. A summary of clinical symptoms associated with nutrient deficiencies is found in Tables F-13 and F-14. Clinical symptoms of peripheral edema and ascites should be monitored to assess fluid and sodium needs. Symptoms of encephalopathy are used to assess tolerance to dietary protein and to alter daily protein intake. The symptoms of hepatic encephalopathy include central nervous system changes ranging from asterixis, or "flapping tremor," loss of coordination,

TABLE 21-3. Clinical Stages of Hepatic Encephalopathy

Stage	Mental Status	Asterixis	EEG
I	Euphoria/depression, mild confusion, slurred speech, disordered sleep	±	Usually normal
II	Lethargy, moderate confusion	+	Abnormal
III	Marked confusion, incoherent speech, sleeping but rousable	+	Abnormal
IV	Coma; may or may not respond to noxious stimuli	−	Abnormal

Reprinted with permission from J.T. Lamont, R.S. Koff, and K.J. Isselbacher. Cirrhosis. In *Harrison's Principles of Internal Medicine* (10th ed.), eds. R.G. Petersdorf et al. New York: McGraw-Hill, 1983, p. 1815.

decreased mental alertness, confusion, and restlessness in the early stages to loss of consciousness, convulsions, and coma in the late stages (6). A summary of the various clinical stages of hepatic encephalopathy is outlined in Table 21-3.

The clinical symptoms of Wernicke's encephalopathy, an alcohol-related disorder associated with thiamin deficiency, differ from those of hepatic encephalopathy. Every patient with a history of alcohol abuse and poor nutritional status should be screened and treated for Wernicke's encephalopathy. Clinical features of this disorder include a triad of ocular abnormalities, especially horizontal nystagmus, ataxia and a global confusional state (7). The global confusional state is manifested by apathy, impaired awareness of the immediate situation, spatial disorientation and an inability to concentrate. Eighty percent of patients with Wernicke's encephalopathy develop Korsakoff's psychosis, which is characterized by amnesia. Wernicke's encephalopathy can be induced by intravenous infusion of glucose in the presence of marginal thiamin stores (8). This is why a parenteral thiamin dose of 50 mg q.d. is usually routinely given to alcoholics during the first few days of admission.

ANTHROPOMETRIC

Body weight is often unreliable in patients with liver disease due to fluid imbalances associated with edema and ascites. Body weight can be increased by as much as 10 kg in cirrhotics with both ascites and peripheral edema. Skinfold measurements are also often unreliable because of edema. Monitoring of daily weight changes and urinary output, and measurement of abdominal girth are often used to assess diuresis in cirrhotic patients with ascites.

BIOCHEMICAL

Several biochemical indices relate to nutritional status and dietary management of the patient with liver disease. Serum levels of nutrients relevant to carbohydrate, protein, and fat metabolism may be altered with liver disease. Hypoglycemia is common in acute liver disease possibly due to impaired glycogenesis, glycogenolysis and gluconeogenesis. Hyperglycemia is often observed with cirrhosis and chronic hepatitis and may be associated with increased glucagon levels and an insensitivity to insulin. Hepatic steatosis, mild steatorrhea (10 g of fat or less per day), and decreased plasma lipoprotein levels are all associated with hepatic necrosis and cirrhosis.

Alterations in plasma parameters of nitrogen metabolism have the most clinical significance. Hepatic synthesis of albumin and clotting factors are reduced in liver disease, resulting in low serum albumin (less than 2.8 g per dl) and low serum transferrin (under 150 mg per dl) values. Reduced albumin levels can lead to edema and ascites, and interference with synthesis of clotting factors can cause problems with blood coagulation and delayed PTT and PT times. In addition, albumin and transferrin levels are not an accurate reflection of the influence of diet on visceral protein status in the patient with liver disease. BUN levels are reduced and ammonia levels are increased in liver disease due to decreased hepatic urea synthesis. Nitrogen balance is generally not accurate when calculated based on UUN levels in patients with liver disease. Total urinary nitrogen, not UUN, should be used when calculating nitrogen balance in these patients. In the patient with ascites, reduced urine output, and lactulose therapy, the calculation of nitrogen balance is not accurate.

Excessive protein intake in a patient with altered nitrogen metabolism due to liver disease can lead to hepatic encephalopathy. The cause of hepatic encephalopathy is thought to be a result of altered protein metabolism, but the exact mechanism is controversial. The distorted amino acid profile of patients with chronic liver disease is suggested to play a role in the development of encephalopathy, and forms the basis of specialized enteral- and parenteral-feeding products. In patients with chronic liver disease, plasma levels of aromatic amino acids, including phenylalanine, tyrosine, and tryptophan, as well as methionine, glutamine, and aspartate, are elevated, and levels of the branched-chain amino acids (BCAA) leucine, isoleucine, and valine are usually depressed.

Plasma levels of vitamins and minerals are often depressed in chronic liver disease. Thiamin deficiency, which is particularly a problem, is associated with reduced RBC transketolase activity and symptoms of peripheral neuropathy. Assays to determine blood levels of vitamins and minerals are summarized in Table F-15. Nutrition-dependent forms of anemia, particularly folate deficiency–megaloblastic anemia and pyridoxine deficiency-sideroblastic anemia, are common in alcoholics. The differential diagnosis of anemia is summarized in Table F-16.

TO TEST YOUR UNDERSTANDING

1. Analyze the alcohol-food record presented in Table 21-2 for the following nutrients (show your calculations):

	Amount
Alcohol	_____ g
Alcohol energy	_____ kcal
Total energy	_____ kcal
% energy as alcohol	_____ %
Protein	_____ g

   b. In what vitamins and minerals is this intake likely to be inadequate?

2. a. Define *ascites* and, in anatomical terms, explain where the fluid accumulates.
   b. Explain how the following factors contribute to the development of ascites and edema in the patient with advanced liver disease:

   (1) Increased portal hydrostatic pressure
   (2) Decreased plasma oncotic pressure
   (3) Direct movement of albumin into the free peritoneal space
   (4) Increased sodium retention mediated by aldosterone secondary to a decreased effective plasma volume

3. Joe Smith is a 40 y.o. alcoholic with a 15-year history of excessive alcohol intake. He lives alone and works as a bookkeeper. Mr. Smith seeks medical attention because of a severe cold and also complains of a sore tongue and loose bowel movements. A slight generalized peripheral edema is noted. Additional data are as follows:

Hgb	11 g/dl
Hct	35%
MCV	110 FL

Serum folate	1.5 ng/ml
RBC folate	70 ng/ml
Serum B_{12}	600 pg/ml
Ht/Wt	5 ft 9 in, 165 #
Albumin	3.0 g/dl

He admits to consuming a pint of vodka and a six-pack of beer per day for the past 10 years. He dislikes most vegetables, eats mainly fried foods, avoids dairy products because of gas and diarrhea, and likes salty foods. Mr. Smith eats mainly convenience foods, especially canned soups, and frequently eats at fast-food restaurants.

The physician prescribes folic acid, 5 mg t.i.d. for 14 days, and a multivitamin-mineral supplement. The physician arranges for Mr. Smith to contact Alcoholics Anonymous (AA) and also asks you to speak with Mr. Smith regarding a low-lactose, low-fat, 3-g-sodium diet.

a. Describe Mr. Smith's anemia and any associated clinical symptoms.

b. Explain why a low-lactose, low-fat, 3-g-sodium diet was prescribed for Mr. Smith.

c. What difficulties would you predict that Mr. Smith would have in following such a diet?

d. Estimate Mr. Smith's daily intake of alcohol. (Show your calculations.)

_____ g alcohol/day
_____ kcal from alcohol/day

e. What interpretation can you make about Mr. Smith's diet in terms of visceral protein status?

DIETARY MANAGEMENT

The goals of nutritional support of patients with hepatic failure include maintenance of adequate nutrition, enhancement of liver regeneration, and the recovery and prevention or amelioration of hepatic encephalopathy (9). Abstinence from alcohol is an essential part of management of alcohol-related liver disease. Modifications of protein, sodium, fluid, fat, and carbohydrate intake are often necessary for dietary management of patients with alcoholic liver disease. Consideration of the texture of the diet is a concern in patients with portal hypertension and esophageal varices. A multivitamin-mineral preparation should be routinely provided for patients with chronic liver disease, especially if it is alcohol-related. Parenteral thiamin is usually given to alcoholics during the first few days of admission (100 to 200 mg b.i.d.). Vitamin K should also be given parenterally to patients with liver disease in whom prothrombin time is depressed.

PROTEIN

The quantity of protein allowed in the diet varies with the degree of hepatic injury. A protein intake that permits positive nitrogen balance and hepatic repair without symptoms of protein intolerance should be given. Severe protein restrictions of 10 g or less per day are generally not necessary and may be harmful if used for more than a few days due to an enhanced net loss of lean body mass. A calorie intake of 35 to 45 kcal per kg per day is needed in order to decrease endogenous protein catabolism to meet energy needs.

We will consider the protein needs of patients with the following stages of liver disease: hepatitis without significant hepatic damage, stable liver disease with cirrhosis, decompensated chronic cirrhosis, and hepatic encephalopathy with protein intolerance.

Patients with hepatitis are often anorectic and nauseated, yet protein and energy needs are generally high. Protein intakes of 1.5 to 2.0 g pro per kg and 3,000 to 4,000 kcal per day are usually provided to allow for hepatic repair. The patient with stable liver disease and underlying cirrhosis can usually tolerate a moderate protein intake of up to 1 g pro per kg per day. With decompensated chronic cirrhosis and mild hepatic encephalopathy (stage I), 0.5 to 0.7 g pro per kg "dry" or usual body weight is often given (10). In patients with protein intolerance and severe hepatic encephalopathy progressing to coma, protein intakes may be reduced to 0 to 20 g per day, and then gradually increased by 5 to 10 g every 2 to 3 days. Lactulose and neomycin therapy are also important for decreasing ammonia production in these patients. An alternative to offering a gradually increasing protein intake is to give BCAA-enriched, low-aromatic-amino-acid formulations. At this point, studies have demonstrated that *some* patients with encephalopathy demonstrate dramatic improvement when BCAA-enriched formulas are used (11). The efficacy of these formulas is the subject of current research.

The decision to offer a certain protein intake to a patient with liver disease is an empirical one. All patients must be monitored for signs of protein intolerance, such as the development of encephalopathy, as discussed earlier, in the nutritional assessment section of this chapter.

The form in which protein is given is also important. Cirrhotic patients may tolerate the protein from dairy and vegetable products better than fleshy animal proteins (12), perhaps because vegetable proteins contain less methionine and fewer aromatic amino acids than do other proteins. They may also change the bacterial flora of the gut. Because of the suggested role of ammonia in the pathogenesis of hepatic encephalopathy, foods that contain preformed ammonia are usually omitted in diets prescribed for these patients. These foods include various cheeses, salami, bacon, ham, ground beef, and gelatin (13).

FLUID AND SODIUM

Fluid and sodium are restricted in order to ameliorate edema and ascites formation. The sodium restriction is generally more severe than that used in renal and cardiovascular disease. Sodium intakes are often limited to 500 mg sodium or less per day in patients with ascites because the use of diuretic drugs must be limited in cirrhotic patients, and also because patients with severe ascites may excrete only 30 mg or less of sodium per day. Fluid may be restricted to a volume equivalent to the previous day's urine output in order to effect a net loss of body water, or it may simply be limited to 1,000 to 1,500 ml per day. Bed rest is another important aspect of treatment for ascites. The objective of fluid and sodium restriction in the patient with ascites is to effect a weight loss of 0.5 to 1.0 kg per day (14). There is a great deal of individual variation in the use of fluid and sodium restriction to manage these patients. Guidelines for planning a fluid- and sodium-restricted diet are included in Chapter 19.

FAT, CARBOHYDRATE, AND TEXTURE

Fat intake may need to be modified in the patient with liver disease in order to ameliorate nausea or steatorrhea. Patients with hepatitis are often nauseated when fat intake exceeds 100 g per day. Most patients with liver disease can tolerate 150 to 200 g of dietary fat per day without adverse effects (10). Patients with severe jaundice and decreased bile excretion may need dietary fat restriction until enterohepatic circulation returns to normal. Severe steatorrhea—that is, greater than 30 g per day of fat in the stools—usually improves with a reduction in fat intake coupled with MCT supplementation. Patients with fat malabsorption frequently need fat-soluble vitamin supplementation.

Carbohydrate intake is generally not a problem in liver disease, with the exception of lactose intake in patients with malabsorption. Small, frequent meals often alleviate the hypoglycemia which accompanies acute hepatic injury. The impaired glucose tolerance observed with chronic liver disease and cirrhosis may be better managed with enteral formulas that are supplemented with glucose polymers.

A modification of dietary texture is needed for the patient with esophageal and gastric varices. A soft diet is thought to avoid damage to the mucosa and resultant gastrointestinal bleeding. A soft, low-fiber diet may cause constipation, however, and straining at the stool can precipitate variceal rupture and hemorrhage. Therefore, a soft, fiber-enriched diet should be encouraged in patients with esophageal varices. Lactulose will also reduce constipation. Meals should be small and frequent, and patients should be advised to eat slowly and chew their food thoroughly.

METHODS OF FEEDING

Oral intake is the preferred method of feeding the patient with liver disease. Unfortunately, anorexia and nausea usually make it difficult to achieve the high-energy (35 to 45 kcal per kg), moderate-protein (1 g per kg), high-vitamin diet needed by most patients with stable liver disease. In these cases, enteral tube feeding or parenteral feeding are used to meet nutrient needs. An algorithm for formulating a nutritional management plan for the patient with liver disease is shown in Figure 21-1.

ENTERAL FEEDING

Tube feeding may either augment limited oral intake or serve as the sole method of feeding in patients with hepatic disease and a functioning GI tract. Standard tube-feeding formulations, such as Isocal, Ensure, or Osmolite, can be used for patients without encephalopathy or significant protein intolerance. If fluid restriction is required, formulas with a caloric density of greater than 1 kcal per ml, including Magnacal, Ensure Plus, or Travasorb STD, may be needed. Nasogastric bolus or continuous-infusion feeding may be used in patients without encephalopathy.

In patients with encephalopathy, specialized tube feedings which can be adjusted to individual tolerance are needed. Quantities of protein, sodium, fluid, and fat can be easily varied with modular feedings. Modular tube feedings are designed using individual components of protein, carbohydrate, lipid, vitamins, and minerals. Another, simpler approach to modular feeding is to dilute a concentrated formula, such as Magnacal, with a carbohydrate (Polycose) and fat (Microlipid) source to achieve a desired composition. Frequent modification of protein intake is needed in encephalopathic patients. A patient may start with a protein intake of 25 to 35 g per day and gradually advance by 5 to 10 g increments to 60 to 80 g of protein per day. Modular formulas facilitate these frequent changes in protein intake. BCAA-enriched formulations may be used in those patients who do not tolerate gradual advancement of formulas with standard amino acid composition; examples of these products include Hepatic-Aid and Travasorb Hepatic. Continuous nasoduodenal tube feeding is indicated in encephalopathic patients to reduce the risk of aspiration.

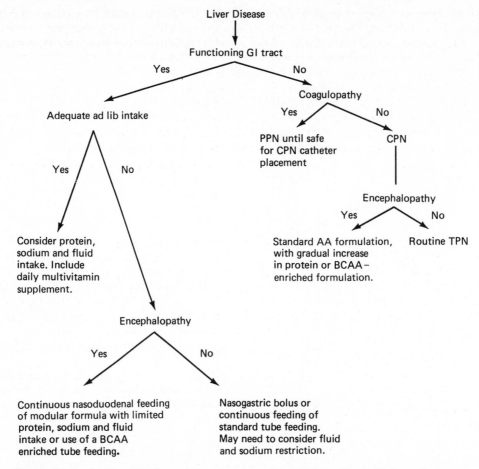

Figure 21-1   An algorithm for nutritional management of the patient with liver disease.

PARENTERAL FEEDING

Parenteral feeding is used in patients with liver disease in the absence of a functioning GI tract. Patients with coagulopathy require peripheral parenteral nutrition (PPN) until normal blood coagulation returns and it is safe to place a central parenteral nutrition (CPN) catheter. Standard total parenteral nutrition (TPN) solutions can be used in patients without encephalopathy. However, these patients need to be monitored carefully for the onset of encephopathy, edema, fluid retention, ascites, glucose intolerance, and electrolyte abnormalities.

Patients with encephalopathy who require TPN present management problems. They are at high risk for sepsis, are often carbohydrate intolerant, and are especially susceptible to the hepatic complications of TPN itself, steatosis, and fibrosis. TPN should be initiated with gradually increasing quantities of protein from standard intravenous amino acid solutions. Protein intake should be increased until estimated protein requirements are met or until encephalopathy intervenes, in which case protein concentration should be reduced. In patients unable to tolerate an adequate protein intake, BCAA-enriched amino acid solutions may be given. These formulations should be used with caution, however, because they are costly and of questionable benefit to the majority of patients.

TO TEST YOUR UNDERSTANDING

4. Recommend an appropriate daily protein intake for the following situations:

g pro/kg usual weight

   a. an individual with chronic cirrhosis who enters the hospital for elective surgery   _____

   b. an otherwise healthy teenager who contracts hepatitis from food prepared by a sick food service worker   _____

   c. a patient with stage I hepatic encephalopathy   _____

5. An alcoholic with stage III hepatic encephalopathy and moderate ascites is admitted. She is started on lactulose. A meat-free, 20-g-pro, 1-g-Na, 2,500-kcal diet with a 1,500-ml fluid restriction is ordered for her. By day 3 of admission, asterixis is less pronounced, and the patient is more alert and speaking more coherently. The physician advances her dietary protein intake to 30 g per day.

   a. Why was a 20-g-pro, meat-free diet initially prescribed?

   b. How well would you predict that this patient would be able to consume her prescribed diet?

   c. What role does lactulose play in the patient's therapy?

   d. What clinical data did the physician use to reach a decision to advance her protein intake?

   e. If the patient had been on a lactose-free tube feeding instead of oral intake, and if diarrhea developed and persisted, would this indicate that the tube feeding was not tolerated? Explain.

6. A 70-kg alcoholic with hepatitis is to receive 2,400 ml per day of Isocal by continuous NG infusion. What is the projected nutrient intake for this patient?

   a. _____ kcal/kg/day

   b. _____ g pro/kg/day

   c. Is this adequate for hepatic repair? _____

7. A patient with alcoholic liver disease usually weighs 154 # (dry weight) but, because of ascites and peripheral edema, now weighs 186 #. The physician initially tries to promote diuresis in this patient by a combination of bed rest, a 500-mg-Na diet, and fluid intake limited to 1 L per day. Weight loss averages ½ # per day, but abdominal girth is reduced by only 1 cm per day on this regimen. The physician decides to add spironolactone, 25 mg q.i.d., to the treatment plan in order to enhance diuresis. This is undertaken cautiously, however, because in patients with end-stage liver disease, a "brisk" diuresis can result in decreased renal function and hypokalemic acidosis, which enhances the development of encephalopathy.

   a. Approximately how much excess fluid is associated with the 32 # increase above usual body weight? (Give answer in liters.)

   b. If the development of hypokalemic acidosis is of concern, why is spironolactone a good diuretic to use?

   c. What rate of daily weight loss might be considered excessive and potentially dangerous in this patient?

8. A modular BCAA-enriched tube feeding is ordered for a patient in hepatic coma. The order for the formula is as follows:

   1,000 ml
   30 g amino acid–high branched chain
   500 mg Na
   2,000 kcal

Your institution stocks the Nutrisource products for such purposes (see Table G-2). The amino acid mixture comes in 15.4 g packets providing 15 g of amino acids (44 percent BCAA) without electrolytes. Calculate a recipe for the prescribed modular tube feeding by completing the following table.

Nutrisource Modules	Amount	CHO (g)	Pro (g)	Fat (g)	Kcal	Na (mEq)
Amino Acids–High Branched Chain	pkg					
Carbohydrate	ml					
Lipid–LCT	ml					
Vitamins	pkg					
Minerals for AA– Electrolyte Restricted	pkg					
NaCl	g					
Total Volume	ml					
Totals:						
% Kcal						

TOPICS FOR FURTHER DISCUSSION

1. What are the nutritional implications of the cardiac and GI complications of alcoholism?

2. Discuss nutritional care in hepatitis.

REFERENCES

1. MEZEY E. Liver disease and nutrition. *Gastroenterology* 74:(1978)770–783.
2. LEEVY, C.M., H. BAKER, W. TENTLOVE, O. FRANK, AND G.R. CHERRICK. B-complex vitamins in liver disease of the alcoholic. *Am. J. Clin. Nutr.* 16:(1965)339–346.
3. Liver disease. In *Nutritional and Metabolic Support of Hospitalized Patients*, eds. M.A. Bernard, D.O. Jacobs, and J.L. Rombeau. Philadelphia: Saunders, 1986, pp. 192–213.
4. ROE, D.A. Nutritional deficiencies and excesses: People at risk. In *Nutrition for Family and Primary Care Practitioners*, eds. A.B. Lasswell, D.A. Roe, and L. Hochheiser. Philadelphia: George F. Stickley Co., 1986, pp. 115–150.
5. DURBEC, J.P. AND H. SARLES. Multicenter survey on the etiology of pancreatic disease. *Digestion* 18:(1978)337–350.
6. LEEVY, C.N., A. THOMPSON, AND T. BAKER. Vitamins and liver injury. *Am. J. Clin. Nutr.* 23:(1970)493–499.
7. REULER, J.B., D.E. GIRARD, AND T.G. COONEY. Wernicke's encephalopathy. *N. Eng. J. Med.* 312:(1985)1035–1039.
8. SCHENKER, S., G.I. HENDERSON, A.M. HOYUMPA, AND D.W. MCCANDLESS. Hepatic and Wernicke's encephalopathies: Current concepts of pathogenesis. *Am. J. Clin. Nutr.* 33:(1980)2719–2726.
9. FISCHER, J.E. AND R.H. BOWER. Nutritional support in liver disease. *Surg. Clin. N. Amer.* 61:(1981)653–660.
10. JACOBS, D.O., M.C. BORAAS, AND J.L. ROMBEAU. Enteral nutrition and liver disease. In *Enteral and Tube Feeding*, eds. J.L. Rombeau and M.D. Caldwell. Philadelphia: Saunders, 1984, pp. 376–402.
11. CHRISTIE, M.L., D.M. SACK, J. POMPOSELLI, AND D. HORST. Enriched branched-chain amino acid formula versus a casein-based supplement in the treatment of cirrhosis. *J.P.E.N.* 9:(1985)671–678.
12. GREENBERGER, N.J., J. CARLEY, AND S. SCHENKER. Effect of vegetable and animal protein diets in chronic hepatic encephalopathy. *Am. J. Dig. Dis.* 22:(1977)845–855.
13. RUDMAN, D., R.B. SMITH, A. SALAM, W.D. WARREN, J.T. GALAMBOS, AND J. WENGER. Ammonia content of food. *Am. J. Clin. Nutr.* 26:(1970)487–490.
14. LAMONT, J.T., R.S. KOFF, AND K.J. ISSELBACHER. Cirrhosis. In *Harrison's Principles of Internal Medicine* (10th ed.). eds. R.G. Petersdorf, R.D. Adams, E. Braunwald, K.J. Isselbacher, J.B. Martin, & J.D. Wilson. New York: McGraw-Hill, 1983, p. 1815.

ADDITIONAL SOURCES OF INFORMATION

ANTONOW, D.R. AND C.J. MCCLAIN. Nutritional support in alcoholic liver disease. *J.P.E.N.* 9:(1985)566–567.

FISHER, M.M. AND C.C. ROY. *Pediatric Liver Disease*. New York: Plenum, 1983.

Liver and Biliary Disease, eds. R. Wright, G.H. Millward-Sadler, K.G. Alberti, and S. Karran. Philadelphia: Saunders, 1985.

PATTISON, E.M. AND E. KAUFMAN. *Encyclopedic Handbook of Alcoholism*. New York: Gardner Press, 1982.

Symposium: Interactions of Alcohol and Nutrition. *Alcoholism: Clin. Exper. Res.* 7:(1983)2–34.

Symposium on ethyl alcohol and disease, ed. M.C. Geokas. *Med. Clin. N. Amer.* 68:(1984)1–255.

CASE STUDY IX   ALCOHOLIC LIVER DISEASE

Part I: Presentation
Present Illness: Mr. A.A. is an anxious 35 y.o. who presents to his physician's office with complaints of loss of appetite, abdominal pain, blood-tinged vomitus, and general malaise for the past 10 days.
Past Medical History: Unremarkable except for a stated daily consumption of a 6-pack of beer and 1 to 2 shots of whiskey for 10 years. No medications or nutritional supplements.
Social History: Married with two children, age 7 and 10 years. Self-employed as a computer software expert.
Examination: Jaundiced white male with hepatomegaly; 5 ft, 10 in; 82 kg; medium frame. BP 120/70; P 65, regular; R 15; T 101° F.

Laboratory: Hgb 13 mg/dl; Hct 45%
MCV = 106 FL
TIBC = 500 µg/dl
Albumin = 3.1 g/dl

Prothrombin time—prolonged
Hepatic enzymes: SGOT = 1,200 U/ml
SGPT = 1,000 U/ml
Alkaline phosphatase = 45 King-Armstrong U
Bilirubin = 17.0 mg/dl
Serum amylase = 300 Somogyi units/dl
Urinary amylase/24 hr = 3,000 Somogyi units
Lipase = 1.0 Cherry-Crandall U/ml

Impression/Plan: Alcoholic hepatitis. Pancreatitis and gastritis are also possible diagnoses, but 24-hr urinary amylase excretion indicates that pancreatic function is WNL. Admit to hospital for additional diagnostic tests and treatment of hepatitis. Diet Rx: 3,000 kcal, 150 g protein, plus a daily multivitamin-mineral supplement.

QUESTIONS

You ask Mr. A.A. to complete the Alcohol Intake Questionnaire in Table 21-1. You then obtain a 24-hr alcohol-food record from Mr. A.A. based on a typical "drinking" day. To check the accuracy of the alcohol-food record, you also elicit food-frequency intake information. Mr. A.A.'s 24-hr alcohol-food record is as follows:

6:00 AM	1 shot whiskey		2 oz potato chips
7:00 AM	8 oz orange juice		2 beers (12 oz cans)
	1 fried egg	5:00 PM	4 beers
	2 slices toast with butter and jelly	7:00 PM	1 chicken leg (thigh and drumstick)
	2 c coffee (black)		½ c mashed potato with gravy
10:00 AM	1 c coffee (black)		½ c peas and carrots
	1 doughnut		½ c chocolate ice cream
12:30 PM	1 tuna sandwich	9:00–11:00 PM	3 shots whiskey and water

1. Estimate Mr. A.A.'s daily alcohol intake based on the alcohol-food record just presented.

_____ g alcohol/day
_____ kcal from alcohol/day

2. Which alcohol intake information is probably the most reliable, yours or the data presented under "Presentation"? Explain.

3. How does Mr. A.A.'s alcohol-food record relate to the possible diagnosis of
   a. pancreatitis

   b. gastritis

4. What three aspects of Mr. A.A.'s dietary intake might affect his hematological status?
   1.

   2.

   3.

5. a. Why is a high-calorie-high-protein diet ordered for Mr. A.A.?

b. Why might Mr. A.A. have trouble consuming this diet?

c. How might you ensure that Mr. A.A. receives his prescribed nutrient intake?

Part II: Decompensated Chronic Cirrhosis

Ten years later, Mr. A.A. is brought to the local hospital Emergency Room by the police, who have found him wandering around downtown. He appears unkempt, smells of alcohol, and is noted to have impaired mental status.

Social History: Mr. A.A.'s business went bankrupt 3 years ago, and his wife divorced him shortly afterward. His drinking has been steadily increasing during the past 5 years. He presently lives alone in an apartment and supports himself with part-time computer programming work at a local bank.

Examination: RUQ pain secondary to hepatomegaly, abdominal tenderness with ascites, peripheral edema, and mild asterixis. Present weight 78 kg. Usual weight 73 kg.

Laboratory Studies:

Hgb = 11 mg/dl; Hct = 35%
MCV = 105 FL

Albumin = 2.5 g/dl
Prothrombin time—prolonged
SGOT = 450 U/ml
SGPT = 300 U/ml

Impression/Plan: Probable alcoholic cirrhosis with impending delirium tremens (DTs). Admit for alcoholic detoxification and liver biopsy.

Orders: Thiamin 100 mg IV b.i.d. × 3 days
Lactulose
Librium for DTs
Strict bed rest with cloth restraints
Daily multivitamin-mineral supplement

Diet: Lactose-free tube feeding of 1,200-ml total volume to provide 1 g Na, 0.5–0.7 g pro/kg, and 35–45 kcal/kg. Administer via continuous drip #8 French nasoduodenal silastic feeding tube.

QUESTIONS

6. Calculate Mr. A.A.'s nutrient needs according to his usual or dry weight and the diet Rx. Provide a rationale for each of the four dietary parameters.

Rationale

a. Protein _____ g

b. Kcals _____

c. Fluid _____ ml

d. Sodium _____ mg

7. Your hospital does not carry a tube-feeding formula that meets Mr. A.A.'s diet Rx. The decision is made to modify a high-kcal formula. Show the procedure for doing this by completing parts a–e.
a. Which formula would you use? Why?

_____ ml of _____ = _____ kcal
_____ g pro
_____ mg Na

b. Which two carbohydrate sources could you use?

_____ or _____

Which one is most appropriate for the diet Rx? Why?

_____ =   _____ kcal
                                      _____ g pro
                                      _____ mg Na

e?

_____ =   _____ kcal
                                      _____ g pro
                                      _____ mg Na

_____ (formula)
_____ (CHO)
_____ (lipid)

_____ g pro _____ mg Na _____ ml volume

and minerals, or is a supplement needed?

8. Calculate a Nutrisource modular tube feeding, based on a usual weight of 73 kg, as follows: 1,200 ml, 1 g Na, 0.6 g pro/kg, 40 kcal/kg. Provide one-half the lipid as LCT and one-half as MCT to enhance absorption. Nutrisource Protein is supplied in packages providing 19.8 g of powder, 15 g protein, and 2.3 mEq Na. One package of Nutrisource Minerals for Protein formulas contains 43 mEq of Na. Consult Table G-2 for additional information on the composition of Nutrisource modules.

Nutrisource Modules	Amount	CHO (g)	Pro (g)	Fat (g)	Kcal	Na (mEq)
Protein powder, pkg						
Carbohydrate, ml						
Lipid—MCT, ml						
Lipid—LCT, ml						
Vitamins, pkg						
Minerals for Protein, pkg						
Total volume distilled water, ml						
Totals:						
% Calories:						

9. During the course of his hospitalization, Mr. A.A. progresses to a medically stable condition. He is alert with an appropriate mental status; asterixis is not present. He has returned to his usual weight of 73 kg. After Mr. A.A.'s prothrombin time improves, a liver biopsy is performed. The liver biopsy indicates hepatic steatosis with alcoholic cirrhosis. Mr. A.A. is advised to stop all intake of alcohol and is referred to the local Alcoholics Anonymous group. What diet would you recommend that he be given on discharge?

Part III: Decompensated Chronic Cirrhosis with Portal Hypertension and Encephalopathy

Five years later, Mr. A.A. presents to the E.R. with a life-threatening upper-GI bleed. He appears jaundiced and severely malnourished, has spider angiomata over the face and arm, and is markedly confused, with incoherent speech. He is also ataxic and demonstrates horizontal nystagmus and 3+ asterixis. Severe ascites and peripheral edema are present. Present weight = 75 kg, bilirubin = 20 mg/dl, SGOT = 100 U/ml, SGPT = 93 U/ml, BUN = 45 mg/dl, and creatinine = 1.1 mg/dl.

Impression/Plan: Stage III encephalopathy with documented cirrhosis in an alcoholic who has a 25-year history of alcohol abuse. Suspect esophageal varices secondary to portal hypertension. Esophagoscopy/gastroscopy to verify source of GI bleed. Possible Wernicke's encephalopathy, which will be treated with 50 mg thiamin IVq.d.× 3 days. Lactulose and multivitamins daily. Diet Rx: 2,500-kcal, 20-g pro, 500-mg Na, soft diet with 700 ml fluid restriction when stabilized.

QUESTIONS

10. a. Why is a soft diet with such a severe protein restriction ordered for Mr. A.A.? Why would a tube feeding not be used?

b. What type of protein would you include in the diet plan? Explain.

c. Using Form EE, calculate a meal plan for the prescribed diet.

d. Write a sample menu on Form FF from the plan in Part C.

11. What pertinent clinical symptoms and/or laboratory abnormalities does Mr. A.A. demonstrate in the following areas? (Do not duplicate symptoms in several categories.) What general therapy is used for each area?

	Symptom	Therapy
a. Hepatic encephalopathy		
b. Wernicke's encephalopathy		
c. Portal hypertension		
d. Cirrhosis/hepatic dysfunction		

12. Mr. A.A.'s mental status improves and his encephalopathy progresses to Stage I–II. Diuresis brings him down to a weight of 62 kg, and the fluid restriction is liberalized to 1,200 ml/day. At this point, his protein intake is increased by 5 g every 2 to 3 days. However, he is unable to tolerate a total protein intake greater than 30 g without a deterioration in mental status. When you last spoke with Mr. A.A., when he was receiving a 40-g protein diet, he said that he enjoyed "the lovely Thanksgiving meal"—in July.

Your assessment is that Mr. A.A. is unable to tolerate a maintenance intake of protein to prevent further catabolism of LBM. You suggest to the physician that a BCAA-supplemented formula be gradually introduced into Mr. A.A.'s diet.

You decide to use Travasorb Hepatic formula (see Table G-3), with a gradually increasing intake up to 500 ml/day. If Mr. A.A. receives 500 ml/day of Travasorb Hepatic and also 30 g pro/day from solid foods, what will his total daily intake of protein be?

a. g pro/day from 500 ml Travasorb Hepatic =   _____ g

   g pro/day from diet =   30 g

   _____ Total g pro/day

Form EE

University Medical Center
Protein, Fat, Sodium, and Fluid-Restricted Diet

Prescribed: Pro _____ g;   Fat _____ mg;   Na _____ mg;
              Fluid _____ ml;   _____ kcal
              _____ % HBV = _____ g HBV protein

List	Amount	Pro g	Fat mg	Na mg	Fluid ml	Kcal
Egg						
Meat, Low Na						
High Na						
Dairy						
SUBTOTAL						
Bread, etc.						
Low Na						
Regular						
Vegetable #1						
#2						
#3						
#4						
Fruit #1						
#2						
#3						
Fats, Regular						
Unsalted						
Sweets						
Salt List						
Miscellaneous						
TOTAL						

Meal Plan:

BREAKFAST	Serving	Pro	Fat	Na	Fluid	Kcal
# _____ Fruit						
Meat list, High Na						
Low Na						
Egg						
Bread, Regular						

Low Na _____
Dairy _____
Fats, Regular _____
Low Na _____
Misc. _____

_____

SUBTOTAL _____

LUNCH
Meat list, High Na _____
Low Na _____
Bread list, Regular _____
Low Na _____
_____ Veg list _____
_____ Veg list _____
_____ Fruit list _____
Dairy list _____
Fats, Regular _____
Low Na _____
Misc. _____

_____

SUBTOTAL _____

DINNER
Meat list, High Na _____
Low Na _____
Bread list, Regular _____
Low Na _____
_____ Veg list _____
_____ Veg list _____
_____ Fruit list _____
Dairy list _____
Fats, Regular _____
Low Na _____
Misc. _____

_____

SUBTOTAL _____

SNACKS AND SUPPLEMENTS _____

_____

GRAND TOTAL _____

b. Based on a dry weight of 62 kg, what will his protein intake be in _____ g pro/kg?

c. Explain why the protein in the BCAA supplement would be more likely to be tolerated by this patient.

13. Summarize your assessment and recommendations in a SOAP note.

Form FF

Nonselect Menu

Diet _____

Breakfast	Lunch	Dinner

_____ Margarine
_____ Milk—no fat, low
  fat, whole
Coffee, Tea, Sanka
Salt, Salt Substitute
Pepper
Sugar, Sugar Substitute

Snacks:

_____ Margarine
_____ Milk—no fat, low
  fat, whole
Coffee, Tea, Sanka
Salt, Salt Substitute
Pepper
Sugar, Sugar Substitute

Snacks:

_____ Margarine
_____ Milk—no fat, low
  fat, whole
Coffee, Tea, Sanka
Salt, Salt Substitute
Pepper
Sugar, Sugar Substitute

Snacks:

22

Nutritional Care of the Critically Ill Patient

Critically ill patients are in the acute stages of trauma or disease. These individuals require specialized medical management and nutritional support in order to sustain life. Critical illness can occur in a variety of disease states and conditions, including gastrointestinal, cardiac, hepatic, or renal disease, cancer, burns, trauma, sepsis, and associated surgeries. The degree of stress associated with an illness is an indication of the level of nutritional support which may be needed. Third degree burns, trauma, and sepsis are considered to be the most catabolic or stressful injuries, requiring large calorie intakes to maintain body weight.

Appetite and the ability to digest and absorb food is generally poor, while energy and protein requirements are high in the critically ill patient due to hypermetabolism. Thus, the maintenance of an adequate nutrient intake presents a real challenge for the nutritional care specialist. Nutritional support for the critically ill patient frequently involves the use of supplemental feeding, tube feeding, parenteral feeding, or a combination of these feeding techniques.

In this chapter we will focus on the following areas: nutritional assessment of the critically ill patient, multiple-organ system failure and nutritional support of the critically ill pulmonary patient, nutrition and burn trauma, and nutrition and the cancer patient. The related chapters in your text should be consulted for a review of the metabolic alterations associated with critical illness.

NUTRITIONAL ASSESSMENT

Nutritional assessment of the critically ill patient follows the general principles of anthropometric, biochemical, clinical, and dietary evaluation outlined in Chapters 4 and 5. Many of the standard nutritional assessment tests are affected by stress, however, making their interpretation difficult.

The timing of the nutritional assessment is an important consideration in the critically ill patient (1). An initial assessment within 5 days of admission usually coincides with the peak metabolic response to injury and is thus of limited value, other than in identifying the high-risk patient and in establishing an estimate of calorie and nutrient needs. The stress response to injury usually subsides by the fifth to tenth postinjury day, allowing for a more complete and meaningful "postcatabolism" nutritional assessment. Serial assessment of nutritional status is important during convalescence to adjust nutritional intake as requirements subside with time and healing.

The clinical course of a patient's illness and the degree of stress imposed on the patient determine his nutritional needs. For example, the patient who develops a fistula or becomes septic after surgery is more stressed and requires greater nutritional support than the patient who experiences an uncomplicated postoperative recovery period. Another example would be a patient undergoing therapy for cancer who requires surgery compared to an individual who undergoes the same surgery without a recent history of serious illness. If a comprehensive nutritional assessment cannot be completed on a critically ill patient, an examination of the history of the patient's illness often forms the basis for determination of nutritional needs.

The nutritional evaluation of the critically ill patient will be considered from the standpoint of the following: an initial postinjury assessment and estimation of nutrient needs, a more in-depth postcatabolism evaluation, and long-term serial assessment of the adequacy of the nutritional care plan.

INITIAL POSTINJURY ASSESSMENT

Many of the common anthropometric measurements cannot be used in the five-day postinjury period. A statement of usual preinjury body weight from the patient or family is probably the most useful. Roy and

328

colleagues (2) suggest that percentage of usual body weight is a valid predictor of surgical risk in individual patients. In Roy's sample of 46 high-risk surgical patients, no complications or deaths occurred when the percentage of usual body weight was 94 percent or greater. Measurement of triceps skinfold and arm circumference can provide information on somatic protein and subcutaneous fat stores. However, many serious accidents involve injuries to the upper arm, thus often making these measurements impossible to perform.

During the first few days postinjury, catecholamine production and the glucagon-to-insulin ratio increase catabolism and alter results of various standard biochemical tests used to assess nutritional status (3). For example, the creatinine-height index (CHI) is initially invalid because creatinine excretion is elevated by trauma and stress, and creatinine excretion becomes an indicator of the degree of catabolism rather than of depletion of somatic protein stores (4). Measurement of serum concentrations of transport proteins such as albumin, transferrin. prealbumin, and retinol-binding proteins is also invalid. The sudden increase in protein catabolism that occurs in stress decreases serum concentrations of these proteins. Evaluation of visceral protein status by measurement of serum concentration of transport proteins may not respond to nutritional intervention for up to 20 days postinjury (5). Other factors that will alter serum protein concentrations include administration of blood products (such as albumin, fresh frozen plasma, or whole blood) and iron deficiency (which will induce transferrin synthesis).

Even though serum albumin levels and total lymphocyte count are altered in stress, depressed levels of these parameters have been correlated with increased morbidity and mortality and the need for immediate aggressive nutritional support (6). Since serum albumin and CBC tests are standard orders for most injured patients, they are usually available in the medical record and can be viewed as *rough* indicators of nutritional risk in the postinjury period.

Indicators of immunocompetence, such as lymphocyte count and delayed cutaneous hypersensitivity testing, are also affected by stress and injury. The presence of a large wound or burn may reduce lymphocytes in the serum, and sepsis can cause an elevation in the WBC count so that the absolute total lymphocyte count is invalid (1). Anergy has been associated with trauma, burn injury, and surgery (7).

In summary, the following test results are altered as a result of stress or injury: increased excretion of creatinine, increased WBC count, anergy to skin tests, and decreased serum concentration of transport proteins. Meaningful measures of nutritional status in the immediate postinjury period are primarily limited to anthropometric measurements, a few biochemical determinations, and dietary information, as summarized in Table 22-1.

TABLE 22-1. Initial Nutritional Assessment in the Postinjury Period*

Procedure	Interpretation
Anthropometric	
% usual body weight	Consider a body weight of less than 94% of preinjury weight as suggestive of an increased risk of morbidity and mortality.
Triceps skinfold and arm circumference	If injury permits.
Biochemical	
Serum albumin	Gives a rough indicator of nutritional risk when the history of recent weight change is also considered.
Total lymphocyte count	
Clinical	
History of present illness	May be the only information available; patient may be unable to communicate, and the medical record or family may be the only source of information.
Dietary	
Diet history	Evaluate patient's ability to tolerate various types of nutritional therapies—oral supplement, tube feeding, TPN, or a combination of these as influenced by the extent and location of injury.
24-hour recall	

*0–5 days

The initial postinjury assessment should include an estimate of energy and nutrient requirements and an evaluation of the patient's ability to tolerate various feeding regimens. Feeding regimens for the critically ill patient may include oral intake, tube feeding, TPN, use of a supplemental feeding, or any combination of these approaches. Chapters 11, 12, and 13 include information on indications and procedures for these nutritional support techniques.

Various methods can be used to assess the energy needs of the critically ill patient. The Harris-Benedict equation can be used to calculate BEE with adjustment for an activity and injury factor, as explained in Chapter 4. For the critically ill patient, however, application of an injury factor to the equation may overestimate energy needs, when compared to true energy needs as measured by indirect calorimetry (8). Provision of excessive calories can be especially critical in the patient with respiratory failure, as will be discussed later in this chapter. Chapter 13 includes a discussion of determination of energy and protein needs for critically ill patients who frequently require TPN, and Table 13-3 presents an alternative method for the estimation of energy needs when anthropometric data are not available.

POSTCATABOLISM ASSESSMENT

A more comprehensive and accurate nutritional assessment can be completed once the initial period of peak catabolism subsides and the patient becomes more anabolic. By the sixth to tenth postinjury day, the stress response usually diminishes, with a reduction in the level of catecholamines and the glucagon-to-insulin ratio. Blood volume is usually restored by this time, and massive fluid shifts are generally resolved. In many severe illnesses, such as third-degree burns, trauma, and sepsis, the catabolic phase may last longer than 10 days. Bistrian (9) has described a *catabolic index* (CI) based on urinary urea excretion to assess the stress response to an injury. The CI is calculated as follows:

$$CI = UUN - \tfrac{1}{2}\text{ dietary nitrogen} + 3 \quad (22\text{-}1)$$

where UUN (urinary urea nitrogen) and dietary nitrogen are in g per day. It is interpreted as follows: CI of 0 = no significant stress, CI of 1–5 = mild stress, and CI of >5 = moderate to severe stress. The calculation of the CI compares actual nitrogen excretion with expected nitrogen excretion. The equation assumes that 50 percent of dietary nitrogen is utilized, 50 percent is converted to urea, and 3 g, known as the obligatory nitrogen loss, is excreted even if the patient consumes no protein. Thus, the extent to which the measured UUN exceeds 50 percent of nitrogen intake is an index to assess the degree of stress imposed by an illness. A postcatabolism nutritional assessment could be performed when the CI is less than 5, suggesting that the stress response has subsided.

The postcatabolism nutritional assessment may include the standard components of anthropometric, biochemical, clinical, and dietary information as presented in Chapters 4 and 5.

SERIAL NUTRITIONAL ASSESSMENT

The best continuing evaluation of adequacy of the nutritional care plan consists of a monitoring of daily calorie and nutrient intake coupled with a recording of changes in body weight. Serial evaluation of body weight should be compared with usual preinjury, or postcatabolism, weight to eliminate the effect of fluid resuscitation. A weight change greater than 1 pound per day, or 0.5 kg per day, suggests fluid imbalance that will usually negate the interpretation of serum protein concentration values.

The usual components of a comprehensive nutritional assessment can be repeated on a serial basis. It is also important to reevaluate protein and energy requirements during recovery, as requirements will decrease with time and healing.

Indicators of lean body mass, such as arm muscle circumference and creatinine-height index, are not highly sensitive to changes in somatic protein sources and need be measured no more than every 10 days. If the patient is immobile and physical therapy is not given, lean body mass will probably not increase in spite of aggressive nutritional support (1).

Immunocompetence usually returns after 7 to 10 days in anergic patients when nutritional support is given. A poor prognosis may be anticipated when anergy persists despite aggressive nutritional support.

Nitrogen retention, which reflects adequacy of protein intake, can be estimated by measuring urea nitrogen in a 24-hour urine collection and calculating nitrogen balance using equation 4-29. However, this formula does not take into account abnormal extrarenal nitrogen losses such as commonly occur with burns, extensive soft tissue damage, fistulas, or severe vomiting or diarrhea. The formula can thus underestimate nitrogen losses in critically ill patients who experience abnormal nitrogen losses, and can result in an invalid value for nitrogen retention. Monitoring of daily weight change and of fluctuations in plasma albumin and transferrin levels every 10 to 14 days will help indicate adequacy of protein intake in cases in which calculation of nitrogen balance is not feasible (1).

TO TEST YOUR UNDERSTANDING

1. Rank the following conditions according to the degree of stress and need for nutritional support; 1 = most stressful, in need of aggressive nutritional support, and 5 = least.

   a. A healthy, young, well-nourished patient is scheduled for an elective surgical procedure. _____

   b. A well-nourished patient with recently discovered cancer is admitted to begin aggressive chemotherapy. _____

   c. A 14-year-old male with third-degree burns over 20 percent of his body is admitted to the burn unit. _____

   d. A middleaged moderately wasted patient with severe emphysema is admitted with pneumonia. _____

   e. An otherwise healthy patient with multiple injuries enters the intensive care unit. _____

2. Tell why the following parameters of nutritional assessment are not of value in the described situations.

a. A young comatose male with fractures of both arms secondary to a motorcycle accident, and who has recently received 2 units of whole blood.

Midarm muscle circumference
Dietary interview
Serum transport proteins

b. A septic patient on TPN with a draining abdominal fistula.

Nitrogen balance based on urinary urea excretion
Total lymphocyte count
Daily serum albumin levels

c. A burn victim 5 days postinjury.

Body weight
Creatinine-height index
Delayed cutaneous hypersensitivity testing

3. A trauma victim who has undergone several surgeries for compound fractures is now 8 days postinjury. The patient has an intake of 100 g of protein per day with a 24-hr UUN excretion of 20 g per day.
   a. Calculate the patient's CI.
   b. Would it be appropriate to perform a postcatabolism nutritional assessment at day 8 postinjury for this patient? Explain.

4. You are monitoring the nutritional status of a young woman who has recovered from many of the injuries sustained in a car accident, but who is still comatose. The patient receives 1,600 kcal per day from Osmolite in an intermittent tube feeding. How do you monitor the patient's long-term nutritional status in the following areas:

   a. Overall adequacy of nutrient intake
   b. Lean body mass
   c. Visceral protein

MULTIPLE-ORGAN SYSTEM FAILURE

Patients who survive the immediate effects of severe trauma and those who develop postoperative complications may experience a syndrome known as *multiple organ system failure* (MOSF). MOSF may include a functional collapse of the following systems (10):

1. The lungs, resulting in acute respiratory distress syndrome (ARDS)
2. The kidneys, resulting in acute oliguric renal failure
3. The liver, resulting in cholestatic jaundice and hepatocyte failure
4. The GI tract, resulting in ileus and stress ulceration

MOSF is frequently seen with septic complications following surgery. An individual is more susceptible to MOSF if underlying factors that decrease the body's functional capacity are present. These factors may include nutritional depletion, systemic disease, immune deficits, chronic illness, and a history of smoking or alcohol abuse. Guidelines for the nutritional management of GI, renal, and liver failure which may occur in MOSF are discussed in Chapters 15, 16, 17, 19, and 21.

In the following section we will discuss nutritional therapy for the patient with pulmonary failure, as critically ill patients frequently experience this complication.

THE CRITICALLY ILL PULMONARY PATIENT

Respiratory or pulmonary failure is a clinical diagnosis confirmed by alterations in arterial blood gases (ABGs). *Acute respiratory failure* occurs when the partial pressure of oxygen in arterial blood (PaO_2) is less than 60 mm Hg, and the $PaCO_2$ is greater than 50 mm Hg with an arterial pH of less than 7.30 (11). Normal values are as follows: PaO_2 of 80 to 100, $PaCO_2$ of 35 to 45 mm Hg, and pH of 7.35 to 7.45. Acute respiratory failure is most commonly seen in critical illness or with chronic obstructive pulmonary disease (COPD). *COPD* refers to a group of diseases, including chronic bronchitis and emphysema, which are characterized by irreversible airway obstruction resulting in resistance to airflow during expiration. COPD is the most common form of chronic respiratory illness and the primary cause of death from lung disease (12).

MECHANICAL VENTILATION

The patient with respiratory failure requires mechanical ventilation in order to maintain a blood level of oxygen that meets tissue needs. In order to place a patient on a respirator or mechanical ventilator, intubation or establishment of an airway via the trachea to the lungs is required. The common means of establishing an airway for mechanical ventilation are placement of an orotracheal tube or a nasotracheal tube. A tracheostomy is used when a patient requires a longer course of mechanical ventilation. Adequate oxygenation on a respirator is accomplished by manipulation of the concentration of inspired oxygen (FIO_2) and use of positive end-expiratory pressure (PEEP). PEEP prevents alveolar collapse and enables a lower FIO_2 to be used.

MALNUTRITION AND PULMONARY FUNCTION

The basic problem in respiratory failure is insufficient oxygenation of the tissues coupled with retention of carbon dioxide. With increasing calorie intake and the oxidation of nutrients, both oxygen demand and carbon dioxide production are increased. On the other hand, discontinuation of, or a great reduction in, feeding decreases oxygen demand and carbon dioxide production and reduces the burden on the respiratory system. However, malnutrition further compromises respiratory insufficiency and should be avoided, especially in the ventilator-dependent patient (13).

With malnutrition, the muscles of breathing—that is, the diaphragmatic, intercostal, and accessory muscles—are catabolized for energy, resulting in a decrease in inspiratory capacity. The decrease in serum albumin level which occurs with inadequate protein intake, if sufficiently severe, may cause a decrease in oncotic pressure, leading to pulmonary edema. The central nervous system control of respiration can be impaired by the hypoxia which accompanies starvation.

Malnutrition also depresses clearance of bacteria from the lungs and predisposes to pulmonary infection, to which pulmonary patients are already susceptible. In fact, pneumonia is the most frequent immediate cause of death in starvation. Lung surfactant production is reduced in malnutrition, which can result in decreased compliance, pulmonary collapse, and pneumonia. All these factors suggest that adequate nutritional support is especially important to maintain normal pulmonary function.

RESPIRATORY QUOTIENT

The *respiratory quotient* (RQ) is defined as the ratio of carbon dioxide produced to oxygen consumed. The higher the RQ, the more carbon dioxide is produced to be expired, and the greater the demand on the respiratory system. The RQ is an indication of the type of substrate being metabolized for energy. Protein, carbohydrate, and fat have characteristic RQs when

TABLE 22-2. Respiratory Quotient of Metabolic Fuels

Substrate	Respiratory Quotient (RQ)*
Carbohydrate	
glucose oxidation	1.00
Fat	
triglyceride oxidation	0.71
triglyceride synthesis from:	
glucose	8.70
triglyceride	1.00
amino acids	0.74
Protein	
amino acid oxidation	0.80
Mixed Diet	
carbohydrate, protein, and fat	0.825

*RQ = ratio of the amount of CO_2 expired to the amount of O_2 inspired. An RQ of greater than 1 is considered medically dangerous.

metabolized. Recall the equation for the oxidation of glucose:

$$C_6H_{12}O_6 + 6O_2 \rightarrow 6CO_2 + 6H_2O$$

Thus, 6 molecules of oxygen are used to produce 6 molecules of carbon dioxide. The RQ of glucose oxidation is thus 6/6, or 1.0, a higher amount of carbon dioxide production than is seen with other nutrients. Fat is oxidized with an RQ of 0.7 and is associated with a lesser degree of carbon dioxide production than glucose, while protein has an intermediate RQ value of 0.80. The RQ of a mixed diet is approximately 0.825.

It is also possible for the RQ to be higher than 1, putting an even greater strain on the respiratory system. Triglyceride synthesis from carbohydrate is associated with an RQ greater than 1. Table 22-2 summarizes the RQ of various metabolic fuels.

Increased carbon dioxide production caused by either excessive administration of total calories or adequate administration of total calories composed primarily of glucose will increase the workload of the lungs. When excess calories are reduced or fat replaces carbohydrate as a calorie source, production of carbon dioxide is decreased, and the demands on pulmonary function are also decreased.

WEANING FROM THE RESPIRATOR

Weaning a patient from a respirator is a gradual process which eventually leads to the patient's breathing independently. The PEEP must be 5 cm of H_2O or less before weaning can start, as breathing against PEEP requires extra effort during expiration. The FIO_2 is decreased at a rate of 5 to 10 percent per hour, and PEEP is also gradually decreased.

Two approaches are commonly used in weaning from mechanical ventilation (11). The classical weaning approach involves removing the patient from the ventilator for progressively longer intervals. Another approach involves the use of synchronized intermittent mandatory ventilation (SIMV), which allows the patient to breathe independently as the ventilator delivers a preset number of machine breaths in synchrony with the patient's breaths (8). SIMV serves as a form of graduated active exercise for the respiratory muscles. The patient's progress is evaluated by ABG determinations throughout the weaning process.

Nutritional support plays an important role in weaning a patient from a respirator. In one report (13), 86 percent of ventilator-dependent patients who had received some degree of nutritional support, compared to only 22 percent of those patients who had received only 5 percent dextrose in water, were able to be weaned from mechanical ventilation.

Provision of a calorie level above the maintenance requirement will result in increased carbon dioxide production and difficulty in weaning a patient from a ventilator. For the nutritionally depleted patient on a respirator, such as commonly occurs with COPD, it is sometimes considered to be preferable to continue the patient on the respirator for a longer period, providing a higher level of caloric support for repletion. This allows for restoration of lean body mass, including the muscles of respiration. As a result, respiratory function would be improved and weaning from the respirator would be facilitated.

For both the nutritionally depleted patient and the hypermetabolic patient, a consideration of calorie level and proportion of calories as glucose is essential to facilitate weaning. Monitoring of ABG determinations and RQ values, if available, during the weaning process can be used as a guideline for making changes in the nutrient intake.

NUTRIENT REQUIREMENTS

Energy requirements of the respirator patient can be estimated using the Harris-Benedict equation and an activity and injury factor as previously discussed. Another, simpler method for estimating energy needs is to provide 25 to 35 kcal per kg per day for maintenance and 45 kcal per kg per day for anabolism or maintenance during a catabolic state (8). (See Table 22-3.)

The proportion of calories to be provided as fat or carbohydrate is an important consideration in the respirator-dependent patient. To reduce carbon dioxide production, lipid should provide 30 to 60 percent of total calorie intake. As discussed in Chapter 13, glucose infusion should not exceed 4 to 6 mg per kg per min, especially when the patient is hypermetabolic. A protein intake of 1.5 g per kg per day or 0.2 g N per kg per day is usually adequate. A protein intake of 2.0 to 2.5 g protein per kg may be needed in patients experiencing severe stress due to sepsis, trauma, or burns. Excess protein intake should be avoided when attempting to wean a patient from mechanical ventilation. Patients receiving high protein intakes have been observed to have an increased ventilatory drive, resulting in dyspnea or shortness of breath (8).

Adequate provision of minerals, vitamins, and trace

TABLE 22-3.   Estimated Nutrient Requirements for the Critically Ill Pulmonary Patient

Energy
   25–35 nonprotein kcal/kg/day for maintenance
   45 nonprotein kcal/kg/day for anabolism and maintenance in conditions of severe stress
   30%–60% kcal as lipid, maximum infusion of 4–6 mg/kg/min of dextrose
Protein
   1.5 g protein/kg/day (0.2 g nitrogen/kg/day) or approximately 15% of total calories
   2.0–2.5 g protein/kg/day in conditions of severe stress

elements is also important. Phosphate depletion can result in respiratory failure due to decreased levels of 2,3-diphosphoglycerate concentration in red blood cells. This decrease in 2,3-diphosphoglycerate concentration can cause an increase in oxyhemoglobin affinity and a decrease in oxygen delivery to tissues. Inclusion of phosphate in intravenous solutions in the amounts outlined in Chapter 13 will supply adequate levels of phosphate. Commercial tube feedings or a varied dietary intake will also meet phosphate needs. Table 22-3 summarizes the estimated nutrient requirements for the critically ill pulmonary patient.

METHODS OF NUTRITIONAL SUPPORT

Enteral or parenteral feeding can be used to provide nutritional support for the ventilator-dependent patient. Nutritional support is instituted after the patient has stabilized on mechanical ventilation. Many patients become agitated when first placed on a ventilator and require morphine sulfate for sedation. The morphine can often result in reduced intestinal motility and paralytic ileus.

Parenteral Feeding

TPN is required when the patient has a paralytic ileus or when maximal rest of the intestinal tract is indicated. A nearby tracheostomy can increase septic risk at a subclavian catheter insertion site. Special dressings may be used to protect the catheter insertion site, or the catheter may be tunneled under the skin away from the tracheostomy.

Enteral Feeding

Enteral feedings, rather than TPN, should be used when the gut is functioning. The long-term tracheostomy patient is usually able to eat via the oral route, but may have difficulty swallowing. In ventilator-dependent patients with an orotracheal or nasotracheal tube and a functioning gut, tube feeding is necessary. Tracheal tube cuffs should be inflated during feeding to seal off the trachea and reduce the risk of aspiration. Bolus feeding of formulas is associated with a higher incidence of vomiting, reflux, and aspiration. Continuous feeding or intermittent gravity drip is preferred in the patient on a respirator if tube feeding is necessary.

Consuming a large meal can result in exertion, abdominal distention, and considerable dyspnea for a pulmonary patient. Resting before and after meals may help with fatigue. If the patient is able to eat orally, six small meals per day may minimize respiratory distress. The patient should also be instructed to eat slowly and be given soft, easy-to-chew foods to avoid overexertion during meal times.

Transitional Feeding

Patients maintained on a respirator frequently experience several transitions in feeding technique. These transitions may include a change from parenteral to enteral nutrition, with either ad libitum intake or tube feedings. A transition from TPN to tube feeding is probably the most common type of parenteral to enteral transition in respirator patients. At a later point, most patients maintained on tube feedings eventually consume ad libitum meals with discontinuation of their tube feedings. If a respirator patient is changed from TPN to oral ad libitum intake, an important consideration is the texture of the diet. A soft diet is usually better tolerated because the patient will probably be suffering from a sore throat, which often occurs with intubation for a period of time.

A common rule can be applied to discontinuation of the "old" feeding method—that is, the patient should be receiving at least half of estimated calorie needs by the new feeding method before the old one is discontinued. This ensures that the patient does not experience a significant interruption in nutrient delivery. A calorie count of oral food intake or verification via intake and output sheets of the actual amount of tube feeding received by the patient is needed to determine nutrient intake with the new feeding method.

When a patient is changed from TPN to tube feeding, the site and rate of infusion and the composition of the infusate must be considered. Factors affecting the choice of infusion site—nasogastric, nasoduodenal, or nasojejunal, to name a few—and of rate of infusion—bolus, intermittent, or continuous—are discussed in detail in Chapter 12. The tube feeding should initially be given at half strength. It should also be a lactose-free formula that is low in osmolality (not greater than 600 mOsm per L) and residue because mucosal atrophy and decreased digestive enzyme synthesis occur when enteral feedings are eliminated for more than a week. The tube feeding should be gradually increased and the TPN simultaneously decreased by a comparable volume and energy content. Specific recommendations for initiating a tube feeding and monitoring the tube-fed patient are presented in Chapter 12. In advancing a tube feeding, it is important to avoid simultaneously increasing the volume and the concentration of the formula.

TO TEST YOUR UNDERSTANDING

5. A 50-year-old male is admitted to the emergency room (ER) following a motor vehicle accident. The patient has a history of alcoholism and has smoked two packs of cigarettes per day for the past 20 years. He weighs 55 kg and is 5 ft, 10 in tall. The patient undergoes surgery shortly after admission to the ER. By the third postoperative day, evidence of pulmonary edema and sepsis is present. The patient is started on 24 percent oxygen delivered by a face mask. The following parameters are noted in the chart:

Mental status: disoriented
P: 150
R: 45
BP 170/100
ABG on 24 percent oxygen:
   pH = 7.25
   $PaCO_2$ = 68 mm Hg
   PaO_2 = 43 mm Hg

The patient is diagnosed as having acute respiratory failure. He is intubated and placed on a mechanical ventilator set to provide full ventilatory support. Representative ABGs obtained once the patient is settled on mechanical ventilatory support with 40 percent oxygen are as follows: pH = 7.42, $PaCO_2$ = 53 mm Hg, and PaO_2 = 71 mm Hg.
   a. Suggest three factors that most likely contributed to the patient's acute respiratory failure.
   b. Why was the patient disoriented and why did he demonstrate an elevated heart and respiratory rate before being intubated and placed on mechanical ventilation?
6. a. Rank the following enteral feeding products from highest (1) to lowest (7) percent of total kcals from fat. (Use Appendix G as a reference.)

Ranking

_____Vivonex Standard

_____Ensure

_____Isocal

_____Criticare HN

_____Osmolite

_____Pulmocare

_____Traumacal

b. Which of these formulas could be used as an enteral feeding for a respiratory patient who requires at least 35 percent of total kcals as fat?

7. a. What does the RQ indicate?

b. Can the RQ be used to assess the degree of hypermetabolism that a patient is experiencing? Answer yes or no, and explain your answer.

8. The following situations are associated with difficulty in weaning from mechanical ventilation. Explain how nutrition may affect the weaning process in each case.

a. A cachectic patient with a 10-year history of COPD develops acute bacterial pneumonia and is placed on mechanical ventilation. The patient develops an ileus secondary to morphine sedation and is maintained on peripheral TPN. The solution infused includes 250 ml per day 10 percent fat emulsion and 1 L per day composed of 5 percent amino acids and 10 percent dextrose. A serum phosphorus value of 2.0 mg/dl is determined at the time of weaning.

b. A young, otherwise healthy near-drowning victim is placed on mechanical ventilation and maintained with a tube feeding that provides 45 kcal per kg per day. The RQ is greater than 2.0.

c. A patient is receiving 30 kcal per kg per day of Vivonex tube feeding while being maintained on mechanical ventilation. The RQ is 1.0.

9. A patient on a respirator has been maintained on TPN for the past 15 days. His GI tract is now functioning and the physician asks that you make recommendations to initiate tube feeding. Circle your choices and explain why in the following areas:

a. Tube placement: nasogastric, nasoduodenal, or nasojejunal. Why?

b. Method of infusion: bolus, intermittent, or continuous. Control of infusion rate: hand control or peristaltic pump or pressure clip. Why?

c. Choice of formula: Isocal, Vivonex, Compleat B, or Meritene. Why?

d. Strength, rate: ½ str, 100 ml per hr; full str, 50 ml per hr; ½ str, 25–50 ml per hr; full str, 25 ml per hr. Why?

e. What clinical signs will you watch for to evaluate tolerance of the tube feeding?

f. When should the TPN be discontinued?

BURNS

A severe burn is an extremely catabolic injury, resulting in higher nutritional requirements than any other condition. Burns are associated with increased risk of sepsis, and multiple surgical procedures are usually required during recovery. Both these factors compound the stress and further increase nutrient requirements. In addition, gastrointestinal dysfunction and anorexia may interfere with food intake in the burn patient, and frequent modifications in feeding regimens and techniques are required. Thus, vigorous nutritional support of the burn patient is essential for wound healing and survival.

NUTRITIONAL ASSESSMENT

Assessment of the nutritional status of a burn victim is subject to the same limitations as assessment of the critically ill patient. Massive fluid resuscitation in the first 24 hours after the burn often results in increases in body weight of up to 12 to 15 percent. Preinjury body weight, rather than present body weight, becomes the baseline value in the burn patient. The site of the burn often interferes with anthropometric measurements used to assess somatic protein stores. In addition, frequent infusion of blood products negates the use of plasma transport proteins to assess visceral protein stores in the burn patient.

Monitoring of calorie intake and changes in body weight compared to preinjury weight throughout the recovery period is the most valid approach to monitoring the adequacy of nutrient intake. Limiting weight loss to 10 percent of preinjury weight should be a primary goal of nutritional therapy in the burn patient.

NUTRIENT REQUIREMENTS

In patients suffering burn injury, calorie requirements are directly proportional to the extent of the injury. Protein requirements are also a function of the extent of burn injury, as protein is lost through the burn wound itself. Formulas are available for calculating energy and protein requirements on the basis of burn size. Curreri and colleagues (14) suggest use of the following formulas to estimate the calorie and protein requirements of burn patients:

Adults:

$$\text{Kcal/24 hr} = (25 \text{ kcal} \times \text{kg body wt}) + (40 \text{ kcal} \times \% \text{ body surface area burned}) \quad \text{(22-2)}$$

$$\text{Protein, g/24 hr} = (1 \text{ g/kg of body weight}) + (3 \text{ g} \times \% \text{ body surface area burned}) \quad \text{(22-3)}$$

Children (1 year or older):

$$\text{Kcal/24 hr} = (60 \text{ kcal} \times \text{kg body wt}) + (35 \text{ kcal} \times \% \text{ body surface area burned}) \quad \text{(22-4)}$$

$$\text{Protein, g/24 hr} = (3 \text{ gm} \times \text{kg body wt}) + (1 \text{ gm} \times \% \text{ body surface area burned}) \quad \text{(22-5)}$$

Another approach is to provide a calorie intake of twice the predicted BEE and 1.5 to 2.5 g protein per kg per day for patients who have sustained burns affecting more than 20 to 30 percent total body surface area. (2). The calculated methods just described of establishing energy requirements in the burn patient are, at best, good estimates. These formulas may overestimate energy requirements in the burn patient. Because calorie requirements change throughout recovery from a burn, with skin grafting and wound closure, they should be periodically reassessed.

Some studies suggest that vitamin and mineral requirements increase with burn injury. Vitamin C is usually supplemented to provide 1.0 to 1.5 g per day, and zinc is frequently provided at a level of 2 to 3 times the RDA. There is some evidence to suggest that the requirements for niacin, biotin, pyridoxine, thiamin, and folate are increased with burns. With the exception of vitamin C and zinc, commercial tube feedings and supplemented parenteral-feeding solutions will provide an adequate intake of vitamins and minerals for the burn victim. If the patient is consuming an oral diet, a daily multiple vitamin-mineral supplement should be included.

METHODS OF NUTRITIONAL SUPPORT

The real challenge of providing nutritional care to a burn victim is in devising feeding regimens that can provide large calorie and protein intakes. A variety of feeding techniques are usually incorporated into the nutritional care plan of a burn patient. Most serious burns initially result in a postinjury paralytic ileus. The ileus usually resolves within 48 to 72 hours after admission. At this time, a high-calorie, high-protein diet can be initiated. If a patient is able to eat, a protein-calorie supplement is often required to achieve an adequate nutrient intake. After the first few weeks the appetite usually improves, reducing the need for supplementation.

Enteral Feeding

Patients with burns covering more than 30 percent of the body surface area are seldom voluntarily able to ingest enough food to meet energy needs. For these individuals, tube feeding is required in order to provide an adequate calorie intake or to augment oral intake. In patients with burns of the face and mouth, an adequate oral intake is difficult to achieve, and tube feeding is essential. A tube feeding with a calorie density of 1.5 to 2.0 kcal per ml is usually indicated to achieve the calorie goal in burn patients. A tube feeding with an elemental formula may be useful in patients who have burns on the buttocks and thighs, in order to reduce contamination from stool. Carbohydrate intake should not exceed 4 to 6 mg per kg per min in the burn patient, as discussed in Chapter 13. Because of the high carbohydrate content of most tube feedings, a modular tube feeding may be needed in those burn victims who require over 5,000 kcal per day.

Parenteral Feeding

Parenteral feeding is used when a persistent or recurrent paralytic ileus occurs or when enteral feedings are inadequate. Access sites for a TPN catheter can be limited when a burn covers a large area of the body. Of greatest concern is the increased risk of sepsis in burn patients when TPN is used. Special precautions must be observed when changing dressings at the catheter site. Despite the risk of infection, TPN is frequently used, either alone or in combination with enteral feeding, because nutritional support is essential for these patients' survival.

TO TEST YOUR UNDERSTANDING

Mr. G., a 32 y.o. industrial chemist, was severely burned over much of the trunk, arms, and back in an accident at the chemical plant where he works. After emergency first-aid at the plant, he was transported by ambulance to the University Hospital Burn Center. Mr. G. was admitted to the Burn Center in shock.

Physical Exam: Patient is experiencing pain, but no respiratory distress. Unburned skin is pale and cool. 5 ft, 10 in; 165 # (preinjury); BP 90/60; P 110, weak and thready; R 22 and regular.

Laboratory: The following laboratory tests were ordered: CBC, blood type and cross-match, broad-spectrum screening panel (Table E-11), ABGs, and UA.

Impression: 30 percent BSA second- and third-degree burns over lower part of the face, neck, arms, hands, and upper thighs.

Plan: IV therapy was initiated with Ringer's lactate. A Foley catheter was inserted, and urinary output, P, and BP were monitored hourly. Mr. G. was NPO for the first 48 hours of hospitalization. A nasogastric tube was passed to the stomach for decompression. Maalox was given every 2 hours through the tube.

As soon as the shock was under control, Mr. G.'s wounds were washed with soap and saline, debrided, and dressed with silver sulfadiazine using a fine-mesh gauze. He was given a tetanus shot, and 600,000 U of procaine penicillin were administered every 12 hours.

After 3 days, Mr. G.'s urinary output was 40 to 50 ml per hour, and peristalsis had resumed. NG feedings of 50 ml per hour ½-strength Ensure Plus were initiated. These were advanced to 100 ml per hour full strength Ensure Plus. Mr. G. was encouraged to eat whatever he could.

10. a. Why was Mr. G. NPO for the first 48 hours after admission to the hospital?
    b. Why was an NG tube necessary for decompression?

11. Calculate Mr. G.'s calorie and protein requirements by the following methods. Show your calculations.
    a. Curreri formulas

    _____ kcal
    _____ g protein

    b. Kcals = 2 × BEE, protein = 2.5 gm/kg/day

    _____ kcal
    _____ g protein

    c. Kcals = 50 kcal/kg, protein = establish using a nonprotein kcal to N ratio of 150:1.

    _____ kcal
    _____ g protein

    d. Discuss the accuracy with which these methods predict true calorie requirements for the burn patient.

12. What is the best method of determining whether calorie and protein intake are adequate for a burn patient?

13. Assume that Mr. G. is trying to eat orally despite the burns on his face and hands. He manages to consume approximately 600 kcal per day during meal times. How could his Ensure Plus tube feeding be changed in order to provide approximately 3,000 additional kcal per day and not interfere with his intake at meal times?

14. Assume that Mr. G is undergoing skin grafting and is generally recovering from his burn injury. By 28 days postburn, his weight is 68 kg and he is no longer receiving a tube feeding. Plan a menu for Mr. G. that includes three meals and three snacks, and provides approximately 3,600 kcal and 170 g protein per day. Use the menu for day _____ (day to be assigned by your instructor) and any appropriate supplemental feeding.

NUTRITIONAL CARE OF THE CANCER PATIENT

The nutritional care of cancer patients often involves the use of several different feeding techniques and a wide variety of dietary modifications. The diverse nature of nutritional problems and the high frequency of anorexia makes the delivery of nutritional care to cancer patients one of the most challenging and demanding areas of work for a nutritional care specialist.

In this section we will focus on nutritional assessment of the cancer patient, the common nutritional problems experienced by patients undergoing cancer therapy, and dietary approaches to help solve these common nutritional problems.

NUTRITIONAL ASSESSMENT

In addition to a general nutritional assessment, as described in Chapter 4, the following information is needed to assess the nutrient needs of a cancer patient (3):

1. Site and type of tumor
2. Surgery—type, extent, and findings
3. Chemotherapy—type, dose level, and duration
4. Radiation—site, dose level, duration, and the effect of treatment on gastrointestinal tract function

A careful assessment of the patient's ability to tolerate an oral intake is also needed; this would include the following:

1. the physical ability to ingest food—chewing and swallowing ability, dryness, and soreness or inflammation of oral mucosa secondary to tumor or therapy
2. specific food tolerances—anorexia, appetite fluctuation, nausea and vomiting, allergies, food preferences and aversions, taste changes, and relation of food tolerance to treatments
3. bowel habits—diarrhea, steatorrhea, constipation, and presence of an ostomy.

A careful assessment of a patient's specific dietary intolerances and response to cancer therapy will allow for the development of an individualized nutritional care plan. An individualized approach to each patient's specific food intolerances is one of the most important aspects of successful nutritional management of the cancer patient.

EFFECTS OF CANCER THERAPY

Surgery, radiation therapy, and chemotherapy produce a wide variety of effects that influence eating patterns. Anorexia, nausea, vomiting, diarrhea, loss of taste, aversion to certain foods, and subsequent weight loss are commonly seen with all three types of therapy.

Location and extent of a surgical procedure determine the appropriate modified diet to use. For example, nasogastric tube feeding is required following head and neck surgery, a dumping diet is needed after a gastrectomy, and TPN may be required after radical intestinal surgery.

Radiation therapy is a localized treatment which usually damages normal tissues surrounding the tumor. Irradiation of the oropharyngeal area results in changes in taste buds and taste perception. Reduced salivation, sore throat, dysphagia, and dental deterioration compound eating problems in these patients. Teeth may become overly sensitive to cold, heat, and sweet flavors. Irradiation of the abdomen and pelvis may produce diarrhea, malabsorption, stenosis, and obstruction. A diet restricted in gluten, lactose, fat, and residue may be needed.

Chemotherapy will accentuate preexisting anorexia. Mucositis, stomatitis, esophagitis, severe diarrhea, and an increasing number of food aversions are common. Food aversion is worsened when strongly fla-

TABLE 22-4. Ways to Alleviate Symptoms from Cancer Treatment That Affect Eating Comfort

Symptom	Recommendation
Stomatitis	Avoid spicy and acid foods. Try bland, soft, and liquid diets served at room temperature. Use mouth rinses with local anesthetics, such as lidocaine HCl (e.g., Xylocaine Viscous) before meals.
Mucositis	Use warm saline solution
Xerostomia	Lubricate with food—gravy, butter, margarine, milk, beer, bouillon. Try sugarless gum and sugarless lemon drops. Use synthetic saliva.
Nausea and vomiting	Wrap ice packs around neck. Avoid liquids with meals. Eat cold foods rather than hot. Try small frequent meals. Patients without stomatitis should try lemons or dill pickles. Use antiemetics before meals.
Diarrhea	Use antidiarrheals, such as Lomotil or Kaopectate.

Adapted from Gormican, A. Influencing food acceptance in anorexic cancer patients. *Postgraduate Medicine* 68:(1980) 145–152.

vored foods are served *before* chemotherapy or radiation therapy. Offering blandly flavored foods before treatment may reduce the frequency of food aversions (15).

Approaches to alleviate some of the common food-related problems associated with cancer therapy are summarized in Table 22-4. Chapter 7 discusses dietary modifications for the management of nausea.

FOOD PREFERENCES

Several generalizations can be made about food preferences in cancer patients. There is an increased sensitivity to the tastes of sweet and bitter, resulting in an aversion to sweet foods and hot meats. Tart foods, fruits, vegetables, and most dairy products are better accepted. Liquid beverages and supplements are also popular. In general, cancer patients seem to prefer cold foods or foods served at room temperature to hot foods that formerly were favorites.

TO TEST YOUR UNDERSTANDING

15. A description of common problems experienced by patients undergoing cancer therapy follows. Suggest diet modifications you might recommend in each case.
    a. A patient with ovarian cancer receives radiation to the abdominal area. She experiences diarrhea and vomiting for the first few days after every treatment.
    b. A patient receiving chemotherapy for breast cancer develops mucositis and stomatitis.
    c. A patient undergoes surgery for head and neck cancer and then receives radiation to the oropharyngeal area. Tube feeding is used initially, but when oral intake eventually resumes, the patient experiences a general lack of taste associated with eating.

REFERENCES

1. Jensen, T.G. Determination of nutritional status in critical care. *J. Am. Diet. Assoc.* 84:(1984)1345–1348.

2. Roy, L.B., P.A. Edwards, and L.H. Barr. The value of nutritional assessment in the surgical patient. *J.P.E.N.* 9:(1985)170–172.

3. Quality Assurance Committee of the Dietitians in Critical Care Dietetic Practice Group. *Suggested Guidelines for Nutrition Management of the Critically Ill Patient.* Chicago: The American Dietetic Association, 1984.

4. Gray, G.E. and L.K. Gray. Anthropometric measurements and their interpretation: Principles, practices, and problems. *J. Am. Diet. Assoc.* 77:(1980)534–539.

5. Forse, R.A. and H.M. Shizgal. Serum albumin and nutritional status. *J.P.E.N.* 4:(1980)450–454.

6. Seltzer, M.H., H.S. Fletcher, and B.A. Slocum. Instant nutritional assessment in the intensive care unit. *J.P.E.N.* 5:(1981)70–72.

7. Towmey, P., D. Siegler, and J. Rombeau. Utility of skin testing in nutritional assessment: A critical review. *J.P.E.N.* 6:(1982)50–58.

8. Deitel, M., V.P. Williams, and T.W. Rice. Nutrition and the patient requiring mechanical ventilatory support. *J. Am. Coll. Nutr.* 2:(1983)25–32.

9. Bistrian, B.R. A simple technique to estimate severity of stress. *Surg. Gynecol. Obstet.* 148:(1979)675–678.

10. Borzotta, A.P. and H.C. Polk. Multiple-system organ failure. *Surg. Clin. N. Amer.* 63:(1983)315–336.

11. Shapiro, B.A. Airway pressure therapy for acute restrictive pulmonary pathology. In *Textbook of Critical Care,* eds. W.C. Shoemaker, W.L. Thompson, and P.R. Holbrook. Philadelphia: Saunders, 1984, pp. 224–236.

12. American Lung Association. Epidemiology. In *Chronic Obstructive Pulmonary Disease.* New York, 1977, pp. 18–25.

13. Barrocas, A., R. Tretola, and A. Alonso. Nutrition and the critically ill pulmonary patient. *Resp. Care* 28:(1983)50–60.

14. Curreri, P.W., D. Richmond, J. Marvin, and C.R. Baxter. Dietary requirements of patients with major burns. *J. Am. Diet. Assoc.* 65:(1974)415–417.

15. Gormican, A. Influencing food acceptance in anorexic cancer patients. *Postgraduate Medicine* 68:(1980)145–152.

CASE STUDY X   THE CRITICALLY ILL PATIENT

Part I: Presentation

Ms. C. is a 50 y.o. telephone operator who is admitted to University Hospital with a 2-week history of constipation, decreased appetite, nausea, vomiting, and progressive abdominal distention.

Past medical history: Remarkable for 10 years of hypertension, moderate alcohol consumption, and 30 years of smoking two packs of cigarettes per day.

Physical exam: Unremarkable except for a pelvic mass discovered on bimanual examination. Subsequent evaluation by barium enema demonstrated an obstructed sigmoid colon at 35 cm.

Impression: Colon cancer.

Plan: The patient is scheduled for surgery on the third day of hospitalization for tumor resection and temporary colostomy.

The patient's immediate postop period is characterized by hypotension and tachycardia. By the second postop day, she has developed frank pulmonary edema and evidence of sepsis. On the third postop day, the patient is intubated and placed on a ventilator due to deteriorating pulmonary status. Central parenteral feeding is started on the fourth postop day. A nutritional consult is requested from the Nutrition Support Team. The consult reads "Advise on appropriate CPN regimen for 50 y.o. septic female, s/p CA surgery with ARDS."

[handwritten: acute respitory distress symptom]   *[handwritten: status postop]*

QUESTIONS

1. You are the dietitian member of the hospital Nutrition Support Team, which also includes a surgeon, a nurse, and a pharmacist. You visit Ms. C., who is intubated with an orotracheal tube, review her medical record, and speak with her daughter. You complete an initial postinjury nutritional assessment based on the following available information: 5 ft, 6 in; 135 # (usual), 120 # (preinjury); serum albumin 2.5 mg/dl; WBC 25,000/ml.

    a. You estimate a calorie and protein intake sufficient to minimize further loss of body weight in this severely stressed patient based on her preinjury weight. Show your calculations.

    _____ nonprotein kcal/kg = _____ nonprotein kcal/day

    _____ g protein/kg = _____ g protein/day.

    b. After discussing the case with the Nutrition Support Team pharmacist, you establish recommendations for composition and delivery of CPN using a total fluid volume of 2.5 L. Summarize your observations and recommendations in a SOAP note.

Part II: Transition from CPN to Tube Feeding

Ms. C.'s condition deteriorates, requiring surgical reexploration of the abdomen with drainage of an abdominal abscess. A tracheostomy is placed and she remains on mechanical ventilation. After 20 days of hospitalization, the ileus resolves and tube feeding is initiated. Body weight has decreased from 120 # to 110 #. A nutritional consult is again requested. The consult reads "Advise on appropriate tube feeding for anabolism in pt presently maintained on CPN and mechanical ventilation."

QUESTIONS

2. Why is the goal of nutritional therapy now anabolism rather than maintenance, as it was during the postinjury period?

[handwritten: Patient stable now, during postop catabolism occured, cannot be prevented. Now that the trauma has ended it is time to rebuild lost tissue. To regain the wt that has been lost, under IBW.]

3. Based on present body weight, what level of energy and protein would you recommend? Show your calculation...

_____ nonpro kcal/kg = _1766-1826_ nonpro kcal/day

_1.2-1.5_ g protein/kg = _60-75_ g protein/day

4. a. Suggest two specific tube feedings that you might recommend and provide a rationale for each.

b. How much of each of these tube feedings would be needed per day in order to meet the *nonprotein* calorie and protein requirements determined in question 3? Show your calculations.

Tube Feeding	ml/day	nonpro kcal/day	g pro/day
(1)			
(2)			

5. In the transition from CPN to tube feeding in this patient, a nasoduodenal feeding tube would most likely be placed and the patient would be initiated on half-strength formula.
a. Why would half-strength formula be used initially?

b. What advantage would a nasoduodenal feeding have over nasogastric feeding? What aspects of tube-feeding regimens are important with nasoduodenal feeding?

c. What characteristics of tube-feeding administration are important to consider in nasoduodenal feeding?

d. Suggest a possible transition schedule for changing the patient from CPN to nasoduodenal tube feeding using _____ formula.

Day	CPN rate	TF rate	TF strength	TF kcal

e. List five clinical parameters that you will monitor to ensure adequacy and tolerance of the tube feeding.

Part III: Weaning from the Respirator and Initiation of Oral Feeding

The patient's clinical status gradually improves. After 40 days of hospitalization, the serum albumin concentration is 3.0 mg/dl and body weight is 117 #. At this time, several unsuccessful attempts are made to wean Ms. C. from the ventilator.

QUESTIONS

6.   Discuss what role Ms. C.'s nutritional support may play in the failure to wean her from mechanical ventilation.

7.   Assume that Ms. C. is successfully weaned from the ventilator and oral feeding is started. How would you initiate and monitor the transition from tube feeding to oral feeding?

Appendix A:
Recommended Nutrient Intakes

Table A-1. Food and Nutrition Board, National Academy of Sciences–National Research Council Recommended Daily Dietary Allowances[a]

	Age (years)	Weight (kg)	Weight (lb)	Height (cm)	Height (in)	Protein (g)	Fat-Soluble Vitamins Vitamin A (μg RE)[b]	Vitamin D (μg)[c]	Vitamin E (mg α-TE)[d]
Infants	0.0–0.5	6	13	60	24	kg × 2.2	420	10	3
	0.5–1.0	9	20	71	28	kg × 2.0	400	10	4
Children	1–3	13	29	90	35	23	400	10	5
	4–6	20	44	112	44	30	500	10	6
	7–10	28	62	132	52	34	700	10	7
Males	11–14	45	99	157	62	45	1000	10	8
	15–18	66	145	176	69	56	1000	10	10
	19–22	70	154	177	70	56	1000	7.5	10
	23–50	70	154	178	70	56	1000	5	10
	51+	70	154	178	70	56	1000	5	10
Females	11–14	46	101	157	62	46	800	10	8
	15–18	55	120	163	64	46	800	10	8
	19–22	55	120	163	64	44	800	7.5	8
	23–50	55	120	163	64	44	800	5	8
	51+	55	120	163	64	44	800	5	8
Pregnant						+30	+200	+5	+2
Lactating						+20	+400	+5	+3

[a]The allowances are intended to provide for individual variations among most normal persons as they live in the United States under usual environmental stresses. Diets should be based on a variety of common foods in order to provide other nutrients for which human requirements have been less well defined.

[b]Retinol equivalents. 1 retinol equivalent = 1 μg retinol or μg β carotene.

[c]As cholecalciferol. 10 μg cholecalciferol = 400 IU of vitamin D.

[d]α-tocopherol equivalents. 1 mg d-α tocopherol = 1 α-TE.

Table A-1.   *(Continued)*

Water-Soluble Vitamins							Minerals					
Vitamin C (mg)	Thiamin (mg)	Riboflavin (mg)	Niacin (mg NE)[e]	Vitamin B-6 (mg)	Folacin[f] (μg)	Vitamin B-12 (μg)	Calcium (mg)	Phosphorus (mg)	Magnesium (mg)	Iron (mg)	Zinc (mg)	Iodine (μg)
35	0.3	0.4	6	0.3	30	0.5[g]	360	240	50	10	3	40
35	0.5	0.6	8	0.6	45	1.5	540	360	70	15	5	50
45	0.7	0.8	9	0.9	100	2.0	800	800	150	15	10	70
45	0.9	1.0	11	1.3	200	2.5	800	800	200	10	10	90
45	1.2	1.4	16	1.6	300	3.0	800	800	250	10	10	120
50	1.4	1.6	18	1.8	400	3.0	1200	1200	350	18	15	150
60	1.4	1.7	18	2.0	400	3.0	1200	1200	400	18	15	150
60	1.5	1.7	19	2.2	400	3.0	800	800	350	10	15	150
60	1.4	1.6	18	2.2	400	3.0	800	800	350	10	15	150
60	1.2	1.4	16	2.2	400	3.0	800	800	350	10	15	150
50	1.1	1.3	15	1.8	400	3.0	1200	1200	300	18	15	150
60	1.1	1.3	14	2.0	400	3.0	1200	1200	300	18	15	150
60	1.1	1.3	14	2.0	400	3.0	800	800	300	18	15	150
60	1.0	1.2	13	2.0	400	3.0	800	800	300	18	15	150
60	1.0	1.2	13	2.0	400	3.0	800	800	300	10	15	150
+20	+0.4	+0.3	+2	+0.6	+400	+1.0	+400	+400	+150	[h]	+5	+25
+40	+0.5	+0.4	+5	+0.5	+100	+1.0	+400	+400	+150	[h]	+10	+50

[e]1 NE (niacin equivalent) is equal to 1 mg of niacin or 60 mg of dietary tryptophan.

[f]The folacin allowances refer to dietary sources as determined by *Lactobacillus casei* assay after treatment with enzymes (conjugases) to make polyglutamyl forms of the vitamin available to the test organism.

[g]The recommended dietary allowance for vitamin B-12 in infants is based on average concentration of the vitamin in human milk. The allowances after weaning are based on energy intake (as recommended by the American Academy of Pediatrics) and consideration of other factors, such as intestinal absorption.

[h]The increased requirement during pregnancy cannot be met by the iron content of habitual American diets nor by the existing iron stores of many women; therefore the use of 30–60 mg of supplemental iron is recommended. Iron needs during lactation are not substantially different from those of nonpregnant women, but continued supplementation of the mother for 2–3 months after parturition is advisable in order to replenish stores depleted by pregnancy.

From Committee on Dietary Allowances, Food and Nutrition Board–National Research Council. *Recommended Dietary Allowances* (9th rev. ed.). Washington, D.C.: National Academy Press, 1980. Used with permission.

Table A-2. Mean Heights and Weights and Recommended Energy Intake[a]

Category	Age (Years)	Weight (kg)	Weight (lb)	Height (cm)	Height (in)	Energy Needs (with Range) (kcal)		Energy Needs (with Range) (MJ)[b]
Infants	0.0–0.5	6	13	60	24	kg × 115	(95–145)	kg × 0.48
	0.5–1.0	9	20	71	28	kg × 105	(80–135)	kg × 0.44
Children	1–3	13	29	90	35	1300	(900–1800)	5.5
	4–6	20	44	112	44	1700	(1300–2300)	7.1
	7–10	28	62	132	52	2400	(1650–3300)	10.1
Males	11–14	45	99	157	62	2700	(2000–3700)	11.3
	15–18	66	145	176	69	2800	(2100–3900)	11.8
	19–22	70	154	177	70	2900	(2500–3300)	12.2
	23–50	70	154	178	70	2700	(2300–3100)	11.3
	51–75	70	154	178	70	2400	(2000–2800)	10.1
	76+	70	154	178	70	2050	(1650–2450)	8.6
Females	11–14	46	101	157	62	2200	(1500–3000)	9.2
	15–18	55	120	163	64	2100	(1200–3000)	8.8
	19–22	55	120	163	64	2100	(1700–2500)	8.8
	23–50	55	120	163	64	2000	(1600–2400)	8.4
	51–75	55	120	163	64	1800	(1400–2200)	7.6
	76+	55	120	163	64	1600	(1200–2000)	6.7
Pregnancy						+300		
Lactation						+500		

[a]The data in this table have been assembled from the observed median heights and weights of children, together with desirable weights for adults for the mean heights of men (70 in) and women (64 in) between the ages of 18 and 34 years as surveyed in the U.S. population (HEW/NCHS data).

The energy allowances for the young adults are for men and women doing light work. The allowances for the two older age groups represent mean energy needs over these age spans, allowing for a 2 percent decrease in basal (resting) metabolic rate per decade and a reduction in activity of 200 kcal/day for men and women between 51 and 75 years, 500 kcal for men over 75 years, and 400 kcal for women over 75 years. The customary range of daily energy output is shown in parentheses for adults and is based on a variation in energy needs of ±400 kcal at any one age, emphasizing the wide range of energy intakes appropriate for any group of people.

Energy allowances for children through age 18 are based on median energy intakes of children of these ages followed in longitudinal growth studies. The values in parentheses are 10th and 90th percentiles of energy intake to indicate the range of energy consumption among children of these ages.

[b]MJ = megajoule

From *Recommended Daily Allowances* (9th rev. ed.). Washington, D.C., National Academy Press, 1980. Used with permission.

Table A-3. Estimated Safe and Adequate Daily Dietary Intakes of Selected Vitamins and Minerals[a]

		Vitamins		
	Age (Years)	Vitamin K (µg)	Biotin (µg)	Pantothenic Acid (mg)
Infants	0–0.5	12	35	2
	0.5–1	10–20	50	3
Children and Adolescents	1–3	15–30	65	3
	4–6	20–40	85	3–4
	7–10	30–60	120	4–5
	11+	50–100	100–200	4–7
Adults		70–140	100–200	4–7

		Trace Elements[b]					
	Age (Years)	Copper (mg)	Manganese (mg)	Fluoride (mg)	Chromium (mg)	Selenium (mg)	Molybdenum (mg)
Infants	0–0.5	0.5–0.7	0.5–0.7	0.1–0.5	0.01–0.04	0.01–0.04	0.03–0.06
	0.5–1	0.7–1.0	0.7–1.0	0.2–1.0	0.02–0.06	0.02–0.06	0.04–0.08
Children and Adolescents	1–3	1.0–1.5	1.0–1.5	0.5–1.5	0.02–0.08	0.02–0.08	0.05–0.1
	4–6	1.5–2.0	1.5–2.0	1.0–2.5	0.03–0.12	0.03–0.12	0.06–0.15
	7–10	2.0–2.5	2.0–3.0	1.5–2.5	0.05–0.2	0.05–0.2	0.10–0.3
	11+	2.0–3.0	2.5–5.0	1.5–2.5	0.05–0.2	0.05–0.2	0.15–0.5
Adults		2.0–3.0	2.5–5.0	1.5–4.0	0.05–0.2	0.05–0.2	0.15–0.5

		Electrolites		
	Age (Years)	Sodium (mg)	Potassium (mg)	Chloride (mg)
Infants	0–0.5	115–350	350–925	275–700
	0.5–1	250–750	425–1275	400–1200
Children and Adolescents	1–3	325–975	550–1650	500–1500
	4–6	450–1350	775–2325	700–2100
	7–10	600–1800	1000–3000	925–2770
	11+	900–2700	1525–4575	1400–4200
Adults		1100–3300	1875–5625	1700–5100

[a]Because there is less information on which to base allowances, these figures are not given in the main table of RDA and are provided here in the form of ranges of recommended intakes.

[b]Since the toxic levels for many trace elements may be only several times usual intakes, the upper levels for the trace elements given in this table should not be habitually exceeded.

From *Recommended Daily Allowances* (9th rev. ed.). National Academy Press, Washington, D.C., 1980. Used with permission.

Table A-4. Summary Examples of Recommended Nutrient intakes for Canadians

Age	Sex	Weight (kg)	kcal/kg[b]	Protein (g/day)[c]	Vitamin A (RE/day)[d]	Vitamin D (μg/day)[e]	Vitamin E (mg/day)[f]
					Fat-Soluble Vitamins		
Months[a]							
0–2	Both	4.5	120–100	11[h]	400	10	3
3–5	Both	7.0	100–95	14[h]	400	10	3
6–8	Both	8.5	95–97	17[h]	400	10	3
9–11	Both	9.5	97–99	18	400	10	3
Years							
1	Both	11	101	19	400	10	3
2–3	Both	14	94	22	400	5	4
4–6	Both	18	100	26	500	5	5
7–9	M	25	88	30	700	2.5	7
	F	25	76	30	700	2.5	6
10–12	M	34	73	38	800	2.5	8
	F	36	61	40	800	2.5	7
13–15	M	50	57	50	900	2.5	9
	F	48	46	42	800	2.5	7
16–18	M	62	51	55	1,000	2.5	10
	F	53	40	43	800	2.5	7
19–24	M	71	42	58	1,000	2.5	10
	F	58	36	43	800	2.5	7
25–49	M	74	36	61	1,000	2.5	9
	F	59	32	44	800	2.5	6
50–74	M	73	31	60	1,000	2.5	7
	F	63	29	47	800	2.5	6
75+	M	69	29	57	1,000	2.5	6
	F	64	23	47	800	2.5	5
Pregnancy (additional)							
1st Trimester			100	15	100	2.5	2
2d Trimester			300	20	100	2.5	2
3d Trimester			300	25	100	2.5	2
Lactation (additional)			450	20	400	2.5	3

[a]Recommended intakes during periods of growth are taken as appropriate for individuals representative of the midpoint in each age group. All recommended intakes are designed to cover individual variations in essentially all of a healthy population subsisting upon a variety of common foods available in Canada.

[b]Figures for energy are estimates of average requirements for expected patterns of activity. For nutrients not shown, the following amounts are recommended: thiamin, 0.4 mg/1,000 kcal (0.48 mg/5,000 kJ); riboflavin, 0.5 mg/1,000 kcal (0.6 mg/5000 kJ); niacin, 7.2 NE/1,000 kcal (8.6 NE/5,000 kJ); vitamin B_6, 15 μg, as pyridoxine, per gram of protein; phosphorus, same as calcium.

[c]The primary units are expressed per kilogram of body weight. The figures shown here are only examples.

[d]One retinol equivalent (RE) corresponds to the biological activity of 1 μg of retinol, 6 μg of β-carotene or 12 μg of other carotenes.

[e]Expressed as cholecalciferol or ergocalciferol.

[f]Expressed as d-α-tocopherol, relative to which β- and γ-tocopherol and α-tocotrienol have activities of 0.5, 0.1 and 0.3 respectively.

Table A-4.   (*Continued*)

	Water-Soluble Vitamins			Minerals			
Vitamin C (mg/day)	Folacin (µg/day)[c,g]	Vitamin B$_{12}$ (µg/day)	Calcium (mg/day)	Magnesium (mg/day)[c]	Iron (mg/day)	Iodine (µg/day)	Zinc (mg/day)
20	50	0.3	350	30	0.4[i]	25	2[j]
20	50	0.3	350	40	5	35	3
20	50	0.3	400	50	7	40	3
20	55	0.3	400	50	7	45	3
20	65	0.3	500	55	6	55	4
20	80	0.4	500	70	6	65	4
25	90	0.5	600	90	6	85	5
35	125	0.8	700	110	7	110	6
30	125	0.8	700	110	7	95	6
40	170	1.0	900	150	10	125	7
40	180	1.0	1000	160	10	110	7
50	150	1.5	1100	210	12	160	9
45	145	1.5	800	200	13	160	8
55	185	1.9	900	250	10	160	9
45	160	1.9	700	215	14	160	8
60	210	2.0	800	240	8	160	9
45	175	2.0	700	200	14	160	8
60	220	2.0	800	250	8	160	9
45	175	2.0	700	200	14[k]	160	8
60	220	2.0	800	250	8	160	9
45	190	2.0	800	210	7	160	8
60	205	2.0	800	230	8	160	9
45	190	2.0	800	220	7	160	8
0	305	1.0	500	15	6	25	0
20	305	1.0	500	20	6	25	1
20	305	1.0	500	25	6	25	2
30	120	0.5	500	80	0	50	6

[g]Expressed as total folate.

[h]Assumption that the protein is from breast milk or is of the same biological value as that of breast milk and that between 3 and 9 months adjustment for the quality of the protein is made.

[i]It is assumed that breast milk is the source of iron up to 2 months of age.

[j]Based on the assumption that breast milk is the source of zinc for the first 2 months.

[k]After the menopause the recommended intake is 7 mg/day.

Adapted from *Recommended Nutrient Intakes for Canadians.* Ottawa: Canadian Government Publishing Centre, 1983. Used with permission of Health and Welfare–Canada.

Table A-5. Estimated Amino Acid Requirements

| Amino Acid | Requirement/kg of Body Wt (mg/day) | | | Amino Acid Pattern for High-Quality Protein (mg/g of Protein)[a] |
	Infant (4–6 mo)	Child (10–12 yr)	Adult	
Histidine	33	?	?	17
Isoleucine	83	28	12	42
Leucine	135	42	16	70
Lysine	99	44	12	51
Total S-containing amino acids	49	22	10	26
Total aromatic amino acids	141	22	16	73
Threonine	68	28	8	35
Tryptophan	21	4	3	11
Valine	92	25	14	48

[a]Two g/kg of body weight/day of protein of the quality listed in column 4 would meet the amino acid needs of the infant.

From *Recommended Daily Allowances*, (9th rev. ed.). Washington, D.C., National Academy Press, 1980. Used with permission.

Appendix B:
Tables of Food Values

Table B-1. "Rough" Food Value Table for Crude Assessment of Vitamin and Mineral Content of Diets

IRON
8 mg in
  ½ c Cream of Wheat or Malt-O-Meal
  26 oz commercial infant formula, fortified
7 mg in
  6 T infant cereal (dry)[ab]
5 mg in
  ½ c prune juice
  2 oz beef liver
3 mg in
  3 oz cooked beef, pork (not ham), turkey
  ½ c raisins
  ½ c cooked cereal
  ⅔ c ready-to-eat cereal
  1 waffle
  1 slice pizza
  1 tortilla
  1 T molasses
2 mg or more in
  ¾ c cooked leafy greens, asparagus
  1 c leafy greens, raw
  ½ c dry beans, split peas
  3 oz shellfish, ham
  2 eggs
  3½ T strained liver (infant)
  7 T strained meat (not liver) (infant)
1 mg in
  9 T strained infant dinner ("high meat")
  9 T strained green vegetables (infant)
0.5 mg in
  1 slice whole-grain or enriched bread
  ½ c fruit or vegetable, other than dark greens
  1 T peanut butter
  2 dried prunes or apricot halves
  9 T strained fruit (infant)
  9 T strained vegetables (except green) (infant)
  9 T strained vegetables with meat "dinners" (infant)
CALCIUM
300 mg in
  1 c of milk or buttermilk (8 oz)
  1 c yogurt (8 oz)
250 mg in
  1 oz Swiss cheese
  ½ c red salmon (with bone)

Table B-1. *(Continued)*

CALCIUM
200 mg in
  1 oz Cheddar cheese
  1 c raw oysters (13–19)
150 mg in
  1 oz American processed cheese
  ½ c dark greens (except spinach, chard, beet greens)
100 mg in
  ⅓ c cottage cheese
  ½ c ice cream or ice milk
  ½ c spinach
300 mg calcium in rest of diet
PHOSPHORUS
300 mg in
  2 oz sardines, beef liver
200 mg in
  1 c whole milk or yogurt
  3 oz turkey
  1 oz cheese
  ½ c cauliflower
150 mg in
  1 oz cooked calf liver
  ½ c beans, kidney or white, cooked
  ⅓ c cottage cheese
100 mg in
  1 egg
75 mg in
  1 oz broiled cod, halibut
  1 oz cooked lean pork or beef
  1 T peanuts, roasted or butter
  ½ c lima beans; peas, cooked
50 mg in
  1 slice bread
  ½ c fruit
  ½ c other vegetables
MAGNESIUM
70 mg in
  ½ c cooked dry beans
  ½ c dark leafy greens
50 mg in
  1 oz nuts
  2 T peanut butter
30 mg in
  3 oz fish or shellfish
  1 T wheat germ

(continued)

350

Table B-1. *(Continued)*

MAGNESIUM
30 mg in
  1 c cooked pasta
  1 c milk
20 mg in
  1 slice whole-wheat bread
15 mg in
  3 oz meat
  1 oz Cheddar cheese
  ½ c other vegetables
ZINC
2.0 mg in
  3 oz roast beef
  3 oz pork liver
1.0 mg in
  1 egg
  1 c milk
  3 oz other meat, poultry, fish
  ¾ c legumes, cooked
  1 oz whole-grain dry cereal
  ¾ c whole-grain cooked cereal
  1 T wheat germ
0.5 mg in
  1 oz cheese
  1 slice whole-grain bread
  ½ c cooked rice or peas
VITAMIN A
15,000 IU in
  1 oz liver (cooked) (beef, lamb, or pork)
8,000 IU in
  ½ c carrots, sweet potato, spinach, pumpkin (cooked)
5,000 IU in
  ½ c dark leafy greens—spinach, turnip, mustard, etc. (cooked)
  ½ c winter squash
  ½ c cantaloupe
  10 dried apricot halves
  1/16 watermelon
  1½ T strained liver (infant)
  9 T strained dark leafy or orange vegetable (infant)
2,000 IU in
  ½ c broccoli (cooked)
  ½ c canned apricots
1,000 IU in
  ½ c tomatoes or tomato juice or 1 small tomato
  ½ c peaches (raw)
  ½ c leaf lettuce, watercress
  ½ c apricot nectar
500 IU in
  ½ c head lettuce
  ½ c light green vegetables (green beans, peas, asparagus, limas, etc.)
  1½ c milk (12 oz)
  1½ oz Cheddar cheese
  1 T butter or margarine
  2 waffles
  1 slice pizza
  1 c ice cream
  9 T strained other vegetables (infant)
  4½ T strained vegetable with meat "dinners" (infant)
200 IU in
  9 T strained fruit (infant)
THIAMINE
1.25 mg in
  1 T Brewer's yeast
0.3 mg in
  1 oz pork
  2 oz other meat

0.1 mg in
  ½ c whole-grain or fortified cereal
  2 eggs
THIAMINE
0.1 mg in
  ¼ c dried beans (cooked)
  ¼ c enriched rice (cooked)
  1 slice whole-grain or enriched bread
  ½ c enriched macaroni, spaghetti, noodles (cooked)
0.07 mg in
  ½ c vegetables
  1 c milk
0.06 mg in
  ½ c fruit
ASCORBIC ACID
50 mg in
  ½ c orange or juice
  ½ c grapefruit or juice
  1 c tomato (raw or canned)
  1 c cabbage or cauliflower (raw or cooked)
  1 c dark leafy greens—spinach, mustard, etc. (cooked)
  ½ c broccoli or brussel sprouts (cooked)
  ½ med. sweet pepper (raw)
  1 c cantaloupe or other melon
  1 c strawberries
20–40 mg in
  1 potato, baked or boiled
  ½ c rutabaga, cooked
  1 sweet potato, cooked in skin
10 mg in
  ½ c other vegetables (cooked or raw)
  4½ T strained fruit (infant)
  9 T strained vegetable (infant)
5 mg in
  ½ c other fruit (cooked or raw)
RIBOFLAVIN
1 mg in
  1 oz liver
  3½ T strained liver (infant)
0.4 mg in
  1 c milk (8 oz)
  1 c yogurt (8 oz)
  1 c oysters (raw) (13–19)
0.3 mg in
  ½ c cottage cheese
  1 T Brewer's yeast
0.1 mg in
  1 c dried beans (cooked)
  1 oz Cheddar cheese
  1 egg
  ½ c dark greens (spinach, turnip, mustard, etc.)
  ½ waffle
  1 slice pizza
  3½ T strained meat, except liver (infant)
  9 T strained dinner, "high meat" (infant)
0.05 mg in
  1 oz meat, fish, poultry
  1 slice whole-grain or enriched bread
  ½ c cereal, whole-grain or enriched
  ½ c cooked or raw vegetable
  ½ c pineapple, pineapple juice
  9 T strained vegetables (infant)
0.03 mg in
  ½ c cooked, raw, or frozen fruit
NIACIN (Note that tryptophan, contained in any complete protein, may also be a source of niacin
14 mg or more in
  3 oz liver

(continued)

(continued)

Table B-1.   (Continued)

NIACIN
10 mg or more in
   3 oz tuna, chicken, turkey
   ½ c peanuts
6 mg or more in
   3 oz salmon
3.0–5.5 mg in
   3 oz beef, lamb, pork
   1 c niacin-enriched cereals
   1 T Brewer's yeast
   2 T peanut butter
1.5 mg in
   1 c enriched pasta products
   2 slices enriched or whole-grain bread
   1 medium potato
   ½ c green peas
VITAMIN B_6
0.5 mg in
   3 oz beef liver
   1 small banana
0.2–0.3 mg in
   3 oz meat, poultry, fish
   ¾ c legumes, cooked
   1 T wheat germ
   1 medium potato
   ½ c tomato juice
   ½ c cooked corn
0.1 mg in
   1 c milk
   ½ c broccoli, cauliflower, Brussels sprouts, spinach
   ½ c whole pineapple or juice
VITAMIN E
2.0 IU or more in
   1 oz nuts
   1 T vegetable oil
   ¾ c leafy greens, cooked
   1 c leafy greens, raw
   1 T wheat germ
FOLIC ACID (Values are for total folacin)
300 µg in
   1 T Brewer's yeast
50–70 µg in
   ½ c orange juice
   1 orange
   ½ c spinach, beets, or broccoli, cooked
   ¼ cantaloupe
   1 c diced beans, cooked
   ½ c peanuts, roasted
25 µg in
   1 egg
   ½ c peas
   ½ c grapefruit or tomato juice
VITAMIN B_{12}
50 µg in
   2 oz fried beef liver
2 µg in
   3 oz beef or lamb
   1 oz fish or shellfish
1 µg in
   3 oz chicken
   1 egg
   ½ c cottage cheese
   1 c milk
0.5 µg in
   3 oz pork
   2 oz Cheddar cheese

[a]Same nutrient values are used for homemade or commercial infant foods.

[b]Approximate quantities in commercial infant food jars—Strained meat: 7 T; Strained fruit, vegetables, and "dinners": 9 T.

Table B-2.   Fiber Content of Foods

Food	Fiber (g/100 g)	
	Dietary	Crude
Cereal products		
Arrowroot	—	
Barley, boiled	2.2	—
Bran, wheat	44.0	9.1
Flour, whole wheat	9.6	2.3
Flour, white	3.2	0.3
Flour, self-rising	3.7	0.4
Macaroni, raw	—	0.3
Macaroni, boiled	—	0.1
Oatmeal	0.8	
Rice, polished, raw	2.4	0.3
Rice, boiled	0.8	0.1
Rye flour (100%)	—	2.0
Sago raw	—	
Semolina, raw	—	
Soya flour, full fat	11.9	2.4
Spaghetti, raw	—	
Spaghetti, boiled	—	0.3
Spaghetti, canned, in tomato sauce	—	0.1
Tapioca, raw	—	0.1
Breakfast cereals		
40% Bran flakes	26.7	4.4
Corn Flakes	11.0	0.7
Grape Nuts	7.0	
Puffed Wheat	15.4	2.0
Shredded Wheat	12.3	2.3
Bread		
Whole wheat	8.5	1.6
Brown	5.1	
White	2.7	0.2
Toasted	2.8	0.3
Dried crumbs	3.4	
Rolls, brown, crusty	5.9	1.6
Rolls, brown, soft	5.4	
Rolls, white, crusty	3.1	0.2
Rolls, white, soft	2.9	0.2
Rolls, starch reduced	2.0	
Other baked goods		
Crisp bread, rye	11.7	2.2
Matzo	3.9	
Shortbread	2.1	0.2
Wafers, filled	1.6	0.1
Fruits		
Apples, flesh only	1.4	0.6
Apricots, fresh, raw	2.1	0.6
Apricots, dried, raw	24.0	3.0
Apricots, dried, stewed without sugar	8.9	
Apricots, canned	1.3	0.6
Avocados	2.0	1.6
Bananas, raw	1.8	0.5
Cherries, raw	1.2	0.2
Cranberries, raw	4.2	1.4
Currants, dried	6.5	
Dates, dried	8.7	2.3
Dates, dried, with pits	7.5	
Figs, green, raw	2.5	1.2
Figs, dried, raw	18.5	5.6
Fruit salad, canned	1.1	0.4
Grapes, black, raw	0.4	0.6
Grapes, white, raw	0.9	0.5
Grapefruit, raw	0.6	0.2
Grapefruit, canned	0.4	0.2
Lemon juice, fresh	0	Trace
Mandarin oranges, canned	0.3	0.1

(continued)

Table B-2. *(Continued)*

Fruits

Mangoes, raw	1.5	0.9
Mangoes, canned	1.0	
Melons		
Cantaloupe, raw	1.0	0.3
Watermelon, raw	—	0.3
Nectarines, raw	2.4	0.4
Olives, in brine	4.4	1.3
Oranges, peeled	29	0.5
Orange juice, fresh	0	0.1
Peaches, raw	2.3	0.6
Peaches, dried, raw	14.3	3.1
Peaches, canned	1.0	0.4
Pears, raw, flesh only	2.4	1.8
Pears, canned	1.7	0.8
Pineapple, fresh	1.2	0.4
Pineapple, canned	0.9	0.3
Plums, raw	1.5	
Prunes, dried, raw	16.1	1.6
Prunes, stewed, no sugar	8.1	0.8
Raisins, dried	6.8	0.9
Raspberries, raw	7.4	3.0
Rhubarb, stewed, no sugar	2.4	
Strawberries, raw	2.2	1.3
Tangerines, raw	1.9	0.5

Nuts

Almonds	14.3	2.6
Brazil nuts	7.7	3.1
Chestnuts	6.8	1.1
Hazelnuts	6.1	3.0
Coconut, fresh	13.6	4.0
Coconut, desiccated	23.5	3.9
Peanuts, fresh	8.1	2.4
Peanuts, roasted, salted	9.3	2.0
Peanut butter, smooth	7.6	1.9
Walnuts	5.2	14.8

Vegetables and legumes

Artichokes, globe, boiled	—	2.4
Asparagus, boiled	1.5	0.7
Beans, French, boiled	3.2	1.1
Beans, runner, raw	3.4	
Beans, broad, boiled	4.2	
Beans, red kidney, raw	7.3	4.2
Beans, baked, canned	7.3	
Bean sprouts, canned	3.0	0.7
Broccoli, boiled	4.1	1.5
Brussels sprouts, boiled	2.9	1.6
Cabbage, red, raw	3.4	1.0
Cabbage, white, raw	2.8	0.8
Cabbage, boiled	2.8	
Carrots, old, raw	2.9	1.0
Carrots, boiled	3.1	1.0
Carrots, young, boiled	3.7	1.0
Carrots, canned	3.7	1.0
Cauliflower, raw	2.1	1.0
Cauliflower, boiled	1.8	1.0
Celery, raw	1.8	0.6
Celery, boiled	2.2	0.6
Cucumber, raw	0.4	0.3
Eggplant, raw	2.5	
Endive, raw	2.2	0.9
Leeks, raw	3.1	1.3
Leeks, boiled	3.9	
Lentils, raw	11.7	3.9
Lentils, split, boiled	3.7	1.2
Lettuce, raw	1.5	0.5

(continued)

Table B-2. *(Continued)*

Vegetables and Legumes

Mushrooms, raw	2.5	0.8
Okra, raw		
Onions, raw	2.1	0.6
Onions, boiled	1.3	0.6
Parsley, raw	9.1	1.5
Parsnips, boiled	2.5	2.0
Peas, fresh, raw	5.2	2.0
Peas, fresh, boiled	5.2	2.0
Peas, frozen, raw	7.8	1.9
Peas, frozen, boiled	12.0	1.9
Peas, canned, garden	6.3	2.3
Peas, dried, boiled	4.8	0.4
Peas, split, dried, raw	11.9	1.2
Peas, split, dried, boiled	5.1	0.4
Peppers, green, raw	0.9	1.4
Peppers, green, boiled	0.9	1.4
Potatoes, old, raw	2.1	0.5
Potatoes, boiled	1.0	0.5
Potatoes, mashed, with		
margarine and milk	0.9	0.4
Potatoes, baked	2.5	0.6
Potatoes, fried	3.2	
Potatoes, new, boiled, with		
skin	2.0	0.5
Potatoes, new, canned	2.5	0.2
Potatoes, instant powder	16.5	1.6
Potatoes, instant powder,		
reconstituted	3.6	0.3
Potato chips	3.2	1.6
Radishes, raw	1.0	0.8
Rutabagas, raw	2.4	
Spinach, boiled	6.3	0.6
Spring greens, boiled	3.8	
Sweet corn, on the cob,		
boiled	4.7	0.7
Sweet corn, canned, kernels	5.7	0.8
Sweet potatoes, raw	2.5	0.7
Sweet potatoes, boiled	2.3	0.7
Tomatoes, raw	1.4	0.5
Tomatoes, canned	0.9	0.4
Turnips, raw	2.2	0.9
Turnips, boiled	2.2	0.9
Turnip tops, boiled	3.9	0.8
Watercress, raw	3.3	0.7
Yam, raw	4.1	0.9
Yam, boiled	3.9	
Squash		
Summer, raw		0.6
Summer, boiled		0.6
Zucchini, raw		0.6
Zucchini, boiled		0.6
Winter, all varieties		
Raw		1.4
Baked		1.8
Boiled, mashed		1.4

Beverages

Cocoa (dry)	43.27
Chocolate drink	8.20
Coffee essence	0.79

Adapted from Southgate, D.A.T., B. Bailey, E. Collinson, and A. F. Wacker. A guide to calculating intakes of dietary fiber. *J. Human Nutr.* 30:(1976) 303–313; Paul, A. and D.A.T. Southgate. *McCance and Widowson's The Composition of Foods* (4th ed.). New York: Elsevier/North Holland, 1978; *Composition of Foods* (Agricultural Handbook No. 456). Washington, D.C., USDA, 1975.

Table B-3.   Ratios of Polyunsaturated Fat to Saturated Fat in Fats and Nuts

	Sample Brand	P/S Ratio[a]
Vegetable Oils (nonhydrogenated)		
Safflower	Hollywood, Saffola	8.19
Sunflower	Sunflo Pure Sunflower Oil	6.37
Corn	Mazola, Numade	4.62
Soybean	CHB	4.02
Soybean/Cottonseed	Wesson, Kraft Pure Vegetable	3.50
Sesame		2.70
Cottonseed	Wesson Institutional	1.90
Peanut	Planter's Popcorn	1.60
Olive		0.20
Palm or coconut		<0.20
Margarine		
Corn oil, soft tub	Mrs. Filberts' 100% Corn Oil Soft, Parkay Soft	2.2
Safflower, stick	Saffola, Hain	1.8
Soybean and cottonseed, soft tub		1.7
Corn oil, stick	Mazola	1.4
Soybean and cottonseed, stick		0.9
Nuts[b]		
Walnut, black		8.0
Walnut, English		5.9
Pinenut		—
Beechnut		—
Pecan		2.9
Chestnut		—
Almond		2.3
Filberts		—
Peanuts		1.6
Brazil nut		1.5
Pistachio		0.95
Cashew		0.8
Macadamia		0.2

[a]Ratio of polyunsaturated to saturated fat.

[b]Listed in decreasing order of polyunsaturation.

Adapted from Reeves, J. B. *Composition of foods: Fats and Oils, Raw, Processed, Prepared* (Handbook 8-4). Washington, D.C.: Science and Education Administration, U.S. Department of Agriculture, 1979.

Table B-4.   Average Cholesterol Content of Selected Foods Foods

Food	Amount	Cholesterol (mg)
Beef, lean	3.5 oz	100
Butter	1 T	31
Cheeses	1 oz	25
Ice cream, vanilla	1 c	59
Milk, whole	1 c	34
2% fat	1 c	18
Chicken, without skin	3.5 oz	85
Egg	1 egg	273
Fish, fresh	3.5 oz	75
Lamb	3.5 oz	70
Mayonnaise	1 T	8
Turkey, without skin	3.5 oz	75
Shellfish		
Oysters/Clams	3 oz	42
Crab	½ c	85
Shrimp	½ c	128
Lobsters	3.5 oz	200

Adapted from J.A. Pennington & H.N. Church, *Bowes & Church Food Values of Portions Commonly Used* (14th ed.). Philadelphia: Lippincott, 1985.

Table B-5.   Fat Portion Exchange List[a]

Food	Amount
Fat and Oils	
Polyunsaturated Fats	
Margarine, soft, tub-packed	1 t
diet	1 T
Mayonnaise, regular	1 ½ t
diet	1 T
Salad dressing (regular, with vegetable oil)	2 t
(low-cal, with vegetable oil)	2 T
Sunflower seeds, sesame seeds, pumpkin kernels	1 T
Vegetable oil (corn, sunflower, safflower, soybean, sesame)	1 t
Walnuts, almonds, pecans	1 T or 5 nuts
Other Fats	
Avocado	2 T
Bacon fat, lard	1 t
Butter	1 t
Whipped butter	2 t
Coconut	½ oz
Cream cheese	1 T
Oil (olive, palm, coconut, peanut)	1 t
Olives	4
Peanut butter	2 t
Sour cream	2 T
Eggs	
Yolk or whole	1
Dairy Products	
Milk	
Whole milk (regular, homogenized)	½ c
2% milk, low-fat chocolate milk	1 c
1% milk, buttermilk (99% fat-free)	2 c
Evaporated whole milk	¼ c
Yogurt	
Regular	½ c
Low-fat (4g fat/c)	1 c
Skim (2 g fat/c)	2 c

(continued)

Table B-5. *(Continued)*

Food	Amount
Cream	
Half and half	3 T
Whipping cream, fluid	1 T
whipped	2 T
Light cream	1 ½ T
Nondairy creamer	3 T
Desserts	
Ice cream	⅓ c
Ice milk	1 c
Milk shake	½ c
Tofutti	½ c
Cheese	
American, blue, brick, Cheddar, Cheshire, Colby, Fontina, Gjetost, Gruyere, Monterey, Muenster, Roquefort	½ oz
Brie, Edam, Gouda, Jarlsberg, Limberger, provolone, Romano, Swiss	2.3 oz
Camembert, mozzarella (low moisture), Neufchatel	¾ oz
Cottage cheese, 1% milk fat	2 c
2 % milk fat	1 c
4% milk fat	½ c
Meat and Poultry[b]	
Bacon	1 oz
Beef, corned	½ oz
creamed, chipped	
lean (choice grade, trimmed of all separable fat)	1 ½ oz
Round steak	3 oz
Chuck roast or steak	2 ½ oz
Stew; sirloin, tenderloin or T-bone steak	2 oz
Ground beef (10% fat)	1 ½ oz
Rib roast or steak	1 oz
Bologna: beef	½ oz slice
pork or turkey	1 oz. slice
Canadian bacon	2 oz
Chicken (broilers or fryers), roasted	
without skin: breast	1 breast
drumstick	2
thigh	1 (2 oz)
wing	3
with skin: breast	¼ to ⅓
drumstick	1
thigh	½
Duck, without skin	2 oz
Ham, cured, regular (11% fat)	1 ½ oz
fresh, lean	3 oz
Lamb: loin chops, lean	2 oz
roast leg, lean	3 oz
Liver	3 oz
Pepperoni	½ oz
Pork: loin chop, lean	¾ chop
roasted blade butt or picnic, lean	2 oz
roasted, lean and marbled	1 oz

(continued)

Table B-5. *(Continued)*

Food	Amount
Meat and Poultry[b]	
Sausage: pork links	½ oz
Turkey breast (without skin)	2 oz
Veal (except breast)	3 oz
Fish and Other Seafood[b]	
Cod, flounder, haddock, lobster (spiny), scallops, sea bass (white), sole, and tuna (canned in water)	Unlimited
Halibut[c], perch[c], (Atlantic redfish or yellow), pike, pollack, red and gray snapper, shrimp (canned)	16 oz
Catfish	6 oz
Crabs	10 oz
Halibut (Greenland)[c]	2 oz
Herring, Atlantic	2 oz
Pacific or lake	7 oz
Smoked or kippered	1 ½ oz
King mackerel	6 oz
Mackerel, Atlantic	1 ½ oz
canned	2 oz
Perch, Pacific[c]	12 oz
white (Southern)	4 ½ oz
Salmon, Atlantic or Chinook	1 oz
chum or pink	2 oz
silver, red, or smoked	2 oz
Sardines	2 oz
Tuna, canned in oil	2 oz
Protein Alternatives	
Legumes, cooked	
Lima beans, split peas	6 c
Black beans, brown beans, lentils, mung beans, pinto beans	5 c
Black-eyed peas, cowpeas, kidney beans, navy beans, commmon white beans	4 c
Chick peas	1 c
Soybeans	½ c
Tofu	2 to 3 oz
Tempeh	2 to 3 oz
Bread and Starch Group (high-fat snacks and desserts)	
Baking powder biscuit	1
Brownies	¾ oz
Cake	1 oz
Corn chips, potato chips	½ oz
Crackers	5
Croissants, Danish, eclairs	⅓ of one
Doughnuts	¾
French fries, onion rings	7
Pancakes, waffles, French toast, muffins	1

[a]This exchange list is not suited for use in planning diets for patients with diabetes mellitus. One exchange equals 5 g of fat.

[b]Weight after cooking with no added fat.

[c]Different fish with the same name sometimes have different amounts of fat.

Appendix C:
Diabetic Exchange Lists*

Table C-1. Composition of Diabetic Exchanges

Exchange	Approximate Measures	Weight (g)	Composition			Calories
			Pro (g)	Fat (g)	CHO (g)	
Milk, nonfat	1 c	240	8	Trace	12	90
1%	1 c	240	8	2	12	100
2%	1 c	240	8	5	12	120
whole	1 c	240	8	8	12	150
Vegetable	½ c	100	2	—	5	25
Fruit	Varies	Varies	—	—	15	60
Bread/starch	1 slice (other items vary)	25	3	Trace	15	80
Meat or substitute						
low fat	1 oz	30	7	3	—	55
medium fat	1 oz	30	7	5	—	75
high fat	1 oz	30	7	8	—	100
Fat	1 t (other items vary)	5		5	—	45

*Tables 1 to 9 are adapted from *Exchange Lists for Meal Planning* (1986) prepared by Committees of the American Dietetic Association and the American Diabetes Association, Inc., in cooperation with the Public Health Service, U.S. Department of Health, Education, and Welfare; *Diet Manual Utilizing a Vegetarian Diet Plan* (rev. ed.), Loma Linda, Calif.: Seventh-Day Adventist Dietetic Association, 1975; *Modern Nutrition in Health and Disease* (6th ed.), eds. R.S. Goodhart and M.E. Shils. Philadelphia: Lea & Febiger, 1980; *Manual of Clinical Dietetics,* University of California, Los Angeles, 1977; *Mayo Clinic Diet Manual* (5th ed.), eds. C.M. Pemberton and C.F. Gastineau. Philadelphia: Saunders, 1981, and Chicago Dietetic Association. *Manual of Clinical Dietetics* (2d ed.). Philadelphia: Saunders, 1981.

Table C-2.   Milk Exchanges*a*

Type	Amount
Nonfat fortified milk[b]	
Skim or nonfat milk	1 c
Powdered (nonfat dry, before adding liquid)	⅓ c
Evaporated skim milk, canned	½ c
Buttermilk (made from skim milk)	1 c
Yogurt (made from skim milk; plain, unflavored)	1 c
Low-fat fortified milk	
1% fat fortified milk	1 c
2% fat fortified milk	1 c
Acidophilus 2% milk	1 c
Yogurt (made from 2% fortified milk; plain, unflavored)	1 c
Whole milk	
Whole milk	1 c
Evaporated whole milk, canned	½ c
Buttermilk (made from whole milk)	1 c
Yogurt, plain, unflavored, made from whole milk	1 c
Soy milk, unsweetened (add ½ bread exchange)	1 c

*a*Composition: One exchange of each of the three types of milk includes:

	Carbohydrate (g)	Protein (g)	Fat (g)	Calories
Nonfat	12	8	trace	90
Lowfat (1%)	12	8	2	100
Lowfat (2%)	12	8	5	120
Whole	12	8	8	150

[b]Italic type indicates nonfat.

Table C-3.   Vegetable Exchanges*a*

Artichoke[b] *(½ medium)*	*Beet*	*Pea pods, snow peas*
Asparagus	*Chard*	*Rutabaga*
Bean sprouts	*Collards*	*Sauerkraut*
Beets	*Dandelion*	*String beans, green or yellow*
Broccoli	*Kale*	*Summer squash*
Brussels sprouts	*Mustard*	*Tomato, (one large)*
Cabbage	*Spinach*	*Turnips*
Carrots or juice	*Turnip*	*Vegetable/tomato juice*
Cauliflower	*Jicama*	
Chayote	*Kohlrabi*	*Water chestnuts*
Eggplant	*Leeks*	*Wax beans*
Green pepper	Mushrooms, cooked	*Zucchini,* cooked
Greens:	*Okra*	
	Onions	

Note: Starchy vegetables are found in the bread/starch exchanges.

*a*One exchange is ½ c of cooked vegetables or vegetable juice or 1 cup of raw vegetables unless otherwise noted. Composition: One exchange = 2 g protein, 5 g carbohydrate, 25 kcal, and 2–3 g of dietary fiber.

[b]Italic type indicates nonfat.

Table C-4. Fruit Exchanges[a]

Fruit	Amount	Fruit Juices and Drinks	Amount
Apple,[b] 2 in. diam.	1	Apple juice	½ c
Applesauce		Apricot nectar	⅓ c
(unsweetened)	½ c	Blackberry juice	½ c
Apricots, fresh	4 medium	Cider	½ c
Apricots, canned	4 halves		
Apricots, dried	7 halves	Cranberry juice, low calorie	1 c
Banana, 9 inch	½	Cranberry juice, regular	⅓ c
Berries (raw)		Del Monte fruit drinks	½ c
Blackberries	¾ c	Gatorade	1 c
Blueberries	¾ c	Grapefruit or Grape instant breakfast drinks	
Gooseberries	1 c	(powder)	3 t
Loganberries	¾ c	Grapefruit juice	½ c
Raspberries	1 c	Grape juice	⅓ c
Strawberries	1¼ c	Hawaiian Punch, low calorie	1 c
Cherries, raw	12 large	Hi-C fruit drinks	½ c
Cherries, canned	½ c		
Dates	2½ med	Orange juice	½ c
Figs, fresh, 2 in.	2	Peach nectar	⅓ c
Figs, dried	1½	Pear nectar	⅓ c
Fruit cocktail, canned	½ c	Pineapple juice	½ c
Grapefruit	½, or ¾ c sections	Prune juice	⅓ c
Grapes	15 small	Tang (powder)	3 t
Kiwi, large	1		
Mango	½ small		
Melon			
Cantaloupe, 5 in.	⅓ small, 1 c cubes		
Honeydew, Casaba	⅛ medium, 1 c cubes		
Watermelon	1¼ c		
Nectarine, 1½ in. diam.	1		
Orange, 2½ in. diam.	1		
Papaya	1 c		
Peach, 2¾ in. diam.	1		
Peaches, canned	2 halves		
Pear, fresh	1 small or ½ large		
Pear, canned	2 halves		
Persimmon, native	2 medium		
Pineapple, canned	⅓ c		
Pineapple, raw	¾ c		
Plums	2 medium		
Pomegranate	½ medium		
Prunes	3 medium		
Raisins, uncooked	2 T		
Tangerine, 2½ in. diam.	2		

[a]Composition: One exchange = 15 g carbohydrate, 60 kcal, and 2 g of dietary fiber for fresh, frozen or dried fruits.
[b]Italic type indicates low fat.

Table C-5. Bread Exchanges^a (plus Cereals and Starchy Vegetables)

Food	Amount
Bread^b	
White (including French, Italian)	1 slice
Whole wheat	1 slice
Rye or pumpernickel	1 slice
Cocktail rye	3 slices
Raisin	1 slice
Bagel, small	½
Bread sticks, 4 × ½ in.	2
English muffin, small	½
Plain roll, bread	1
Holland Rusk	2
Frankfurter roll	½
Hamburger bun	½
Syrian or Pita bread, 6 inch	½
Dried bread crumbs	3 T
Tortilla, 6-inch, not fried	1
Boston Brown Bread, 3 inch × ½ inch	1 slice
Cereal	
Bran cereals, concentrated; shredded wheat	⅓ c
Flaked bran cereals	½ c
Unsweetened flaked cereals	¾ c
Puffed cereal (unfrosted)	1½ c
Cereal (cooked)	½ c
Grape Nuts	3 T
Dried legumes	
Beans, peas, lentils (dried and cooked)	⅓ c
Baked beans, no pork (canned)	¼ c
Starchy vegetables	
Corn	½ c
Corn on cob	1 small
Lima beans	½ c
Parsnips	⅔ c
Peas, green (canned or frozen)	½ c
Plaintain, cooked	½ c
Potato, white, baked, 3 oz.	1
Potato (mashed)	½ c
Pumpkin	¾ c
Winter squash, acorn or butternut	¾ c
Yam or sweet potato	⅓ c
Prepared foods	
Biscuit, 2-inch diameter (omit 1 fat exchange)	1
Corn bread, 2 inch × 2 inch × 1 inch (omit 1 fat exchange)	1
Corn muffin, 2-inch diameter (omit 1 fat exchange)	1
Crackers, round, butter type (omit 1 fat exchange)	6
Muffin, plain small (omit 1 fat exchange)	1
Pancake, 5 inch × ½ inch (omit 1 fat exchange)	1
Popover, 2–3 inches (omit 1 fat exchange)	1
Potatoes, french fried, length 2–3 ½ inch (omit 1 fat exchange)	10
Potato, corn or other chips (omit 2 fat exchanges)	1 oz
Taco shell (omit 1 fat exchange)	2
Waffle, 5 inch × ½ inch (omit 1 fat exchange)	1
Flour, wheat	2½ T
Rye flour	3 T
Tapioca, dry	2 T
Barley, millet	½ c
Grits, hominy (cooked)	½ c
Pasta, cooked (spaghetti, noodles, macaroni, etc.)	½ c
Popcorn (popped, no fat added, large kernel)	3 c
Rice, white or brown (cooked)	⅓ c
Rice, glutinous	¼ c
Wheat germ	3 T
Crackers	
Arrowroot	3
Graham, 2½ inch square	3

(continued)

Table C-5. *(Continued)*

Food	Amount
Crackers	
Matzo, 4 inch × 6 in	¾ oz.
Oyster	24
Pretzels, 3⅛ long × ½ inch diameter	¾ oz.
Rye wafers, 2 inch × 3½ inch	4
Saltines	6
Other (for occasional use only)	
Cookies, 1¾ in. diam. (omit 1 fat exchange)	2
Frozen fruit yogurt	⅓ c
Ginger Snaps	3
Granola (omit 1 fat exchange)	¼ c
Granola bar, small (omit 1 fat exchange)	1
Ice cream, any flavor (omit 2 fat exchanges)	½ c
Sherbet, any flavor	¼ c
Vanilla wafers, small (omit 1 fat exchange)	6

^aComposition: One exchange = 3 g protein, 15 g carbohydrate, a trace of fat, and 80 kcal. Whole grain products average about 2 g of dietary fiber per serving.

^bItalic type indicates low fat.

Table C-6. Meat Exchanges (lean, medium-fat, and high-fat)^a

Type	Description	Amount
Lean Meat (one exchange = 7 g protein, 3 g fat)		
Beef^b	Baby beef (very lean), chipped beef, chuck, flank steak, London broil, sandwich steaks, tenderloin, plate ribs, plate skirt steak, bottom round, all cuts rump, spare ribs, tripe	1 oz
Pork	Leg (whole rump, center shank), ham, smoked (center slices), Canadian bacon	1 oz
Veal	Leg, loin, rib, shank, shoulder	1 oz
Game	Opossum, rabbit, squirrel, venison	1 oz
Poultry	Meat (without skin) of chicken, turkey, cornish hen, guinea hen, pheasant	1 oz
Fish	Any fresh or frozen	1 oz
	Drained canned salmon, tuna, mackerel, crab, and lobster	¼ c
	Clams, oysters, scallops, shrimp	5 or 1 oz
	Sardines (drained)	3
Cheeses containing less than 5% butterfat		1 oz
Cottage cheese, dry and 2% butterfat		¼ c
Egg whites		3
95% fat-free cold cuts		1 oz
Egg substitute with less than 55 kcal/¼ c		¼ c
Medium-Fat Meat (one exchange = 7 g protein, 5 g fat)		
Beef	Ground (15% fat), roasts and steaks, corned beef (canned), rib eye, round	1 oz
Pork	Loin (all cuts tenderloin), chops, roasts, shoulder arm (picnic), shoulder blade, Boston butt	1 oz
Lamb	Most products	1 oz
Veal	Cutlet	1 oz
Poultry	Chicken with skin, duck, goose, and ground turkey	1 oz
Fish	Tuna, drained, or salmon, drained	¼ c

(continued)

Table C-6. *(Continued)*

Type	Description	Amount
Cheese	Mozzarella, ricotta, farmer's cheese, Neufchatel, Parmesan, Camembert, Edam, Liederkranz	1 oz
Legumes	Soybeans	⅓ c
	Soybean curd	½ block
	Tofu	4 oz
Liver, heart, kidney, and sweetbreads (high in cholesterol)		1 oz
Cottage cheese, creamed		¼ c
Egg (high in cholesterol)		1
High-Fat Meat (one exchange = 7 g protein, 8 g fat)		
Beef	Brisket, corned beef (brisket), ground beef (more than 20% fat), hamburger (commercial), chuck (ground, commercial), roasts (rib), steaks (club, rib, Porterhouse, New York strip, T-bone), most prime beef	1 oz
Lamb	Ground	1 oz
Pork	Spare ribs, loin (back ribs), pork (ground), country style ham, deviled ham, hocks, feet, sausage	1 oz
Cheeses	Cheddar types, American, blue, Roquefort, brick, gorgonzola, gouda, Gruyere, limberger, Muenster, Swiss	1 oz
Peanut butter		1 T
Legumes	Peanuts (omit ½ bread, 2 fat exchanges)	4 T
	Pumpkin seeds (omit 1½ fat exchanges)	8 t
	Sesame seeds and sunflower seeds (omit 2½ fat exchanges)	4 T
	Hummus (omit 1 bread exchange)	4 T
	Pignolia nuts (omit ½ vegetable and 1 fat exchange)	6 T
Cold cuts, 4½ inch × ⅛ inch slices		1 slice
Frankfurter (omit additional fat exchange)		1 small

[a]Trim off all visible fat.

[b]Italic type indicates lean (low-fat) meats.

Table C-7 Fat Exchanges[a]

Fat Source	Amount
Margarine, soft in tub or sticks[b,c]	1 t
Avocado (4-inch diameter)[d]	⅛
Oil: corn, cottonseed, safflower, soy, sunflower	1 t
Oil, olive[d]	1 t
Oil, peanut[d]	1 t
Olives[d]	10 small or 5 large
Almonds[d]	6 whole
Pecans[d]	2 whole
Peanuts[d]	20 small or 10 large
Walnuts	2 whole
Nuts, other[d]	1 T
Margarine, diet	1 T
Butter	1 t
Bacon fat	1 t
Bacon crisp	1 strip
Cream	
Light	2 T

(continued)

Table C-7 *(Continued)*

Fat Source	Amount
Sour	2 T
Heavy	1 T
Cream cheese	1 T
French dressing	1 T
Italian dressing	1 T
Lard	1 t
Mayonnaise	2 t
Salad dressing, reduced calorie	1 T
Salad dressing, mayonnaise type	2 t
Salt pork	¼ oz

[a]Composition: One exchange = 5 g fat and 45 kcal.

[b]Italic type indicates polyunsaturated fat.

[c]High content of polyunsaturated fat if made with corn, cottonseed, safflower, soy, or sunflower oil.

[d]Fat content is primarily monounsaturated.

Table C-8. Free Foods[a]

Condiments	Garlic, fresh
Catsup (1 T)	Powder
Horseradish	Herbs
Mustard	Hot pepper sauce
Pickles, dill, unsweetened	Lemon
Salad dressing, low-calorie (2 T)	Lemon juice
	Lemon pepper
Taco sauce (1 T)	Lime
Vinegar	Lime juice
Drinks	Mint
Bouillon or broth without fat low sodium	Onion powder
	Oregano
Carbonated drinks, sugar-free	Paprika
Carbonated water	Pepper
Club soda	Pimento
Cocoa powder, unsweetened (1 T)	Spices
	Soy sauce, regular
Coffee/tea	Low sodium ("lite")
Drink mixes, sugar-free	Wine, cooking (¼ c)
Tonic water, sugar-free	Worcestershire sauce
Fruit	*Sweet Substitutes*
Cranberries, unsweetened (½ c)	Candy, hard, sugar-free
	Gelatin, sugar-free
Rhubarb, unsweetened (½ c)	Gum, sugar-free
	Jam/jelly, sugar-free (2t)
Salad Greens	Pancake syrup, sugar-free
Endive	(1–2 T)Sugar substitutes
Escarole	(saccharine, aspartame)
Lettuce	Whipped topping (2 T)
Romaine	
Spinach	*Vegetables (raw, 1 c)*
Seasonings	Cabbage
Basil (fresh)	Celery
Celery seeds	Chinese cabbage (bok choy)
Chili powder	Cucumber
Chives	Green onion
Cinnamon	Hot peppers
Curry	Mushrooms
Dill	Radishes
Flavoring extracts (almond, butter, lemon, peppermint, vanilla, etc.)	Zucchini

[a]Composition: Contain less than 20 calories per serving. Foods without a specified serving size may be eaten as desired. Foods with a specific serving size should be limited to 2 to 3 servings per day.

Table C-9. Combination Foods^a

Food	Amount	Exchanges
Casserole, homemade	1 cup (8 oz.)	2 starch, 2 medium-fat meat, 1 fat
Cheese pizza, thin crust	¼ of 15 oz. or ¼ of 10"	2 starch, 1 medium-fat meat, 1 fat
Chili with beans (commercial)	1 cup (8 oz.)	2 starch, 2 medium-fat meat, 2 fat
Chow mein (without noodles or rice)	2 cups (16 oz.)	1 starch, 2 vegetable, 2 lean meat
Macaroni and cheese	1 cup (8 oz.)	2 starch, 1 medium-fat meat, 2 fat
Soup		
Bean	1 cup (8 oz.)	1 starch, 1 vegetable, 1 lean meat
Chunky, all varieties	10¾ oz. can	1 starch, 1 vegetable, 1 medium-fat meat
Cream (made with water)	1 cup (8 oz.)	1 starch, 1 fat
Vegetable or broth	1 cup (8 oz.)	1 starch
Spaghetti and meatballs (canned)	1 cup (8 oz.)	2 starch, 1 medium-fat meat, 1 fat
Sugar-free pudding (made with skim milk)	½ cup	1 starch
Beans if used as a meat substitute		
Dried beans, peas, lentils	1 cup (cooked)	2 starch, 1 lean meat

^aThis list gives average exchange values for some typical mixed or combination foods.

Table C-10. Diabetic Exchange Equivalents of Selected Alcoholic Beverages

Beverages	Serving Size oz	Comments	Exchange Value
Beer^a	12 oz		
Regular			1 bread, 2 fat
Light			2 fat
Extra light			1 ½ fat
Near beer			1 bread
Cider, fermented	6 oz		1 ½ fat
Wine			
Table red, rosé, or dry white	4 oz	*Red*—Burgundy, Cabernet Sauvignon, Claret, Gamay Beaujolais, Merlot. White—Chablis, Chardonnay, dry Chenin blanc, French Colombard, dry Riesling, dry Sauterne, dry Sauvignon, blanc, white burgundy, also dry rosé.	2 fat
Sweet^a	4 oz		2 fat, ⅓ bread
Light	4 oz		1 fat
Sparkling			
Champagne	4 oz	Dry	2 fat
Sweet kosher	4 oz		2 fat, 1 bread
Dessert Wines			
Sherry	2 oz		1 ½ fat
Sweet^a	2 oz	Sweet sherry, port, muscatel	1 ½ fat, ½ bread
Vermouth			
Dry	3 oz		2 fat
Sweet^a	3 oz		2 fat, 1 bread
Liquors			
Distilled spirits, 80 proof	1.5 oz	Whiskey, scotch, gin, vodka, rum	2 fat
Daiquiri	3.5 oz.		½ bread, 2 fat
Manhattan	3.5 oz		½ bread, 3 fat
Martini	3.5 oz		3 fat
Old-Fashioned	4 oz		½ bread, 3 ½ fat
Tom Collins	10 oz		½ bread, 3 ½ fat
Brandy, Cognac	1 oz	Dry	1 ½ fat
Liqueurs, cordials^a (anisette, benedictine, creme de menthe, curacao)	—	Sugar content up to 50%. Alcohol content 20%–50% by volume.	½ bread, 1 fat

^aBeer, sweet wines, liqueurs, and cordials are best avoided because of their high carbohydrate content.

Appendix D:
Medical Terminology

Table D-1. Vocabulary

Root Words	Meaning
Arterio-	Artery
Adeno-	Gland
Andro-	Men
Ano-	Anus
Antr-	Cavity, cave
Arthro-	Joint
-blast	Immature form, sprout, germ
Broncho-	Bronchus
Canc-, carc-	Malignant tumor
Cardi-, cardio-	Heart
Chole-	Bile
Cholecysto-	Gallbladder
Choledocho-	Bile duct
Chondro-	Cartilage
Col-	Colon
Corp-	Body, mass
Crani-, cranio-	Skull
Cyano-	Blue
Cysto-	Bladder; any fluid-filled sac
Cyto-	Cell
Derm-, dermato-	Skin
Duodeno-	Duodenum
Em-	Blood
Encephalo-	Brain, skull
Entero-	Intestine
Erythro-	Red
Esophago-	Esophagus
Esthe-	Feeling, sensation
Fis-	Cleavage, split
For-	Opening, aperture
Forn-	Arch, vault
Gastr-	Stomach
Glosso-	Tongue
Gynec-	Women (especially women's reproductive organs)
Hem-, hemat-	Blood
Hepato-	Liver
Hist-	Tissue
Hydr-	Water
Hyster-, hystero-	Uterus
Idio-	Unknown, strange, peculiar
Ileo-	Ileum

(continued)

Table D-1. *(Continued)*

Root Words	Meaning
Jejuno-	Jejunum
Laryngo-	Larynx
Leuc-, leuk-	White
Lipo-	Fat
Lith-	Stone
Lymph-	Waterlike
Malac-	Softening
Mea-	Passage
Meg-	Large, great, strong
Menin-	Membrane
Morph-	Form, shape
My-, myo-	Muscle
Myelo-	Marrow
Naso-	Nose
Necro-	Dead
Neph-, nephro-	Kidney
Neuro-	Nerve
Oligo-	Few, scant
Oophor-	Ovary
Ophthalm-	Eye
Os-, oss-, ost-, osteo-	Bone
-osis	Disease
Ot-	Ear
Ovar-	Ovary
Pancreato-	Pancreas
Parieto-	Wall
Path-	Disease
Ped-	Child, feet
Pneumo-, Pneumon-	Lung
Poly-	Many, much
Proct-	Anus, rectum
Pseud-	False
Pulm-	Lung
Pyel-, pyelo-	Pelvis
Py-, pyo-	Pus
Pyr-	Fever, fire
Recto-	Rectum
Reni-, reno-	Kidney
Retic-, reticulo-	Netlike
Rhino-	Nose
Salping-	Tube
Sang-	Blood
Sclero-	Hard

(continued)

Table D-1. (*Continued*)

Root Words	Meaning
Seb-	Hard fat
Sept-	Thin wall
Septic-	Poison
Sinu-	Curved, hollow
Sta-	Stand
Stomato-	Mouth
Tox-, toxic-	Poison
Tracheo-	Trachea
Uretero-	Ureter
Urethro-	Urethra
Utero-	Uterus
Vari-	Bent, stretched
Veni-, veno-	Vein

Modifiers	Meaning
A-	Without, from
Ab-, abs-	From
Ad-	To, toward, at
-algia	Pain in
Am-, ambi-, amphi-	Around
-asis	Affected with, disease
Ante-	Before, forward
Anti-	Against, opposite
Brachy-	Short
Brady-	Slow
-cele	Hernia of
Circum-	Around
-cleisis	Closure of
Con-	With
-cyte	Cell
De-	Down, from, away
Demi-	Half
Dextro-	Right
Dia-	Through
Dis-	Apart
-duct	Lead, guide
-dynia	Pain in
Dys-	Difficult, painful
E-	From, out of, without
Ec-	Out
-ectasis	Dilation of
Ecto-	Without, outside, external
-ectomy	Excision of
-ectopy	Displacement of
Ek-	From, out of, without
Em-	In
-emesis	Vomiting
-emia	In blood
En-	In
Endo-, ento-	Within
Epi-	On, against
-esthesia	Feeling, sensation
Eu-	Well, abundant, easy
Ex-	From, out of, without
Exo-	Outside, beyond
Extra-	Outside, beyond
-genesis, -genic	Producing, forming
Hemi-	Half
Hyper-	Over, above, beyond, excessive
Hypo-	Under, deficiency of
Im-, in-	In, into, not
Infra-	Below, beneath
Inter-	Between
Intra-	Within, during
-itis	Inflammation of

(continued)

Table D-1. (*Continued*)

Modifiers	Meaning
Lev-, levo-	Left
-lith	Stone
-lysis, -lytic	Destructive
Mal-	Bad
Meso-	Middle, between
-oid	Formed like
-oma	Tumor
-osis	Disease
Pan-	All, every
Para-	Beside
-pathy	Disease
-penia	Without, lack of
Peri-	Around
-phagia	To eat
-phobia	Fear of
-pnea	Breathing air
-poiesis	To produce
Poly-	Many
Post-	After
Pre-, pro-	Before
Privia-	Without, lack of
-ptosis	Falling of
Quad-, quar-	Four
Re-	Again
Retro-	Backward
-rrhagia	Bursting from
-rrhaphy	Sewing of
-rrhea	Flowing
-rrhexis	Rupture of
-scopy	Viewing of
Semi-	Half
-spasm	Spasm of
-stenosis	Narrowing of
-stomy	Making a mouth
Sub-	Under, below
Super-	Over, above
Supra-	Above
Tachy-	Swift, fast
-tomy	Cutting of
Trans-	Above, beyond, through, across
-trismus	Spasm of
-trophy	Growth or mutation

From Zeman, Frances J. *Clinical Nutrition and Dietetics*, New York: Macmillan, 1983, pp. 619–621.

Table D-2. Abbreviations Used in Medical Records

a	Before
A	Artery
A, Asmt	Assessment
AAA	Abdominal aortic aneurysm
A&B	Apnea and bradycardia
Ab	Antibody; abortion; antibiotic
Abd	Abdomen, abdominal
ABG	Arterial blood gases
a.c.	Before meals, *ante cibum*
ACTH	Adrenocorticotropic hormone
ad lib	As needed or desired
A.D.C. VAN DISSEL	Mnemonic for Admit, Diagnosis, Condition, Vitals, Activity, Nursing procedures, Diet, Ins and outs, Specific drugs, Symptomatic drugs, Extras, Labs

(continued)

Table D-2. (*Continued*)

ADH	Antidiuretic hormone
ADL	Activities of daily living
AE	Above elbow
AEIOU TIPS	Mnemonic for Alcohol, Encephalopathy, Insulin, Opiates, Uremia, Trauma, Infection, Psychiatric, Syncope
AF	Afebrile, aortofemoral, or atrial fibrillation
AFB	Acid-fast bacilli
AFP	Alpha-fetoprotein
AI	Aortic insufficiency
A/G	Albumin/globulin ratio
AKA	Above-knee amputation
Alb	Albumin
ALL	Acute lymphocytic leukemia
AML	Acute myelogenous leukemia
Amts	Amounts
Amb	Ambulate
AOB	Alcohol on breath
AODM	Adult-onset diabetes mellitus
AP	Angina pectoris; anterior-posterior; abdominal-perineal
ARF	Acute renal failure
AS	Aortic stenosis
ASCVD	Atherosclerotic cardiovascular disease
ASD	Atrial septal defect
ASAP	As soon as possible
ASHD	Arteriosclerotic heart disease
ASO	Antistreptolysin O
AV	Atrioventricular
A-V	Arteriovenous
a&w	Alive and well
B I&II	Billroth I and II
BBB	Bundle branch block
BCAA	Branched-chain amino acids
BE	Barium enema
BEE	Basal energy expenditure
BF	Breast feeding
b.i.d., b.d.	Twice daily
BJ	Bone and joint
BK	Below knee
BKA	Below-knee amputation
BM	Bone marrow; bowel movement
BMI	Body mass index
BMR	Basal metabolic rate
BOM	Bilateral otitis media
BP	Blood pressure
BPM	Beats per minute
BRP	Bathroom privileges
BS	Bowel sounds; breath sounds
BT	Bedtime
BUN	Blood urea nitrogen
Bx	Biopsy
c	Cup
c̄	With
ca	Approximately
Ca, Ca^{++}	Calcium
CA	Cancer
CAA	Crystalline amino acids
CAD	Coronary artery disease
CAT, CT	Computerized (axial) tomography
CBC	Complete blood count
CC	Chief complaint
CCU	Coronary care unit; clean catch urine
CF	Cystic fibrosis
CHD	Coronary heart disease
CHF	Congestive heart failure
CHI	Creatinine-height index

(continued)

Table D-2. (*Continued*)

chol	Cholesterol
CHO	Complex carbohydrate
CI	Cardiac index
cm	Centimeter
CMI	Cell-mediated immunity
CML	Chronic myelogenous leukemia
CNS	Central nervous system
C/O	Complains of
CO	Cardiac output
COAD	Chronic obstructive airway disease
COLD	Chronic obstructive lung disease
COPD	Chronic obstructive pulmonary disease
CPK	Creatine phosphokinase
CPN	Central parenteral nutrition
CRF	Chronic renal failure
CrCl	Creatinine clearance
CSF	Cerebrospinal fluid
cv	Cardiovascular
CVA	Cerebrovascular accident
CVP	Central venous pressure
CVR	Cardiovascular-renal
CVS	Cardiovascular system
CXR	Chest X ray
DAT	Diet as tolerated
DBW	Desirable body weight
D/C	Discontinue; discharge; direct current
DCH	Delayed cutaneous hypersensitivity
decaf	Decaffeinated
def.	Deficiency
dex	Dexter (right)
DIC	Disseminated intravascular coagulation
dil	Dilate
DKA	Diabetic ketoacidosis
dl	Deciliter
DM	Diabetes mellitus
DOB	Date of birth
DOE	Dyspnea on exertion
DTR	Deep tendon reflexes
Dx	Diagnosis
D$_5$LR	5% dextrose in lactated Ringer's solution
D$_5$W	5% dextrose in water
ECG, EKG	Electrocardiogram
EAA	Essential amino acids
EEG	Electroencephalogram
ENT	Ear, nose, and throat
EENT	Eye, ear, nose, and throat
EFA (D)	Essential fatty acid (deficiency)
e.g.	For example
elec.	Electrolytes
elim.	Eliminate, elimination
esp.	Especially
EtOH	Ethanol, ethyl alcohol
ESRD	End-stage renal disease
FBS	Fasting blood sugar
FFA	Free fatty acids
FH	Family history
fl	Fluid
FMH	Family medical history
FTT	Failure to thrive
F/U	Follow-up
FUO	Fever of unknown origin
Fx	Fracture
g	Gram
G	Gravida
GA	General appearance
GB	Gallbladder
GC	Gonococcus; gonorrhea
GE	Gastroenteritis

(continued)

Table D-2. *(Continued)*

gest	Gestation
GFR	Glomerular filtration rate
GI	Gastrointestinal
gluc	Glucose
Gt	A drop
gr	Grain
gtts	Drops
GTT	Glucose tolerance test
GU	Genitourinary
GYN	Gynecology
H&H	Hemoglobin & hematocrit
Hgb	Hemoglobin
HBP	High blood pressure
HBV	High biological value
HC	High calorie
HCG	Human chorionic gonadotropin
Hct	Hematocrit (*See* PCV)
HCVD	Hypertensive cardiovascular disease
HEENT	Head, eyes, ears, nose, and throat
H&N	Head and neck
HOB	Head of bed
H/O	History of
H&P	History and physical
Hp	Hemiplegia
HLP	Hyperlipidemia
HPI	History of present illness
HR	Heart rate
HS	At bedtime, *hora somni*
HTN, HPN	Hypertension
ht	Height
I	Infant
IBW	Ideal body weight
ICU	Intensive care unit
ID	Identification
IDDM	Insulin-dependent diabetes mellitus
i.e.	That is
IHD	Ischemic heart disease
IM	Intramuscular
IMP	Impression
I&O	Intake and output
I.P.	Intraperitoneal
IRDM	Insulin-resistant diabetes mellitus
IV	Intravenous
IVC	Intravenous cholangiogram
IVP	Intravenous pyelogram
Jc	Juice
JODM	Juvenile-onset diabetes mellitus
kg	Kilogram
KOR	Keep-open rate
KUB	Kidney, ureter, bladder
KVO	Keep vein open
L	Liter, left
LBW	Low birth weight, low biological value
LDH	Lactic acid dehydrogenase
LE	Lupus erythematosus
LLE	Left lower extremity
LLL	Left lower lobe (lung)
LLQ	Left lower quadrant
LLSB	Left lower sternal border
LML	Left middle lobe (lung)
LMD	Local medical doctor
LMP	Last menstrual period
LOC	Loss of consciousness
LOM	Limitation of motion
LP	Lumbar puncture
LPN	Licensed practical nurse
LS	Lumbosacral; low salt
LSB	Left sternal border
LUE	Left upper extremity

l&w	Living and well
lytes	Electrolytes
MAC	Midarm circumference
MAFA	Midarm fat area
MAMA	Midarm muscle area
MAMC	Midarm muscle circumference
MBF	Meat-base formula
MCH	Mean cell hemoglobin
mEq	Milliequivalent
MH	Menstrual history
MI	Mitral insufficiency, myocardial infarction
ml	Milliliter
mm	Millimeter
mmol	Millimole
mos.	Months
mOsm	Milliosmole
MCH	Mean cell hemoglobin
MCHC	Mean cell hemoglobin concentration
MCL	Midclavicular line
MCT	Medium-chain triglyercide
MCV	Mean cell volume
meds	Medications
MP	Metatarsal-phalangeal
mg	Milligram
MS	Mitral stenosis; multiple sclerosis; morphine sulfate
MVI	Multivitamin injection
N, NML, Nl	Normal
NAD	No acute distress; no active disease
NCAT	Normocephalic atraumatic
NCD	Normal childhood disease
NED	No evidence of disease
NERD	No evidence of return disease
ng	Nanogram
NG	Nasogastric
NIDDM	Non-insulin-dependent diabetes mellitus
NKA	No known allergies
NKDA	No known drug allergies
NPN	Nonprotein nitrogen
NPO	Nothing by mouth, *non per os*
NR	Not remarkable
NS	Normal saline; neurosurgery
NSR	Normal sinus rhythm
N&V	Nausea and vomiting
OB	Obstetrics
OBW	Optimal body weight
OC	Oral contraceptives
OCG	Oral cystogram
OD	Overdose; right eye
OK	Okay, suitable
OOB	Out of bed
O&P	Ova and parasites
OR	Operating room
OS	Left eye
OU	Both eyes
oz	Ounce
Para	Pregnancies; paraplegic
pc	After eating, *post cibum*
PC	Present complaint
PCM	Protein-calorie malnutrition
PCV	Packed cell volume (hematocrit)
PDA	Patent ductus arteriosus
PDR	*Physician's Desk Reference*
PE	Pulmonary embolus
pg	picogram
PG	Pregnant, pregnancy
PH	Past history
PI	Present illness; pulmonary insufficiency

(continued)

Table D-2   *(Continued)*

PID	Pelvic inflammatory disease
PKU	Phenylketonuria
PMD	Private medical doctor
PMH	Past medical history
PMN	Polymorphonuclear leukocyte (neutrophil)
po	By mouth, given orally
P.O.	Postoperative
POD	Postoperative day
PP	Patient profile
PPN	Peripheral parenteral nutrition
pr	By rectum, given rectally
PR	Pulse rate
prn	Whenever necessary
Pro	Protein
Pt	Patient
PT	Physical therapy; prothrombin time
PTA	Prior to admission
PTH	Parathormone
PTT	Partial thromboplastin time or prothrombin time
PUFAs	Polyunsaturated fatty acids
PUD	Peptic ulcer disease
PVD	Peripheral vascular disease
PZI	Protamine zinc insulin
q	Every
q.d.	Every day
qh	Every hour
q.i.d.	Four times daily
q.o.d.	Every other day
q2h, q3h	Every 2 hours, every 3 hours
quad	Quadriplegic
r.b.c.	Red blood cells
RBC	Red blood cell count
RCM	Right costal margin
RDAs	Recommended dietary allowances
RLE	Right lower extremity
RLL	Right lower lobe
RLQ	Right lower quadrant
RO, R/O	Rule out
ROM	Range of motion
ROS	Review of systems
RTA	Renal tubular acidosis
RTC	Return to clinic
RUE	Right upper extremity
RUL	Right upper lobe (lung)
RUQ	Right upper quadrant
rx	Take
Rx	Prescription, treatment
s̄	Without
SAA	Synthetic amino acids
S&A	Sugar and acetone
SBS	Short bowel syndrome
SCr	Serum creatinine
SG	Swan-Ganz (catheter)
SGA	Small for gestational age
SGOT	Serum glutamic oxaloacetic transaminase
SGPT	Serum glutamic pyruvic transaminase
SH	Social history
sig	Label
SL	Sublingual
SLE	Systemic lupus erythematosus
SOAP	Mnemonic for Subjective, Objective, Assessment, Plan

SOB	Short of breath
SOBOE	Short of breath on exertion
sos	If necessary
S/P	Status postoperatively
SQ	Subcutaneous, given subcutaneously
S&S	Signs and symptoms
stat	At once, immediately
sub	Substitute
SUN	Serum urea nitrogen
Sx	Symptoms
T	Tablespoon
t	Teaspoon
T&A	Tonsillectomy and adenoidectomy
TB	Tuberculosis
TBLC	Term birth, living child
TDE	Total daily energy expenditure
temp	Temperature
TF	Tube feeding; transferrin
TG, Trig.	Triglycerides
TIA	Transient ischemic attack
TIBC	Total iron-binding capacity
t.i.d.	Three times daily
TKO	To keep open
TLC	Total lymphocyte count; tender loving care; total lung capacity
TPN	Total parenteral nutrition
TPR	Temperature, pulse, and respiration
TSF	Triceps skinfold
TSH	Thyroid stimulating hormone
TV	Tidal volume
Tx	Treatment
UA, U.A.	Urine analysis; uric acid
UBW	Usual body weight
UCD	Usual childhood diseases
UGI	Upper gastrointestinal
UNA	Urea nitrogen appearance
URI	Upper respiratory (tract) infection
US	Ultrasound
UTI	Urinary tract infection
UUN	Urinary urea nitrogen
Vag	Vaginal
VC	Vital capacity
V&P	Vagotomy and pyloroplasty
Vit.	Vitamin(s)
VMA	Vanillylmandelic acid
vs	Versus
VS	Vital signs
VSS	Vital signs stable
w.b.c.	White blood cells
WBC	White blood cell count
WDWN	Well developed, well nourished
WNL	Within normal limits
w/o	Without
W/U	Workup
w/v	Weight per volume
yrs	Years
y.o.	Years old
#	Pounds
2°	Secondary to
24°	24 hours
37°	37 degrees
↑	High, increased, elevated
↓	Low, decreased, depressed

(continued)

Appendix E:
Normal Laboratory Values

Table E-1. *Normal Hematologic Values*

Acid hemolysis test (Ham)	No hemolysis
Alkaline phosphatase, leukocyte	Total score 14–100
Bleeding time	
Ivy	Less than 5 min
Duke	1–5 min
Carboxyhemoglobin	Up to 5% of total
Cell counts	
Erythrocytes: Males	4.6–6.2 million/mm^3
Females	4.2–5.4 million/mm^3
Children (varies with age)	4.5–5.1 million/mm^3

Leukocytes		
Total	5000–10,000/mm^3	
Differential	*Percentage*	*Absolute*
Myelocytes	0	0/mm^3
Band neutrophils	3– 5	150– 400/mm^3
Segmented neutrophils	54–62	3000–5800/mm^3
Lymphocytes	25–33	1500–3000/mm^3
Monocytes	3– 7	285– 500/mm^3
Eosinophils	1– 3	50– 250/mm^3
Basophils	0– 0.75	15– 50/mm^3

(Infants and children have greater relative numbers of lymphocytes and monocytes)

Platelets	150,000–350,000/mm^3
Reticulocytes	25,000– 75,000/mm^3
	0.5–1.5% of erythrocytes
Clot retraction, qualitative	Begins in 30–60 min
	Complete in 24 hr
Coagulation time (Lee-White)	5–15 min (glass tubes)
	19–60 min (siliconized tubes)
Cold hemolysin test (Donath-Landsteiner)	No hemolysis

Corpuscular values of erythrocytes
(Values are for adults; in children, values vary with age)

MCH (mean corpuscular hemoglobin)	27–31 pg
MCV (mean corpuscular volume)	80–105 µ^3
MCHC (mean corpuscular hemoglobin concentration)	32–36%
Euglobulin lysis time	2–6 hr at 73°C.
Factor VIII and other coagulation factors	50–150% of normal

(continued)

Table E-1 *(Continued)*

Fibrin split products (Thrombo-Wellco test)	Negative at > 1:4 dilution
Fibrinogen	200–400 mg/dL
Fibrinolysins	0
Hematocrit	
Males	40–54 ml/dL
Females	37–47 ml/dL
Newborn	49–54 mg/dL
Children (varies with age)	35–49 ml/dL
Hemoglobin	
Males	14.0–18.0 g/dL
Females	12.0–16.0 g/dL
Newborn	16.5–19.5 g/dL
Children (varies with age)	11.2–16.5 g/dL
Hemoglobin, fetal	Less than 1% of total
Hemoglobin A$_{1c}$	3–5% of total
Hemoglobin A$_2$	1.5–3.0% of total
Hemoglobin, plasma	0–5.0 mg/dL
Methemoglobin	0.03–0.13 g/dL
Osmotic fragility of erythrocytes	Begins in 0.45–0.39% NaCl
	Complete in 0.33–0.30% NaCl
Activated partial thromboplastin time	35–45 sec.
Prothrombin consumption	Over 80% consumed in 1 hr
Prothrombin content	100% (calculated from prothrombin time)
Prothrombin time (one stage)	12.0–14.0 sec
Sedimentation rate	
Wintrobe: Males	0–5 mm in 1 hr
Females	0–15 mm in 1 hr
Westergren: Males	0–15 mm in 1 hr
Females	0–20 mm in 1 hr

(May be slightly higher in children and during pregnancy)

Thromboplastin generation test	Compared to normal control

Bone marrow, differential cell count	*Range*	*Average*
Myeloblasts	0.3– 5.0%	2.0%
Promyelocytes	1.0– 8.0%	5.0%
Myelocytes: Neutrophilic	5.0–19.0%	12.0%
Eosinophilic	0.5– 3.0%	1.5%
Basophilic	0.0– 0.5%	0.3%

(continued)

Table E-1 *(Continued)*

Metamyelocytes	13.0–32.0%	22.0%
Polymorphonuclear neutrophils	7.0–30.0%	22.0%
Polymorphonuclear eosinophils	0.5– 4.0%	2.0%
Polymorphonuclear basophils	0.0– 0.7%	0.2%
Lymphocytes	3.0–17.0%	10.0%
Plasma cells	0.0– 2.0%	0.4%
Monocytes	0.5– 5.0%	2.0%
Reticulum cells	0.1– 2.0%	0.2%
Megakaryocytes	0.03– 3.0%	0.4%
Pronormoblasts	1.0– 8.0%	4.0%
Normoblasts	7.0–32.0%	18.0%

Tables E-1 through E-10 have been reprinted with permission from *Textbook of Surgery* (12th ed.), ed. David C. Sabiston. Philadelphia: Saunders, 1981.

Table E-2. Normal Blood, Plasma, and Serum Values*

Acetone, serum	
Qualitative	Negative
Quantitative	0.3–2.0 mg/dL
Adrenocorticotropin (ACTH), plasma	10–80 pg/ml
Aldolase, serum	0.8–3.0 mIU/ml (30°)
	(Sibley-Lehninger)
Amino acid nitrogen, serum	4–6 mg/dL
Ammonia nitrogen, blood	75–196 µg/dL
plasma	56–122 µg/dL
Amylase, serum	80–160 Somogyi
	units/dL
Anion gap	8–16 mEq/L
Ascorbic acid	See Vitamin C
Bile acids, serum	0.3–3.0 mg/dL
Bilirubin, serum	
Direct	0.1–0.4 mg/dL
Indirect	0.2–0.7 mg/dL
	(Total minus direct)
Total	0.3–1.1 mg/dL
Calcium, serum	4.5–5.5 mEq/L
	(9.0–11.0 mg/dL)
	(Slightly higher in children)
	(Varies with protein concentration)
Calcium, serum, ionized	2.1–2.6 mEq/L
	(4.25–5.25 mg/dL)
Carbon dioxide content, serum	24–30 mEq/L
	Infants: 20–28 mEq/L
Carbon dioxide tension (Pco_2), blood	35–45 mm Hg
Carotene, serum	50–300 µg/dL
Ceruloplasmin, serum	23–44 mg/dL
Chloride, serum	96–106 mEq/L
Cholesterol, serum	
Total	150–250 mg/dL
Esters	68–76% of total cholesterol
Cholinesterase, serum	0.5–1.3 pH units
RBC	0.5–1.0 pH units
Copper, serum	
Male	70–140 µg/dL
Female	85–155 µg/dL
Cortisol, plasma	6–23 µg/dL
Creatine, serum	0.2–0.8 mg/dL
Creatine phosphokinase, serum	
Male	0–50 ml U/ml (30°)
	(Oliver-Rosalki)

Table E-2. *(Continued)*

Female	0–30 ml U/ml (30°)
	(Oliver-Rosalki)
Creatine phosphokinase isoenzymes, serum	
CPK-MM	Present
CPK-MB	Absent
CPK-BB	Absent
Creatinine, serum	0.7–1.5 mg/dL
Cryoglobulins, serum	0
Fatty acids, total, serum	190–420 mg/dL
Ferritin, serum	20–200 ng/ml
Fibrinogen, plasma	200–400 mg/dL
Folic acid, serum	7–16 ng/ml
Follicle stimulating hormone, (FSH), plasma	
Males	4–25 mIU/ml
Females	4–30 mIU/ml
Postmenopausal	40–250 mIU/ml
Glucose (fasting)	
blood	60–100 mg/dL
plasma or serum	70–115 mg/dL
Growth hormone, serum	0–10 ng/ml
Haptoglobin, serum	40–170 mg/dL
Hydroxybutyric dehydrogenase, serum	0–180 mIU/ml (30°)
	(Rosalki-Wilkinson)
	114–290 units/ml
	(Wroblewski)
17-Hydroxycorticosteroids, plasma	8–18 µg/dL
Immunoglobulins, serum	
IgG	800–1500 mg/dL
IgA	50–200 mg/dL
IgM	40–120 mg/dL
Insulin, plasma (fasting)	5–25 microunits/ml
Iodine, protein bound, serum	3.5–8.0 µg/dL
	(May be slightly higher in infants)
Iron, serum	75–175 µg/dL
Iron binding capacity, total, serum	250–410 µg/dL
saturation	20–55%
17-Ketosteroids, plasma	25–125 µg/dL
Lactic acid, blood	6–16 mg/dL
Lactic dehydrogenase, serum	0–300 ml U/ml (30°)
	(Wroblewski modified)
	150–450 units/ml
	(Wroblewski)
	80–120 units/ml
	(Wacker)
Lactate dehydrogenase isoenzymes, serum	
LDH_1	22–37% of total
LDH_2	30–46% of total
LDH_3	14–29% of total
LDH_4	5–11% of total
LDH_5	2–11% of total
Lipase, serum	0–1.5 units (Cherry-Crandall)
Lipids, total, serum	450–850 mg/dL
Luteinizing hormone (LH), serum	6–18 mIU/ml
Males	5–22 mIU/ml
Females, premenopausal	3 times baseline
midcycle	Greater than 30 mIU/ml
Magnesium, serum	1.5–2.5 mEq/L
	(1.8–3.0 mg/dL)
Nitrogen, nonprotein, serum	15–35 mg/dL
Osmolality, serum	285–295 mOsm/L
Oxygen, blood	
Capacity	16–24 vol % (varies with Hgb)

(Continued)

(Continued)

Table E-2. *(Continued)*

Content: arterial	15–23 vol %
venous	10–16 vol %
Saturation: arterial	94–100% of capacity
venous	60–85% of capacity
Tension, Po, Arterial	75–100 mm Hg
P_{50} blood	26–27 mm Hg
pH, arterial, blood	7.35–7.45
Phenylalanine, serum	Less than 3 mg/dL
Phosphatase, acid, serum	1.0–5.0 units (King-Armstrong)
	0–7.0 milliunits/ml (IU)
Phosphatase, alkaline, serum	5.0–13.0 units/dl (King-Armstrong)
	30–85 milliunits/ml (IU)
	(Values are higher in children)
Phosphate, inorganic, serum	3.0–4.5 mg/dL
	(Children: 4.0–7.0 mg/dL)
Phospholipids, serum	6–12 mg/100 ml as lipid phosphorus
Potassium, serum	3.5–5.0 mEq/L
Proteins, serum	
Total	6.0–8.0 g/dL
Albumin	3.5–5.5 g/dL
Globulin	2.5–3.5 g/dL
Electrophoresis	
Albumin	3.5–5.5 g/dL
	52–68% of total
Globulin	
Alpha$_1$	0.2–0.4 g/dL
	2–5% of total
Alpha$_2$	0.5–0.9 g/dL
	7–14% of total
Beta	0.6–1.1 g/dL
	9–15% of total
Gamma	0.7–1.7 g/dL
	11–21% of total
Pyruvic acid, plasma	1.0–2.0 mg/dL
Sodium, serum	136–145 mEq/L
Sulfates, inorganic, serum	0.8–1.2 mg/dL (as S)
Testosterone, plasma	
Males	275–875 ng/dL
Females	23–75 ng/dL
Pregnant	38–190 ng/dL
Thyroxine, serum	4–11 μg/dL
Thyroxine, free, serum	1.0–2.1 ng/dL
Tri-iodothyronine (T_3), serum	150–250 ng/dL
Thyroxine binding globulin (TBG), serum	10–26 μg/dL
Thyroid stimulating hormone (TSH), serum	0–7 microunits/ml
T_3 uptake, resin (T_3RU)	25–38%
Thyroxine iodine (T_4), serum	2.9–6.4 μg/dL
Transaminase, serum: SGOT	0–19 mIU/ml (30°) (Karmen modified)
	15–40 units/ml (Karmen)
	18–40 units/ml (Reitman-Frankel)
SGPT	0–17 mIU/ml (30°) (Karmen modified)
	6–35 units/ml (Karmen)
	5–35 units/ml (Reitman-Frankel)

(Continued)

Table E-2 *(Continued)*

Triglycerides, serum	0–150 mg/dL
Urea, blood	21–43 mg/dL
plasma or serum	24–49 mg/dL
Urea nitrogen, blood (BUN)	10–20 mg/dL
plasma or serum	11–23 mg/dL
Uric acid, serum	
Male	2.5–8.0 mg/dL
Female	1.5–6.0 mg/dL
Vitamin A, serum	20–80 μg/dL
Vitamin B$_{12}$, serum	200–800 pg/ml
Vitamin C, blood	0.4–1.5 mg/dL

*For some procedures the normal values may vary depending upon the methods used.

Table E-3. Normal Urine Values

Acetone and acetoacetate	0	
Aldosterone	3–20 μg/24 hrs	
Amino acid nitrogen	50–200 mg/24 hrs	
	(Not over 1.5% of total nitrogen)	
Ammonia nitrogen	20–70 mEq/24 hrs	
Amylase	35–260 Somogyi units/hr	
Bence Jones protein	Negative	
Bilrubin (bile)	Negative	
Calcium		
Low Ca diet (Bauer-Aub)	Less than 150 mg/24 hrs	
Usual diet	Less than 250 mg/24 hrs	
Catecholamines		
Epinephrine	Less than 10 μg/24 hrs	
Norepinephrine	Less than 100 μg/24 hrs	
Total free catecholamines	4–126 μg/24 hrs	
Total metanephrines	0.1–1.6 mg/24 hrs	
Chloride	110–250 mEq/24 hrs	
	(Varies with intake)	
Chorionic gonadotrophin	0	
Copper	0–30 μg/24 hrs	
Creatine		
Male	0–40 mg/24 hrs	
Female	0–100 mg/24 hrs	
	(Higher in children and during pregnancy)	
Creatinine	15–25 mg/kg of body weight/24 hrs	
Cystine or cysteine, qualitative	Negative	
Delta aminolevulinic acid	1.3–7.0 mg/24 hrs	

Estrogens	Male	Female
Estrone	3–8	4–31
Estradiol	0–6	0–14
Estriol	1–11	0–72
Total	4–25	5–100

	(Units above are μg/24 hrs)
	(Markedly increased during pregnancy)
Glucose (reducing substances)	Less than 250 mg/24 hrs
Gonadotrophins, pituitary	10–50 mouse units/24 hrs
	(Increased after menopause)
Hemoglobin and myoglobin	Negative

(continued)

Table E-3   *(Continued)*

Hemogentisic acid, qualitative	Negative
17-hydroxycorticosteroids	
Male	3–9 mg/24 hrs
Female	2–8 mg/24 hrs
	(Varies with method used)
5-Hydroxyindole-acetic acid (5-HIAA)	
Qualitative	Negative
Quantitative	Less than 16 mg/24 hrs
17-Ketosteroids	
Male	6–18 mg/24 hrs
Female	4–13 mg/24 hrs
Metanephrines (see Catecholamines)	
Osmolality	38–1400 mOsm/kg water
pH	4.6–8.0, average 6.0
	(Depends on diet)
Phenylpyruvic acid, qualitative	Negative
Phosphorus	0.9–1.3 g/24 hrs
	(Varies with intake)
Porphobilinogen	
Qualitative	Negative
Quantitative	0–0.2 mg/100 ml
	Less than 2.0 mg/24 hrs
Porphyrins	
Coproporphyrin	50–250 µg/24 hrs
Uroporphyrin	10–30 µg/24 hrs
Potassium	25–100 mEq/24 hrs
	(Varies with intake)
Pregnanetriol	Less than 2.5 mg/24 hrs in adults
Protein	
Qualitative	0
Quantitative	10–150 mg/24 hrs
Sodium	130–260 mEq/24 hrs
	(Varies with intake)
Specific gravity	1.003–1.030
Sugar	0
Titratable acidity	20–40 mEq/24 hrs
Urobilinogen	Up to 1.0 Ehrlich unit/2 hrs (1–3 PM)
	0–40 mg/24 hrs
Vanillylmandelic acid (VMA)	1–8 mg/24 hrs

Table E-4.   Normal Values for Gastric Analysis

	Concentration Mean ± 1 S.D.	Output Mean ± 1 S.D.
Basal gastric secretion (one hour)		
Male	25.8 ± 1.8 mEq/L	2.57 ± 0.16 mEq/hr
Female	20.3 ± 3.0 mEq/L	1.61 ± 0.18 mEq/hr
After histamine stimulation		
Normal	Mean output = 11.8 mEq/hr	
Duodenal ulcer	Mean output = 15.2 mEq/hr	
After maximal histamine stimulation		
Normal	Mean output 22.6 mEq/hr	
Duodenal ulcer	Mean output 44.6 mEq/hr	
Diagnex blue (Squibb): Anacidity	0–03 mg in 2 hrs	
Doubtful	0.3–0.6 mg in 2 hrs	
Normal	Greater than 0.6 mg in 2 hrs	
Volume, fasting stomach content	50–100 ml	
Emptying time	3–6 hr	
Color	Opalescent or colorless	
Specific gravity	1.006–1.009	
pH (adults)	0.9–1.5	

Table E-5.   Normal Values for Feces

Bulk	100–200 g/24 hrs
Dry matter	23–32 g/24 hrs
Fat, total	Less than 6.0 g/24 hrs
Nitrogen, total	Less than 2.0 g/24 hrs
Urobilinogen	40–280 mg/24 hrs
Water	Approximately 65%

Table E-6.   Normal Values for Serologic Procedures

Anti-hyaluronidase	Less than 1:200. Significant if rising titer can be demonstrated at weekly intervals.
Anti-streptolysin O titer	Normal up to 1:128. Single test usually has little significance. Rise in titer or persistently elevated titer is significant.
Bacterial agglutinins	Significant only if rise in titer is demonstrated or if antibodies are absent.
Complement fixation tests	Titers of 1:8 or less are usually not significant. Paired sera showing rise in titer of more than two tubes are usually considered significant.
C3 Test	80–140 mg/100 ml
C4 Test	11–75 mg/100 ml
C reactive protein (CRP)	Negative
Heterophile titer	Less than 1:56
Proteus OX-19 agglutinins	1:80 Negative
	1:160 Doubtful
	1:320 Positive
R. A. test (latex)	1:40 Negative
	1:80 –1:160 Doubtful
	1:320 Positive
Rose test	1:10 Negative
	1:20–1:40 Doubtful
	1:80 Positive
Tularemia agglutinins	1:80 Negative
	1:160 Doubtful
	1:320 Positive

Table E-7.   Toxicology

Arsenic, blood	3.5–7.2 µg/dL
Arsenic, urine	Less than 100 µg/24 hrs
Barbiturates, serum	0
	Coma level: Phenobarbital approximately 11 mg/dL; most other barbiturates 1.5 mg/dL
Bromides, serum	0
	Toxic levels above 17 mEq/L
Carbon monoxide, blood	Up to 5% saturation
	Symptoms occur with 20% saturation
Dilantin, blood or serum	Therapeutic levels 1–11 µg/ml
Ethanol, blood	Less than 0.005%
Marked intoxication	0.3–0.4%
Alcoholic stupor	0.4–0.5%
Coma	Above 0.5%
Lead, blood	0–40 µg/dL
Lead, urine	Less than 100 µg/24 hrs

(continued)

Table E-7   (Continued)

Lithium, serum	0
	Therapeutic levels 0.5–1.5 mEq/L
	Toxic levels above 2 mEq/L
Mercury, urine	Less than 10 μg/24 hrs
Salicylate, plasma	0
Therapeutic range	20–25 mg/dL
Toxic range	Over 30 mg/dL
Death	45–75 mg/dL

Table E-8.   Pancreatic (Islet) Function Tests

Glucose tolerance tests	Patient should be on a diet containing 300 g of carbohydrate per day for 3 days prior to test.
Oral	After ingestion of 100 g of glucose or 1.75 g glucose/kg body weight, blood glucose is not more than 160 mg/dL after 60 minutes, 140 mg/dL after 90 minutes, and 120 mg/dL after 120 minutes. Values are for blood: serum measurements are approximately 15% higher.
Intravenous	Blood glucose does not exceed 200 mg/dL after infusion of 0.5 g of glucose/kg body weight over 30 minutes. Glucose concentration falls below initial level at 2 hours and returns to preinfusion levels in 3 hours or 1 hour. Values are for blood: serum measurements are approximately 15% higher.
Cortisone-glucose tolerance test	The patient should be on a diet containing 300 g of carbohydrate per day for 3 days prior to test. At 8½ and again 2 hours prior to glucose load patient is given cortisone acetate by mouth (50 mg if patient's ideal weight is less than 160 lb, 62.5 mg if ideal weight is greater than 160 lb.). An oral dose of glucose 1.75 g/kg body weight, is given and blood samples are taken at 0, 30, 60, 90, and 120 minutes. Test is considered positive if true blood glucose exceeds 160 mg/dL at 60 minutes, 140 mg/dL at 90 minutes, and 120 mg/dL at 120 minutes. Values are for blood: serum measurements are approximately 15% higher.

Table E-9.   Renal Function Test

Clearance tests (corrected to 1.73 sq meters body surface area)

Glomerular filtration rate (G.F.R.) Inulin clearance, Mannitol clearance, or Endogenous creatinine clearance	{ Males 110–150 ml/min { Females 105–132 ml/min
Renal plasma flow (RPF) p-Aminohippurate (PAH), or Diodrast	{ Males 560–830 ml/min { Females 490–700 ml/min
Filtration fraction (FF) $$FF = \frac{GFR}{RPF}$$	{ Males 17–21% { Females 17–23%

Table E-9   (Continued)

Urea clearance (C_q)	Standard 40–65 ml/min Maximal 60–100 ml/min
Concentration and dilution	Specific gravity > 1.025 on dry day Specific gravity < 1.003 on water day
Maximal Diodrast excretory capacity T_{M_O}	Males 43–59 mg/min Females 33–51 mg/min
Maximal glucose reabsorptive capacity T_{M_C}	Males 300–450 mg/min Females 250–350 mg/min
Maximal PAH excretory capacity $T_{M_{PAH}}$	80–90 mg/min
Phenolsulfonphthalein excretion (PSP)	25% or more in 15 min 40% or more in 30 min 55% or more in 2 hrs After injection of 1 ml PSP intravenously

Table E-10.   Gastrointestinal Absorption Tests

d-Xylose absorption test	After an 8 hour fast 10 ml/kg body weight of a 5% solution of d-xylose is given by mouth. Nothing further by mouth is given until the test has been completed. All urine voided during the following 5 hours is pooled, and blood samples are taken at 0, 60, and 120 minutes. Normally 26% (range 16–33%) of ingested xylose is excreted within 5 hours, and the serum xylose reaches a level between 25 and 40 mg/100 ml after 1 hour and is maintained at this level for another 60 minutes
Vitamin A absorption test	A fasting blood specimen is obtained and 200,000 units of vitamin A in oil is given by mouth. Serum vitamin A level should rise to twice fasting level in 3 to 5 hours.

Table E-11.   Typical Test Panels[a]

Preliminary Screening (SMA 6)	**Hemogram**
Bicarbonate (CO_2)	Hemoglobin
Sodium	Hematocrit
Potassium	Red cells
Chloride	White cells
Blood urea nitrogen (BUN)	Differential
Blood glucose	Neutrophils, segmented
(Reported in patient's chart as follows:	Neutrophils, nonsegmented
	Lymphocytes
	Monocytes
	Eosinophils
	Basophils
	Atypical lymphocytes
	Other
	RBC morphology
	Platelets:
Health Survey Screening	morphology
Albumin	count
Alkaline phosphatase	Mean corpuscular volume (calc)
SGOT	
Bilirubin (total)	Mean corpuscular hemoglobin (calc)

e.g.

	Na	Cl	BUN
	K	HCO₃	Glucose
	142	102	10
	4.0	28	102)

(continued)   (continued)

Table E-11 *(Continued)*

Blood urea nitrogen (BUN)
Calcium
Cholesterol
Glucose
Lactic dehydrogenase (LDH)
Phosphorus
Protein total

Uric acid
Routine Urinanalysis
Color
Appearance

Specific gravity
pH
Albumin, qualitative
Glucose, qualitative
Ketone bodies, qualitative
Bilirubin, qualitative
Occult blood
Casts
Organisms
Mucus
Epithelial cells
Crystal
White blood cells
Red blood cells

**Broad Spectrum Screening
(SMA 20)**
Albumin
Alkaline phosphatase
Bicarbonate (CO_2)
Bilirubin, total
  direct
  indirect
Blood urea nitrogen (BUN)
BUN/creatinine ratio
Calcium
Ionized calcium (est)
Chloride
Cholesterol
Creatinine
Globulin
Glucose
Lactic dehydrogenase (LDH)
Inorganic phosphorus
Potassium
Serum glutamic oxaloacetic
  transaminase (SGOT)
Serum glutamic pyruvic
  transaminase (SGPT)
Sodium
Total protein

Mean corpuscular hemoglobin
  concentration (calc)
(Some of the above values
  above are reported in the
  patient's chart as follows:
  Hgb Segs/Bands/Lymphs/
  Monos/Basos/Eos
WBC—MCV-MCH-MCHC
Hct Platelet count
e.g. 10.2 40S, 20B, 30L, 6M,
  1B, 3E

11,000 ---- 80/27/32
  30.4 286,000
A complete blood count (CBC)
  usually includes Hgb, Hct,
  RBC, WBC, MCV, MCH,
  MCHC)

(continued)

Table E-11 *(Continued)*

Triglycerides
Uric acid
Anion gap (calc)

Lipid panel
Cholesterol, total
Cholesterol, LDL
Cholesterol, HDL
Cholesterol, VLDL
LDL:HDL ratio
Triglycerides
VLDL:triglycerides ratio
Lipoprotein electrophoresis
Phospholipids
Total lipids
Glucose

CHD Risk Profile
HDL
Cholesterol, total
Triglycerides
Glucose

Hypertension Panel
Renal panel
Blood gases:
  pH
  pCO_2
  Bicarbonate
Cholesterol
Glucose
LDH
Triglycerides

Liver Panel
Alkaline phosphatase
Bilirubin, total
  direct
LDH
LDH isozymes
SGOT (AST)
SGPT (ALT)
Protein, total
Protein electrophoresis
Urine bile pigment
Albumin
Globulin

Pancreatic Panel
Serum amylase
Serum lipase
Urine amylase

Acute heart panel
Creatinine phosphokinase
  (CPK)
Hydroxybutyric
  dehydrogenase (HBD)
Lactate dehydrogenase (LDH)
LDH isozymes

Potassium
SGOT

Renal Panel
BUN
Creatinine
Creatinine clearance
Calcium
Chloride
Phosphorus
Potassium
Protein, total
Protein electrophoresis
Sodium
Urine specific gravity
Urine culture

Diabetes Mellitus Panel
Glucose
Glucose tolerance (if not
  contraindicated)
Serum ketones
Triglycerides
Urine glucose/24 hours
Urine ketones

Diabetes Management Profile
Glucose
Hemoglobin A_{1c}

[a]Test panels are the result of the development of automated analytical instruments. It is common for the physician to order an automated panel of tests, rather than ordering individual tests. The contents of some typical test panels are shown in this table.

Appendix F:
Nutritional Assessment Data

Table F-1. 1983 Metropolitan Height and Weight Tables

Men					*Women*					
Height		Small Frame	Medium Frame	Large Frame	Height		Small Frame	Medium Frame	Large Frame	
Feet	Inches				Feet	Inches				
5	2	128–134	131–141	138–150	4	10	102–111	109–121	118–131	
5	3	130–136	133–143	140–153	4	11	103–113	111–123	120–134	
5	4	132–138	135–145	142–156	5	0	104–115	113–126	122–137	
5	5	134–140	137–148	144–160	5	1	106–118	115–129	125–140	
5	6	136–142	139–151	146–164	5	2	108–121	118–132	128–143	
5	7	138–145	142–154	149–168	5	3	111–124	121–135	131–147	
5	8	140–148	145–157	152–172	5	4	114–127	124–138	134–151	
5	9	142–151	148–160	155–176	5	5	117–130	127–141	137–155	
5	10	144–154	151–163	158–180	5	6	120–133	130–144	140–159	
5	11	146–157	154–166	161–184	5	7	123–136	133–147	143–163	
6	0	149–160	157–170	164–188	5	8	126–139	136–150	146–167	
6	1	152–164	160–174	168–192	5	9	129–142	139–153	149–170	
6	2	155–168	164–178	172–197	5	10	132–145	142–156	152–173	
6	3	158–172	167–182	176–202	5	11	135–148	145–159	155–176	
6	4	162–176	171–187	181–207	6	0	138–151	148–162	158–179	

Weights at ages 25–59 based on lowest mortality. Weight in pounds according to frame (in indoor clothing weighing 5 lbs. for men and 3 lbs. for women; shoes with 1″ heels).

Source of basic data: 1979 Build Study, Society of Actuaries and Association of Life Insurance Medical Directors of America, 1980. Reproduced with permission from Metropolitan Life Insurance Company.

Table F-2.   An Approximation of Frame Size

Height in 1" heels	Elbow Breadth
Men	
5'2"–5'3"	2½"–2⅞"
5'4"–5'7"	2⅝"–2⅞"
5'8"–5'11"	2¾"–3"
6'0"–6'3"	2¾"–3⅛"
6'4"	2⅞"–3¼"
Women	
4'10"–4'11"	2¼"–2½"
5'0"–5'3"	2¼"–2½"
5'4"–5'7"	2⅜"–2⅝"
5'8"–5'11"	2⅜"–2⅝"
6'0"	2½"–2¾"

Reproduced with permission from Metropolitan Life Insurance Company.

Table F-3.   Evaluation of Weight Change

Time	Significant Weight Loss (% of change)	Severe Weight Loss (% of change)
1 wk	1–2	>2
1 mo.	5	>5
3 mo.	7.5	>7.5
6 mo.	10	>10

Reprinted with permission from Blackburn, G.L., B.R. Bistrian, B.S. Maini, et al., Nutritional and metabolic assessment of the hospitalized patient. *J.P.E.N.* 1: (1977) 15.

Table F-4.   Weight (lb) For Height (in) Males

Height in inches	Percentile	18–24	25–34	35–44	45–54	55–64	65–74
62 inches	50	130	141	143	147	143	143
	15	102	109	115	118	113	116
	5	85	91	98	100	96	100
63 inches	50	135	145	148	152	147	147
	15	107	113	120	123	117	120
	5	90	95	103	105	100	104
64 inches	50	140	150	153	156	153	151
	15	112	118	125	127	123	124
	5	95	100	108	109	106	108
65 inches	50	145	156	158	160	158	156
	15	117	124	130	131	128	129
	5	100	106	113	113	111	113
66 inches	50	150	160	163	164	163	160
	15	122	128	135	135	133	133
	5	105	110	118	117	116	117
67 inches	50	154	165	169	169	168	164
	15	126	133	141	140	138	137
	5	109	115	124	122	121	121
68 inches	50	159	170	174	173	173	169
	15	131	138	146	144	143	142
	5	114	120	129	126	126	126
69 inches	50	164	174	179	177	178	173
	15	136	142	151	148	148	146
	5	119	124	134	130	131	130
70 inches	50	168	179	184	182	183	177
	15	140	147	156	153	153	150
	5	123	129	139	135	136	134
71 inches	50	173	184	190	187	189	182
	15	145	152	162	158	159	155
	5	128	134	145	140	142	139
72 inches	50	178	189	194	191	193	186
	15	150	157	166	162	163	159
	5	133	139	149	144	146	143
73 inches	50	183	194	200	196	197	190
	15	155	162	172	167	167	163
	5	138	144	155	149	150	147
74 inches	50	188	199	205	200	203	194
	15	160	167	177	171	173	167
	5	143	149	160	153	156	151

Reproduced with permission from Ross Laboratories, Columbus, Ohio 43216.

Table F-5. Weight (pounds) For Height (inches) Females

Height in inches	Percentile	Age group in years					
		18–24	25–34	35–44	45–54	55–64	65–74
57 inches	50	114	118	125	129	132	130
	15	85	85	89	94	97	100
	5	68	65	67	73	77	82
58 inches	50	117	121	129	133	136	134
	15	88	88	93	98	101	104
	5	71	68	71	77	81	86
59 inches	50	120	125	133	136	140	137
	15	91	92	97	101	105	107
	5	74	72	75	80	85	89
60 inches	50	123	128	137	140	143	140
	15	94	95	101	105	108	110
	5	77	75	79	84	88	92
61 inches	50	126	132	141	143	147	144
	15	97	99	105	108	112	114
	5	80	79	83	87	92	96
62 inches	50	129	136	144	147	150	147
	15	100	103	108	112	115	117
	5	83	83	86	91	95	99
63 inches	50	132	139	148	150	153	151
	15	103	106	112	115	118	121
	5	86	86	90	94	98	103
64 inches	50	135	142	152	154	157	154
	15	106	109	116	119	122	124
	5	89	89	94	98	102	106
65 inches	50	138	146	156	158	160	158
	15	109	113	120	123	125	128
	5	92	93	98	102	105	110
66 inches	50	141	150	159	161	164	161
	15	112	117	123	126	129	131
	5	95	97	101	105	109	113
67 inches	50	144	153	163	165	167	165
	15	115	120	127	130	132	135
	5	98	100	105	109	112	117
68 inches	50	147	157	167	168	171	169
	15	118	124	131	133	136	139
	5	101	104	109	112	116	121

Reproduced with permission from Ross Laboratories, Columbus, Ohio 43216.

Table F-6. Standards for Anthropometric Measurements

Sex	Triceps Skinfold (mm)	Arm Circumference (cm)	Arm Muscle Circumference (cm)
Male	12.5	29.3	25.3
Female	16.5	28.5	23.2

Reprinted with permission from Blackburn, G.L., B.R. Bistrian, B.S. Maini, et al., Nutritional and metabolic assessment of the hospitalized patient. *J.P.E.N.* 1: (1977) 15.

Table F-7. Interpretation of Nutritional Assessment Values[a]

	Deficit			
Observation[a]	None	Mild	Moderate	Severe
TSF (% of standard)	>90	90–51	50–30	<30
MAMC (% of standard)	>90	90–81	80–70	<70
CHI (% of standard)	>90	90–81	80–71	70–60
Serum albumin (g/dl)	>3.5	<3.5–3.2	<3.2–2.8	<2.8
Transferrin (mg/dl)	>200	<200–180	<180–160	<160
TIBC (μg/dl)	>214	<214–182	<182–152	<152
Total lymphocytes (per mm^3)	>1,500	1,500–1,201	1,200–800	<800

[a]TSF = thickness of triceps skinfold; MAMC = midarm muscle circumference; CHI = creatinine-height index; TIBC = total iron-binding capacity.

Values compiled from Blackburn, G.L., B.R. Bistrian, B.S. Maini, et al., Nutritional and metabolic assessment of the hospitalized patient. *J.P.E.N.* 1: (1977) 11–22; and Blackburn, G.L., Nutritional assessment: An overview. *Clin. Consult. Nutr. Support* 1: (1981) 10.

From Zeman, F.J. *Clinical Nutrition and Dietetics.* New York: Macmillan, 1983, p. 29. Used by permission of the publisher.

Table F-8. Percentiles for Triceps Skinfold (mm)[a]

Age Group	n	5	10	25	50	75	90	95	n	5	10	25	50	75	90	95
	Males								*Females*							
1–1.9	228	6	7	8	10	12	14	16	204	6	7	8	10	12	14	16
2–2.9	223	6	7	8	10	12	14	15	208	6	8	9	10	12	15	16
3–3.9	220	6	7	8	10	11	14	15	208	7	8	9	11	12	14	15
4–4.9	230	6	6	8	9	11	12	14	208	7	8	8	10	12	14	16
5–5.9	214	6	6	8	9	11	14	15	219	6	7	8	10	12	15	18
6–6.9	117	5	6	7	8	10	13	16	118	6	6	8	10	12	14	16
7–7.9	122	5	6	7	9	12	15	17	126	6	7	9	11	13	16	18
8–8.9	117	5	6	7	8	10	13	16	118	6	8	9	12	15	18	24
9–9.9	121	6	6	7	10	13	17	18	125	8	8	10	13	16	20	22
10–10.9	146	6	6	8	10	14	18	21	152	7	8	10	12	17	23	27
11–11.9	122	6	6	8	11	16	20	24	117	7	8	10	13	18	24	28
12–12.9	153	6	6	8	11	14	22	28	129	8	9	11	14	18	23	27
13–13.9	134	5	5	7	10	14	22	26	151	8	8	12	15	21	26	30
14–14.9	131	4	5	7	9	14	21	24	141	9	10	13	16	21	26	28
15–15.9	128	4	5	6	8	11	18	24	117	8	10	12	17	21	25	32
16–16.9	131	4	5	6	8	12	16	22	142	10	12	15	18	22	26	31
17–17.9	133	5	5	6	8	12	16	19	114	10	12	13	19	24	30	37
18–18.9	91	4	5	6	9	13	20	24	109	10	12	15	18	22	26	30
19–24.9	531	4	5	7	10	15	20	22	1,060	10	11	14	18	24	30	34
25–34.9	971	5	6	8	12	16	20	24	1,987	10	12	16	21	27	34	37
35–44.9	806	5	6	8	12	16	20	23	1,614	12	14	18	23	29	35	38
45–54.9	898	6	6	8	12	15	20	25	1,047	12	16	20	25	30	36	40
55–64.9	734	5	6	8	11	14	19	22	809	12	16	20	25	31	36	38
65–74.9	1,503	4	6	8	11	15	19	22	1,670	12	14	18	24	29	34	36

[a]Data collected from whites in the United States Health and Nutrition Examination Survey I (1971–1974).

Reproduced from Frisancho, A.R. New norms of upper limb fat and muscle areas for assessment of nutritional status. *Am. J. Clin. Nutr.* 34 (1981) 2540. © *Am. J. Clin. Nutr.* American Society for Clinical Nutrition.

Table F-9. Thickness of Triceps and Subscapular Skinfolds at 1 to 36 Months of Age

Age (months)	Percentiles	Triceps (mm) Males	Triceps (mm) Females	Subscapular (mm) Males	Subscapular (mm) Females
1	2.5	2.9	3.5	3.1	3.8
	10	4.0	4.5	4.2	4.9
	25	4.7	5.2	4.8	5.4
	50	5.3	5.8	5.6	6.2
	75	6.2	6.7	6.5	7.0
	90	7.0	7.6	7.5	7.9
	97.5	8.1	8.3	8.3	9.0
3	2.5	4.5	5.0	3.5	4.7
	10	6.0	6.2	4.9	5.9
	25	6.8	7.2	5.8	6.9
	50	8.1	8.2	6.9	8.0
	75	9.2	9.2	8.1	8.6
	90	10.3	10.5	9.0	9.4
	97.5	11.7	11.8	10.7	11.1
6	2.5	6.3	6.7	3.8	4.0
	10	7.8	8.2	5.5	5.9
	25	8.6	9.0	6.2	6.9
	50	9.7	10.4	7.1	8.1
	75	11.1	11.3	8.4	8.9
	90	11.8	12.7	10.1	10.3
	97.5	13.5	13.9	11.0	12.4
9	2.5	6.0	6.7	3.4	4.7
	10	7.5	7.9	5.3	6.0
	25	8.7	8.8	6.0	6.7
	50	9.9	10.1	7.1	7.6
	75	11.2	11.3	8.5	8.8
	90	12.5	12.5	9.7	10.1
	97.5	14.0	13.5	11.4	11.1
12	2.5	6.2	6.4	3.8	4.5
	10	7.8	7.6	5.3	6.0
	25	8.6	8.7	6.0	6.5
	50	9.8	9.8	7.2	7.5
	75	11.1	11.2	8.6	8.7
	90	12.2	12.2	9.6	9.8
	97.5	13.8	13.6	11.0	10.9
18	2.5	6.4	6.8	3.9	4.2
	10	7.7	7.9	5.3	5.7
	25	8.6	8.9	6.0	6.2
	50	9.9	10.3	6.8	7.1
	75	11.4	11.3	7.9	8.0
	90	12.2	12.3	9.3	9.0
	97.5	13.6	13.6	10.3	10.2
24	2.5	5.8	6.5	3.0	3.9
	10	7.4	8.3	4.6	5.3
	25	8.5	8.9	5.4	5.6
	50	9.8	10.1	6.5	6.5
	75	11.6	11.6	7.4	7.3
	90	13.1	12.8	8.3	8.4
	97.5	14.2	14.1	10.2	9.5
36	2.5	6.6	6.4	2.9	2.6
	10	7.8	8.2	4.5	4.7
	25	9.0	9.4	5.0	5.2
	50	9.8	10.3	5.5	6.1
	75	11.0	11.5	6.4	7.2
	90	12.2	12.5	7.1	8.6
	97.5	13.4	14.4	8.9	10.6

(continued)

Adapted from Karlberg, P., et al. The development of children in a Swedish urban community: A prospective longitudinal study. III. Physical growth during the first three years of life. *Acta. Pediatr. Scand.* 187(1968)48; courtesy of *Acta. Pediatr. Scand.* in Palmer, S. and S. Ervall, eds. *Pediatric Nutrition in Developmental Disorders,* 1978. Courtesy of Charles C Thomas, Publisher, Springfield, Ill.

Table F-10. Percentiles of Upper Arm Circumference and Estimated Upper Arm Muscle Circumference[a]

Age Group	Midarm Circumference (mm)							Midarm Muscle Circumference (mm)						
	5	10	25	50	75	90	95	5	10	25	50	75	90	95
Males														
1–1.9	142	146	150	159	170	176	183	110	113	119	127	135	144	147
2–2.9	141	145	153	162	170	178	185	111	114	122	130	140	146	150
3–3.9	150	153	160	167	175	184	190	117	123	131	137	143	148	153
4–4.9	149	154	162	171	180	186	192	123	126	133	141	148	156	159
5–5.9	153	160	167	175	185	195	204	128	133	140	147	154	162	169
6–6.9	155	159	167	179	188	209	228	131	135	142	151	161	170	177
7–7.9	162	167	177	187	201	223	230	137	139	151	160	168	177	190
8–8.9	162	170	177	190	202	220	245	140	145	154	162	170	182	187
9–9.9	175	178	187	200	217	249	257	151	154	161	170	183	196	202
10–10.9	181	184	196	210	231	262	274	156	160	166	180	191	209	221
11–11.9	186	190	202	223	244	261	280	159	165	173	183	195	205	230
12–12.9	193	200	214	232	254	282	303	167	171	182	195	210	223	241
13–13.9	194	211	228	247	263	286	301	172	179	196	211	226	238	245
14–14.9	220	226	237	253	283	303	322	189	199	212	223	240	260	264
15–15.9	222	229	244	264	284	311	320	199	204	218	237	254	266	272
16–16.9	244	248	262	278	303	324	343	213	225	234	249	269	287	296
17–17.9	246	253	267	285	308	336	347	224	231	245	258	273	294	312
18–18.9	245	260	276	297	321	353	379	226	237	252	264	283	298	324
19–24.9	262	272	288	308	331	355	372	238	245	257	273	289	309	321
25–34.9	271	282	300	319	342	362	375	243	250	264	279	298	314	326
35–44.9	278	287	305	326	345	363	374	247	255	269	286	302	318	327
45–54.9	267	281	301	322	342	362	376	239	249	265	281	300	315	326
55–64.9	258	273	296	317	336	355	369	236	245	260	278	295	310	320
65–74.9	248	263	285	307	325	344	355	223	235	251	268	284	298	306
Females														
1–1.9	138	142	148	156	164	172	177	105	111	117	124	132	139	143
2–2.9	142	145	152	160	167	176	184	111	114	119	126	133	142	147
3–3.9	143	150	158	167	175	183	189	113	119	124	132	140	146	152
4–4.9	149	154	160	169	177	184	191	115	121	128	136	144	152	157
5–5.9	153	157	165	175	185	203	211	125	128	134	142	151	159	165
6–6.9	156	162	170	176	187	204	211	130	133	138	145	154	166	171
7–7.9	164	167	174	183	199	216	231	129	135	142	151	160	171	176
8–8.9	168	172	183	195	214	247	261	138	140	151	160	171	183	194
9–9.9	178	182	194	211	224	251	260	147	150	158	167	180	194	198
10–10.9	174	182	193	210	228	251	265	148	150	159	170	180	190	197
11–11.9	185	194	208	224	248	276	303	150	158	171	181	196	217	223
12–12.9	194	203	216	237	256	282	294	162	166	180	191	201	214	220
13–13.9	202	211	223	243	271	301	338	169	175	183	198	211	226	240
14–14.9	214	223	237	252	272	304	322	174	179	190	201	216	232	247
15–15.9	208	221	239	254	279	300	322	175	178	189	202	215	228	244
16–16.9	218	224	241	258	283	318	334	170	180	190	202	216	234	249
17–17.9	220	227	241	264	295	324	350	175	183	194	205	221	239	257
18–18.9	222	227	241	258	281	312	325	174	179	191	202	215	237	245
19–24.9	221	230	247	265	290	319	345	179	185	195	207	221	236	249
25–34.9	233	240	256	277	304	342	368	183	188	199	212	228	246	264
35–44.9	241	251	267	290	317	356	378	186	192	205	218	236	257	272
45–54.9	242	256	274	299	328	362	384	187	193	206	220	238	260	274
55–64.9	243	257	280	303	335	367	385	187	196	209	225	244	266	280
65–74.9	240	252	274	299	326	356	373	185	195	208	225	244	264	279

[a]Data collected from whites in the United States Health and Nutrition Examination Survey I (1971–1974).

Reproduced from Frisancho, A.R. New norms of upper limb fat and muscle areas for assessment of nutritional status. *Am. J. Clin. Nutr.* 34(1981)2540. © *Am. J. Clin. Nutr.*, American Society for Clinical Nutrition.

Table F-11. Percentiles for Estimates of Upper Arm Fat Area and Upper Arm Muscle Area[a]

Age Group	Arm Muscle Area Percentiles (mm²)							Arm Fat Area Percentiles (mm²)						
	5	10	25	50	75	90	95	5	10	25	50	75	90	95
Males														
1–1.9	956	1,014	1,133	1,278	1,447	1,644	1,720	452	486	590	741	895	1,036	1,176
2–2.9	973	1,040	1,190	1,345	1,557	1,690	1,787	434	504	578	737	871	1,044	1,148
3–3.9	1,095	1,201	1,357	1,484	1,618	1,750	1,853	464	519	590	736	868	1,071	1,151
4–4.9	1,207	1,264	1,408	1,579	1,747	1,926	2,008	428	494	598	722	859	989	1,085
5–5.9	1,298	1,411	1,550	1,720	1,884	2,089	2,285	446	488	582	713	914	1,176	1,299
6–6.9	1,360	1,447	1,605	1,815	2,056	2,297	2,493	371	446	539	678	896	1,115	1,519
7–7.9	1,497	1,548	1,808	2,027	2,246	2,494	2,886	423	473	574	758	1,011	1,393	1,511
8–8.9	1,550	1,664	1,895	2,089	2,296	2,628	2,788	410	460	588	725	1,003	1,248	1,558
9–9.9	1,811	1,884	2,067	2,288	2,657	3,053	3,257	485	527	635	859	1,252	1,864	2,081
10–10.9	1,930	2,027	2,182	2,575	2,903	3,486	3,882	523	543	738	982	1,376	1,906	2,609
11–11.9	2,016	2,156	2,382	2,670	3,022	3,359	4,226	536	595	754	1,148	1,710	2,348	2,574
12–12.9	2,216	2,339	2,649	3,022	3,496	3,968	4,640	554	650	874	1,172	1,558	2,536	3,580
13–13.9	2,363	2,546	3,044	3,553	4,081	4,502	4,794	475	570	812	1,096	1,702	2,744	3,322
14–14.9	2,830	3,147	3,586	3,963	4,575	5,368	5,530	453	563	786	1,082	1,608	2,746	3,508
15–15.9	3,138	3,317	3,788	4,481	5,134	5,631	5,900	521	595	690	931	1,423	2,434	3,100
16–16.9	3,625	4,044	4,352	4,951	5,753	6,576	6,980	542	593	844	1,078	1,746	2,280	3,041
17–17.9	3,998	4,252	4,777	5,286	5,950	6,886	7,726	598	698	827	1,096	1,636	2,407	2,888
18–18.9	4,070	4,481	5,066	5,552	6,374	7,067	8,355	560	665	860	1,264	1,947	3,302	3,928
19–24.9	4,508	4,777	5,274	5,913	6,660	7,606	8,200	594	743	963	1,406	2,231	3,098	3,652
25–34.9	4,694	4,963	5,541	6,214	7,067	7,847	8,436	675	831	1,174	1,752	2,459	3,246	3,786
35–44.9	4,844	5,181	5,740	6,490	7,265	8,034	8,488	703	851	1,310	1,792	2,463	3,098	3,624
45–54.9	4,546	4,946	5,589	6,297	7,142	7,918	8,458	749	922	1,254	1,741	2,359	3,245	3,928
55–64.9	4,422	4,783	5,381	6,144	6,919	7,670	8,149	658	839	1,166	1,645	2,236	2,976	3,466
65–74.9	3,973	4,411	5,031	5,716	6,432	7,074	7,453	573	753	1,122	1,621	2,199	2,876	3,327
Females														
1–1.9	885	973	1,084	1,221	1,378	1,535	1,621	401	466	578	706	847	1,022	1,140
2–2.9	973	1,029	1,119	1,269	1,405	1,595	1,727	469	526	642	747	894	1,061	1,173
3–3.9	1,014	1,133	1,227	1,396	1,563	1,690	1,846	473	529	656	822	967	1,106	1,158
4–4.9	1,058	1,171	1,313	1,475	1,644	1,832	1,958	490	541	654	766	907	1,109	1,236
5–5.9	1,238	1,301	1,423	1,598	1,825	2,012	2,159	470	529	647	812	991	1,330	1,536
6–6.9	1,354	1,414	1,513	1,683	1,877	2,182	2,323	464	508	638	827	1,009	1,263	1,436
7–7.9	1,330	1,441	1,602	1,815	2,045	2,332	2,469	491	560	706	920	1,135	1,407	1,644
8–8.9	1,513	1,566	1,808	2,034	2,327	2,657	2,996	527	634	769	1,042	1,383	1,872	2,482
9–9.9	1,723	1,788	1,976	2,227	2,571	2,987	3,112	642	690	933	1,219	1,584	2,171	2,524
10–10.9	1,740	1,784	2,019	2,296	2,583	2,873	3,093	616	702	842	1,141	1,608	2,500	3,005
11–11.9	1,784	1,987	2,316	2,612	3,071	3,739	3,953	707	802	1,015	1,301	1,942	2,730	3,690
12–12.9	2,092	2,182	2,579	2,904	3,225	3,655	3,847	782	854	1,090	1,511	2,056	2,666	3,369
13–13.9	2,269	2,426	2,657	3,130	3,529	4,081	4,568	726	838	1,219	1,625	2,374	3,272	4,150
14–14.9	2,418	2,562	2,874	3,220	3,704	4,294	4,850	981	1,043	1,423	1,818	2,403	3,250	3,765
15–15.9	2,426	2,518	2,847	3,248	3,689	4,123	4,756	839	1,126	1,396	1,886	2,544	3,093	4,195
16–16.9	2,308	2,567	2,865	3,248	3,718	4,353	4,946	1,126	1,351	1,663	2,006	2,598	3,374	4,236
17–17.9	2,442	2,674	2,996	3,336	3,883	4,552	5,251	1,042	1,267	1,463	2,104	2,977	3,864	5,159
18–18.9	2,398	2,538	2,917	3,243	3,694	4,461	4,767	1,003	1,230	1,616	2,104	2,617	3,508	3,733
19–24.9	2,538	2,728	3,026	3,406	3,877	4,439	4,940	1,046	1,198	1,596	2,166	2,959	4,050	4,896
25–34.9	2,661	2,826	3,148	3,573	4,138	4,806	5,541	1,173	1,399	1,841	2,548	3,512	4,690	5,560
35–44.9	2,750	2,948	3,359	3,783	4,428	5,240	5,877	1,336	1,619	2,158	2,898	3,932	5,093	5,847
45–54.9	2,784	2,956	3,378	3,858	4,520	5,375	5,974	1,459	1,803	2,447	3,244	4,229	5,416	6,140
55–64.9	2,784	3,063	3,477	4,045	4,750	5,632	6,247	1,345	1,879	2,520	3,369	4,360	5,276	6,152
65–74.9	2,737	3,018	3,444	4,019	4,739	5,566	6,214	1,363	1,681	2,266	3,063	3,943	4,914	5,530

[a]Data collected from whites in the United States Health and Nutrition Examination Survey I (1971–1974).

Reproduced from Frisancho, A.R. New norms of upper limb fat and muscle areas for assessment of nutritional status. *Am. J. Clin. Nutr.* 34(1981)2540. © *Am. J. Clin. Nutr.*, American Society for Clinical Nutrition.

Table F-12. Normal 24-hour Creatinine Excretion (mg/24 hours)

Height (cm)	Children aged 0–9 years	Males	Females
50.0	36		
53.5	45		
56.9	55		
60.4	66		
64.4	79		
66.4	85		
69.6	96		
73.8	113		
76.3	124		
80.7	143		
84.7	165		
88.5	189		
94.1	231		
98.0	264		
102.2	290		
105.6	308		
108.7	337		
113.2	385		
117.2	408		
121.5	478		

(continued)

Table F-12. *(Continued)*

Height (cm)	Children aged 0–9 years	Males	Females
124.5	528		
126.0	557		
129.0	617		
130.0		448	525
135.0		480	589
140.0		556	653
145.0		684	717
150.0		812	781
155.0		940	845
160.0		1,068	909
165.0		1,196	
170.0		1,324	
175.0		1,452	

The usual creatinine excretion rate is 20–26 mg/kg/day in men, and 14–22 mg/kg/day in women.

Adapted from Viteri, F.E. and J. Alvarado. The creatinine-height index: Its use in the estimation of the degree of protein depletion and repletion in protein-calorie malnourished children. *Pediatrics* 46:(1970)696–706; Graystone, J.E. Creatinine excretion during growth. In Cheek, D.B. *Human Growth, Body Composition, Cell Growth, Energy and Intelligence.* Philadelphia: Lea & Febiger, 1968, pp. 182–197.

Table F-13. Clinical Evaluation of Nutritional Status

	Clinical Findings	*Deficiency*	*Differential Diagnosis*
Skull	In infants: bossing of the skull over ossification centers, delayed closure of anterior fontanelle	Vitamin D, calcium	Syphilis, sickle-cell disease, positional deformity, hydrocephalus
	Decreased head circumference	Protein-calorie	
Hair	Dry, wirelike, easily pluckable, brittle, depigmented, sparse	Protein-calorie	
	Impaired keratinization (hair is "steely")	Copper	
	Hair loss	Zinc, biotin, protein, essential fatty acids	
Skin	Malar pigmentation (darkened pigment over malar eminences)	Calories, B complex, especially niacin	Melasma in pregnancy or from oral contraceptives, Addison's disease
	Nasolabial seborrhea	Niacin, riboflavin, B_6	
	Ecchymosis	Vitamin C	Hematologic disorders (thrombocytopenia), trauma, liver disease, anticoagulant overdose, orthostatic purpura, Fabry's disease, emboli, stasis, clotting factor deficiency
	Perifollicular petechiae	Vitamin K	
	Follicular hyperkeratosis (skin is rough, surrounding skin is dry)	Vitamin A	Fungus infection, perifolliculitis or scurvy, keratosis pilaris, Darier's disease
	Xerosis (skin is dry, with fine flaking)	Vitamin A, essential fatty acids	Aging, environmental drying, hypothyroidism, uremia, poor hygiene, ichthyosis
	Hyperpigmentation (seen more frequently on hands and face)	Niacin, folic acid, B_{12}	Addison's disease, environmental factors, trauma
	Scrotal dermatitis	Riboflavin, zinc	Fungus infection
	Pellagrous dermatitis (lesions are symmetric and in areas exposed to the sun)	Niacin	Chemical injury, sunburn, thermal burn
	Thickened skin at pressure points (predominantly in belt area)		
	Delayed wound healing	Zinc, vitamin C, protein	

(continued)

Table F-13.　(Continued)

	Clinical Findings	Deficiency	Differential Diagnosis
Eyes	Circumcorneal injection (bilateral)	Riboflavin	
	Xerophthalmia (conjunctiva is dull, lusterless, exhibits a striated or rough surface)	Vitamin A	
	Bitot's spots (small circumscribed, dull, dry lesions usually seen on the lateral aspect of the bulbar conjunctiva)	Vitamin A	Pterygium
	Keratomalacia	Vitamin A	
	Night blindness	Vitamin A	
	Xanthomatosis, hyperlipidemia, and hypercholesterolemia leading to localized deposits of lipids	Excess intake of fat with elevated serum lipoproteins	
Lips	Cheilosis (lips may be swollen)	Niacin, riboflavin	Herpes simplex, arid or arctic environmental exposure
	Angular fissures (corners of mouth broken or macerated)	Niacin, riboflavin, iron, B_6	Herpes, syphilis
Gums	Bleeding gums (spongy)	Vitamin C	Dilantin toxicity, periodontal disease
Teeth	Dental caries	Fluoride	Poor oral hygiene
	Mottled enamel	Excess fluoride	Staining from tetracyclines
Tongue	Glossitis (red, painful tongue—may be fissured)	Folic acid, niacin, riboflavin, B_{12}, B_6, iron	Uremia, antibiotics, malignancy, aphthous stomatitis, monilial infection
	Atrophy of filiform papillae (low or absent)	Niacin, folic acid, B_{12}, iron	Non-nutritional anemias
	Hypertrophy of fungiform papillae	General malnutrition	Dietary irritants
	Pale, atrophic tongue	Iron, folic acid, B_{12}, niacin, riboflavin, B_6	Non-nutritional anemias
Exocrine	Parotid enlargement	Protein (?)	Mumps
Endocrine	Goiter	Iodine	Thyroglossal duct cyst, bronchial cleft cysts and tumors, hyperthyroidism, thyroiditis, thyroid carcinoma
Oral	Dysgeusia (disorderd taste)	Zinc	Cancer therapy
	Hypogeusia (loss of taste acuity)		
Nails	Koilonychia (spoon nails; nails are thin, concave)	Iron	Cardiac or pulmonary disease
Cardiac	Cardia enlargement, tachycardia	Thiamine, iron	
Abdominal	Hepatomegaly	Chronic malnutrition	Liver disease
Skeletal	Rickets (bowed legs, deformities may also be seen in pelvic bones)	Calcium, phosphates, vitamin D	Renal rickets, malabsorption, congenital deformity
	Costochondral beading (?)	Calcium, vitamin D	
	Scorbutic rosary (costochondral junctions may have sharp edges caused by epiphyseal separation)	Vitamin C	
	Epiphyseal swelling secondary to epiphyseal hyperplasia (in rickets, secondary to tenderness and swelling caused by hemorrhage)	Vitamin D, calcium, vitamin C	Renal disease, malabsorption, congenital deformity
Neurologic	Absence of tendon reflexes (bilateral)	Thiamine, B_{12}	Peripheral neuropathy from other causes
	Absence of vibratory sense (bilateral)		
	Calf tenderness	Thiamine	
	Pseudoparalysis (movement restricted because of pain)	Vitamin C	Hypokalemia
Extremities	Calf tenderness	Thiamine	Muscle strain, trauma, other causes of peripheral neuropathy, deep venous thrombosis
	Bilateral edema of lower extremities	Protein (occurs late in deficiency)	Congestive heart failure, renal failure, protein-losing enteropathy
Growth	Nutritional dwarfism, subcutaneous fat loss	Calories, protein	
	Dwarfism, hypogonadism	Zinc	

Reproduced with permission from Walker, W.A. and K.M. Hendricks. *Manual of Pediatric Nutrition*. Philadelphia: Saunders, 1985.

Table F-14.   Clinical Examination in Nutritional Deficiencies and Excesses

	Major Physiologic Functions	Deficiency Signs	Excess Signs	Important Food Sources
Nutrient				
Protein	Constitutes part of the structure of every cell; regulates body processes as part of enzymes, some hormones, body fluids, and antibodies that increase resistance to infection; provides nitrogen and has a caloric density of 4 kcal/g	Dry, depigmented, easily pluckable hair; bilateral, dependent edema, cirrhosis, fatty liver, decreased visceral proteins; skin is dry with pellagroid dermatoses in severe cases	Azotemia, acidosis, hyperammonemia	Meat, poultry, fish, legumes, eggs, cheese, milk and other dairy products, nuts, breast milk, infant formula
Carbohydrate	Supplies energy at an average of 4 kcal/g of glucose (sparing protein) and is the major energy source for CNS function; unrefined, complex carbohydrates supply fiber that aids in normal bowel function	Seizures	May cause diarrhea	Breads, cereals, crackers, potatoes, corn, simple sugars (sugar, honey), fruits and vegetables, milk, breast milk, infant formula
Fat	Concentrated calorie source at an average 9 kcal/g; constitutes part of the structure of every cell; supplies essential fatty acids and provides and carries fat-soluble vitamins (A, D, E, K)	Essential fatty acid deficiency: dry, scaly skin, poor weight gain, hair loss	Atherosclerosis may be affected by excessive intakes of certain dietary fats; altered blood lipid levels	Shortening, oil, butter, margarine, protein-rich foods (meat, dairy, nuts), breast milk, infant formula
Fat-Soluble Vitamins				
Vitamin A (serum carotene)	Formation and maintenance of skin and mucous membranes; necessary for the formation of rhodopsin (the photosensitive pigment of the rods governing vision in dim light), and regulation of membrane structure and function	Night blindness, degeneration of the retina, xerophthalmia, follicular hyperkeratosis, poor growth, keratomalacia, Bitot's spots	Fatigue, malaise, lethargy, abdominal pain, hepatomegaly, alopecia, headache with increased intracranial pressure, vomiting	Carrots, liver, green vegetables, sweet potatoes, butter, margarine, apricots, melons, peaches, broccoli, cod liver oil, breast milk, infant formula
Vitamin D	Promotes intestinal absorption of calcium and phosphate, renal conservation of calcium and phosphorus	Rickets, osteomalacia, costochondral beading, epiphyseal enlargement, cranial bossing, bowed legs, persistently open anterior fontanelle	Hypercalcemia, vomiting, anorexia, irritability, azotemia, diarrhea, convulsions	Cod liver oil, fish, eggs, liver, butter, fortified milk, sunlight (activation of 7-dehydrocholesterol in the skin), infant formula
Vitamin E	Acts as an antioxidant and free radical scavenger to prevent peroxidation of polyunsaturated fatty acids in the body; enhances absorption and utilization of vitamin A	Hemolytic anemia in the premature and newborn, enhanced fragility of red blood cells, increased peroxidative hemolysis	None known	Oils high in polyunsaturated fatty acids, milk, eggs, breast milk, infant formula
Vitamin K	Necessary for prothrombin and the three blood-clotting factors VII, IX, and X; half of the vitamin K in humans is of intestinal origin, synthesized by gut flora; necessary for bone mineralization	Hemorrhagic manifestations (especially in newborns), cirrhosis	Hemolytic anemia, nerve palsy	Green leafy vegetables, fruits, cereals, dairy products, soybeans, breast milk, infant formula

(continued)

Table F-14. *(Continued)*

	Major Physiologic Functions	Deficiency Signs	Excess Signs	Important Food Sources
Water-Soluble Vitamins				
Vitamin C	Forms collagen cross-linkages of proline hydroxylase, thus strengthening tissue and improving wound healing and resistance to infection; aids utilization of iron; is a water-soluble antioxidant and thus protects other lipid-soluble vitamins	Joint tenderness, scurvy (capillary hemorrhaging), impaired wound healing, acute periodontal gingivitis, petechiae, purpura	Increased incidence of renal oxalate stones	Heat-labile; broccoli, papaya, orange, mango, grapefruit, strawberries, tomatoes, potatoes, leafy vegetables, breast milk, infant formula
Thiamine (B_1)	Aids in energy utilization as part of a coenzyme component to promote the utilization of carbohydrate; promotes normal functioning of the nervous system; coenzyme for oxidative carboxylation of 2-keto acids	Beriberi, neuritis, edema, cardiac failure, anorexia, restlessness, confusion, loss of vibration sense and deep tendon reflexes, calf tenderness	None known	Pork (lean), and nuts, whole grain and fortified cereal products, breast milk, infant formula
Riboflavin (B_2)	Functions primarily as the reactive portion of flavoproteins concerned with biologic oxidations (cellular metabolism)	Cheilosis, glossitis, photophobia, angular stomatitis, corneal vascularization, scrotal skin changes, seborrhea, magenta tongue	None known	Dairy products, liver, almonds, lamb, pork, breast milk, infant formula
Niacin	Aids in energy utilization as part of a coenzyme (NAD+ and NADP+) in fat synthesis, tissue respiration, and carbohydrate utilization; aids digestion and fosters normal appetite; synthesized from the amino acid tryptophan	Pellagra (dermatitis, diarrhea, dementia, death), cheilosis, angular stomatitis, inflammation of mucous membranes, weakness	Dilation of the capillaries, vasomotor instability, "flushing" (utilization of muscle glycogen, serum lipids, mobilization of fatty acids during exercise)	Liver, meat, fish, poultry, peanuts, fortified cereal products, yeast, breast milk, infant formula
Pyridoxine (B_6)	Coenzyme component for many of the enzymes of amino acid metabolism	Convulsions, loss of weight, abdominal distress, vomiting, hyperirritability, depression, confusion, hypochromic and macrocytic anemia	None known	Fish, poultry, meat, wheat, breast milk, infant formula
Folacin	Utilized in carbon transfer and thus nucleotide synthesis	Megaloblastic anemia, stomatitis, glossitis	None known	Liver, leafy vegetables, fruit, yeast, breast milk, infant formula
Cobalamin (B_{12}; intrinsic factor required)	Cobalamin-containing coenzymes function in the degradation of certain odd-chain fatty acids and in the recycling of tetrahydrofolate	Megaloblastic anemia, neurologic deterioration	None known	Animal products, breast milk, infant formula
Biotin	Component of several carboxylating enzymes; plays an important role in the metabolism of fat and carbohydrate	Anorexia; nausea; vomiting; glossitis; depression; dry, scaly dermatitis; thin hair; loss or eyebrows	None known	Liver, kidney, egg yolk, breast milk, infant formula
Pantothenic Acid	Component of coenzyme A; plays a role in release of energy from carbohydrates and in synthesis and degradation of fatty acids	Infertility, abortion, slowed growth, depression	None known	Meat, fish, poultry, whole grains, legumes, breast milk, infant formula
Minerals				
Calcium	Essential for calcification of bone (matrix forma-	Osteomalacia, osteoporosis	Hypercalcemia (vomiting, anorexia)	Dairy products (i.e., milk, cheese), sardines,

(continued)

Table F-14.   (Continued)

	Major Physiologic Functions	Deficiency Signs	Excess Signs	Important Food Sources
	tion); assists in blood clotting; functions in normal muscle contraction and relaxation and in normal nerve transmission			oysters, salmon, herring, greens, breast milk, infant formula
Phosphorus	Important intracellular anion; involved in many chemical reactions within the body; necessary for energy turnover (ATP)	Weakness, anorexia, malaise, bone pain, growth arrest	Hypocalcemia (when parathyroid gland not fully functioning)	Dairy products, fish, legumes, pork, breast milk, infant formula
Magnesium	Essential part of many enzyme systems; important for maintaining electrical potential in nerves and muscle membranes and for energy turnover	Tremor, convulsions, hyperexcitability (hypocalcemic tetany)	Sedation	Widely distributed, especially in food of vegetable origin; breast milk, infant formula
Trace Elements				
Iron	Part of hemoglobin molecule; prevents nutritional anemia and fatigue; increases resistance to infection; functions as a part of enzymes involved in tissue respiration	Anemia, malabsorption, irritability, anorexia, pallor, lethargy	Hemosiderosis, hemochromatosis	Red meats, liver, dried beans and peas, enriched farina, breast milk, iron-fortified infant formula, infant cereal
Zinc	Constituent of enzymes involved in most major metabolic pathways (specifically nucleic acid synthesis for cellular growth and repair)	Growth failure, skin changes, delayed wound healing, hypogeusia, sexual immaturity, hair loss, diarrhea	Acute gastrointestinal upset, vomiting	Whole grains, legumes, beef, lamb, pork, poultry, nuts, seeds, shellfish, eggs, some cheeses, breast milk, infant formula
Iodine	Component of thyroid hormones triiodothyronine and thyroxine, important in regulation of cellular oxidation and growth	Goiter, depressed thyroid function, cretinism	Thyroid suppression (thyrotoxicosis)	Iodized table salt, salt water, fish, shellfish (content of most other foods geographically dependent), breast milk, infant formula
Copper	Constituent of proteins and enzymes, some of which are essential for the proper utilization of iron	Anemia (hemolytic), neutropenia, bone disease	Excess accumulation in the liver, brain, kidney, cornea	Oysters, nuts, liver, kidney, corn-oil margarine, dried legumes
Manganese	Essential part of several enzyme systems involved in protein and energy metabolism and in the formation of mucopolysaccharides	Impaired growth, skeletal abnormalities, lowered reproductive function, neonatal ataxia	In extremely high exposure of contamination: severe psychiatric and neurologic disorders	Nuts, whole grains, dried fruits, fruits, vegetables (nonleafy)
Fluoride	The main target organs of fluoride in humans are the enamel of teeth and bones, where fluoride is incorporated into the crystalline structure of hydroxyapatite and produces increased caries resistance	Poor dentition, caries, osteoporosis	Mottling, brown staining of teeth (in excess of 4 ppm); fluorosis occurs after prolonged (10–20 yrs) ingestion of 20–80 mg/day	Fluoridated water; depends on the geochemical environment and therefore amount in foods varies widely
Chromium	Maintenance of normal glucose metabolism, cofactor for insulin	Disturbed glucose metabolism (lower glucose tolerance caused by insulin resistance)		Brewer's yeast, meat products, cheeses

(continued)

Table F-14.   (*Continued*)

	Major Physiologic Functions	Deficiency Signs	Excess Signs	Important Food Sources
Selenium	Functions as a part of the enzyme glutathione peroxidase, which protects cellular components from oxidative damage	Cardiomyopathy, probably secondary to oxidative damage	In animals, blindness, abdominal pain, lack of vitality	Seafoods, kidney, liver, meat, grains (depending on growing area)
Molybdenum	Essential for the function of flavin-dependent enzymes involved in the production of uric acid and in the oxidation of aldehydes and sulfites	Not described in humans	Acts as an antagonist to the essential element copper; goutlike syndrome associated with elevated blood levels of molybdenum, uric acid, and xanthine oxidase	Varies considerably, depending on growing environment; main contributions come from meat, grains, and legumes

Reproduced with permission from Walker, W.A. and K.M. Hendricks. *Manual of Pediatric Nutrition.* Philadelphia: Saunders, 1985.

Table F-15.   Current Guidelines for Laboratory Evaluation of Nutritional Status

Nutrient and Units	Age of Subject (yrs)	Criteria of Status		
		Deficient	Marginal	Acceptable
Visceral Protein				
Serum albumin (g/dl)[a]	<1		<2.5	2.5+
	1–5		<3.0	3.0+
	6–16		<3.5	3.5+
	16+	<2.8	2.8–3.4	3.5+
	Pregnant	<3.0	3.0–3.4	3.5+
Hematological Indices				
Hemoglobin (g/dl)[a]	1 wk			13–20
	1 mo			≥14
	6–23 mo	<9.0	9.0–9.9	10.0+
	2–5	<10.0	10.0–10.9	11.0+
	6–12	<10.0	10.0–11.4	11.5+
	13–16 M	<12.0	12.0–12.9	13.0+
	13–16 F	<10.0	10.0–11.4	11.5+
	16+ M	<12.0	12.0–13.9	14.0+
	16+ F	<10.0	10.0–11.9	12.0+
	Pregnant			
	2nd trimester	<9.5	9.5–10.9	11.0+
	3rd trimester	<9.0	9.0–10.5	10.5+

(*continued*)

Table F-15. (Continued)

Nutrient and Units	Age of Subject (yrs)	Criteria of Status		
		Deficient	Marginal	Acceptable
Hematocrit (packed cell volume in %)[a]	1 wk			43–66
	1 mo			>50
	3 mo			>35
	6 mo–5 yr			>38
	6–12	<30	30–35	36+
	13–16 M	<37	37–39	40+
	13–16 F	<31	31–35	36+
	16+ M	<37	37–43	44+
	16+ F	<31	31–37	33+
	Pregnant	<30	30–32	33+
Mean corpuscular hemoglobin (μg)	All ages			27–35
Mean corpuscular hemoglobin concentration (%)	All ages			32–36
Mean corpuscular volume (μm^3)	All ages			80–94
Serum iron (μg/dl)[a]	<2 yr	<30		30+
	2–5	<40		40+
	6–12	<50		50+
	12+ M	<60		60+
	12+ F or pregnant	<40	40	40+
Transferrin saturation (%)[a]	<2	<15.0		15.0+
	2–12	<20.0		20.0+
	12+ M	<20.0		20.0+
	12+ F or pregnant	<15.0	15	15.0+
Vitamins				
Serum ascorbic acid (mg/dl)[a]	All ages	<0.1	0.1–0.19	0.2+
Plasma vitamin A (μg/dl)[a]	All ages	<10	10–19	20+
Plasma carotene (μg/dl)[a]	All ages	<20	20–39	40+
	Pregnant		40–79	80+
Serum folic acid (ng/ml)[b]	All ages; pregnant	<2.0	2.1–5.9	6.0+
Serum vitamin B$_{12}$ (pg/ml)[b]	All ages; pregnant	<100	100	100+
Thiamine in urine (μg/g of creatinine)[a]	1–3	<120	120–175	175+
	4–5	<85	85–120	120+
	6–9	<70	70–180	180+
	10–15	<55	55–150	150+
	16+	<27	27–65	65+
	Pregnant	<21	21–49	50+
Riboflavin in urine (μg/g of creatinine)[a]	1–3	<150	150–499	500+
	4–5	<100	100–299	300+
	6–9	<85	85–269	270+
	10–16	<80	70–199	200+
	16+	<27	27–79	80+
	Pregnant	<30	30–89	90+
RBC transketolase-TPP effect (ratio)[b]	All ages	25+	15–25	<15
RBC glutathione reductase-FAD effect (ratio)[b]	All ages	1.2+		<1.2
Tryptophan load (mg xanthurenic acid excreted)[b]	Adults (Dose: 100 mg/kg body weight)	6 hr 25+ 24 hr 75+		<25 <75
Urinary pyridoxine (μg/g of creatinine)[b]	1–3	<90		90+
	4–6	<80		80+
	7–9	<60		60+
	10–12	<40		40+
	13–15	<30		30+
	16+	<20		20+

(continued)

Table F-15. *(Continued)*

Nutrient and Units	Age of Subject (yrs)	Criteria of Status		
		Deficient	*Marginal*	*Acceptable*
Urinary N'methyl nicotinamide (mg/g of creatinine)[a]	All ages Pregnant	<0.2 <0.8	0.2–5.59 0.8–2.49	0.6+ 2.5+
Urinary pantothenic acid (μg)[b]	All ages	<200		200+
Vitamin E (serum tocopherol) (mg/dl)	Birth 2 mo 2–12 yr Adults			0.22 0.33 0.72 0.85
Transaminase index (ratio)[b] EGOT EGPT	 Adult Adult	 2.0+ 1.25+		 <2.0 <1.25

M = male subjects; F = female subjects; RBC = red blood cells; TPP = thiamine pyrophosphate; FAD = flavin adenine dinucleotide; EGOT = erythrocyte glutamic oxaloacetic transaminase; EGPT = erythrocyte glutamic pyruvic transaminase.

[a] Adapted from the Ten-State Nutritional Survey.

[b] Criteria may vary with methodology.

Compiled from *Critical Resources in Clinical Laboratory Sciences*, eds. J.W. King and W.R. Faukner. Cleveland: CRC Press, 1973, p. 116; Ney, D. Nutritional assessment. In *Manual of Pediatric Nutrition*, eds. D.G. Kelts and E.G. Jones. Boston: Little, Brown, 1984, p. 119.

Table F-16. Laboratory Tests in the Differential Diagnosis of Anemias

Type of Anemia	Hgb	Hct	MCV	Serum Iron	TIBC	Transferrin Saturation	Ferritin	Marrow Hemosiderin	Sideroblasts	RBC	Retic	Other
Iron deficiency	D*	D	D	D	I	D	D	D	D	N	D	Hypochromic, microcytic, or normocytic
Vitamin B_{12}	D	D	I	I	D or N	I, D, or N	N	I	I	D	D or N	Macrocytic, megaloblastic, hypersegmented neutrophils, low-serum B_{12}, thrombocytopenia, leukopenia
Folic acid	D	D	I	I	D or N	I, D, or N	D	I	I	D	D or N	Macrocytic, megaloblastic, normal or slightly low B_{12}, decreased red cell folate
Vitamin E	D	D	I or N	I	D	N	N	I	I	D	I	Hemolytic anemia, low serum vitamin E, increased RBC, hemolysis, normochromic, normocytic
Anemia of chronic disease	D	D	N	D	D	D	N	N or I	D	D	D	Usually normocytic, normochromic, may be hypochromic, microcytic
Anemia of chronic infection	D	D	N or D	D	D	D or N	I or N	I, N, or D	D	D	D	Normochromic and normocytic, may be hypochromic and microcytic

*D: decreased; N: normal; I: increased.

Reproduced with permission from Walker, W.A. and K.M. Hendricks. *Manual of Pediatric Nutrition*. Philadelphia: Saunders, 1985.

Table F-17. Normal Value (mg/dl) for Total Cholesterol

Age (Years)	White Males				Age (Years)	White Females (Non-sex hormone users)			
		Percentiles					Percentiles		
	Mean	5	50	95		Mean	5	50	95
0–4	155	114	151	203	0–4	156	112	156	200
5–9	160	121	159	203	5–9	164	126	163	205
10–14	158	119	155	202	10–14	160	124	158	201
15–19	150	113	146	197	15–19	157	120	154	200
20–24	167	124	165	218	20–24	164	122	160	216
25–29	182	133	178	244	25–29	171	128	168	222
30–34	192	138	190	254	30–34	175	130	172	231
35–39	201	146	197	270	35–39	184	140	182	242
40–44	207	151	203	268	40–44	194	147	191	252
45–49	212	158	210	276	45–49	203	152	199	265
50–54	213	158	210	277	50–54	218	162	215	285
55–59	214	156	212	276	55–59	231	173	228	300
60–64	213	159	210	276	60–64	231	172	228	297
65–69	213	158	210	274	65–69	233	171	229	303
70+	207	151	205	270	70+	228	169	226	289

Tables F-17 through F-20 have been reproduced with permission from U.S. Department of Health and Human Services, Public Health Service, National Institute of Health, Lipid Metabolism Branch, NHBLI; the Lipid Research Clinic. *Population Studies Data Book*, Vol. 1. Bethesda, Md.: NIH Publication No. 80-1527, 1980.

Table F-18. Normal Values (mg/dl) for Total Triglycerides

Age (Years)	White Males				Age (Years)	White Females (Non-sex hormone users)			
		Percentiles					Percentiles		
	Mean	5	50	95		Mean	5	50	95
0–4	56	29	51	99	0–4	64	34	59	112
5–9	56	30	51	101	5–9	60	32	55	105
10–14	66	32	59	125	10–14	75	37	70	131
15–19	78	37	69	148	15–19	72	39	66	124
20–24	100	44	86	201	20–24	72	36	64	131
25–29	116	46	95	249	25–29	75	37	65	145
30–34	128	50	104	266	30–34	79	39	69	151
35–39	145	54	113	321	35–39	86	40	73	176
40–44	151	55	122	320	40–44	98	45	82	191
45–49	152	58	124	327	45–49	105	46	87	214
50–54	152	58	124	320	50–54	115	52	97	233
55–59	141	58	119	286	55–59	125	55	106	262
60–64	142	58	119	291	60–64	127	56	105	239
65–69	137	57	113	267	65–69	131	60	112	243
70+	130	58	111	258	70+	132	60	111	237

Table F-19. Normal Values (mg/dl) for LDL-Cholesterol

Age (Years)	*White Males* Mean	Percentiles 5	50	95	Age (Years)	*White Females (Non-sex hormone users)* Mean	Percentiles 5	50	95
0–4	—	—	—	—	0–4	—	—	—	—
5–9	93	63	90	129	5–9	100	68	98	140
10–14	97	64	94	132	10–14	97	68	94	136
15–19	94	62	93	130	15–19	95	60	93	135
20–24	103	66	101	147	20–24	98	—	98	—
25–29	117	70	116	165	25–29	106	70	103	151
30–34	126	78	124	185	30–34	109	67	108	150
35–39	133	81	131	189	35–39	119	76	116	172
40–44	136	87	135	186	40–44	125	77	120	174
45–49	144	98	141	202	45–49	130	80	127	187
50–54	142	89	143	197	50–54	146	90	141	215
55–59	146	88	145	203	55–59	152	95	148	213
60–64	146	83	143	210	60–64	156	100	151	234
65–69	150	98	146	210	65–69	162	97	156	223
70+	143	88	142	186	70+	149	96	146	207

Table F-20. Normal Values (mg/dl) for HDL-Cholesterol

Age (Years)	*White Males* Mean	Percentiles 5	50	95	*White Females (Non-sex hormone users)* Mean	Percentiles 5	50	95
5–9	55.5	38	54	74	53.0	36	52	73
10–14	55.0	37	55	74	52.0	37	52	70
15–19	46.0	30	46	63	52.0	35	51	73
20–24	45.0	30	45	63	52.0	—	50	—
25–29	45.0	31	44	63	56.0	37	55	81
30–34	45.5	28	45	63	55.0	38	55	75
35–39	43.0	29	43	62	55.0	34	52	82
40–44	44.0	27	43	67	57.0	33	55	87
45–49	45.0	30	45	64	58.0	33	56	86
50–54	44.0	28	44	63	60.0	37	59	89
55–59	48.0	28	46	71	59.0	36	58	86
60–64	51.5	30	49	74	62.0	36	60	91
65–69	51.0	30	49	78	60.5	34	60	89
70+	50.0	31	48	75	60.0	33	60	91

Appendix G:
Formula Feeding Products

Table G-1. Oral Supplementary Feedings

Product (ml to provide 100% RDA)	Composition (Source)			Caloric Density (kcal/ml)	Lactose	Residue	Notes
	Carbohydrate (g/100 kcal)	Protein (g/100 kcal)	Fat (g/100 kcal)				
Citrotein[a] (powder) (1,180)	18.25 (Maltodextrins, sucrose)	6.25 (Egg albumin)	0.26 (Soy oil, monoglycerides, diglycerides)	0.66	No	Low	Protein and vitamin supplement to clear-liquid diet. 263.4 g dry weight needed to give 1,000 kcal. 3.1 mEq Na/dl; 1.8 mEq K/dl. Nonpro C:N ratio = 76:1. Gluten-free; 480–515 mOsm/kg
Delmark Eggnog[b]	13 (Nonfat dry milk, maltodextrins, sugar)	5.25 (Nonfat dry milk, egg white, egg yolk solids)	3.0 (Cottonseed oil, soy oil, egg yolk)	1.16	Yes		
Delmark Milkshake[b]	12.5 (Sugar, maltodextrins, ice cream mix)	3.8 (Egg, milk)	3.85 (Vegetable oil)	0.95	Yes		
Dietene[a]	15.75 (Nonfat milk, sucrose)	8.75 (Nonfat milk)	0.2	0.8	Yes		Add powder to milk
dp High p.e.r. Protein[c]	2.0	20.6	1.0	2.58 kcal/g			Protein supplement; low electrolyte; 258 g dry weight to give 1,000 kcal
Duocal[d]	15.5 (Maltodextrins)	0	4.7 (Vegetable; 34% MCT; 23% linoleate)	4.7	No	Low	Energy supplement; low electrolyte; 100 g = 28 mg Na, 3.5 mg K
Gevral[e]	6.68 (Lactose, sucrose)	17.1 (Calcium caseinate)	0.57 (Milk fat)	0.653	Yes	Low	Protein-calorie supplement; artificial flavors; 284.8 dry weight to give 1,000 kcal
Lolactene[a]	13 (Corn syrup solids, sucrose)	6.6 (Caseinate)	2.3 (Vegetable oil, monoglycerides, diglycerides)	0.8	Low	None	1,150 ml gives 1,000 kcal
Lonalac[f]	30 (Lactose)	21 (Casein)	49 (Coconut oil)	0.67	High	Low	Low sodium (4 mg/dl), high potassium, high protein; do not reconstitute with water *high* in Na content
MCT Duocal[d]	15.7 (Maltodextrins)	0	4.94 (82.5% MCT; 12.5% linoleate; 5% LCT vegetable oil)	4.7	No	Low	Energy supplement; 100 g = 175 mg Na, 6.0 mg K

Product	Carbohydrate source (g)	Protein source (g)	Fat source (g)		Lactose	Residue	Comments
Nutrex Broth[g]	87 (Corn syrup solids)	13 (Calcium and sodium caseinate)	0	1.39	No	None	Clear soup; C:N = 203; nonpro kcal:N = 175; osmolality = 350 mOsm/kg; Powder to mix with water; Flavors: chicken, beef, vegetable. PER = 2.5
Nutrex CLD[g]	12.9 (Sucrose)	11.4 (Egg white solids, gelatin)	0	0.95	No	Low	Clear gel. Semisolid; PER = 2.95. 680 mOsm/kg. Powder to mix with water; 6 flavors
Nutrex Drink[g]	20.0 (Corn syrup; sucrose)	5.3 (Egg white solids)	0	0.71	No	Low	Clear liquid. PER = 2.92. 450 mOsm/kg. Powder to mix with water; 6 flavors.
Nutrex Protamine (1200)[g]	15.0 (Corn syrup; sucrose)	3.1 (Calcium & sodium caseinate; soy protein)	3.0 (Corn oil)	1.27	No	Low	Full-liquid diet. PER = 2.62. 450 mOsm/kg. Powder to mix with water; 3 flavors
Ross SLD[h] (powder) (1,200)	19.5 (Sucrose; hydrolyzed cornstarch)	5.35 (Egg white solids)	0.1	0.7	No	Low	Clear-liquid supplement; C:N ratio 92:1; 550 mOsm/kg; 3.6 mEq Na/dl 2.1 mEq K/dl
Sustacal Pudding[f]	53 (Nonfat milk; sucrose)	11 (Milk)	36 (Soy oil)	48/oz	Yes	Low	Vanilla, chocolate, butterscotch. C:N = 226:1; nonpro C:N = 200:1; RSL = 46.2 mOsm/5 oz serving; Na 120 mg/serving

Note: The composition of these products is subject to change. Current product literature should be consulted before use. This table is not intended to be comprehensive.

[a]Sandoz
[b]Delmark
[c]General Mills
[d]Scientific Hospital Supplies
[e]Lederle Laboratories
[f]Mead Johnson Nutritional
[g]Nutrex
[h]Ross

393

Table G-2. Sources of Single Nutrients

Product (form)	Composition (Source)			Caloric Density	Osmolality (mOsm/kg)	Lactose	Residue	Notes
	Carbohydrate (g/100 kcal)	Protein (g/100 kcal)	Fat (g/100 kcal)					
Protein sources								
Case[a] (powder)	0	23.78 (Calcium caseinate)	0.54 (Butterfat)	3.7 kcal/g		No	Low	Add to liquid or food; provides no vitamins; 270 g dry weight gives 1,000 kcal; low sodium
Dialamine[b] (powder)	17.22	6.9 (Amino acids)	Trace	3.6 kcal/g	918 at 1:5 dilution	No		For oral or tube feeding in chronic renal failure; contains all essential amino acids + cystine + histidine; gluten-free; orange-flavored; tartrazine-free. 100 g powder = 168 mg Na, 9.2 mg K
Maxipro HBV[b] (powder)	Trace	22.56 (Whey protein, amino acids)	1.02	3.9 kcal/g	165 at 1:5 dilution	Trace		For oral or tube feeding; 100 g = 230 mg Na, 450 mg K; gluten-free
Nutrisource Protein[c] (powder)	1.75	18.75 (Delactosed lactalbumin; egg white solids)	2.1	4.02 kcal/g		No		Use only as part of modular tube feeding; PER = 3.0; 76 g pro/100 g
Nutrisource Amino Acids[c] (powder)	0	24.87 (Free amino acids)	0	3.9 kcal/g		No		Use only as part of modular tube feeding; PER = 3.1; 97 g pro/100 g
Nutrisource Amino Acids—High Branched Chain[c] (powder)	0	24.87 (Free amino acids)	0	3.9 kcal/g		No		Use only as part of modular tube feeding; 44% branched-chain amino acids
Promix[d] (powder)	2.27	22.7 (Whey protein)	1.1	3.52 kcal/g		No		Add to liquid foods; provides no vitamins
ProMod[e]	0	18.9 (Whey protein)	0			No		Unflavored; add to liquid foods
Propac[f] (powder)	1.25	19.2 (Whey protein)	20	4.0 kcal/g		Yes		Add to liquid foods; provides no vitamins

Carbohydrate sources

Product	Carbohydrate (g)	Protein (g)	Fat (g)	kcal	mOsm			Comments
Cal Power[c] (liquid)	27.2 (Deionized corn syrup)	0.06	0	1.8 kcal/ml		No		High osmolality; 8 fluid oz carton = 30 mg Na, 3 mg K; for oral or tube feeding; 550 g liquid gives 1,000 kcal
Controlyte[c] (powder)	14.3 (Cornstarch hydrolysate)	Trace	4.8 (Soy oil)	2.0 kcal/ml (or 5.0 kcal/g)	598	No	Low	For oral or tube feedings; calorie source; add to liquid or food; high osmolality; low protein; 14 oz can = 60 mg Na, 16 mg K; 198 g dry weight gives 1,000 kcal
Hy-Cal[g] (liquid)	24.41	0.01	0.01	2.5 kcal/ml	2,781	No	Low	Oral supplement; high osmolality; 4 oz bottle = 16 mg Na, 0.7 mg K; 407 ml liquid gives 1,000 kcal
Liquid Carbohydrate Supplement[d]	25 (Glucose polymers)	0	0	2.5 kcal/ml		No	Low	
Liquid Maxijul[b] (liquid)	26.7 (Maltodextrins)	0	0	1.87 kcal/ml	400	No	Low	50% Maxijul powder in water; 100 ml = 23 mg Na, 0.4 mg K
Maxijul[b] (powder)	25.6 (Maltodextrins)	0	0	3.75 kcal/g	525 in 40% solution	No	Low	For oral use; calorie source; 100 g = 46 mg Na, 3.9 mg K
Maxijul LE[b] (powder)	25.6 (Maltodextrins)	0	0	3.75 kcal/g	525 in 40% solution	No	Low	For oral use; calorie source; 100 g = 0.23 mg Na, 0.4 mg K
Pure Carbohydrate Supplement[d] (powder)	25 (Glucose polymers)	0	0	4.0 kcal/g		No	Low	
Moducal[a] (liquid or powder)	25 (Maltodextrins)	0	0	2.0 kcal/ml (liquid) 3.8 kcal/g (powder)	725 (liquid)	No	Low	Calorie source; 206 mOsm in 60 g/250 ml distilled water
Nutrisource Carbohydrate[c] (liquid)	25 (Deionized corn syrup solids in water)	0	0	3.2 kcal/ml		No	Low	Deionized for minimum electrolyte content. For modular tube feeding only.

(continued)

Table G-2. *(Continued)*

Product (form)	Composition (Source) Carbohydrate (g/100 kcal)	Protein (g/100 kcal)	Fat (g/100 kcal)	Caloric Density	Osmolality (mOsm/kg)	Lactose	Residue	Notes
Pedialyte[e]	25	0	0	0.2 kcal/ml				80 g carbohydrate/100 ml; Calorie & electrolyte source
Polycose[e] (liquid or powder)	25 (Hydrolyzed cornstarch)	0	0	2.0 kcal/ml (liquid) 3.8 kcal/g (powder)	570	No	Low	Calorie supplement; 4 oz bottle = 72 mg Na, 3 mg K; 4 oz powder = 436 mg Na, 19 mg K; 250 g dry weight gives 1,000 kcal
Sumacal[f] (powder or liquid)	25 (Maltodextrins)	0	0	4.0 kcal/g	680	No	Low	Calorie supplement; 12 oz bottle = 150 mg Na, 40 mg K
Sumacal Plus[f] (powder)	3.2	0	0	2.5 kcal/g	890	No	Low	Calorie supplement; low electrolyte
Lipid sources								
Calogen[b] (liquid)	0	0	11.1 (Arachis oil)	4.5 kcal/ml		No	Low	LCT; 100 ml = 20.7 mg Na, 19.6 mg K; 77% linoleate
High Fat Supplement[c] (powder)	6.6 (Corn syrup solids)	0.8	7.7 (Partly hydrogenated coconut oil)	6.12 kcal/g		No	Low	Contains trace amounts of Ca, P, and Na
Lipomul-Oral[h]	0.11	0.01	11.11 (Corn oil)	6.0 kcal/ml		No	Low	Oral supplement; 1 oz. (2 T) = 20 mg Na, 0.8 mg K; 166.7 ml gives 1,000 kcal; 8.3 kcal/g
Liquigen[b] (liquid)	0	0	7.69 (MCT oil)	4.0 kcal/ml		No	Low	MCT; 100 ml = 39.1 mg Na, 27.4 mg K; linoleate-free
MCT Oil[a] (liquid)	0	0	12.05 (Coconut oil fraction)	7.7 kcal/ml	Negligible	No		Oral supplement; 60% C8 & 24% C10 fatty acids; low electrolyte; 120.5 g liquid gives 1,000 kcal
Microlipid[f] (liquid)	0	0	11.11 (Soy, corn, or safflower oil)	4.5 kcal/ml	80	No	Low	Oral supplement; low electrolyte; P:S ratio 7.3:1; 73.7% linoleate

Nutrisource Lipid Medium-Chain Triglyceridesᶜ	0	11.9 (Coconut oil)	2.01 kcal/ml		No	Low	Electrolyte-free; for modular tube feeding only. 2 g LCT + 22 g MCT/100 ml emulsion Linoleate-free
Nutrisource Lipid Long-Chain Triglyceridesᵇ (liquid)	0	11.1 (Soy oil)	2.16 kcal/ml		No	Low	Electrolyte-free; P:S ratio 2.4:1.0; for modular tube feeding only; linoleate = 49%

Electrolyte sources

Lytrenᵃ (powder)	25.3	0	0.333 kcal/g	290	No	Low	Electrolyte source (mEq/L): 30 Na; 25 K; 4 Ca; 4 Mg; 36 citrate; 4 SO_4; 25 Cl; 5 PO_4. Provides some kcals; useful in prevention of metabolic defects due to diarrhea; 268 g dry weight or 3,333 ml standard dilution gives 1,000 kcal
Reosolⁱ	25.0	0	0	290	No	Low	Electrolyte source (mEq/L): 50 Na; 20 K; 50 Cl; 4 Ca; 4 Mg; 34 citrate. 24 g fat/100 ml.

Micronutrient sources

Nutrisource Vitaminsᶜ	(See manufacturer's literature for composition)
Nutrisource Minerals for Protein Formulasᶜ	(Provides 100% of NRC-RDA for essential vitamins in each 10 g packet. For use in modular tube feeding.)
Nutrisource Minerals for Protein Formulas—Electrolyte Restrictedᶜ	(Provides 100% of NRC-RDA for essential minerals in each 24 g packet *if used with 3 packets* of Nutrisource Protein; also provides safe levels of trace elements.)
Nutrisource Minerals for Amino Acid Formulasᶜ	(Is essentially sodium-, potassium-, and chloride-free. Provides 100% of NRC-RDA of other minerals plus trace elements *if used with 3 packets of Nutrisource Protein.*)
Nutrisource Minerals for Amino Acid Formulas—Electrolyte Restrictedᶜ	(Provides 100% of NRC-RDA for essential minerals in each 24 g packet plus trace elements if used with Nutrisource Amino Acids or Amino Acid–High Branched Chain packets.)
	(Is essentially sodium-, potassium-, and chloride-free. Provides 100% of NRC-RDA of other minerals plus trace elements when used with Nutrisource Amino Acids or Amino Acids–High Branched Chain packets.)

Note: The composition of these products changes frequently. Current product literature should be consulted before use. This table is not intended to be comprehensive.

ᵃMead Johnson Nutritional
ᵇScientific Hospital Supplies
ᶜSandoz
ᵈNavaco Laboratories
ᵉRoss Laboratories
ᶠChesebrough-Pond
ᵍBeecham Laboratories
ʰThe Upjohn Company
ⁱWyeth

Table G-3.   Complete Liquid Formula Diets

Product (form) (Kcal to meet vitamin RDA)	Composition (Source)		
	Carbohydrate (% of kcal)	Protein (% of kcal)	Lipid (% of kcal)
Hydrolyzed protein-based			
Aminex[h] (liquid) (2,000)	82.2 (Maltodextrins, modified starch)	15.3 (Free amino acids)	2.5 (Safflower oil)
Criticare HN[a] (liquid) (1,887)	83 (Maltodextrins; modified cornstarch)	14 (Hydrolyzed casein; 60% free amino acids, 40% small peptides)	3 (Safflower oil)
Elemental 028[b] (powder)	76.5 (Glucose polymer; sucrose)	10 (Crystalline amino acids)	14.5 (Arachis oil)
Isotein HN[j] (powder) (1,776)	52 (Maltodextrin, monosaccharide)	23 (Delactosed lactalbumin)	30 (Corn oil, MCT)
Newtrition High Nitrogen[n] (liquid) (1,240)	52 (Maltodextrin)	19 (Sodium and calcium caseinate; soy isolate)	29 (MCT; corn oil)
Newtrition Isotonic[n] (liquid) (1,900)	56 (Maltodextrin)	14 (Sodium and calcium caseinate; soy isolate)	30 (MCT; corn oil)
Nutramigen[a]	52 (Sucrose; tapioca starch)	13 (Hydrolyzed casein)	35 (Corn oil)
Nutrex Besure[h] (powder) (1,887)	54.5 (Corn syrup solids, sucrose)	14 (Sodium and calcium caseinate, soy isolate)	31.5 (Hydrogenated soy oil, mono- and diglycerides)
Nutrex Protamin[h] (powder) (1,180)	60.3 (Corn syrup solids, sucrose)	12.6 (Caseinate)	27.1 (Corn oil, lecithin)
Pepti-2000[g] (powder) (1,600)	79.5 (Maltodextrin)	16.07 (Hydrolyzed lactalbumin)	8.5 (MCT; corn oil)
Pre-Fortison[g] (liquid) (1,600)	48 (Maltodextrin)	16 (Sodium and calcium caseinate)	36 (Corn oil)
Pregestimil[a] (powder)	54 (Corn syrup solids; tapioca starch)	11 (Hydrolyzed casein; amino acids)	35 (Corn oil; MCT oil)
Travasorb[c] (liquid) (1,900)	54.5 (Sucrose; corn syrup solids)	14 (Casein; soy isolate)	31.5 (Corn oil; soy oil)
Travasorb STD[c] (powder) (2,100)	81.1 (Oligosaccharides)	6.9 (Hydrolyzed lactalbumin; L-methionine)	12 (MCT; sunflower oil)
Travasorb HN[c] (powder) (2,000)	70 (Oligosaccharides)	18 (Hydrolyzed lactalbumin; L-methionine)	12 (MCT; sunflower oil)
Vipep[d]	68 (Corn syrup solids; sucrose; cornstarch; potassium gluconate; tapioca flour)	10 (20% amino acids; 80% short-chain peptides)	22 (MCT Oil; corn oil)
Vital HN[e] (powder) (1,500)	74 (Sucrose; hydrolyzed cornstarch)	16.7 (Partially hydrolyzed whey, meat, soy; amino acids)	9.3 (Safflower oil; MCT)
Vivonex Standard[f] (powder) (1,800)	90.5 (Glucose and oligosaccharides)	8.2 (Crystalline L-amino acids)	1.3 (Safflower oil)
Vivonex HN[f] (powder) (3,000)	81.5 (Glucose and oligosaccharides)	17.7 (Crystalline L-amino acids)	0.78 (Safflower oil)
Vivonex TEN[f] (powder) (2,000)	82.2 (Maltodextrin and modified starch)	15.3 (Amino acids)	2.5 (Safflower oil)
Isolates of intact protein; Non-milk-based			
Enrich[e] (liquid) (1,390)	55.0 (Hydrolyzed cornstarch; sucrose; soy polysaccharide)	14.5 (Caseinate; soy)	30.5 (Corn oil)
Ensure[e] (liquid) (1,890)	54.5 (Hydrolyzed cornstarch; sucrose)	14 (Sodium and calcium caseinate; soy isolate)	31.5 (Corn oil)

Electrolytes (mEq/dl at usual dilution)		Caloric Density (kcal/ml at usual dilution)	Osmolality (mOsm/kg) (Flavors)	Lactose	Residue	Notes
Sodium	Potassium					
2.0	2.0	1.0	600	0	Low	C:N ratio = 149:1
2.7	3.4	1.06	650	0	Low	For oral or tube feeding; C:N ratio = 148:1. RSL = 23 mOsm/100 kcal
2.61	2.39	0.5 at 1:5 dilution	450 (at 1:5 dilution) unflavored; 720 (orange)	0	Low	For oral or tube feeding; C:N ratio = 220:1. All values are 1:5 dilution
2.7	2.7	1.2	0 300	0	Low	C:N ratio = 86:1
2.6	2.6	1.24	300	0	Low	C:N ratio = 104:1
2.6	2.6	1.06	300	0	Low	C:N ratio = 154:1
1.38	1.76	0.68	479	0	Low	For oral or tube feeding; infant formula; galactose-free; useful in management of allergy, galactosemia; RSL = 13 mOsm/dl
3.7	4.0	1.06	450	0	Low	C:N ratio = 153:1
0.74	4.36	1.3	450	0	Low	C:N ratio = 174:1
2.9	2.9	1.0	490	0	Low	C:N ratio = 131:1
1.5	1.5	0.5	150	0	Low	C:N ratio = 131:1
1.38	1.9	0.65 (Infants) 1.5 (Adults)	348	0	Low	For oral feeding; infant feeding; RSL 13 mOsm/dl in formulas containing 20 kcal/oz: useful in management of malabsorption disorders
3.2	3.25	1.06	488	0	Low	C:N ratio = 154:1
4.0	2.99	1.35	450 (Unflavored) 500 (Orange) 600 (Beef broth)	0	Low	For oral or tube feeding; C:N ratio = 363:1
4.0	2.99	1.06	560	0	Low	For oral or tube feeding; C:N ratio = 154.1
3.26	2.18	1.0	520	0	Low	
2.03	3.41	1.0	460 (Various flavors)	0	Low	C:N ratio = 125:1
2.04	3.0	1.0	550 (Unfl.) 678 (Beef broth) 610 (Orange, grape, strawberry) 580 (Tomato)	0	Low	For oral or tube feeding; C:N ratio = 281:1
2.3	3.0	1.0	810 (Unfl.) 920 (Beef broth) 850 (Orange, grape, strawberry) 910 (Tomato)	0	Low	For oral or tube feeding; C:N ratio = 125:1
2.0	2.0	1.0	630 (Vanilla, strawberry, orange-pineapple, lemon-lime)	0	Low	For oral or tube feeding; 52:48 essential to nonessential amino acids; 33% BCAA; 6% aromatic amino acids; C:N ratio = 149:1
3.7	4.0	1.10	480 (Vanilla)	0	High	5.0 g fiber (soy polysaccharide) per 8 fluid oz; 15 mg/L of cholesterol. Use 10F tube or larger if gravity fed. RSL = 344 mOsm/L; C:N ratio = 148:1
3.7	4.0	1.06	450 (Flavor packets available)	0	Low	For oral or tube feeding; C:N ratio = 153:1

(continued)

Table G-3.   *(Continued)*

Product (form) (Kcal to meet vitamin RDA)	Composition (Source)		
	Carbohydrate (% of kcal)	Protein (% of kcal)	Lipid (% of kcal)
Ensure HN[e] (liquid) (1,320)	53.2 (Corn syrup; sucrose)	16.7 (Caseinate; soy isolate)	30.1 (Corn oil)
Ensure Plus[e] (liquid) (1,600)	53.3 (Corn syrup; sucrose)	14.7 (Sodium and calcium caseinate; soy isolate)	32 (Corn oil)
Ensure Plus HN[e] (liquid) (947)	53.3 (Corn syrup; sucrose)	16.7 (Caseinate; soy isolate)	30.0 (Corn oil)
Entrition[m] (liquid) (2,000)	54.5 (Maltodextrins)	14 (Sodium and calcium caseinate)	31.5 (Corn oil)
Fortical[g] (liquid) (1,060)	48 (Maltodextrin; sucrose)	16 (Caseinate)	60 (Corn oil)
Fortison L.S.[g] (liquid) (1,600)	48 (Maltodextrin)	16 (Caseinate)	40 (Corn oil)
Isocal[a] (liquid) (1,320)	50 (Maltodextrins)	13 (Sodium and calcium caseinate; soy isolate)	37 (Soy oil; MCT)
Isocal HCN[a] (liquid) (1,500)	45 (Corn syrup)	15 (Caseinate)	40 (70% soy oil; 30% MCT Oil)
Isolife[m] (liquid) (2,000)	55 (Hydrolized corn syrup)	15 (Whey and soy proteins)	30 (Corn oil, MCT)
Magnacal[g] (liquid) (1,000)	50 (Maltodextrins; sucrose)	14 (Sodium and calcium caseinate)	36 (Soy oil)
Nutrex Encare with Fiber[h] (1,200)	66 (Corn syrup solids; sucrose)	11 (Egg white solids; calcium caseinate)	23 (Soy oil)
Nutri-Aid[i] (2,075)	53.7 (Corn syrup solids; sucrose)	14.8 (Caseinate)	31.5 (Corn oil; monoglycerides; diglycerides)
Nutri-1000 LF[d]	38 (Sucrose; corn syrup)	15 (Caseinate; soy isolate)	47 (Corn oil)
Osmolite[e] (liquid) (1,320)	54.6 (Hydrolyzed cornstarch)	14.0 (Sodium and calcium caseinate; soy isolate)	31.4 (MCT Oil; corn oil; soy oil)
Osmolite HN[e] (liquid) (1,890)	53.3 (Hydrolyzed cornstarch)	16.7 (Caseinate; soy isolate)	30 (50% MCT; 50% soy & corn oil)
Portagen[a] (powder) (960)	45 (Corn syrup solids; sucrose; lactose)	14 (Sodium caseinate)	41 (95% MCT Oil; 5% corn oil)
Precision HN[j] (powder) (2,850)	82.2 (Maltodextrin; sucrose)	16.7 (Egg albumin; caseinate)	1.1 (Soy oil)
Precision Isotonic[j] (powder) (1,560)	60 (Sucrose; glucose; oligosaccharides)	11.8 (Egg albumin)	28.2 (Soy oil)
Precision LR[j] (powder) (1,710)	89.2 (Sucrose; maltodextrins)	9.5 (Egg albumin)	1.3 (Soy oil)
ProSobee[a]	40 (Glucose polymers)	12 (Soy isolate; L-methionine)	48 (Soy oil; coconut oil)
Renu[g] (liquid) (2,000)	50 (Maltodextrins; sucrose)	14 (Soy isolate; L-methionine; caseinate)	36 (Soy oil)
Resource[j] (Instant Crystals) (1,896)	54.5 (Maltodextrins; sucrose)	14 (Caseinate; soy isolate)	31.5 (Soy oil)
Travasorb[c] (1,900)	54.5 (Sucrose; corn syrup solids)	14 (Caseinate; soy isolate)	31 (Corn oil; soy oil)
Travasorb HN[c] (powder) (2,000)	70 (Glucose oligosaccharides)	18 (Hydrolyzed lactalbumin)	12 (MCT; safflower oil)
Travasorb MCT[c] (powder) (2,000)	50 (Corn syrup solids)	20 (Lactalbumin; caseinate)	30 (80% MCT Oil; 20% safflower oil)
Travasorb MCT Liquid Diet[c] (1,333)	50 (Maltodextrin)	20 (Casein; lactalbumin)	30 (Safflower oil, MCT)
TwoCal HN[e] (liquid) (950)	43.2 (Hydrolyzed cornstarch)	16.7 (Caseinate)	40.1 (Corn oil; MCT)
Isolates of intact proteins: Milk-based			
Carnation Instant Breakfast[k] (+8 oz whole milk) (1,480)	51 (Corn syrup solids; sucrose; lactose)	22.1 (Milk; nonfat dry milk; sodium caseinate; whey)	26.3 (Milk fat)

Electrolytes (mEq/dl at usual dilution)		Caloric Density (kcal/ml at usual dilution)	Osmolality (mOsm/kg) (Flavors)	Lactose	Residue	Notes
Sodium	Potassium					
4.05	4.0	1.06	470	0	Low	For oral or tube feeding; C:N ratio = 125.1
5.0	5.4	1.5	600 (Flavor packets available)	0	Low	For oral feeding; for tube feeding with caution only; C:N ratio = 146:1
5.15	4.65	1.50	650	0	Low	For oral or tube feeding; C:N ratio = 125:1
3.05	3.07	1.0	300	0	Low	Tube feeding in 1 L ready-to-use pouch; C:N ratio = 154:1
4.4	4.4	1.5	410	0	Low	C:N ratio = 131:1
0.9	3.4	1.0	240	0	Low	C:N ratio = 131:1
2.3	3.4	1.06	300	0	Low	For tube feeding; RSL = 210 mOsm/qt; C:N ratio = 167:1
3.5	3.6	2.0	690	0	Low	For tube feeding; RSL = 383 mOsm/qt; C:N ratio = 145:1
3.1	2.6	1.0	300	0	Low	C:N ratio = 144:1
4.3	3.2	2.0	590	0	Low	For oral or tube feeding; C:N ratio = 154:1
0.74	4.4	1.46	460 (Vanilla; chocolate; strawberry)	0	4 g per sv.	For oral feeding; full-liquid diet. C:N ratio = 232; nonpro kcal:N = 208. Added fiber
3.04	3.07	1.1	290/L (Vanilla; chocolate; strawberry)	0	Low	C:N ratio = 167:1. For oral or tube feeding
2.3	3.9	1.0	380 (Chocolate; vanilla)	0	Low	For tube feeding
2.4	2.59	1.06	300	0	Low	For tube feeding; C:N ratio = 153:1
4.05	4.0	1.06	310	0	Low	For tube feeding; C:N ratio = 125:1
2.0	3.2	0.68 (Infants) 1.0 (Adults)	320	<0.3 per qt	Low	For oral or tube feeding; useful in fat malabsorption; RSL = 15 mOsm/dl; nonpro C:N ratio = 153:1
4.26	2.33	1.05	525	0	Low	For oral or tube feeding; C:N ratio = 125:1
1.97	2.46	0.96	300 (Vanilla; orange)	0	Low	For oral or tube feeding; C:N ratio = 183:1
3.04	2.26	1.11	500–545 (Cherry; lemon; lime; orange)	0	Low	For oral or tube feeding; C:N ratio = 239:1
1.3	2.1	0.68	200	0	Low	For oral feeding; ready-to-use or concentrated; infant formula; lactose free; sucrose free; useful in management of allergy, lactose or sucrose intolerance, galactosemia, gluten sensitivity; RSL = 13 mOsm/dl
2.2	3.2	1.0	300	0	Low	For oral or tube feeding; C:N ratio = 154:1
3.68	4.05	1.06	450 (Vanilla; chocolate)	0	Low	For oral feeding; crystalline to mix with water. C:N ratio = 154:1
3.22	3.25	1.06	488 (Vanilla; black walnut; eggnog)	0	Low	For oral or tube feeding; C:N ratio = 154:1
4.0	3.0	1.0	560	0	Low	C:N ratio = 126:1
1.52	2.6	1.0	312	0	Low	C:N ratio = 102:1
2.28	2.56	1.5	488	0	Low	C:N ratio = 100:1
4.58	5.94	2.0	700	0	Low	For oral or tube feeding. C:N ratio = 126:1. Use tube 12F or higher if gravity fed
4.2–5.2	5.7–7.7	1.06	677–715	9.51	Low	C:N ratio = 89:1

(continued)

Table G-3. *(Continued)*

Product (form) *(Kcal to meet vitamin RDA)*	Composition (Source)		
	Carbohydrate (% of kcal)	Protein (% of kcal)	Lipid (% of kcal)
Enteral 400[b] (liquid)	57.6 (Glucose polymer)	11.6 (Whey isolate)	35.3 (Arachis oil; 24.8% MCT oil)
Isotein HN[j] (powder) (1,770)	52 (Maltodextrins; monosaccharides)	23 (Delactosed lactalbumin; casein)	25 (75% soy oil; 25% MCT)
Meritene Liquid[j] (1,250)	45 (Lactose; corn syrup solids; sucrose)	26 (Nonfat milk)	29 (Milk fat)
Meritene Powder[j] (1,100) (prepared with whole milk)	45 (Lactose; sucrose; corn syrup; fructose)	26 (Milk; casein)	29 (Whole milk)
Nutri-1000[d]	38 (Sucrose; lactose; corn syrup solids)	15 (Milk; caseinate; soy isolate)	47 (Corn oil)
Nutri-1000 LF[c]	38 (Corn syrup solids; sucrose)	15 (Calcium and sodium caseinate; soy isolate)	47 (Corn oil; soy oil)
Sustacal Liquid[a] (1,080)	55 (Sucrose; corn syrup solids)	24 (Skim milk; sodium and calcium caseinate; soy isolate)	21 (Soy oil)
Sustacal HC[a] (liquid) (1,200) (1 packet + whole milk to make 4 kcal/ml)	50 (Corn syrup solids; sucrose)	16 (Caseinates)	34 (Soy oil)
Sustacal Powder[a] (800)	54 (Lactose; sucrose; corn syrup solids)	24 (Nonfat milk)	22 (Milk)
Sustagen[a] (powder) (1,050)	68 (Corn syrup; lactose; sucrose)	24 (Milk; casein)	8 (Powdered whole milk)
Blenderized formulas			
Carnacal #145[k]	48 (Corn syrup solids; sucrose; pureed green beans; pureed peaches)	16 (Pureed beef; nonfat dry milk; modified whey powder; soy protein isolate)	36 (Soy oil)
Citrotein[j] (powder) (1,180)	18.25 (Maltodextrins; sucrose)	6.25 (Egg albumin)	0.26 (Soy oil, monoglycerides; diglycerides)
Compleat Regular Formula[j] (liquid) (1,500)	48 (Maltodextrins; lactose; vegetable and fruit puree; orange juice)	16 (Beef puree; milk)	36 (Corn oil; beef; milk)
Compleat Modified[j] (liquid) (1,500)	54 (Hydrolyzed cereal solids; fruit and vegetable purees)	16 (Beef; calcium caseinate)	30 (Corn oil; beef)
Formula 2[d]	49 (Lactose; sucrose; vegetable; orange juice; farina)	15 (Nonfat dry milk; beef; egg yolks; casein)	36 (Beef; corn oil; egg yolk)
Vitaneed[gf] (liquid) (2,000)	50 (Pureed vegetables and fruit; maltodextrins)	14 (Pureed beef; caseinate)	36 (Soy oil)
Special-Purpose formulas			
Amin-Aid[i] (powder)	74.8 (Maltodextrins; sucrose)	4 (Essential amino acids; histidine)	21.2 (Soy oil)
Hepatic Aid II[j] (powder)	57.3 (Maltodextrins; sucrose)	15 (Free amino acids)	36.2 (Soy oil)
Pulmocare[e] (liquid) (946)	28.4 (Hydrolyzed cornstarch; sucrose)	16.7 (Sodium and calcium caseinate)	55.2 (Corn oil)
Stresstein[j] (powder) (2,000)	57 (Maltodextrins)	23 (Free L-amino acids)	20 (60% MCT; 40% soy oil)
Traum-Aid HBC[i] (powder) (3,000)	66.4 (Maltodextrins)	22.4 (50% amino acids as BCAA)	11.2 (4.5 MCT; 6.7 soy)

Electrolytes (mEq/dl at usual dilution)		Caloric Density (kcal/ml at usual dilution)	Osmolality (mOsm/kg) (Flavors)	Lactose	Residue	Notes
Sodium	Potassium					
2.7	2.99	1.0	330 at 1:4 dilution	Low	Low	For oral or tube feeding; C:N ratio = 193:1; 100 ml = 62.5 mg Na, 116.6 mg K
2.7	2.74	1.2	300	0	Low	Nonpro C:N ratio = 86:1
4.1	3.83	0.96	505 (Vanilla)	5.7	Low	For oral or tube feeding; also available as powder; C:N ratio = 79:1
47.8	71.8	1.0	690 (Vanilla; also chocolate, eggnog, milk chocolate)			C:N ratio = 71:1
2.3	3.9	1.06	500 (Chocolate; vanilla)	Milk-based	Low	
3.13	4.06	1.06		1	Low	
4.1	5.4	1.0	625 (Vanilla) 700 (Chocolate)	0	Low	For oral feeding; for tube feeding with caution; RSL = 364 mOsm/qt; also available as powder or pudding; C:N ratio = 79:1
3.7	3.8	1.5	650 (Vanilla; eggnog)	0		For oral feeding; C:N ratio = 134:1
5.35	8.7	1.33	899			C:N ratio = 80:1
5.5	8.65	1.7	N/A			C:N ratio = 77:1
		1.0	625			Ready to use
3.1	1.8	0.66	480–515	0	Low	Protein & vitamin supplement to clear-liquid diet; 263.4 g dry weight gives 1,000 kcal; C:N ratio = 76:1
2.9	3.6	1.07	300	2.4	Moderate	C:N ratio = 131:1
5.6	3.6	1.07	405	0	Moderate	C:N ratio = 131:1
2.6	4.5	1.0	435–510	3.75	Moderate	For tube feeding; orange flavor; 2,000 ml meets RDA
2.2	3.2	1.02	310	0	Moderate	C:N ratio = 154:1
<0.5	<0.2	1.95	700	0	Low	Indicated for renal disease; also available as pudding; no added vitamins; 213 g dry weight or 489 ml standard dilution gives 1,000 kcal; C:N ratio = 640:1
<1.5	<0.6	1.2	560	0	Low	Indicated for hepatic disease; 46% BCAA; also available as pudding; no added vitamins or electrolytes; C:N ratio = 340:1
5.7	4.88	1.5	490	0		Indicated in ventilator dependency; for oral or tube feeding. Should be limited to 1.7 × caloric need or less; C:N ratio = 125:1
2.83	2.82	1.2	910	0	Low	Indicated for severe metabolic stress. 44% BCAA; C:N = 97:1. For tube feeding
2.3	3.0	1.0	760 (Grape; lemon creme; berry)		Low	For oral or tube feeding; C:N ratio = 102:1

(continued)

Table G-3.   *(Continued)*

Product (form) *(Kcal to meet vitamin RDA)*	Composition (Source)		
	Carbohydrate (% of kcal)	Protein (% of kcal)	Lipid (% of kcal)
Traum-Aid HN[i]	71.9 (Maltodextrins; sucrose)	17.3 (Amino acids; 60% BCAA)	10.8 (Soy; MCT)
TraumaCal[a] (liquid) (2,000)	38 (Corn syrup; sucrose)	22 (Calcium caseinate)	38 (70% soy oil; 30% MCT Oil)
Travasorb Hepatic[c] (powder) (2,100)	77.4 (Glucose oligosaccharides; sucrose)	10.6 (Crystalline amino acids)	12 (MCT Oil; sunflower oil)
Travasorb Renal[c] (powder) (2,100)	81.1 (Glucose oligosaccharides; sucrose)	6.9 (Crystalline amino acids; EEA, histidine, arginine, and others)	12 (MCT Oil; sunflower oil)
MSUD Diet Powder[a]	54	8	38
Product 3200 AB[a] (powder)	52	13 (Casein hydrolysate)	35
Product 3200 K[a] (powder)	39	12 (Soy protein isolate)	49
Product 80056[a] (powder)	59	0	41
Product 3232A[a]	52 (Tapioca starch as stabilizer; add 59 g carbohydrate/qt)	13 (Casein hydrolysate)	35 (MCT Oil)

(continued)

Electrolytes (mEq/dl at usual dilution)		Caloric Density (kcal/ml at usual dilution)	Osmolality (mOsm/kg) (Flavors)	Lactose	Residue	Notes
Sodium	Potassium					
2.3	2.1	1.0	800 (Grape; lemon creme; berry)	0	Low	Indicated for catabolic states; for oral or tube feeding; lemon creme flavor contains tetrazine
5.2	3.6	1.5	550	0	Low	For oral or tube feeding. High in BCAA (1.25 g/100 kcal); C:N ratio = 90:1
1.00	2.2	1.1	690 (Eggnog; custard; chocolate; apricot; strawberry)	0	Low	For hepatic disease; 50% BCAA; low in AAA; C:N ratio = 211:1
0 (approx)	0	1.35	590 (Apricot; strawberry)	0	No	For renal disease; C:N ratio = 340:1; no fat-soluble vitamins; no electrolytes
1.15	1.79	0.68				Free of BCAA; for use in management of maple-syrup urine disease
1.38	1.76	0.68				Low-phenylalanine, low-tyrosine food powder for management of tyrosinemia; with 16 mg phenylalanine/100 kcal & 9 mg tyrosine/100 kcal
1.15	1.49	0.68				Infant formula for management of homocystinuria; contains 34 mg methionine/kcal
	1.02					A protein-free formula base providing carbohydrate and fat to which amino acids and sodium must be added; for management of rare amino acid metabolic disorders
1.38	1.76	0.68				A protein hydrolysate formula base to be used in management of disaccharidase deficiency, impaired glucose transport, or fructose utilization; values given assume addition of 59 g carbohydrate per qt

Note: The composition of these products changes frequently. Current product literature should be consulted before use. This table is not intended to be comprehensive. C:N ratios are *nonprotein* kcal to nitrogen.

MCT = medium-chain triglycerides; BCAA = branched-chain amino acids; AAA = aromatic amino acids; EAA = essential amino acids

[a]Mead Johnson Nutritional

[b]Scientific Hospital Supplies

[c]Travenol Laboratories

[d]Cutter Laboratories (Kabi-Vitrum)

[e]Ross Laboratories

[f]Norwich-Eaton Pharmaceuticals

[g]Chesebrough-Pond

[h]Nutrex

[i]Kendall McGaw

[j]Sandoz

[k]Carnation

[l]Biosearch

[m]Navaco

[n]Knight Medical

Appendix H:
Conversion Factors

Table H-1. Units of Measurement

1. *Metric system weights*
    - 1 kilogram = 1,000 grams (g)
    - 1 milligram = 0.001 g
    - 1 microgram = 10^{-6} g or μ
    - 1 nanogram = 10^{-9} g or mμ
    - 1 picogram = 10^{-12} g or μμ
    - 1 femtogram = 10^{-15} g or mμμ
2. *Metric and avoirdupois systems of volume (fluid)*
    - 1 liter (L)   = 1,000 milliliters (ml) or 1.06 quarts (qt)
    - 1 milliliter = 1,000 microliters (μl)
3. *Conversion factors*
    - 1 kg = 2.2046 pounds (usually rounded to 2.2)
    - 1 fl oz = 29.573 ml (usually rounded to 30)
    - Degrees Celsius = (°F − 32) × 5⁄9
    - Degrees Fahrenheit = (°C × 9⁄5) + 32
    - Parts per million (ppm) to
        percent:

1ppm	= 0.0001%
10ppm	= 0.001%
100ppm	= 0.01%
1,000ppm	= 0.1%
10,000ppm	= 1%

(continued)

Table H-1.   *(Continued)*

Milliequivalents (mEq) to milligrams:
    mEq × atomic weight/valence = mg
    e.g.: (30 mEq Na × 23)/1 = 690 mg Na
Milligrams to milliequivalents:
    (mg/atomic weight) × valence = mEq
    e.g.: (1,482 mg K/39) × 1 = 38 mEq K
Milliequivalents (mEq) to millimoles (mmol)
    mEq ÷ valence = mmol
    e.g.: (5.0 mEq Ca^{++})/2 = 2.5 mmol Ca^{++}
Milligrams to millimoles
    mg ÷ molecular weight = mmol
    e.g.: (10 mg Ca^{++})/40 = 0.25 mmol
For other values, use these atomic weights:

		Atomic weight	Valence
Calcium	Ca	40	2
Chlorine	Cl	35.4	1
Magnesium	Mg	24.3	2
Phosphorus	P	31	2
Potassium	K	39	1
Sodium	Na	23	1
Sulfur	S	32	2
Zinc	Zn	65.37	2

Appendix I:
Revised Daily Food Guide
Food Groups

Table I-1. Daily Food Guide Food Groups

PROTEIN FOODS include both animal and vegetable foods. Animal protein foods supply protein, iron, riboflavin, niacin, vitamins B6 and B12, phosphorus, zinc, and iodine. Vegetable protein foods supply folacin, magnesium, and thiamin, in addition to the nutrients just mentioned for animal protein foods.

Animal-protein foods

A serving is 2 oz (60 g) unless otherwise noted

Beef (ground, cube, roast, or chop)	
Clams	4 large or 9 small
Eggs	2 medium
Fish (fillet or steak)	
Fish sticks	3 sticks
Frankfurters	2
Lamb (ground, cube, roast, or chop)	
Luncheon meat	3 slices
Organ meats:	
heart, kidney, liver, tongue	
Oysters	8–12 medium
Pork, ham (ground, roast, or chop)	
Poultry:	
chicken, duck, turkey	
Rabbit	
Sausage links	4 links
Shellfish:	
crab, lobster, scallops, shrimp	
Spareribs	6 medium ribs
Tuna fish	
Veal (ground, cube, roast, or chop)	

Vegetable-protein foods

Beans are the best choice from vegetable-protein foods. A serving of beans contains more vitamins and minerals than a serving of nuts or seeds. A serving is 1 cup cooked unless otherwise stated.

Canned beans (garbanzo, kidney, lima, pork and beans)	1 cup (240 ml)
Dried beans and peas	1 cup (240 ml)
Nut butters (cashew butter, peanut butter, etc.)	¼ cup (60 ml)
Nuts	½ cup (120 ml)
Sunflower seeds	½ cup (120 ml)
Tofu (soybean curd)	1 cup (240 ml)

MILK AND MILK PRODUCTS are the best food sources of calcium. In addition, these foods supply protein, phosphorus, vitamins A, D, E, B6, and B12, riboflavin, magnesium, and zinc. For some people, milk and milk products serve as primary sources of protein in the diet.

(continued)

Table I-1. *(Continued)*

A serving is 8 oz (1 cup or 240 cc) unless otherwise noted.

Cheese (except camembert, cream)	1 slice (1½ oz or 45 g)
Cheese spread	4 T (60 ml)
Cocoa made with milk	1¼ cups (10 oz or 300 ml)
Cottage cheese	1⅓ cups (320 ml)
Custard (flan)	
Ice cream	1½ cups (360 ml)
Ice milk	1¼ cups (10 oz or 300 ml)
Milk	
buttermilk	
chocolate (not drink)	
evaporated	½ cup (4 oz or 120 ml)
goat	
low fat	
nonfat	
nonfat (made from dry milk powder)	
nonfat dry milk powder	⅓ cup (80 ml)
whole	
Milkshake	
Pudding	
Soups made with milk	1½ cups (12 oz or 360 ml)
Yogurt (plain)	

BREADS AND CEREALS supply thiamin, niacin, riboflavin, iron, phosphorus, and zinc. This food group is divided into two parts: whole-grain items and enriched products. The enriched breads, cereals, and pastas provide significantly lower amounts of magnesium, zinc, and fiber. For this reason, patients should be urged to choose whole-grain products.

Whole-grain items

Bread: cracked, whole wheat, or rye	1 slice
Cereal, hot: oatmeal (rolled oats), rolled wheat, cracked wheat, wheat and malted barley	½ cup cooked (120 ml)
Cereal, ready-to-eat: puffed oats, shredded wheat, wheat flakes, granola	¾ cup (180 ml)
Rice (brown)	½ cup cooked (120 ml)
Wheat germ	1 T (15 ml)

Enriched items

Bagel	1 small

(continued)

Table I-1. *(Continued)*

Bread (all except those listed above)	1 slice
Cereal, hot: cream of wheat, cream of rice, farina, cornmeal, grits	½ cup cooked (120 ml)
Cereal, ready-to-eat (all except those listed above)	¾ cup (180 ml)
Crackers	4
Macaroni, noodles, spaghetti	½ cup cooked (120 ml)
Pancake, waffle	1 medium (5 inch or 13 cm diameter)
Rice (white)	½ cup cooked
Roll, biscuit, muffin, dumpling	1
Tortilla	1 (6 inch or 15 cm diameter)

VITAMIN C–RICH FRUITS AND VEGETABLES supply ascorbic acid. Fresh, frozen, or canned forms may be used although vitamin C content of canned products is lower.
A serving is ¾ cup (180 ml) unless otherwise noted.

Vegetables

Bok choy	
Broccoli	1 stalk
Brussels sprouts	3–4
Cabbage	
Cauliflower	
Chili peppers (green or red)	¼ cup
Greens: collard, kale, mustard, turnip	
Peppers (green or red)	½ medium
Tomatoes	2 medium
Watercress	

Fruits

Cantaloupe	½ medium
Grapefruit	½ large
Guava	½ small
Mango	1 medium
Orange	1 medium
Papaya	½ small
Strawberries	
Tangerine	2 large

Juices

Fruit juices and drinks with vitamin C added	
Grapefruit	½ cup (4 oz or 120 ml)
Orange	½ cup (4 oz or 120 ml)
Pineapple	1½ cups (12 oz or 360 ml)
Tomato	1½ cups (12 oz or 360 ml)

DARK GREEN VEGETABLES are an excellent source of folacin. In addition, these foods supply vitamins A, E, and B6, riboflavin, iron, and magnesium. Cooking temperatures destroy folacin, so eat dark green vegetables raw whenever possible.
A serving is 1 cup (240 ml) raw or ¾ cup (180 ml) cooked.

Asparagus	Escarole
Bok choy	Greens: beet, collard, kale, mustard, turnip
Broccoli	Lettuce (dark leafy: red leaf, romaine)
Brussels sprouts	Scallions
Cabbage	Spinach
Chicory	Swiss chard
Endive	Watercress

(continued)

Table I-1. *(Continued)*

OTHER FRUITS AND VEGETABLES include yellow fruits and vegetables which supply significant amounts of vitamin A. Other fruits and vegetables also contribute varying amounts of B complex vitamins, vitamin E, magnesium, zinc, phosphorus, and also fiber. A serving is ½ cup (120 ml) unless otherwise noted.

Fruits

Apple	1 medium
Apricot	2 medium
Banana	1 small
Berries	
Cherries	
Dates	5
Figs	2 large
Fruit cocktail	
Grapes	
Kumquats	3
Nectarine	2 medium
Peach	1 medium
Pear	1 medium
Persimmon	1 small
Pineapple	
Plums	2 medium
Prunes	4 medium
Pumpkin	¼ cup (60 ml)
Raisins	
Watermelon	

Vegetables

Artichoke	1 medium
Bamboo shoots	
Beans (green, wax)	
Bean sprouts	
Beet	
Burdock root	
Carrot	
Cauliflower	
Celery	
Corn	
Cucumber	
Eggplant	
Hominy	
Lettuce (head, boston, bibb)	
Mushrooms	
Nori seaweed	
Onion	
Parsnip	
Peas	
Pea pods	
Potato	1 medium
Radishes	
Summer squash	
Sweet potato	1 medium
Winter squash	
Yam	1 medium
Zucchini	

Adapted from "Eating Right for Your Baby," prepared by the California Department of Health Services.

Appendix J: Ethnic Food Practices

Table J-1. Cultural Dietary Patterns Classified According to the Daily Food Guide

	Chinese	*Japanese*	*Filipino*	*American Indian*	*Black (Afro-American)*
Milk Group	Intake of fluid milk usually limited; ice cream well accepted; flavored milk drinks preferred until taste is developed Limited intake of cheese; younger generations are consuming larger quantities of milk and cheeses	Milk and cheese consumed in larger quantities by the younger generations Ice cream and milk puddings are well accepted	Dairy foods are gaining acceptance and are tolerated Limited intake of milk and cheese Custards similar to Mexican flan Ice cream, flavored milk drinks, fresh white cheese	Most easily tolerate milk products in fermented form or in small quantities throughout the day Buttermilk, yogurt, cottage cheese, and Monterey Jack cheese Nonfat dry milk is used in cooking	Fresh homogenized milk, chocolate milk, buttermilk, evaporated and nonfat dry milk in cooking; ice cream, milk puddings, and custards Cheese (American, Cheddar, cottage, longhorn) Yogurt
Supplementary Source of Calcium	*Tofu* (soybean curd) has significant calcium content.* Canned fish with bones, sardines, small fried fish eaten whole (smelts), dried small fish including bones Various leafy greens (amaranths, kale, Chinese cress, Chinese mustard greens, pickled mustard leaves)	*Tofu* (soybean curd) has significant calcium content* Whole dried fish, including bones	*Tofu* (soybean curd) has significant calcium content* *Alamang* and *bagoong* (fish sauce) *Dilis* (dried fish) *Malunggay* (dark green, leafy vegetables)		Dark green, leafy vegetables (collard greens, mustard greens, and kale) Sardines
Bread-Cereal Group	Large intake of rice, rice cakes, rice noodles, rice flour; wheat products (breads, noodles, spaghetti, macaroni); millet, oats *Won ton* (stuffed noodles) *Bow* (filled buns)	Large quantities of rice and rice products used; *Mochiko* (rice flour) often used; rice cakes, breads, and crackers *Sushi* (rice wrapped in seaweed) *Somen* and *soba* (noodles), millet and barley are commonly used	Rice is the staple food. Some noodles used also. *Won ton* used in soups as in Chinese diet Cooked cereals; various kinds of bread including *Pan de Sal* (white bread) *Mochiko* (rice flour)	Cornmeal and flours made from ground sweet acorn, wheat, or rye; white flour used for *fry bread* (fried biscuit dough); tortillas also popular Cornbread, rice, *bean bread* (shelled bean and cornmeal mixture), *ta fulla* (hominy and cake of bean ashes), *shi-nish-*	Homemade bread, white and whole-wheat breads, biscuits, cornbread (also cornpone, hush puppies, spoon bread, cracklin' bread), pancakes, grits, rice, macaroni, spaghetti Whole-grain cereals and cooked cream of wheat, oatmeal and rice cereals

(continued)

Table J-1. *(Continued)*

			bay and *buh-kway-shee* (fried bread), *bota-cuppa* (Cherokee poached corn and water with sugar), *walakshi* (fruit-flavored cornmeal dumplings)	Dry cereals (corn flakes, rice, or wheat)
Sources of Vitamin A *Napa* (Chinese celery cabbage), *gai choy* (Chinese mustard greens), watercress, *yin choy* (amaranth greens), leaf lettuce. *oong choy* (water convolvulus), *gou gay* (wolfberry leaves), *lo bok* (Chinese turnips) Green peppers, tomatoes, spinach, Chinese chard, carrots, sweet potatoes, pumpkin, coriander, squash, apricots, peaches	Spinach, carrots, tomatoes, yellow squash, sweet potatoes, parsley, Japanese persimmons, mustard greens *Laver, nori, wakame, kombu* (types of seaweed)	*Camotes* (sweet potatoes), tomatoes, squash, *saluyot* (leafy green, slimy vegetable), *malunggay* (dark green leafy vegetable)	Pumpkin and all squash very popular Carrots, onions, potatoes, celery, cabbage, peas Dandelion greens, milkweed Wild and cultivated berries, yellow corn, eaten very commonly	Leafy greens—fresh preferred (collards, mustard, turnip greens, kale, spinach, chard, beet tops); encourage use of the pot liquor (the liquid in which vegetables are cooked) Tomatoes, sweet potatoes, carrots, pumpkins, yellow squash, green peppers, okra, lettuce Melons, peaches
Sources of Vitamin C *Gai lan* (Chinese broccoli), Chinese cabbage, green peppers, fresh tomatoes, watercress, broccoli, spinach, leafy greens, celery, turnips, cauliflower, *daikon* (white radish), *chow yuk* (stir-fried vegetables) Fruits not eaten frequently; more widely used in younger generations. Oranges, papayas, tangerines, melons, guavas, lemons	Fresh tomatoes, broccoli, *napa* (cabbage), *kimchee* (pickled cabbage), *daikon* (white radish), turnips, potatoes (eaten in limited amounts) Oranges	Cabbage, cauliflower, corn, pith of sago palm, potatoes, turnips, avocados *Achara* (papaya and peppers), melons, guavas, jackfruit, limes, mangoes, oranges, papayas, pomelos, strawberries, *naranghita* (tangelo)	Mustard greens, watercress, cabbage, turnips, potatoes (sweet and white) Lemons, oranges, melons, grapefruit, strawberries, dried fruit (wild cherries, berries, and grapes)	Broccoli, turnips, green peppers, cabbage, mustard greens, tomatoes, potatoes (sweet and white) Oranges, grapefruit, melons, lemons, strawberries
Other Vegetables and Fruits Snow peas (Chinese pea pods), Chinese okra, bamboo shoots, soybean sprouts, mung bean sprouts, alfalfa sprouts, taro roots, lotus tubers, dried day lillies, *Black Juda's ear* (high-fiber dry fungus) Eggplant, cucumbers, green beans, mushrooms, onions, leeks Plums, prunes, persimmons, apples, bananas, pears, figs, grapes, pineapples, pomegranates	String beans, onions, eggplant, cucumbers, pickled vegetables (as dessert), mushrooms, celery, *gobo* (burdock), *takenoko* (bamboo shoots), *seri* (Japanese parsley), *renkon* (lotus root), *wasabi* (horseradish) *Mizutaki* (vegetable soup)	Mung beans, bean sprouts, okra, eggplant, celery, onions, radishes, bamboo shoots, *gabi* (root crop), mushrooms, onions *Tamarind* (pod fruit), *ampalaya* (bitter melon), bananas, pineapple	Eggplant, wild tullies (tuber used as vegetable), green peas, green beans, beets, onions, corn, cucumbers, cassava Grapes, apples, pears, bananas	Green peas, green beans, beets, onions, cucumbers, eggplant, corn, radishes Grapes, bananas, pears, fruit cocktail, apples, pineapple

Vegetable-Fruit Group

(continued)

Table J-1. *(Continued)*

Large intake of pork and pork products (sausage, BBQ pork, roast pork, pig knuckles), fish of various kinds (fresh, canned, salted); seafoods (shrimp, crabs, squid, oysters, clams, octopus, abalone) Poultry (chicken, duck); eggs (chicken, duck); organ meats (liver, heart, tongue, maws, kidney, spleen) Peanuts, almonds, walnuts; dried beans (soybeans, black beans, red beans, white beans); *tofu* (soybean curd)	Pork, beef, chicken; large intake of fish and shellfish dishes; *sashimi* (raw fish), *kamaboko* (fish cake) Soybeans, *miso* (fermented soybean), soya cake, *tofu* (soybean curd) Eggs; peanuts, chestnuts; *azuki beans* (red beans), lima beans *Hekka* (seasoned chicken dish)	Fresh and dried fish as well as shellfish are major sources of protein; *dilis* (dried fish) Chicken, duck, pork, beef, *adobo* (pieces of pork and chicken in soy sauce), *relleno* (chicken) *Tortilla* (an omelet) and *lumpia* (egg roll) also popular *Lechon* (barbequed pig) is considered a specialty Organ meats (liver, heart, intestines) Various sausages, ham and cured meats, canned meats Eggs, dried beans, soybeans, garbanzo beans, peanut butter, *tofu* (soybean curd)	When available in hunting areas, wild rabbit, venison, wild geese, duck, groundhog are popular Fresh fish, pork, chicken; eggs eaten in large quantities Dried peas and beans (kidney, pinto, and lentils very common in diet and usually eaten with rice and other grains) *Roe* (fish eggs) Pinenuts, acorns, peanuts, and other nut sources of protein	Large intake of pork (fresh and cured) and pork products such as sausage (mild or hot) Scrapple (pork and cornmeal), cold cuts, organ meats, including chitterlings (pork intestines), kidney, liver, tongue Beef, lamb, tripe, chicken, turkey, duck, goose Game such as rabbit and venison; fresh and canned fish (buffalo, catfish, trout, shellfish, tuna, salmon, mackerel, sardines) Eggs; walnuts, pecans, peanuts; dried peas and beans (black-eyed peas, chickpeas; kidney, pink and red beans, navy beans) Peanut butter Lower-protein, high-fat meat sources (cured bacon—thin slices or slab, pig's feet, pig ears, souse, pork neck bones)

Meat Group (includes Meat, Poultry, Game, Fish, Eggs, Dried Peas and Beans, and Nuts)

*6 oz of tofu contains an amount of calcium comparable to 1 c of milk.

Reproduced with permission from *Extension of Guide to Good Eating*. Sacramento, Calif., Dairy Council of California.

Table J-2. Food Plans for Selected European Ethnic Groups

	Italian	Greek	German/Hungarian	Polish	Czechoslovak
Milk Group	Very little milk used; cheeses popular, *casicavallo; gorgonzola, locatelli, Parmesan, provolone, mozarella, ricotta;* ice cream desserts as *gelati, spumoni,* and *tortoni.*	Cow, goat, or sheep milk (boiled for children); many cheeses, *feta* cheese popular, fermented milk (*yaourti*) for dessert.	Milk, buttermilk, sour milk, or cream used in cooking, cottage, cream, and brick cheese in cheese cake, strudels, and noodle dishes.	Cow or goat milk; sour cream on vegetables, meats, salads; cream in soup; Brick, cottage and cream cheese. Cottage cheese in kuchens and dumplings.	Cow's milk (fresh for children), fermented milk and buttermilk (preferred by adults). Cheeses from sheep's milk preferred. Use in baking.
Bread-Cereal Group	Cornmeal (*polenta*), farina, macaroni, spaghetti and similar *pastas;* crusty Italian white bread, whole wheat bread (*facaccia*); pizza.	Corn, rice, wheat	Barley, farina, rye, *mehl* (Hungarian flour); noodles, dumplings (*spaetzel*), strudel.	Barley, buckwheat, cornmeal, oats, rice, rye, whole wheat, kasha (buckwheat), oats, millet; rice in meats and vegetables; barley and kasha in soup; dark rye bread with every meal.	Corn, rye, wheat. Cornmeal as a mush; white flour in pastry and dumplings; sour rye bread preferred.

(continued)

Table J-2. *(Continued)*

Vegetable-Fruit Group				
Artichokes, string beans, broccoli, cauliflower, celery, chicory, Savoy cabbage, dandelion greens, endive, eggplant, fennel, garlic, mushrooms, peas, peppers, radishes, romaine, spinach, Italian squash, and tomatoes. Greens are served raw with oil and wine, tomatoes are cooked into sauce, soups, or cooked with meat or fish. Fresh, glazed and dried fruits, grapes, pears, plums, melons, quinces, cherries, peaches, figs, dates, apricots, apples, oranges, persimmon, and raisins. Served for dessert.	Cabbage, cauliflower, cucumbers, eggplant, greens, okra, onions, peppers, some potatoes, vine leaves, zucchini, tomatoes, salad greens, oranges, and lemons. Boiled or fried in a small amount of olive oil, served hot or cold, cooked with meat or fish. Lemon juice on salads and cold foods. Apricots, cherries, dates, figs, grapes, melons, nuts, plums, peaches, pears, quinces, and raisins. Served as dessert. Grapes are pressed into wine or dried as raisins.	Cabbage (red and white), carrots, cauliflower, cucumbers, beets, beans, broccoli, kale, kohlrabi, onions, potatoes, sauerkraut, tomatoes, and lettuce. Lettuce with bacon and hot vinegar, red cabbage with bacon sauce, potato salad with herring. Apples, apricots, bananas, cherries, berries, grapes, melons, oranges, quinces, pears, peaches, and prunes for dessert.	Butter beans, cabbage, carrots, cucumbers, kale, lettuce, mushrooms, onions, parsnips, potatoes, sauerkraut, sorrel, radishes, leeks, turnips, beets, and split peas. Cabbage (sauerkraut) and root vegetables primarily. Potatoes at most of the meals. Vegetables cooked with meat (pig's knuckles) and noodles, cabbage, and split peas, stuffed cabbage, potato pancakes, and borscht (beet soup). Apples, apricots, cherries, grapes, pears, plums, prunes, and strawberries in fruit, soup, dried or raw.	Beets, cabbage, carrots, cauliflower, celeriac, kale, leeks, mushrooms, parsnips, potatoes, spinach, turnips, and tomatoes; potatoes and vegetables boiled and served with cream. Cabbage as sauerkraut. Apples, apricots, berries, cherries, pears, plums, and some imported bananas, pineapple, dried fruits, citrus fruits, raw or preserved; dried fruits in baking.
Meat Group				
Beef, lamb, veal, pork, fowl, and sausages, bologna and salami. Small quantity of meat slow simmered, served with sauce, such as tomato sauce, prepared with garlic, onion, green peppers, tomato; or fried. Usually cut up and stewed, fried or ground and cooked with pasta such as chicken cacciatora, veal (cutlet) scallopine, meat balls with tomato sauce; all fish, and clams, mussels, octopus, fresh sardines, squid, and snails; eggs, dried beans, lentils, and peas. Eggs fried plain or with spinach, onions, and peppers; used as thickening agent; and omelet with cheese. Dried beans, lentils, and peas cooked in thick soups such as *minestrone* and *pastafasiole*.	Lamb, some beef, goat, mutton, pork products; poultry; cut into small pieces or ground. Poultry is cooked into broth. Lamb is cooked on skewers or cut up and browned in oil or fat with rice or flour and vegetables. Salt water fish (fresh, smoked, or salted), shellfish, smoked roe, squid, and octopus; fried or steamed with vegetables, used frequently. Eggs, white beans and legumes, boiled, mashed, stewed, and eaten either hot or cold. Soup made of dried beans, onions, celery, and carrots is a national dish. Eggs are popular.	Beef (muscle and organs), pork, veal, bacon, sausage, poultry (especially goose), and game; fresh-water fish and shrimp; in stews served with dumplings or noodles as chicken and anchovies, beef and noodle soup, beans with pork, veal and peas, and crawfish and tomatoes. Eggs, used in noodles, as thickening agent, or as garnish.	Beef, pork (ham), veal (lungs, tongue, tripe, brain, liver, kidneys), fowl, geese, and salami; stews are preferred; all varieties of fish, fresh in summer, pickled in winter; eggs, in soups and dumplings.	Beef, pork (fresh and smoked), veal, poultry; fresh water fish; eggs, in cooking and baking, lentils, yellow peas, kidney and white beans, boiled, cooked in soups or stews, or served as a relish.
Other				
Fats: Olive or cotton seed oil, lard, salt pork. Desserts: Fruit, fancy cakes, chestnuts, gelati (brick ice cream), marzipan (almond	Fats: Olive oil, seed oils, salted black olives, and little butter. Seasonings: Caraway and pumpkin seeds, herbs, honey, nuts (hazel, pignolia, and	Fats: Butter in cooking and meat fats. Desserts: Fruits, cheese cakes and strudels. Seasonings: Caraway seed, horseradish, garlic, onions, paprika,	Desserts: Fruits, cookies, small cakes and pancakes with preserves. Seasonings: Almonds, chili sauce, dried mushrooms,	Fats: Butter for baking, lard in cooking, poultry fat spread on bread. Seasonings: Caraway, poppy, and sesame seeds, garlic, honey,

(continued)

Table J-2. *(Continued)*

cakes), spumone ice cream, and tortoni; served on feast days and special occasions. Seasoning: Aniseed, cloves, garlic, onions, parsley, pepper, salt, thyme, vinegar. Beverages: Coffee with hot milk and sugar, dry wines in cooking and as beverage for adults, and liquors.	pistachio), and sesame; seeds and nuts as snack or dessert. Beverages: Coffee and wine at meals.	peppers, pickles, poppy seed, parsley, and vinegar. Beverages: Tea, coffee, beer, Tokay wine, schnapps, and Hungarian whisky.	horseradish, mace, onions, pickles, poppy seeds, peppers, and saffron. Beverages: Tea, coffee, Polish beer.	dried mushrooms, nuts, and spices. Beverages: Coffee, cocoa, beer (Czech), and wine (Slovak).

(label in left margin: Other)

Table J-3. Typical Diets of Indochinese Refugees in Minnesota

Group	Breakfast	Lunch & Dinner	Snacks
Vietnamese	Soup—"pho"—containing rice noodles, thin slices of beef or chicken, bean sprouts, and greens *or* Boiled eggs and crusty bread *or* Rice and leftover meat Tea or coffee	Rice (prefer long-grain) Fish and/or meat and vegetable dish Fish sauce—"nuoc mam" Clear soup with vegetables and/or meat Tea, coffee, soft drinks, or alcoholic beverages	Fruits Clear soup Rice
Laotian	Rice (prefer sweet, glutinous) Boiled egg, roasted meat, or fish with sauce Tea or coffee	Fish—"padek"—and/or meat stew with hot peppers and other vegetables Rice Cucumber salad Tea, coffee, soft drinks, or alcoholic beverages	Bananas Stew
Cambodian	Soup with meat and noodles or rice Tea or coffee	Rice Fermented fish—"prahoc" Fish sauce—"tuk-trey"—with cabbage, cucumbers, and/or turnips Tea, coffee, soft drinks, or alcoholic beverages	Sweets made from palm sugar Bananas Clear soup
Hmong[a]	(Most adults do not eat breakfast but may eat first meal early in day. Children eat cereal and milk, or egg and American-type bread.)	Chicken, pork, and/or fish, vegetables, and rice or noodles *or* Tofu, rice (short-grain), and vegetables *or* Rice and soup containing meat and vegetables Tea, coffee, juice, or soft drinks	Fruits Commercial baked goods

[a]Most Hmong eat only two daily meals, the menus for which are listed in the lunch and dinner column. Some families eat meals early and other families eat late. Typical times of early first and second meals are 7:00 AM and 3:30 PM; late first and second meals are eaten at 11:00 AM and 6:00 PM.

Reproduced with permission from Splett, P.L. Indochinese refugees in the WIC program. *WIC Currents* 7(1981)7–20.

Appendix K:
Exchange Lists for Protein-, Sodium-, Potassium-Restricted Diets

Table K-1. Average Nutrient Values Summarized for Quick Calculations

Food list	Calories	Protein g	Sodium mg	Potassium mg
High-sodium meat	90	8.0	200	75
Low-sodium meat	60	8.0	30	100
Dairy	Varies	4.0	70	185
Regular bread, cereal, & starch	90	2.0	200	30
Low-sodium bread, cereal, & starch	65	2.0	5	30
Fruit #1	60	0.5	5	100
#2	65	0.6	5	175
#3	70	0.7	5	250
Vegetable #1	15	1.0	10	100
#2	20	1.0	20	170
#3	30	1.0	15	250
#4	50	2.5	20	Varies

Tables K-1 through K-16 from *A Guide to Protein Controlled Diets for Dietitians.* Los Angeles: Los Angeles District of the California Dietetic Association, 1977. Reprinted with permission.

Table K-2. Dairy List

Averages–Calories: Average Varies				Protein: 4.0 g			Sodium: 70 mg			Potassium: 185 mg
Food Item	Measure	Weight g	Kcal	Pro g	Fat g	Cho g	Ca mg	P mg	Na mg	K mg
Cream, half & half	½ c	120	158	3.6	14	5	127	115	49	157
Cream, light whipping	¾ c	180	524	3.9	55	5	124	110	62	173
Cream, heavy whipping	¾ c	180	616	3.7	66	5	116	112	67	134
Ice cream, (10% fat) plain	¾ c	100	202	3.6	11	24	132	100	87	193
Ice cream, (16% fat) rich	¾ c	110	262	3.1	18	24	113	86	81	166
Ice milk, vanilla, hardened	¾ c	100	138	3.9	4	22	132	97	79	199
Milk:										
Whole, (3.3% fat)	½ c	122	75	4.0	4	6	146	114	60	185
Lowfat, (2% fat)	½ c	122	60	4.1	2	6	148	116	61	188
Nonfat (skim)	½ c	122	43	4.2	tr	6	151	124	63	203
Evaporated, whole, cnd	¼ c	63	84	4.3	5	6	164	128	66	191
Chocolate, whole	½ c	125	104	4.0	4	13	140	126	74	208
Chocolate, low fat (2%)	½ c	125	90	4.0	2	13	142	127	75	211
	True Averages		196	3.9					68	184

(continued)

Table K-2.   (*Continued*)

Averages–Calories: Average Varies		Protein: 4.0 g			Sodium: 70 mg			Potassium: 185 mg		
Food Item	Measure	Weight g	Kcal	Pro g	Fat g	Cho g	Ca mg	P mg	Na mg	K mg
Special Milks—Use only on the advice of the dietitian.										
Buttermilk, cultured	½ c	122	50	4.0	1	6	142	110	128	166
Cocoa, hot, homemade with whole milk	½ c	125	109	4.6	4	13	149	135	62	240
Dry, nonfat milk	2 Tbsp	15	54	5.4	tr	8	188	145	80	269
Dry, whole milk	2 Tbsp	16	80	4.2	4	6	146	124	60	213
Goat's milk	½ c	122	84	4.3	5	6	163	135	61	250
Low-fat milk, protein fortified	½ c	123	68	4.9	2	7	176	138	72	224
Nonfat milk, protein fortified	½ c	123	50	4.9	tr	7	176	138	72	223
Low sodium milk	½ c	122	74	3.8	4	5	123	104	3	308
Yogurt, plain, low fat	½ c	133	72	6.0	2	8	207	163	80	265
Yogurt, fruited, low fat	½ c	113	116	5.0	1	22	172	135	66	221

Note: One serving of milk is 4 fluid ounces, not 8 ounces.

Table K-3.   Vegetable List 1

Averages–Calories: 15		Protein: 1.0 g			Sodium: 10 mg			Potassium: 100 mg		
Food Item	Measure	Weight g	Kcal	Pro g	Fat g	Cho g	Ca mg	P mg	Na mg	K mg
Asparagus, fresh, ck	4 med spears	60	12	1.3	0	2	13	30	1	110
Asparagus, cnd, low Na	⅓ c	79	13	1.6	0	2	14	34	2	132
Asparagus, froz, ck	3 med spears	45	11	1.4	0	2	10	30	1	107
Bean snaps, wax, fresh, ck	½ c	65	15	1.0	0	3	31	23	3	95
Beans, froz, French cut, ck, drained	½ c	65	17	1.0	0	4	25	20	2	88
Beans, green, low Na, cnd, drained	½ c	65	15	1.0	0	3	30	17	1	64
Cucumber, raw, pared,	10 slices, ¼" thick	70	10	0.4	0	2	12	13	4	112
Cabbage, raw, shredded	½ c	45	11	0.6	0	2	22	13	9	105
Cabbage, ck, shredded	½ c	72	15	0.8	0	3	32	15	10	119
Cabbage, red, raw, shredded	½ c	45	14	0.9	0	3	19	16	12	121
Cabbage, Chinese, raw, cut 1" pieces	½ c	37	6	0.4	0	1	16	15	8	95
Carrots, cnd, low Na, drained	½ c	77	20	0.6	0	4	24	17	30	93
Cauliflower, fresh, ck	½ c	68	14	1.5	0	3	13	26	7	129
Endive, raw, chopped	½ c	25	5	0.5	0	1	22	19	4	73
Lettuce, all varieties, chopped	½ c	27	4	0.4	0	1	10	7	3	73
Mustard greens, froz, ck	½ c	75	15	1.7	0	2	78	33	8	118
Onion, raw, sliced	½ c	58	22	0.9	0	5	16	22	6	92
Onion, ckd, sliced	½ c	105	31	1.2	0	7	25	31	8	115
Onion, green, chopped, bulb and top	½ c	50	18	0.8	0	4	25	20	2	115
Parsley sprigs, 2½"	10 sprigs	10	4	0.4	0	1	20	6	5	73
Pepper, sweet green, ck 2¾" × 2½"	1 whole	73	13	0.7	0	3	7	12	7	109
	True Averages		14	0.9					6	102

Table K-4. Vegetable List 2

Averages–Calories: 20   Protein: 1.0 g   Sodium: 20 mg   Potassium: 170 mg

Food Item	Measure	Weight g	Kcal	Pro g	Fat g	Cho g	Ca mg	P mg	Na mg	K mg
Bamboo shoots, raw	¼ c	33	9	0.9	0	2	4	19	0	173
Beets, fresh slices, ck	½ c	85	27	1.0	0	6	12	20	37	177
Beets, cnd, low Na	½ c	123	40	1.1	0	10	17	21	56	206
Carrots, fresh, sliced, ck	½ c	73	23	0.7	0	5	24	23	24	162
Cauliflower, raw	½ c	50	14	1.4	0	3	13	28	7	148
Cauliflower, froz, ck	½ c	90	16	1.7	0	3	16	34	9	187
Celery, raw, diced	½ c	60	10	0.6	0	2	24	17	76	205
Celery, diced, ck	½ c	75	11	0.6	0	2	2	17	66	180
Eggplant, diced, ck	½ c	100	19	1.0	0	4	11	21	1	150
Leeks, raw	2–5″ long	50	26	1.1	0	5	26	25	2	173
Mushrooms, raw, sliced	½ c (3–4 small)	35	10	1.0	0	2	2	4	5	145
Mushrooms, cnd, low Na	½ c	100	23	2.0	0	3	8	90	2	196
Mustard greens, leaves, ck drained	½ c	70	16	1.5	0	3	96	23	13	154
Okra, fresh, ck, sliced	½ c	80	23	1.6	0	5	78	33	2	139
Parsnips, diced, ck	⅓ c	52	34	0.8	0	8	24	32	4	192
Peppers, sweet green, raw 2¾″ × 2½″	1 whole	90	16	0.9	0	4	7	16	10	157
Radishes, raw	10 med	50	8	0.5	0	2	14	14	8	145
Rutabagas, sliced, ck	½ c	85	30	0.8	0	7	50	26	4	142
Squash, summer, cubes, ck	½ c	105	14	0.9	0	3	26	26	1	148
Squash, winter, boiled, mashed	⅓ c	82	31	0.9	0	7	16	26	1	211
Turnips, cubed, ck	½ c	78	18	0.6	0	4	27	18	27	145
True Averages			20	1.0					17	168

Table K-5. Vegetable List 3

Averages–Calories: 30   Protein: 1.0 g   Sodium: 15 mg   Potassium: 250 mg

Food Item	Measure	Weight g	Kcal	Pro g	Fat g	Cho g	Ca mg	P mg	Na mg	K mg
Avocado, raw (¼ small)	¼ c	38	63	0.8	6	2	4	16	2	227
Beet greens, ck	½ c	73	13	1.2	0	2	72	18	55	240
Carrot, raw	7″ long	81	30	0.8	0	7	27	26	34	246
Chard, fresh, ck, leaves & stalks	1½ c	73	13	1.3	0	2	53	18	63	233
Potato, pared, diced, or sliced	½ c	78	50	1.5	0	12	5	33	2	221
Pumpkin, boiled	scant ½ c	100	33	1.0	0	8	25	26	2	240
Squash, winter, baked	¼ c	51	32	0.9	0	8	14	24	1	236
Tomato, ck	⅓ c	80	21	1.0	0	4	12	26	3	231
Tomato, raw, unpeeled	1 small	100	20	1.0	0	4	12	25	3	222
Tomato, cnd, low Na	½ c	120	24	1.2	0	5	7	23	3	262
Tomato catsup, low Na	2 T	30	15	0.6	0	4	13	18	2	270
Tomato chili sauce, low Na	2 T	30	20	1.0	0	3	9	27	2	300
True Averages			28	1.0					14	244

Table K-6. Vegetable List 4

Averages–Calories: 50		Protein: 2.5 g		Sodium: 20 mg			Potassium: 200, but varies widely			
Food Item	*Measure*	*Weight g*	*Kcal*	*Pro g*	*Fat g*	*Cho g*	*Ca mg*	*P mg*	*Na mg*	*K mg*
Artichoke, ck	1 med bud	250	(25)[a]	2.8	0	10	51	69	30	301
Broccoli, fresh, ck stalk cut ½″	½ c	78	20	2.4	0	4	78	48	8	207
Broccoli, froz, chopped, ck	½ c	93	24	2.7	0	4	50	52	14	196
Brussels sprouts, fresh, ck	3 sprouts	63	22	2.6	0	3	20	45	6	172
Collard greens, ck leaves and stems	½ c	73	21	2.0	0	4	110	28	18	170
Collard greens, froz, chopped	½ c	85	26	2.5	0	5	150	43	14	202
Corn, fresh, cut off cob	½ c	83	68	2.7	1	16	3	74	0	136
Corn, froz, on cob	½ ear	114	59	2.2	1	13	2	60	0	145
Corn, cnd, low Na whole kernel	½ c	128	73	2.5	1	17	5	62	3	124
Peas, cnd, low Na	⅓ c	83	46	3.0	0	8	13	55	2	80
Peas, froz, ck	⅓ c	53	36	2.7	0	6	10	46	61	72
Peas and carrots, froz, ck	½ c	80	42	2.6	0	8	20	46	67	126
Potato, raw or baked	1–2 ¼″ diam	100	73	2.0	0	16	7	51	3	391
Spinach leaves, fresh, ck	½ c	90	21	2.7	0	3	83	34	45	292
Spinach, froz, chopped, ck	½ c	102	23	3.1	0	4	116	45	53	341
Sweet potato, baked in skin	5″ × 2″	146	161	2.4	1	37	46	66	14	342
Sweet potato, mashed	½ c	127	145	2.2	1	34	41	60	13	310
Turnip greens, froz, ck	½ c	82	19	2.1	0	3	97	32	14	123
Vegetable, mixed, froz	½ c	91	58	2.9	0	12	23	58	48	174
	True Averages		51	2.5					22	205

[a]Calories depend on storage period; vary from 8–44.

Table K-7. Fruit List 1

Averages–Calories: 60		Protein: 0.5 g		Sodium: 5 mg			Potassium: 100 mg			
Food Item	*Measure*	*Weight g*	*Kcal*	*Pro g*	*Fat g*	*Cho g*	*Ca mg*	*P mg*	*Na mg*	*K mg*
Sweetened with sugar or syrup										
Applesauce, cnd	½ c	128	116	0.2	0	30	5	6	2	83
Blueberries, frozen	¾ c	172	182	1.0	0	46	10	19	2	114
Boysenberries, frozen	½ c	72	68	0.6	0	17	12	12	1	75
Figs, cnd	2 small	80	68	0.4	0	18	10	10	2	120
Grape juice, frozen (diluted 1:3)	1 c	250	133	0.5	0	33	8	10	3	85
Grape drink, cnd	1 c	250	135	0.3	0	34	8	10	3	88
Orange/apricot juice drink, cnd	½ c	124	62	0.4	0	16	6	10	1	117
Pear halves, cnd	2 sm halves	96	72	0.2	0	19	4	6	1	80
Pear nectar, cnd	1 c	250	130	0.8	0	33	8	13	3	98
Pineapple chunks, cnd	½ c	128	94	0.4	0	25	14	6	2	122
Pineapple slices, cnd	1 lg or 2 sm slices	105	78	0.3	0	20	12	5	1	101
Pineapple chunks, frozen	½ c	122	104	0.5	0	27	11	5	3	122
Pineapple/grapefruit juice drink, cnd	½ c	125	68	0.2	0	17	6	6	1	78
Pineapple/orange juice drink, cnd	½ c	125	68	0.2	0	17	6	8	1	88
Raspberries, red, frozen	½ c	125	122	0.9	0	31	16	22	2	125

(continued)

Table K-7.   *(Continued)*

Averages–Calories: 60			Protein: 0.5 g			Sodium: 5 mg			Potassium: 100 mg	

Food Item	Measure	Weight g	Kcal	Pro g	Fat g	Cho g	Ca mg	P mg	Na mg	K mg
Unsweetened (No sugar added or packed in water)										
Apple, fresh	1 sm, 2½" diam	115	61	0.2	0	15	7	11	1	116
Apple juice, cnd	½ c	124	58	0.1	0	15	8	11	1	125
Applesauce, cnd	½ c	122	50	0.2	0	13	5	6	2	95
Blackberries, fresh	½ c	72	42	0.8	0	9	23	14	1	122
Blueberries, fresh	¾ c	109	68	0.8	0	16	16	14	1	88
Blueberries, frozen	¾ c	124	68	0.9	0	17	13	16	2	100
Boysenberries, fresh	½ c	72	42	0.8	0	9	23	14	1	122
Boysenberries, cnd	½ c	122	44	0.8	0	11	23	23	1	104
Boysenberries, frozen	½ c	63	30	0.8	0	7	16	15	1	96
Cherries, sweet, fresh	8 lg	60	38	0.9	0	9	12	10	1	104
Cherries, sour, fresh	8 lg	57	30	0.6	0	7	12	10	1	98
Coconut, fresh	1 pc, 2" × 2" × ½"	45	156	1.6	16	4	6	43	10	115
Coconut, fresh, grated	½ c	40	138	1.4	14	4	5	38	9	102
Cranberries, fresh	1 c	95	44	0.4	0	10	13	10	2	78
Figs, fresh	1 med (2" diam)	50	40	0.6	0	10	18	11	1	97
Figs, cnd	2 small	76	36	0.4	0	9	11	11	2	117
Granadilla, fresh (Passion fruit)	1 whole	35	16	0.4	0	4	2	12	5	63
Lemon, fresh, peeled	1 med, 2" diam	110	20	0.8	0	6	19	12	1	102
Lime, fresh, peeled	1 med, 2" diam	80	19	0.5	0	6	22	12	1	69
Loganberries, fresh	½ c	72	44	0.7	0	11	25	12	1	122
Loquats, fresh	2 whole	32	12	0.1	0	3	5	9	1	86
Lychees, fresh	6 whole	90	35	0.5	0	9	4	23	2	92
Orange, fresh	½ sm, (2½" diam)	66	25	0.6	0	6	20	11	1	94
Pear, Bartlett, fresh	½ lg (2½" diam)	90	50	0.6	0	13	6	9	2	106
Pear, D'Anjou, fresh	½ lg (3" diam)	110	61	0.7	0	16	8	11	2	130
Pear halves, cnd	2 small	90	28	0.2	0	7	4	6	1	80
Persimmon, native, fresh	1 small	30	31	0.2	0	8	7	6	1	76
Pineapple, fresh, diced	½ c	78	40	0.3	0	11	13	6	1	113
Pineapple chunks, cnd	½ c	123	48	0.4	0	13	15	6	1	122
Plums, Japanese, fresh	1 med (2" diam)	70	32	0.3	0	8	8	12	1	112
Prunes, dried	2 med	15	33	0.3	0	9	7	10	1	90
Raspberries, red, fresh	½ c	62	35	0.8	0	8	14	14	1	104
Strawberries, fresh	6 lg	60	22	0.4	0	5	12	12	1	98
Tangerine, fresh	1 med (2½" diam)	116	39	0.7	0	10	34	15	2	108
Watermelon, fresh	½ c	80	21	0.4	0	5	6	8	1	80
	True Averages		61 (unsw– 45) (sw–100)	0.5					2	100

Table K-8. Fruit List 2

Averages–Calories: 65		Protein: 0.6 g		Sodium: 5 mg				Potassium: 175 mg		
Food Item	Measure	Weight g	Kcal	Pro g	Fat g	Cho g	Ca mg	P mg	Na mg	K mg
Sweetened with sugar or syrup										
Apricot nectar, cnd	½ c	126	72	0.4	0	18	12	15	1	190
Blackberries, cnd	½ c	128	116	1.0	0	28	27	16	2	140
Cherries, sweet, cnd	½ c	140	104	1.2	0	26	20	16	2	162
Figs, cnd	4 small	113	95	0.5	0	25	15	15	3	169
Fruit cocktail, cnd	½ c	128	97	0.5	0	25	12	16	6	206
Fruit salad, cnd	½ c	128	96	0.4	0	25	10	14	2	171
Grapefruit sections, cnd	½ c	127	89	0.8	0	23	16	18	2	172
Grapefruit juice, cnd	½ c	125	66	0.6	0	16	10	18	1	202
Grapes, cnd, seedless	½ c	128	98	0.6	0	26	10	16	5	134
Peach halves, cnd	2 med halves	162	126	0.6	0	33	6	20	4	210
Peach slices, frozen	½ c	125	110	0.5	0	28	5	16	2	155
Peach nectar, cnd	1 c	248	120	0.5	0	31	10	27	2	194
Plums, purple, cnd	3 lg	140	110	0.5	0	29	12	13	1	189
Strawberries, froz slices	½ c	128	139	0.6	0	35	18	22	2	143
Unsweetened (No sugar added or packed in water)										
Apricots, fresh	2 med	76	37	0.7	0	9	12	7	1	201
Banana, fresh	3" pc	75	44	0.6	0	11	4	14	1	188
Blackberries, cnd	½ c	122	49	1.0	0	11	27	16	1	140
Blackberry juice, cnd	½ c	122	46	0.4	0	10	14	14	1	208
Cherries, sour, cnd	½ c	122	52	1.0	0	13	18	16	2	158
Cherries, sweet, cnd	½ c	135	60	1.1	0	15	18	16	1	162
Coconut water	½ c	120	26	0.4	0	6	24	16	30	176
Dates	4 med	32	88	0.8	0	24	18	20	2	208
Figs, fresh	2 med (2" diam)	100	80	1.2	0	20	36	22	2	194
Figs, cnd	4 small	107	51	0.5	0	13	15	15	3	165
Fruit cocktail, cnd	½ c	122	46	0.5	0	12	11	16	6	206
Fruit salad, cnd	½ c	122	43	0.5	0	11	10	14	1	170
Grapefruit, fresh	½ med 4" diam	268	55	0.7	0	14	22	22	1	185
Grapefruit sections, cnd	½ c	122	36	0.8	0	9	16	17	5	176
Grapefruit juice, fresh	½ c	123	52	0.5	0	14	11	18	1	200
Grapefruit juice, cnd	½ c	124	50	0.6	0	12	10	18	1	200
Grapefruit juice, frozen (diluted 1:3)	½ c	124	50	0.6	0	12	12	21	1	210
Grapes, seedless, fresh	16 or ½ c	80	54	0.5	0	14	10	16	2	138
Grapes, seeded, fresh	16 or ½ c	80	52	0.4	0	13	9	15	2	132
Grapes, seedless, cnd	½ c	122	62	0.6	0	17	10	16	5	135
Grape juice, cnd	½ c	126	84	0.2	0	21	14	15	2	146
Kumquats, fresh	4 med	80	48	0.8	0	13	48	16	4	176
Lemon juice, fresh or cnd	½ c	122	30	0.6	0	10	8	12	1	172
Lime juice, fresh or cnd	¾ c	184	48	0.5	0	16	16	20	2	192
Nectarine, fresh	½ med, 2½" diam	75	44	0.4	0	12	3	16	4	203
Orange sections, fresh	½ c	82	42	1.0	0	10	33	18	1	160
Peach, fresh	1 med (2½" diam)	115	38	0.6	0	10	9	19	1	202
Peach halves, cnd	2 med halves	154	48	0.6	0	12	6	20	4	210
Persimmon, Japanese, fresh	½ med, 2½" diam	100	64	0.6	0	17	5	22	5	146
Pineapple juice, cnd	½ c	125	69	0.5	0	17	19	12	2	186
Pineapple juice, frozen (Diluted 1:3)	½ c	125	65	0.5	0	16	14	10	2	170
Plums, Damson, fresh	6, 1" diam	66	40	0.3	0	11	11	10	1	179
Plums, prune type, fresh	3, 1½" diam	90	63	0.6	0	17	9	15	1	144

(continued)

Table K-8.   *(Continued)*

Averages–Calories: 65			Protein: 0.6 g				Sodium: 5 mg			Potassium: 175 mg
Food Item	*Measure*	*Weight* g	*Kcal*	*Pro* g	*Fat* g	*Cho* g	*Ca* mg	*P* mg	*Na* mg	*K* mg
Plums, purple, cnd	3 med	100	44	0.4	0	11	9	10	2	141
Pomegranate, fresh	½, 3½″ diam	138	48	0.4	0	13	2	6	2	200
Prune juice, cnd	⅓ c	85	66	0.3	0	16	12	17	2	201
Raisins, dried	2 T	18	52	0.4	0	14	12	18	4	138
Raspberries, red, cnd	½ c	122	42	0.8	0	10	18	18	1	138
Strawberries, cnd	½ c	121	26	0.5	0	7	17	17	1	134
	True Averages		65	0.6					3	174
			(unsw– 50)							
			(sw–100)							

Table K-9.   Fruit List 3

Averages–Calories: 70			Protein: 0.7 g				Sodium: 5 mg			Potassium: 250 mg
Food Item	*Measure*	*Weight* g	*Kcal*	*Pro* g	*Fat* g	*Cho* g	*Ca* mg	*P* mg	*Na* mg	*K* mg
Sweetened with sugar or syrup										
Apricot halves, cnd	4 med halves	110	95	0.7	0	24	12	16	1	258
Apricots, froz	½ c	114	111	0.8	0	28	11	22	4	260
Melon balls, froz (cantaloupe & honeydew)	½ c	115	72	0.7	0	18	12	14	10	216
Orange juice, cnd	½ c	125	65	0.9	0	15	12	22	1	248
Rhubarb, ck	½ c	135	190	0.7	0	49	106	20	2	274
Tangerine juice, cnd	½ c	125	63	0.6	0	15	22	18	1	220
Unsweetened (No sugar added or packed in water)										
Apple, fresh	1 lg (3½″ diam)	230	123	0.4	0	31	15	21	2	233
Apple juice, cnd	1 c	248	117	0.2	0	30	15	22	2	250
Apricot halves, cnd	4 med halves	100	38	0.7	0	10	12	16	1	248
Banana, fresh	5″ piece	100	58	0.8	0	15	6	18	1	252
Guava, fresh	1 med	100	62	0.8	0	15	23	42	4	289
Mango, fresh	½ lg	150	76	0.8	0	19	12	15	8	218
Melons:										
Cantaloupe, fresh	1/6–5″ diam	177	26	0.6	0	7	12	14	11	222
Cantaloupe, fresh	12 melon balls	100	30	0.7	0	8	14	16	12	251
Honeydew, fresh	1/12–6 ½″ diam	198	41	1.0	0	10	18	20	15	314
Honeydew, fresh	12 melon balls	100	33	0.8	0	8	14	16	12	251
Orange juice, fresh	½ c	124	56	0.8	0	13	14	21	1	248
Orange juice, cnd	½ c	124	60	1.0	0	14	12	22	1	248
Orange juice, froz (Diluted 1:3)	½ c	124	61	0.8	0	14	12	21	1	252
Papaya, fresh	⅓ med (3½″ diam)	151	40	0.6	0	10	20	16	3	237
Plaintain, fresh	3″ piece	91	78	0.7	0	20	4	20	3	253
Tangerine juice, fresh or cnd	½ c	124	53	0.6	0	12	22	18	1	220
	True Averages		70	0.7					4	248
			(unsw– 60)							
			(sw–100)							

Table K-10. Regular Bread, Cereal, and Starch List

Averages–Calories: 90   Protein: 2.0 g   Sodium: 200 mg   Potassium: 30 mg

Food Item	Measure	Weight g	Kcal	Pro g	Fat g	Cho g	Ca mg	P mg	Na mg	K mg
Breads and crackers										
Animal crackers, plain	10 crackers	26	112	1.7	2	21	14	30	79	25
Baking powder biscuit	avg 1–2″ diam	28	97	2.0	4	14	26	57	224	32
Bread crumbs, dry	3 T	19	74	2.4	1	14	23	26	138	28
Cracked-wheat bread	1 slice	25	66	2.2	1	13	22	32	132	34
Doughnut, cake type, plain	1 small	42	164	1.9	8	22	17	80	210	38
Doughnut, yeast raised	1 small	42	176	2.7	11	16	16	32	99	34
French, Italian, or Vienna bread	1 slice	20	58	1.8	0	11	7	17	117	17
Graham cracker, plain	2 squares	14	55	1.1	1	10	6	21	95	55
Hamburger or hot dog bun, enriched, plain	½ lg	30	89	2.5	2	16	22	26	152	28
Kaiser roll	½ lg	30	94	2.9	1	18	14	28	188	29
Melba toast	4 slices	15	70	1.9	0	12	12	32	140	40
Muffin, plain	1 small	30	86	2.3	1	13	32	45	132	38
Pancakes, homemade	1–4″ diam	27	62	1.9	2	9	27	38	115	33
Pancake from mix	1–4″ diam	27	61	1.9	2	9	58	70	152	42
Parkerhouse roll	2″ roll	28	75	2.1	1	13	9	21	127	23
Rye bread, American	1 slice	25	61	2.3	0	13	19	37	139	36
Sugar wafers	5 wafers	48	230	2.3	9	35	17	38	90	28
Vanilla wafers	10 wafers	40	185	2.2	6	30	16	25	101	29
White bread, enriched	1 slice	25	68	2.2	1	13	21	24	127	26
Zinger, plain, Dolly Madison	1	40	123	1.3	4	26	19	67	132	52
Cooked Cereals (cooked with salt as directed on package):										
Cornmeal, ck	½ c	120	60	1.3	0	13	1	17	132	19
Cream of Rice, ck	½ c	122	62	1.0	0	14	2	16	216	15
Farina (Cream of Wheat) ck	½ c	122	52	1.6	0	11	5	14	176	11
Hominy grits, ck	½ c	122	62	1.4	0	14	1	12	251	14
Malt-O-Meal, ck	½ c	120	67	2.1	0	14	4	34	198	11
Oatmeal, ck	½ c	120	66	2.4	1	12	11	68	262	73
Dry cereals										
Cheerios	½ c	12	52	1.7	1	9	21	50	138	42
Cocoa Krispies	1 c	28	111	1.3	1	25	8	20	189	25
Corn Chex	¾ c	20	78	1.3	0	17	1	8	197	22
Cornflakes	1 c	21	80	1.5	0	18	1	7	209	18
Frosted Flakes	¾ c	28	109	1.4	0	25	1	6	189	19
Honeycomb	1 c	28	110	1.0	0	25	—	—	234	40
Kix	1 c	25	99	2.0	1	20	2	11	275	29
Product 19	¾ c	21	78	1.8	0	17	56	45	218	17
Quisp	1 c	28	122	1.3	3	23	10	27	215	35
Rice Chex	1 c	25	98	1.3	0	22	4	24	211	28
Rice Krispies	¾ c	21	81	1.3	0	18	2	17	197	20
Wheaties	½ c	14	52	1.4	0	11	6	39	196	55
Starches (Cooked with salt as directed on package)										
Self-rising flour, unsifted	2 T	16	51	1.3	0	11	38	67	155	(14)
Macaroni, enriched, ck	⅓ c	47	52	1.6	0	11	4	23	(288)	28
Noodles, enriched, ck	⅓ c	53	67	2.2	1	12	5	31	(289)	23
Popcorn, popped with oil and salt	1 c	9–15	55	0.9	4	5	1	19	175	(36)
Rice, white, ck	½ c	102	112	2.0	0	25	10	28	383	28
Rice, instant, ck	½ c	82	90	1.8	0	10	2	16	225	tr
Spaghetti, enriched, ck	⅓ c	47	52	1.6	0	11	4	23	(216)	28
	True Averages		87	1.8					180	29

Table K-11.   Low-Sodium Bread, Cereal, and Starch List

Average–Calories: 65			Protein: 2.0 g				Sodium: 5 mg			Potassium: 30 mg	
Food Item	Measure	Weight g	Kcal	Pro g	Fat g	Cho g	Ca mg	P mg	Na mg	K mg
Breads and crackers (Low-protein breads are listed in the free list)										
Low-Sod crackers, Cellu	4 sm	20	60	1.2	2	10	4	19	2	40
Low-Sod melba toast, Cellu	4 slices	20	61	2.1	0	12	7	35	3	44
Low-Sod rice wafers, Cellu	4 wafers	20	37	1.0	0	8	1	22	2	24
Low-Sod white bread, avg	1 slice	25	63	2.2	1	11	—	—	6	(30)
Regular corn tortilla	1–6″ diam	30	63	1.5	1	14	60	42	(1)	(36)
Regular matzo cracker	1–6″ diam	20	78	2.1	0	17	—	—	(1)	(24)
Venus Wheat wafers	4 sm	30	72	2.0	2	12	—	—	4	—
Cooked cereals										
Cornmeal, ck	½ c	120	60	1.3	0	13	1	17	1	19
Cream of Rice, ck	½ c	122	62	1.0	0	14	2	16	1	15
Farina (Cream of Wheat) ck	½ c	122	52	1.6	0	11	5	14	1	11
Hominy grits, ck	½ c	122	62	1.4	0	14	1	12	1	14
Malt-O-Meal, ck	½ c	120	67	2.1	0	14	4	34	1	11
Oatmeal, ck	½ c	120	66	2.4	1	12	11	68	2	73
Dry cereals										
Frosted Mini Wheats	3 biscuits	21	81	1.9	0	17	6	38	3	(45)
Puffed Rice	1 c	15	60	0.9	0	13	3	14	1	15
Puffed Wheat	1 c	15	54	2.3	0	12	4	48	1	51
Shredded Wheat, miniatures	⅓ c	16	59	1.6	0	13	7	65	1	58
Low-Sod Cornflakes, VanBrode	1 c	28	109	1.7	0	25	1	—	2	31
Low-Sod Crisp Rice, VanBrode	1 c	28	109	1.6	0	26	7	—	2	26
Starches										
All-purpose flour, unsifted	2 T	17	62	1.8	0	13	4	15	1	16
Macaroni, enriched, ck	⅓ c	47	52	1.6	0	11	4	23	1	28
Noodles, enriched, ck	⅓ c	53	67	2.2	1	12	5	31	2	23
Popcorn, plain, popped with oil, no salt	1 c	6–12	55	0.9	4	5	(1)	(17)	1	(36)
Rice, white, ck	½ c	102	112	2.0	0	25	10	28	1	28
Spaghetti, enriched, ck	⅓ c	47	52	1.6	0	11	4	23	1	28
	True Averages		65	1.6					2	30

Table K-12. Low-Sodium Meat List (cooked without salt)

Averages–Calories: 60				Protein: 8.0 g			Sodium: 30 mg		Potassium: 100 mg	
Food Item	Measure	Weight g	Kcal	Pro g	Fat g	Cho g	Ca mg	P mg	Na mg	K mg
Beef	1 oz	28	67	8.2	3	0	4	61	16	84
Cheese										
Low-Sod Cheddar, Cellu	1 oz	28	110	7.0	9	0	120	—	10	150
Low-Sod Colby, Cellu	1 oz	28	110	7.0	9	0	120	—	5	150
Low-Sod Cottage	¼ c	60	50	7.0	1	2	22	—	22	83
Chicken, without skin	1 oz	28	51	8.7	2	0	4	72	21	107
Duck	1 oz	28	87	6.4	7	0	5	64	23	80
Egg, Chicken, raw	1 whole	50	79	6.1	6	tr	28	90	69	65
Goose, without skin	1 oz	28	66	9.6	3	0	(4)	(115)	35	171
Lamb	1 oz	28	56	7.9	2	0	4	65	20	88
Organ Meats										
Beef heart	1 oz	28	53	8.9	2	tr	2	51	29	66
Beef liver	1 oz	28	64	7.4	3	2	3	133	51	106
Beef tongue	1 oz	30	74	6.4	5	tr	2	34	18	50
Beef tripe	1 oz	28	28	5.3	1	0	36	24	20	2
Calf liver	1 oz	28	74	8.4	4	1	4	152	33	128
Chicken gizzard	¼ c	36	54	9.8	1	tr	3	26	21	77
Chicken liver	1 liver	25	41	6.6	1	1	3	40	15	38
Turkey gizzard	¼ c	36	71	9.8	3	tr	—	—	18	54
Pork, fresh	1 oz	28	64	8.2	4	0	4	80	20	88
Rabbit	1 oz	28	62	8.3	3	0	6	74	12	105
Seafood (fresh or unsalted waterpacked)										
Catfish, freshwater	1 oz	28	29	4.9	1	0	—	—	17	92
Cod	1 oz	28	48	8.1	2	0	9	78	31	115
Halibut	1 oz	28	48	7.1	2	0	5	70	38	149
Flatfish (such as sole)	1 oz	28	22	4.7	0	0	3	55	22	96
Flounder	1 oz	28	57	8.5	2	0	7	98	67	166
Perch, Atlantic	1 oz	28	64	5.4	4	2	9	64	43	81
Red Snapper	1 oz	28	26	5.5	0	tr	4	60	19	90
Salmon, Fresh	1 oz	28	52	7.7	2	0	—	117	33	126
Salmon, cnd, Low-Sod	1 oz	28	44	6.4	2	0	69	96	20	99
Tuna, cnd, Low-Sod	¼ c	40	51	11.2	tr	0	6	76	16	112
Shellfish										
Clams	¼ c or 4–5 sm	57	43	7.2	1	1	39	92	68	103
Oysters	⅓ c or 3–4 sm	80	63	7.6	2	4	72	118	58	97
Shrimp	1 oz	28	64	5.8	3	3	20	54	53	104
Turkey, without skin	1 oz	28	54	8.9	2	0	2	71	37	104
Veal	1 oz	28	68	7.7	4	0	3	61	18	80
	True Averages		59	7.5					29	96

Table K-13.   High-Sodium Meat List

Averages–Calories: 90				Protein: 8.0 g		Sodium: 200 mg			Potassium: 75 mg	

Food Item	Measure	Weight g	Kcal	Pro g	Fat g	Cho g	Ca mg	P mg	Na mg	K mg
Bacon, cured, ck	5 slices	25	152	7.2	12	1	2	55	255	60
Beef, Kidney, ck	¼ c	35	88	11.6	4	tr	6	85	89	114
Cheese, natural										
Blue	1 oz	28	100	6.1	8	1	150	110	396	73
Cheddar	1 oz	28	114	7.1	9	tr	204	145	176	28
Cottage, creamed	2 oz (¼ c)	56	58	7.1	2	2	34	74	228	48
Cottage, low fat, 2%	2 oz (¼ c)	56	51	7.8	1	2	38	85	230	54
Edam	1 oz	28	101	7.1	8	tr	207	152	274	53
Gruyere	1 oz	28	117	8.4	9	tr	287	172	95	23
Monterey	1 oz	28	106	6.9	9	tr	212	126	152	23
Mozzarella	1 oz	28	80	5.5	6	1	147	107	106	19
Parmesan, grated	3 T	15	69	6.2	4	1	207	120	279	15
Provolone	1 oz	28	100	7.2	1	8	214	141	248	39
Swiss	1 oz	28	107	8.1	8	1	272	171	74	31
Corned Beef, cnd	1 oz	28	60	7.1	3	0	6	30	208	17
Custard, baked	½ c	132	152	7.2	7	15	148	155	104	194
Egg substitute, frozen (made from egg white, corn oil, and nonfat dry milk)	¼ c	60	96	6.8	7	2	44	43	120	128
Pork, cured	1 oz	28	59	7.0	3	0	3	56	273	85
Seafood										
Lobster, Northern, fresh	¼ c	36	35	6.8	1	tr	24	69	76	65
Salmon, cnd, drain	¼ c	55	85	11.3	4	0	128	168	231	191
Sardines, 8/can drain	1 oz or 2 med	28	58	6.8	3	—	124	141	233	167
Tuna, cnd, drain	¼ c	40	79	11.5	3	0	3	94	248	79
	True Averages		89	7.6					195	72

Table K-14.   "Protein-Free" List

Food Item	Measure	Weight g	Kcal	Pro g	Fat g	Cho g	Ca mg	P mg	Na mg	K mg
Fats—unsalted										
Butter, unsalted	1 T	14	102	0.1	12	tr	3	2	1	3
Low-Sod French Dressing, Cellu	1 T	14	60	0	6	1	1	tr	6	10
Lard, regular	1 T	14	117	0	13	0	0	0	0	0
Margarine, unsalted	1 T	14	100	0.1	(11)	0	(3)	(2)	1	3
Vegetable oil	1 T	14	120	0	14	0	0	0	0	0
Whipping cream, heavy unwhipped	1 T	15	52	0.3	6	0	10	9	6	11
Low-protein products										
Arrowroot	1 T	8	29	0	0	7	(0)	(0)	tr	1
Cornstarch	¼ c	32	116	0.1	tr	28	0	0	tr	tr
Wheatstarch cookie, average	1 cookie	30	(113)	0.1	—	—	—	—	(5)	(3)
Low-protein bread, average	1 slice	30	112	0.2	(5)	(18)	—	—	10	6
Aproten low-protein products										
Semolino, hot cereal	½ c, ck	100	68	0.1	—	17	—	—	4	2
Annellini and Tagliatelle imitation pasta	½ c, ck	115	105	0.2	0	25	—	—	9	2
Rigatini imitation pasta	½ c, ck	65	59	0.1	—	14	—	—	5	1
Rusks	1 slice	12	50	0.1	—	10	1	6	4	5
Nondairy products										
Coffee-Mate	1 T	2	11	tr	1	1	0	6	4	14
Dessert topping, froz	¼ c	19	60	0.2	5	4	1	2	5	4
Dessert topping, powdered	¼ c prepared	20	32	0.2	2	3	tr	4	8	8
Dessert topping, pressurized	¼ c	18	46	0.2	4	3	1	3	11	3
D'Zerta whipped topping	1 T	15	8	0	1	0	—	—	(2)	(0)

(continued)

Table K-14. *(Continued)*

Food Item	Measure	Weight g	Kcal	Pro g	Fat g	Cho g	Ca mg	P mg	Na mg	K mg
Spices and seasonings										
All dry spices & herbs	Avg serving	—	—	—	—	—	—	—	2	2–50
Diazest, Milani (low-sod beef flavoring)	4 drops	—	0	0	0	0	—	—	1	1
Garlic, fresh	1 clove	2	4	0.2	0	1	1	6	1	16
Liquid Smoke, Wrights	1 t	5	tr	tr	—	—	—	—	tr	tr
Tabasco sauce	½ t	3	tr	tr	—	—	—	—	11	2
Vinegar, distilled	½ c	120	—	—	—	6	—	—	1	18
Sweets										
Cranberry sauce	¼ c	60	101	0.1	0	26	4	3	1	21
Danish dessert	½ c	120	106	0.2	0	26	2	0	11	2
Gum drops	3 lge	30	98	tr	0	25	2	tr	10	1
Hard candy	1 oz	30	109	0	0	28	6	2	9	1
Honey	1 T	20	64	0.1	0	17	1	1	1	11
Jam or preserves, ass't	1 T	20	54	0.1	tr	14	4	2	2	18
Jelly, assorted	1 T	20	49	tr	tr	13	4	1	3	14
Jelly beans	10 beans	30	104	tr	0	26	3	1	3	tr
Sugar, granulated, white	1 T	12	46	0	0	12	0	0	tr	tr
Sugar, powdered, white	1 T	8	31	0	0	8	0	0	tr	tr

Note: The foods in the free list can be added to your basic diet as desired unless the amount allowed is specified.

Table K-15. Miscellaneous List

Food Item	Measure	Weight g	Kcal	Pro g	Fat g	Cho g	Ca mg	P mg	Na mg	K mg
Alcoholic beverages (Use only if approved by physician)										
Beer, average	8 oz	240	101	0.7	0	9	12	72	17	60
Brandy, gin, vodka, rum, whiskey (80 proof)	3 oz	90	194	—	—	tr	—	—	tr	3
Wine, sweet, dessert	4 oz	120	164	tr	0	9	8	—	4	92
Wine, sherry	4 oz	120	164	0.2	0	9	10	—	4	88
Wine, table, average	4 oz	120	100	0.4	0	5	12	12	4	108
Beverages—carbonated										
Bubble Up	8 oz	240	90	0	—	(22)	—	—	33	9
Coca Cola	8 oz	240	110	0	—	(28)	—	—	30	2
Gingerale	8 oz	240	85	0	—	(21)	—	—	22	9
Hires Root Beer	8 oz	240	100	0	—	(25)	—	—	41	3
Pepsi Cola	8 oz	240	110	0	—	(28)	—	—	28	9
Royal Crown Cola	8 oz	240	110	0	—	(28)	—	—	22	4
Simba	8 oz	240	90	0	—	(22)	—	—	40	2
Shasta, club soda	8 oz	240	0	0	0	0	—	—	131	4
Shasta, sugar free, average	8 oz	240	1	0	0	tr	—	—	51	4
Shasta, regular, average	8 oz	240	110	0	0	(27)	—	—	25	4
Shasta, mixes	8 oz	240	85	0	0	(21)	—	—	25	4
Tab, sugar free	8 oz	240	1	0		tr	—	—	33	9
Beverages—Coffee, Tea, Bouillon										
Coffee, regular instant	1 level t	0.8	1	tr	tr	tr	1	3	1	26
Coffee, freeze dried inst	1 level t	0.9	1	tr	tr	tr	2	3	1	29
Coffee, instant, prepared from 2 g powder	6 oz	180	2	tr	tr	tr	4	7	2	65
Coffee, brewed, weak	6 oz	180	(2)	(tr)	(tr)	(tr)	(2)	(3)	(1)	(112)
Postum	6 oz	180	36	0.6	tr	8	(10)	(87)	4	136
Tea	8 oz	240	2	0.1	0	0	5	4	5	60–130
Bouillon, salted	1 cube	4	5	0.8	tr	tr	—	—	960	4
Bouillon, salted powder	1 level t	2	2	0.4	tr	tr	—	—	480	2
Beverages—Fruit Drinks										
Awake (imitation orange juice)	4 oz	124	51	tr	—	(13)	—	—	5	41
Cranberry juice cocktail	8 oz	240	164	0.3	0	42	13	8	3	25
Grape Tang	8 oz	240	120	0	0	28	—	—	110	2
Kool Aid, regular	8 oz	240	100	0	0	25	—	—	1	1
Kool Aid, presweetened	8 oz	240	90	0	0	23	—	—	1	1
Lemon Tang	8 oz	240	100	0	0	26	—	—	30	2
Lemonade, frozen diluted	8 oz	240	107	0.1	tr	28	2	3	1	40

(continued)

Table K-15. *(Continued)*

Food Item	Measure	Weight g	Kcal	Pro g	Fat g	Cho g	Ca mg	P mg	Na mg	K mg
Limeade, frozen diluted	8 oz	240	102	0.1	tr	27	3	3	tr	32
Orange Tang	8 oz	240	100	0	0	26	—	—	<20	42
Start Inst. Bkfst. drink	8 oz	240	100	0	0	26	—	—	(47)	(47)
Tart Orange Tang	8 oz	240	120	0	0	26	—	—	45	tr
Fats—Salted										
Butter, salted	1 T	15	108	0.1	12	tr	3	3	123	3
Bacon, fried crisp	1 slice	8	43	1.9	4	0	1	17	77	18
Cream cheese	2 T	28	99	2.1	10	1	23	30	84	34
French dressing	1 T	14	66	0.1	6	3	2	2	219	13
Margarine, salted	1 T	14	102	0.1	12	0	3	2	140	3
Mayonnaise, regular	1 T	14	101	0.2	12	0	3	4	84	5
Mayonnaise, imitation	1 T	14	40	0	4	1	—	—	95	—
Miracle Whip	1 T	14	70	0	7	2	—	—	90	—
Peanut Butter, regular	1 T	16	94	4.0	8	3	9	61	97	100
Fats—Unsalted										
Low Sod mayonnaise, Cellu	1 T	14	100	0	11	0	2	6	6	26
Peanut Butter, Low Sod Cellu	1 T	15	90	4.0	7.5	2	8	55	1	(87)
Sour cream	2 T	24	52	0.8	5	1	28	20	34	12
Low-protein products										
Low-Protein baking mix, Paygel	¾ c	100	410	0.3	8	83	5	48	55	10
Low-Protein Gelled Dessert, Prono	½ c	—	55	0	0	14	29	0	5	77
Wheatstarch, Paygel	3 T	25	92	0.1	tr	22	2	2	16	3
Wheatstarch, Cellu	¼ c	35	125	0.1	—	—	—	—	12	2
Wheatstarch cookie, Paygel	1 cookie	14	70	0.1	4	10	6	6	28	11
Nondairy products										
Coffee Rich liquid	¼ c	60	96	0.2	6	11	1	24	24	24
Coffee whiteners, liquid (frozen) average	¼ c	60	80	0.6	6	7	4	40	48	116
Coffee whiteners, pwdr, avg	2 T	12	66	0.6	4	7	tr	48	24	96
Cremora, Borden	2 T	12	66	0.6	—	—	—	—	1	10
Dessert Whip, liquid	¼ c	60	164	0.6	—	—	—	—	40	20
Imitation sour cream	¼ c	56	118	1.4	11	4	2	26	58	92
Mocha Mix	¼ c	60	75	0.2	7	4	7	18	43	28
Party Pride Whip, liquid	2 T	30	99	0.6	—	—	—	—	13	1
Poly Rich liquid	¼ c	60	88	0.2	6	8	1	20	12	40
Rich's Whip Topping, whipped	½ c	23	63	0	—	—	—	—	13	tr
Spices, seasonings, and flavorings										
A-1 Sauce	1 T	17	12	0.2	tr	3	—	—	275	49
Catsup, regular	2 T	30	32	0.6	0	8	6	16	312	108
Catsup, Low-Sod, Featherwgt	2 T	30	12	1.0	0	2	6	11	9	224
Chili sauce, regular	2 T	30	32	0.8	tr	8	6	16	402	(112)
Chili sauce, Low-Sod Featherwgt	2 T	30	16	1.0	0	3	5	12	9	154
Green pepper, chopped	1 T	10	2	0.1	tr	0	1	2	2	20
Horseradish, prepared	1 t	5	2	0.1	tr	0	3	2	5	15
Lemon juice, fresh	1 T	15	4	0.1	tr	1	1	2	tr	21
Lime juice, fresh	1 T	15	4	tr	tr	1	1	2	tr	16
Mustard, regular	1 t	5	4	0.2	0	0	4	4	63	7
Mustard, Low Sod, Featherwgt	1 t	5	4	0.2	—	—	3	4	1	24
Onion, fresh, chopped	1 T	15	4	0.2	tr	1	3	4	1	16
Vinegar, cider	½ c	120	17	tr	(0)	7	(7)	(11)	1	120
Worcestershire sauce	1 t	5	4	0.1	0	1	5	3	105	24
Sweets—Chocolate										
Hershey's Choc. Products										
Choc. Kisses	10 pieces	40	217	3.4	14	23	79	85	42	150
Choc. bar, plain	1 oz	28	152	2.2	10	15	55	60	30	105
Choc. bar, almonds	1 oz	28	142	2.4	8	17	42	60	10	75
Krackel bar	1 oz	28	148	2.3	8	15	50	55	35	85
Mr. Goodbar	1 oz	28	153	3.9	10	12	35	70	20	120
Choc. syrup	1 oz	28	69	0.7	tr	16	5	25	15	55
Cocoa powder	1 T	7	28	1.7	1	3	11	52	5	90
Chocolate Chips, semisweet	¼ c	43	216	1.8	15	24	13	64	1	139
Bitter chocolate squares	1 square	28	142	(1.6)	15	8	28	126	1	232

(continued)

Table K-15.   (*Continued*)

Food Item	Measure	Weight g	Kcal	Pro g	Fat g	Cho g	Ca mg	P mg	Na mg	K mg
Sweets—Other										
Canned cake, Low-Sod, Cellu	½ slice	50	191	2.2	12	20	14	57	8	28
Fruit ice, lime	1 c	—	247	0.8	tr	63	tr	tr	tr	6
Gelatin, regular, flavored	½ c	—	71	1.8	0	17	tr	tr	61	—
Gelatin, Low-Sod D'Zerta	½ c	—	8	2.0	0	0	tr	tr ·	10	50
Honey cake, Holland, Low Sod	½ slice	45	132	1.9	tr	33	—	—	15	225
Log Cabin maple-flavored syrup	1 T	20	35	0	0	10	—	—	13	1
Maple syrup, regular	1 T	20	50	—	—	13	20	2	2	35
Marshmallows, white	4 lg	30	92	0.4	tr	23	4	tr	12	1
Popsicles, Kool Pop	1 bar	36	26	tr	(0)	(6)	—	—	12	tr
Sherbet, orange	½ c	96	135	1.1	2	29	52	37	44	99
Sugar, brown, packed	1 T	14	52	0	0	13	12	3	4	47

Note: The foods and beverages in the miscellaneous list are items of general interest that do not fit into any other group. Averages are not given for this list because the figures vary too much.

The items in the miscellaneous list cannot be used freely within the diet. The dietitian must go over the list and point out which items can be included within each dietary prescription.

Table K-16.   Low-Sodium Specialty Items

Food Item	Measure	Weight g	Kcal	Pro g	Fat g	Cho g	Ca mg	P mg	Na mg	K mg
Chili Con Carne, Campbell	½ can	100	155	7.0	7	15	19	118	30	338
Chili Con Carne, Featherweight	½ can	120	150	8.5	6	13	—	—	18	—
Stuffed Dumpling w/chicken	½ can	120	85	6.0	2	9	7	64	29	420
Beef Ravioli, Featherweight	½ can	120	115	4.0	3	18	16	46	68	166
Spaghetti w/meat balls, Featherweight	½ can	120	110	4.0	4	14	1	—	28	—
Beef stew, Featherweight	½ can	120	105	5.5	4	12	7	64	24	178
Chicken stew, Featherweight	½ can	100	80	4.5	2	10	7	45	16	95
Lamb stew, Featherweight	½ can	100	115	4.5	6	12	8	47	23	119
Spanish Rice, Featherweight	½ can	100	70	1.5	1	14	12	39	14	203
Low-Sodium soups (Canned without added salt)										
Bouillon, Featherweight, unsalted, beef	1 cube	4	12	0	1	2	—	—	10	475
Bouillon, Featherweight, unsalted, chicken	1 cube	4	12	0	1	2	—	—	5	502
Chicken noodle, Featherweight	½ can	120	60	3.0	2	8	6	47	26	463
Chunky beef, Campbell	½ can	100	90	5.0	4	8	6	51	35	192
Chunky chicken, Campbell	½ can	100	75	5.0	3	7	6	41	30	93
Green pea soup, Campbell	½ can	100	65	3.0	1	11	12	48	20	62
Green pea soup, Featherweight	½ can	120	90	4.0	1	16	7	104	14	707
Mushroom cream, Campbell	½ can	100	65	tr	5	5	16	16	15	35
Mushroom cream, Featherweight	½ can	120	60	1.0	2	9	—	—	30	—
Tomato, Campbell	½ can	100	50	1.0	1	9	16	14	15	151
Tomato, Featherweight	½ can	120	60	2.0	0	15	7	26	14	798
Turkey noodle, Campbell	½ can	100	30	1.0	1	4	6	20	20	24
Vegetable, Campbell	½ can	100	40	1.0	1	7	9	18	15	84
Vegetable Beef, Campbell	½ can	100	40	2.0	2	4	10	16	25	72
Vegetable Beef, Featherweight	½ can	120	90	4.0	2	14	9	59	24	492
Beef soup base, Cellu	1 t	5.3	20	0.5	1	3	—	—	6	360
Chicken soup base, Cellu	1 t	5.3	25	0.2	1	4	—	—	1	193

Table K-17. High-Salt Items (400 mg sodium or 1 g salt each)

Food Item	Quantity
Meats and meat substitutes	
Hot dog	1 small
Lunchmeat (Omit braunschweiger, liverwurst, or salami	1 oz or 1 slice
Bacon	4 slices
Pork sausage, ham, corned beef	1½ oz
Tuna, regular, canned	1½ oz
Salmon, regular, canned	3 oz
Crab, regular, canned	1½ oz
Cottage cheese	¾ c
Cheese	2 oz
Breads and cereals	
Pretzels, small	20
Pretzels, twisted medium	3
Pretzels, Dutch or soft	1
Vegetables	
Canned vegetables, regular, canned	2 servings
Sauerkraut, regular, canned, drained	⅓ c
Potato chips	20 (or 1 oz)
Soups, canned, diluted with equal vol of water	
Beef broth	⅔ c
Vegetarian vegetable	⅔ c

(continued)

Table K-17 (*Continued*)

Food Item	Quantity
Tomato bisque, Manhattan-style clam chowder, tomato rice, tomato, cream of celery, cream of asparagus, chicken gumbo, golden vegetable noodle-O's	½ c
Cream of mushroom	⅓ c
Seasonings	
Salt	¼ t
Soy sauce	1 t
Worcestershire sauce	4 t
Catsup	7 t
Mustard, prepared	6 t
Chili sauce	6 t
Barbecue sauce	6 t
Salad Dressings	
Tartar sauce or mayonnaise	4⅔ T
Thousand Island Dressing	¼ c
French dressing	2 T
Russian dressing	3 T
Italian dressing	4 t
Relishes	
Pickles, dill large	½
Olives	4 medium, 3 extra large, 2 giant
Pickle relish, sweet	¼ c

Appendix L:
Food Sources of Potassium

Table L-1. Food Sources of Potassium

Food	Description	Measure
5 to 10 mEq/serving		
Vegetables		
Artichoke	Fresh, cooked	One
Asparagus	Fresh or frozen	½ c
Beans, lima	Fresh or frozen, cooked	½ c
Beets	Fresh, cooked	½ c
Broccoli	Fresh or frozen, cooked	½ c
Brussels sprouts	Fresh or frozen	½ c
Cabbage	Raw	1 c
Carrots	Fresh, raw, or cooked	½ c
Cauliflower		1 c
Celery	Raw	1 c
Chard, Swiss	Fresh, cooked	½ c
Corn	Fresh (5″)	1 ear
Cress	Cooked	½ c
Dandelion greens	Cooked	½ c
Eggplant	Baked	½ c
Kale	Fresh, cooked	½ c
Leeks	Raw	¾ c
Lettuce	Raw	½ c
Mushrooms	Fresh, cooked	½ c
Parsnips	Cooked	½ c
Peas	Dried, cooked	½ c
Potato	Cooked	½ c
Pumpkin	Fresh	½ c
Rutabagas	Raw	¾ c
Spinach	Cooked	½ c
Squash, winter	Frozen, cooked	½ c
Sweet potato	Canned	½ c
Tomato	Cooked, canned	½ c
Tomato	Fresh	1 medium
Tomato juice	Canned	½ c
Tomato juice	Low-sodium or fresh, unsalted	½ c
Turnip	Raw	¾ c
Fruits		
Apple juice	Unsweetened, canned or fresh	1 c
Apricots	Fresh	2 medium

(continued)

Table L-1. *(Continued)*

Food	Description	Measure
Apricots	Canned, unsweetened	½ c
Apricots	Dried	4 halves
Banana		1 small
Blackberries	Fresh or frozen	1 c
Cherries		15 large
Fruit cocktail		½ c
Grape juice	Unsweetened, canned or fresh	1 c
Grapefruit	Fresh	½
Grapefruit juice	Unsweetened, canned or fresh	1 c
Grapes, white		1 c
Nectarines	Fresh	2
Orange juice	Unsweetened, fresh or frozen	½ c
Orange, tangerine, mandarin orange	Fresh	1 medium
Peach	Raw	1 medium
Pear	Raw	1 medium
Pineapple	Fresh	1 c
Pineapple juice	Unsweetened, canned or frozen	1 c
Plums	Fresh	4
Prune juice	Unsweetened, canned	½ c
Prunes	Dried	8
Raspberries	Fresh or frozen	1 c
Strawberries	Fresh or frozen	1 c
Watermelon	Raw	2 c
Meats		
Meat, poultry	Cooked	3 oz
Salmon, pink	Canned	3 oz
Shrimp	Fresh or cooked	3½ oz
Tuna	Fresh or canned	½ c
Milk		
Skim, 2%, whole, buttermilk		1 c

(continued)

Table L-1. (*Continued*)

Food	Description	Measure
Miscellaneous		
Brazil nuts		20
Coffee	instant	1 t
Molasses	Brer Rabbit	5 t
10 to 15 mEq/serving		
Vegetables		
Artichokes	Cooked	½ c
Beans	Dried, cooked	½ c
Beet greens	Cooked	½ c
Chard, Swiss	Chopped	2 c
Chard, Swiss	Whole leaves	3 c
Cress, garden	Raw	3 c
Dandelion greens	Raw	1 c
Kale	Fresh, whole leaves	3 c
Kale	Chopped	2 c
Mushrooms	Fresh	10 small, 4 large
Mushrooms	Sliced	½ c
Potatoes	Baked or raw	½ c
Soybeans	Cooked	½ c
Spinach	Raw, chopped	2 c
Fruits		
Avocado		½
Cantaloupe	6" in diameter	¼
Honeydew	7" in diameter	⅛

(*continued*)

Table L-1. (*Continued*)

Food	Description	Measure
Meats		
Cod	Cooked	3½ oz
Flounder	Cooked	3½ oz
Halibut	Cooked	3½ oz
Salmon	Fresh or cooked	3½ oz
Scallops	Cooked	3½ oz
Miscellaneous		
Peanuts	Roasted with skins	45
Walnuts		¾ c
15 to 20 mEq/serving		
Vegetables		
Potato	Baked	1 medium
Turnip greens		1 c
Mustard greens		¾ c
Fruits		
Dates	Dried	15
Figs	Fresh	1 large
Nectarine	Dried	10 large
Peach	Dried	3
Rhubarb	Fresh	1 c
Raisins		1 c
Meats		
Chicken breast		6 oz

Appendix M: Menu Forms

The menus which follow are house diets reproduced from those used in two unrelated hospitals. These may be used to complete some of the exercises in this book, or you may use menus from your own institution.

The following list contains some of the items and describes their contents. Other items are commonly used. If you are not familiar with them, you should consult a standard recipe book. When using menus from your own institution, it may be necessary to consult your recipe file.

GLOSSARY OF MENU ITEMS

Avocado and grapefruit salad: avocado, canned grapefruit, and lettuce leaf

Banana split salad: 3 scoops cottage cheese, split banana and pineapple, orange and prune topping; served with Melba toast

Banana supreme salad: sliced bananas, raisins, walnuts, mayonnaise-whipped cream dressing

Beef pot pie: braised beef, gravy, carrots, peas

Beef stroganoff: braised beef, sour cream gravy, onions. mushrooms, spices

Blueberry bavarian cream: blueberries, gelatin, and whipped cream; blenderized and chilled

Cheeseburger: ground beef, cheddar cheese, lettuce, tomato, sliced pickles

Cheese tuna casserole: chunks of tuna with noodles in cheese sauce

Chef's salad: tossed greens with julienne of ham, cheese, turkey, beets, hard-cooked eggs

Chicken a la king: chunks of chicken, pimento, celery in white sauce

Chicken pot pie: chicken, eggs, milk, baking powder biscuit

Chicken salad plate with fresh fruit: chicken broth, gelatin, mayonnaise, salt, pepper, chicken, fresh green grapes, and slivered almonds

Coleslaw: cabbage, onion, sour cream, mayonnaise, salt, mustard, and pepper

Cottage cheese salads: canned fruit, lettuce underliner, cottage cheese

Cranberry mold: cranberries and gelatin

Crepes with cherries helene: cherries in small French pancakes with custard

Denver sandwich: egg omelet with diced ham, onion, bell pepper, and pimento on toasted bun with catsup

Escalloped potatoes: potato slices in white sauce with onion

Escalloped tomatoes: tomatoes (peeled), onion, flour, salt, pepper, margarine, and milk

Frozen fruit salad: pineapple, cherries, peaches, and pears in gelatin and whipped cream

Fruit compote: blueberries, Queen Anne cherries, fresh melon

Fruited gelatins: gelatin, canned fruit, lettuce underliner

German potato salad: potatoes, bacon bits, sugar, vinegar, bacon drippings, seasoning

Imperial chicken: chicken dipped in bread crumbs with Parmesan cheese, baked

Lamb shish kebob: marinated chunks of lamb, mushrooms, onions, and tomatoes on a skewer

Lasagna: wide noodles layered with Italian meat sauce, ricotta, and parmesan and mozzarella cheese

Macaroni salad: macaroni, mayonnaise, chopped fresh vegetable, hard-cooked egg, mustard

Marinated fresh vegetables: carrots, olives, and peppers in vinegar

Meat loaf: ground beef, onions, bread crumbs

Mexicorn: corn and pimento

O'Brien potatoes: potatoes, onions, green pepper, flour, milk, bread crumbs, butter

Oxtail soup/vegetable soup: beef, carrots, celery, onions, broth, barley or rice or noodles

Quarter broiler: a quarter chicken seasoned with onion, butter, and garlic; baked

Relish plate: carrot, celery, cauliflower, broccoli pieces, olives, dill pickles

Reuben sandwich: corned beef on rye bread with Swiss cheese and sauerkraut

Rice pilaf: white rice with pimento, green peas

Rosy pear salad: fresh apple and canned pear on a lettuce leaf

Seafood symphony salad: crab, shrimp, and tuna on a lettuce bed garnished with hard-cooked egg, asparagus spears, and tomato wedges; served with mayonnaise or Roquefort dressing

Singapore pork: strips of pork, celery, pineapple, and tomatoes in a sweet-sour sauce served over crisp Chinese noodles

Spanish rice: rice with tomato, onion, pimento, green pepper, spices

Stuffed frankfurters: franks split lengthwise, stuffed with 1 oz Cheddar cheese, wrapped with 1 slice bacon; broiled and served on bun

Sweet and sour pork: braised pork cubes, green pepper, onion, soy sauce, spices, pineapple, vinegar, sugar

Tomato stuffed with tuna or shrimp salad: tuna or shrimp, mayonnaise, celery, spices, onions, lettuce underliner

Tossed salad: lettuce, diced radishes, onions, celery, and carrots

Veal goulash: ground veal, shell macroni, stuffed green olives, tomato sauce

Veal parmigiana: veal cutlet topped with Swiss cheese and a mushroom sauce

Waldorf salad: apples, celery, walnuts, mayonnaise, lettuce underliner

---

Name _____	Name _____	Name _____
Room _____	Room _____	Room _____
Diet _____	Diet _____	Diet _____
Date ___Monday A___	Date _____	Date _____

Breakfast	*Lunch*	*Dinner*
Chilled Orange Juice	Bouillon with Saltines	French Onion Soup with Saltines
Rhubarb	Cream of Asparagus Soup with Saltines	Cream of Corn Soup with Saltines
Chilled Apple Juice	Chilled Tomato Juice with Lemon Wedge	
Wheat Hearts		Prime Rib au Jus
Roman Meal	Chicken a la King* in a Patty Shell	Grilled Salmon Steak with Lemon Butter
Rice Krispies	Cold Meat Platter with Macaroni Salad*	
Waffle with Syrup	Baked Winter Squash	Baked Potato with Sour Cream and Chives
		Buttered Lima Beans
Scrambled Egg	Tossed Green Salad* with Italian	Buttered Chopped Chard with Lemon
Soft-cooked Egg	Dressing	
Hard-cooked Egg	Cherry Pie	Coleslaw
Bacon	Vanilla Ice Cream	Rosy Pear Salad*
	Praline Cookies	
		Angel Food Cake
		Sherbet
		Apricots

Toast:			Bread:			Bread:		
White	Whole-Wheat	Rye	White	Whole-Wheat	Rye	White	Whole-Wheat	Rye
Butter	Margarine	Jelly	Butter	Margarine	Jelly	Butter	Margarine	Jelly
Coffee	Decaf.	Tea	Coffee	Decaf.	Tea	Coffee	Decaf.	Tea
Milk	Skim Milk	Buttermilk	Milk	Skim Milk	Buttermilk	Milk	Skim Milk	Buttermilk
Cream	Half & Half	Sugar	Cream	Half & Half	Sugar	Cream	Half & Half	Sugar
Salt	Pepper	Lemon	Salt	Pepper	Lemon	Salt	Pepper	Lemon

Snacks: Snacks: Snacks:

Name _____
Room _____
Diet _____
Date ___Tuesday A___
Breakfast
Chilled Orange Juice
Mandarin Oranges
Chilled Apple Juice

Roman Meal
Farina
Shredded Wheat

Sweet Roll

Poached Egg
Soft-cooked Egg
Hard-cooked Egg
Sausage Links

Toast:
White	Whole-Wheat	Rye
Butter	Margarine	Jelly
Coffee	Decaf.	Tea
Milk	Skim Milk	Buttermilk
Cream	Half & Half	Sugar
Salt	Pepper	Lemon

Snacks:

Name _____
Room _____
Diet _____
Date _____
Lunch
Consommé with Crackers
Vegetable Soup* with Crackers
Chilled Fruit Punch

Tomato Stuffed with Shrimp Salad*
Bratwurst and German Potato* Salad

Buttered Peas

Sliced Tomatoes on Lettuce Leaf

Blueberry Bavarian Cream*
Strawberry Ice Cream
Pears in Syrup

Bread:
White	Whole-Wheat	Rye
Butter	Margarine	Jelly
Coffee	Decaf.	Tea
Milk	Skim Milk	Buttermilk
Cream	Half & Half	Sugar
Salt	Pepper	Lemon

Snacks:

Name _____
Room _____
Diet _____
Date _____
Dinner
Tomato Bouillon with Crackers
Cream of Asparagus Soup with Crackers

Roast Turkey/Cranberry Sauce/Gravy
Lamb Shish Kebob*

Escalloped Potatoes*
Parslied Buttered Carrots

Tossed Salad with Blue Cheese Dressing
   and Crouton Garnish

Cream Puff with Chocolate Topping
Sherbet

Bread:
White	Whole-Wheat	Rye
Butter	Margarine	Jelly
Coffee	Decaf.	Tea
Milk	Skim Milk	Buttermilk
Cream	Half & Half	Sugar
Salt	Pepper	Lemon

Snacks:

Name _____
Room _____
Diet _____
Date ___Wednesday A___
Breakfast
Chilled Orange Juice
Banana Slices with Cream
Chilled Apricot Nectar

Ralston Cereal
Cream of Wheat
Cornflakes

Hotcakes with Syrup

Fried Egg
Soft-cooked Egg
Hard-cooked Egg
Bacon

Toast:
White	Whole-Wheat	Rye
Butter	Margarine	Jelly
Coffee	Decaf.	Tea
Milk	Skim Milk	Buttermilk
Cream	Half & Half	Sugar
Salt	Pepper	Lemon

Snacks:

Name _____
Room _____
Diet _____
Date _____
Lunch
Consommé with Crackers
Oxtail Soup* with Saltines

Cheeseburger* on Sesame Seed Bun
Roast Pork/Applesauce

Buttered Beets
Buttered Mexicorn*

Avocado and Grapefruit Salad* with
   French Dressing

Butterscotch Pecan Pie
Sherbet

Bread:
White	Whole-Wheat	Rye
Butter	Margarine	Jelly
Coffee	Decaf.	Tea
Milk	Skim Milk	Buttermilk
Cream	Half & Half	Sugar
Salt	Pepper	Lemon

Snacks:

Name _____
Room _____
Diet _____
Date _____
Dinner
Bouillon with Crackers
Cream of Celery Soup with Crackers

Quarter Broiled Chicken
Lasagna

O'Brien Potatoes*
Brussels Sprouts

Marinated Fresh Vegetable Salad

Cherry Cheese Cake
Peach Ice Cream
Sliced Freestone Peaches

Bread:
White	Whole-Wheat	Rye
Butter	Margarine	Jelly
Coffee	Decaf.	Tea
Milk	Skim Milk	Buttermilk
Cream	Half & Half	Sugar
Salt	Pepper	Lemon

Snacks:

Name _____
Room _____
Diet _____
Date   Thursday A _____

Breakfast

Chilled Orange Juice
Stewed Prunes
Chilled Cranberry Juice

Oatmeal
Malt-O-Meal
Rice Krispies

Fried Cornmeal Cakes with Syrup

Scrambled Egg
Soft-cooked Egg
Hard-cooked Egg
Canadian Bacon

Toast:

White	Whole-Wheat	Rye
Butter	Margarine	Jelly
Coffee	Decaf.	Tea
Milk	Skim Milk	Buttermilk
Cream	Half & Half	Sugar
Salt	Pepper	Lemon

Snacks:

Name _____
Room _____
Diet _____
Date _____

Lunch

Beef Broth with Crackers
Cream of Mushroom Soup with Crackers
Chilled Pineapple Juice

Chicken Salad Sandwich Plate/Potato
  Chips
Broiled Lamb Chop

Escalloped Tomatoes*
Spinach Souffle

Chocolate Creme Tart
Green Gage Plums

Bread:

White	Whole-Wheat	Rye
Butter	Margarine	Jelly
Coffee	Decaf.	Tea
Milk	Skim Milk	Buttermilk
Cream	Half & Half	Sugar
Salt	Pepper	Lemon

Snacks:

Name _____
Room _____
Diet _____
Date _____

Dinner

Consommé with Crackers
Vegetable Soup* with Crackers

Roast Sirloin of Beef au Jus
Broiled Sea Bass

Oven-browned Potatoes
Peas with Pearl Onions

Celery Heart, Olives, and Radishes
Cranberry Jello Mold*

Cheese Cake
Chocolate Ice Cream
Fresh Apricots

Bread:

White	Whole-Wheat	Rye
Butter	Margarine	Jelly
Coffee	Decaf.	Tea
Milk	Skim Milk	Buttermilk
Cream	Half & Half	Sugar
Salt	Pepper	Lemon

Snacks:

Name _____
Room _____
Diet _____
Date   Friday A _____

Breakfast

Chilled Orange Juice
Half Grapefruit
Chilled Pear Nectar

Roman Meal
Wheat Hearts
Special K Cereal

Coffee Cake

Poached Egg
Soft-cooked Egg
Hard-cooked Egg
Bacon

Toast:

White	Whole-Wheat	Rye
Butter	Margarine	Jelly
Coffee	Decaf.	Tea
Milk	Skim Milk	Buttermilk
Cream	Half & Half	Sugar
Salt	Pepper	Lemon

Snacks:

Name _____
Room _____
Diet _____
Date _____

Lunch

Cream of Asparagus Soup with Crackers
Chicken-Rice Broth with Crackers
Chilled V-8 Juice with Lemon

Denver Sandwich*
Chicken Salad Plate with Fresh Fruit*

Buttered Chopped Spinach with Lemon

Cottage Cheese and Peach Salad

French Roll with Butter

Apple Crisp with Hard Sauce
Strawberry Sundae
Assorted Cookies

Bread:

White	Whole-Wheat	Rye
Butter	Margarine	Jelly
Coffee	Decaf.	Tea
Milk	Skim Milk	Buttermilk
Cream	Half & Half	Sugar
Salt	Pepper	Lemon

Snacks:

Name _____
Room _____
Diet _____
Date _____

Dinner

Bouillon with Crackers

Baked Pork Chop
Meat Loaf*

Browned Rice
Mashed Potatoes and Gravy
Green Beans Sesame

Waldorf Salad*
Lettuce Heart with Thousand Island
  Dressing

Lemon Layer Cake
Jello Jewels with Whipped Cream
Dark Sweet Cherries

Bread:

White	Whole-Wheat	Rye
Butter	Margarine	Jelly
Coffee	Decaf.	Tea
Milk	Skim Milk	Buttermilk
Cream	Half & Half	Sugar
Salt	Pepper	Lemon

Snacks:

Name _____
Room _____
Diet _____
Date ___Saturday A_____
Breakfast
Chilled Orange Juice
Chilled Pineapple Juice
Half Grapefruit

Raisin Bran
Rice Krispies
Puffed Wheat

Poached Egg
Scrambled Egg
Bacon

Toast:
White	Whole-Wheat	Rye
Butter	Margarine	Jelly
Coffee	Decaf.	Tea
Milk	Skim Milk	Buttermilk
Cream	Half & Half	Sugar
Salt	Pepper	Lemon

Snacks:

Name _____
Room _____
Diet _____
Date _____
Lunch
Navy Bean Soup
Chilled Blended Juice

Baked Stuffed Green Pepper—Stuffed with
   Beef, Rice, plus Tomato Sauce
Triple Medley Sandwich Plate—Egg Salad,
   Roast Beef, and Chicken Salad
Mandarin Beef—Thinly Sliced Flank
   Steak, Onions, Celery, Chinese Pea Pods,
   and Ginger

Escalloped Potatoes*
Steamed Rice

Fresh Vegetable Relishes with Dip
Butter Lettuce Salad with Vinaigrette

French Roll with Butter

Fresh Peach
Vanilla Ice Cream
Berry Pie

Bread:
White	Whole-Wheat	Rye
Butter	Margarine	Jelly
Coffee	Decaf.	Tea
Milk	Skim Milk	Buttermilk
Cream	Half & Half	Sugar
Salt	Pepper	Lemon

Snacks:

Name _____
Room _____
Diet _____
Date _____
Dinner
French Onion Soup
Chilled Orange Juice

Baked Pork Chop/Spiced Crabapple with
   Savory Dressing
Broiled Red Snapper with Lemon Wedge
Steak with Tarragon-Mushroom Sauce

Baked Potato
Whipped Squash
French-Cut Green Beans

Jellied Waldorf Salad*
Tossed Salad Greens* with Alfalfa Sprouts

French Roll with Butter

Bartlett Pear Halves
Sherbet
Walnut Cream Cake

Bread:
White	Whole-Wheat	Rye
Butter	Margarine	Jelly
Coffee	Decaf.	Tea
Milk	Skim Milk	Buttermilk
Cream	Half & Half	Sugar
Salt	Pepper	Lemon

Snacks:

Name _____
Room _____
Diet _____
Date ___Sunday A_____
Breakfast
Chilled Orange Juice
Chilled Grape Juice
Chilled Citrus Sections

Oatmeal
Corn Flakes
Raisin Bran
Cream of Wheat
Rice Krispies
Puffed Wheat

Poached Egg
Scrambled Egg
Canadian Bacon

Danish Pastry

Toast:
White	Whole-Wheat	Rye
Butter	Margarine	Jelly
Coffee	Decaf.	Tea
Milk	Skim Milk	Buttermilk
Cream	Half & Half	Sugar
Salt	Pepper	Lemon

Snacks:

Name _____
Room _____
Diet _____
Date _____
Lunch
Vegetable Soup
Chilled Cranberry Juice

Chef's Salad—Mixed Greens, Ham,
   Turkey, Cheese, and Tomato Wedge with
   Italian Dressing
Lasagna*

Green Peas
Lettuce Wedge with Italian Dressing

French Roll with Butter

Sherbet
Chocolate Pie
Baked Custard

Bread:
White	Whole-Wheat	Rye
Butter	Margarine	Jelly
Coffee	Decaf.	Tea
Milk	Skim Milk	Buttermilk
Cream	Half & Half	Sugar
Salt	Pepper	Lemon

Snacks:

Name _____
Room _____
Diet _____
Date _____
Dinner
Cream of Celery Soup
Chicken Consommé

Roast Beef au Jus
Poached Salmon

Baked Potato
Sliced Zucchini
Broccoli Spears

Fresh Spinach Salad with French
   Dressing

Pineapple Chunks
Tangy Lemon Cake

Bread:
White	Whole-Wheat	Rye
Butter	Margarine	Jelly
Coffee	Decaf.	Tea
Milk	Skim Milk	Buttermilk
Cream	Half & Half	Sugar
Salt	Pepper	Lemon

Snacks:

Name _____
Room _____
Diet _____
Date ___Monday B_____
Breakfast
Chilled Orange Juice
Chilled Peach Nectar
Half Grapefruit

Cream of Rice
Product 19

Waffles with Syrup

Scrambled Egg
Crisp Bacon

Danish Pastry
Toasted English Muffin

Toast:
White	Whole-Wheat	Rye
Butter	Margarine	Jelly
Coffee	Decaf.	Tea
Milk	Skim Milk	Buttermilk
Cream	Half & Half	Sugar
Salt	Pepper	Lemon

Snacks:

Name _____
Room _____
Diet _____
Date _____
Lunch
Cream of Mushroom Soup
Relish Plate*

Breaded Veal Cutlets
Cold Meat Plate with Macaroni Salad

Creamed Potatoes
Buttered Corn

Brownies
Ice Cream

Dinner Roll

Bread:
White	Whole-Wheat	Rye
Butter	Margarine	Jelly
Coffee	Decaf.	Tea
Milk	Skim Milk	Buttermilk
Cream	Half & Half	Sugar
Salt	Pepper	Lemon

Snacks:

Name _____
Room _____
Diet _____
Date _____
Dinner
Cranberry Juice
Creamy Cole Slaw

Grilled Dinner Steak
Sweet and Sour Spareribs

Baked Potato
Glazed Carrots

Cherry Cheesecake
Pear Halves

Bread:
White	Whole-Wheat	Rye
Butter	Margarine	Jelly
Coffee	Decaf.	Tea
Milk	Skim Milk	Buttermilk
Cream	Half & Half	Sugar
Salt	Pepper	Lemon

Snacks:

Name _____

Room _____

Diet _____

Date ___Tuesday B_____

Breakfast

Chilled Orange Juice
Chilled Pineapple Juice
Chilled Berries

Oatmeal
Raisin Bran
Cream of Wheat
Rice Krispies
Puffed Wheat

French Toast with Powdered Sugar and
  Syrup

Poached Egg
Scrambled Egg
Crisp Bacon

Buttermilk Biscuit
Doughnut

Toast:

White	Whole-Wheat	Rye
Butter	Margarine	Jelly
Coffee	Decaf.	Tea
Milk	Skim Milk	Buttermilk
Cream	Half & Half	Sugar
Salt	Pepper	Lemon

Snacks:

Name _____

Room _____

Diet _____

Date _____

Lunch

Gazpacho Soup—Chilled Fresh Vegetable
  Soup with Crisp Tortilla Chips
Chilled Grape Juice

Macaroni and Cheese
Salad Bowl—Greens, Chicken, Fresh
  Tomatoes, Avocado, and Cheese with
  Italian Dressing

Broiled Tomato Half
Green Peas
Relishes

Butter Lettuce Salad with Italian
  Dressing

French Roll

Chilled Plums
Ice Cream
Plain Frosted Cupcake

Bread:

White	Whole-Wheat	Rye
Butter	Margarine	Jelly
Coffee	Decaf.	Tea
Milk	Skim Milk	Buttermilk
Cream	Half & Half	Sugar
Salt	Pepper	Lemon

Snacks:

Name _____

Room _____

Diet _____

Date _____

Dinner

Cream of Mushroom Soup
Chilled Tomato Juice

Roast Turkey with Giblet Gravy and
  Cranberry Sauce
Ham Steak with Pineapple Glaze
Sauteed Liver and Onions

Citrus Yams
Asparagus Spears
Whipped Potatoes
Mixed Vegetables

Spring-Fruit Gelatin Salad with Fruit
  Dressing
Crisp Green Salad with Italian Dressing

Chilled Peaches
Sugar Cookies
Lime Bavarian

Dinner Roll

Bread:

White	Whole-Wheat	Rye
Butter	Margarine	Jelly
Coffee	Decaf.	Tea
Milk	Skim Milk	Buttermilk
Cream	Half & Half	Sugar
Salt	Pepper	Lemon

Snacks:

Name _____
Room _____
Diet _____
Date ___Wednesday B___
Breakfast
Chilled Orange Juice
Chilled Prune Juice
Fresh Banana

Special K Cereal
Raisin Bran
Rice Krispies
Puffed Wheat

Coffee Cake

Poached Egg
Cheese Omelet
Canadian Bacon
Crisp Bacon

Toast:

White	Whole-Wheat	Rye
Butter	Margarine	Jelly
Coffee	Decaf.	Tea
Milk	Skim Milk	Buttermilk
Cream	Half & Half	Sugar
Salt	Pepper	Lemon

Snacks:

Name _____
Room _____
Diet _____
Date _____
Lunch
Split Pea and Tomato Chowder
Chilled Apple Juice

Chicken Pot Pie*
Fresh Fruit and Cottage Cheese Platter
    with Lime Dressing
Reuben Sandwich*

Spinach with Lemon
Fresh Vegetable Relishes

Green Salad with Italian Dressing
Marinated Green Bean Salad

Blueberry Muffin

Chilled Apricots
Black Raspberry Yogurt Whip
Gingerbread with Lemon Sauce

Bread:

White	Whole-Wheat	Rye
Butter	Margarine	Jelly
Coffee	Decaf.	Tea
Milk	Skim Milk	Buttermilk
Cream	Half & Half	Sugar
Salt	Pepper	Lemon

Snacks:

Name _____
Room _____
Diet _____
Date _____
Dinner
Louisiana Gumbo Soup—Chicken Base,
    Shrimp, Okra, and Creole Seasoning
Chilled Pineapple Juice

Veal Parmigiana*
Swedish Meatballs—Savory Meatballs in
    a Light Sherry Sauce
Baked Halibut Garnished with Lemon and
    Paprika

Parsley Noodles
Sliced Zucchini
Sauteed Mushrooms with Pimiento

Sliced Tomato and Cucumber Salad with
    Thousand Island Dressing

French Roll

Fresh Diced Pineapple
Peanut Butter Cookies
Banana Cream Pudding

Bread:

White	Whole-Wheat	Rye
Butter	Margarine	Jelly
Coffee	Decaf.	Tea
Milk	Skim Milk	Buttermilk
Cream	Half & Half	Sugar
Salt	Pepper	Lemon

Snacks:

Name _____
Room _____
Diet _____
Date _____ Thursday B _____
Breakfast
Chilled Orange Juice
Chilled Grapefruit Juice
Applesauce

Oatmeal
Raisin Bran
Rice Krispies
Granola

Sweet Roll
Buttermilk Hotcakes with Syrup

Poached Egg
Scrambled Egg
Crisp Bacon

Toast:

White	Whole-Wheat	Rye
Butter	Margarine	Jelly
Coffee	Decaf.	Tea
Milk	Skim Milk	Buttermilk
Cream	Half & Half	Sugar
Salt	Pepper	Lemon

Snacks:

Name _____
Room _____
Diet _____
Date _____
Lunch
Lentil Soup

Breast of Turkey
Toasted Cheese, Bacon, and Tomato
   Sandwich
Seafood Louis—Salad Greens, Shrimp,
   Crab, and Tuna with Louis Dressing

Broccoli Spears
Rice Pilaf*
Potato Chips
Vegetable Relish

Citrus Avocado Salad with Poppyseed
   Dressing
Lettuce Wedge with Blue Cheese Dressing

French Roll

Fresh Apricots
Flan
Lemon Meringue Pie

Bread:

White	Whole-Wheat	Rye
Butter	Margarine	Jelly
Coffee	Decaf.	Tea
Milk	Skim Milk	Buttermilk
Cream	Half & Half	Sugar
Salt	Pepper	Lemon

Snacks:

Name _____
Room _____
Diet _____
Date _____
Dinner
Chicken Rice Soup
Cranberry Juice Cocktail

Roast Beef au Jus
Mushroom Omelet—A Light, Fluffy
   Omelet Filled with Mushrooms and
   Capped with Mornay Sauce
Broiled Lamb Chop with Mint Jelly

Green and Wax Beens with Pimiento
Oven Browned Potatoes
Quartered Beets

Tossed Green Salad* and Garbanzo Beans
   with Thousand Island Dressing

Bing Cherries
Sherbet
Angel Food Cake with Raspberry Filling

Bread:

White	Whole-Wheat	Rye
Butter	Margarine	Jelly
Coffee	Decaf.	Tea
Milk	Skim Milk	Buttermilk
Cream	Half & Half	Sugar
Salt	Pepper	Lemon

Snacks:

Name _____
Room _____
Diet _____
Date ___Friday B_____

Breakfast

Chilled Orange Juice
Chilled Pineapple Juice
Sliced Peaches

Malt-O-Meal
Rice Krispies

Soft-cooked Egg
Scrambled Egg
Crisp Bacon

Danish Pastry
Toasted English Muffin

Toast:

White	Whole-Wheat	Rye
Butter	Margarine	Jelly
Coffee	Decaf.	Tea
Milk	Skim Milk	Buttermilk
Cream	Half & Half	Sugar
Salt	Pepper	Lemon

Snacks:

Name _____
Room _____
Diet _____
Date _____

Lunch

Cream of Celery Soup
Three Bean Salad

Corned Beef and Cabbage
Baked Cod
Sliced Roast Turkey

Whipped Potatoes
Buttered Carrots

Cherry Pie
Sherbet
Frosted Jello Cubes

Bread:

White	Whole-Wheat	Rye
Butter	Margarine	Jelly
Coffee	Decaf.	Tea
Milk	Skim Milk	Buttermilk
Cream	Half & Half	Sugar
Salt	Pepper	Lemon

Snacks:

Name _____
Room _____
Diet _____
Date _____

Dinner

Minestrone Soup

Meat Loaf* with Gravy
Roast Pork with Applesauce
Salami and Cheese Sandwich on Rye

Mashed Potatoes
Spinach Souffle

Green Salad

Dinner Roll with Margarine

Carrot Cake
Ice Cream

Bread:

White	Whole-Wheat	Rye
Butter	Margarine	Jelly
Coffee	Decaf.	Tea
Milk	Skim Milk	Buttermilk
Cream	Half & Half	Sugar
Salt	Pepper	Lemon

Snacks:

Name _____
Room _____
Diet _____
Date ___Saturday B_____

Breakfast

Chilled Orange Juice
Chilled Apricot Nectar
Stewed Prunes

Cream of Rice
All-Bran

Fried Egg
Soft-cooked Egg
Grilled Ham Slice

Danish Pastry
Toasted English Muffin

Toast:

White	Whole-Wheat	Rye
Butter	Margarine	Jelly
Coffee	Decaf.	Tea
Milk	Skim Milk	Buttermilk
Cream	Half & Half	Sugar
Salt	Pepper	Lemon

Snacks:

Name _____
Room _____
Diet _____
Date _____

Lunch

Chicken Noodle Soup
Layered Peach Cheese Salad

Chile Rellenos
Baked Veal Cutlet
Egg Salad Sandwich

Broccoli Parmesan
Buttered Peas
Spanish Rice*

Dinner Roll

Frosted Coconut Cake
Ice Cream

Bread:

White	Whole-Wheat	Rye
Butter	Margarine	Jelly
Coffee	Decaf.	Tea
Milk	Skim Milk	Buttermilk
Cream	Half & Half	Sugar
Salt	Pepper	Lemon

Snacks:

Name _____
Room _____
Diet _____
Date _____

Dinner

Tomato Juice
Deviled Eggs

New England Pot Roast
Stuffed Cabbage Rolls

Parslied Potatoes
Buttered Green Beans

Dinner Roll

Baked Apples
Jello Jewels

Bread:

White	Whole-Wheat	Rye
Butter	Margarine	Jelly
Coffee	Decaf.	Tea
Milk	Skim Milk	Buttermilk
Cream	Half & Half	Sugar
Salt	Pepper	Lemon

Snacks:

Name _____
Room _____
Diet _____
Date ___Sunday B___

Breakfast

Chilled Orange Juice
Chilled Prune Juice
Sliced Banana

Cream of Wheat
Special K Cereal

Ham Omelet
Poached Egg

Danish Pastry
Toasted English Muffin

Toast:
White	Whole-Wheat	Rye
Butter	Margarine	Jelly
Coffee	Decaf.	Tea
Milk	Skim Milk	Buttermilk
Cream	Half & Half	Sugar
Salt	Pepper	Lemon

Snacks:

Name _____
Room _____
Diet _____
Date _____

Lunch

French Onion Soup
Fresh Fruit Cup

Roast Turkey with Dressing, Gravy, and
   Cranberry Sauce
Tomato Stuffed with Shrimp Salad*

Whipped Potatoes
Buttered Asparagus
Mixed Vegetables

Dinner Roll with Margarine

Vanilla Pudding with Topping
Sherbet
Jello Cubes

Bread:
White	Whole-Wheat	Rye
Butter	Margarine	Jelly
Coffee	Decaf.	Tea
Milk	Skim Milk	Buttermilk
Cream	Half & Half	Sugar
Salt	Pepper	Lemon

Snacks:

Name _____
Room _____
Diet _____
Date _____

Dinner

Apricot Nectar

Beef Stroganoff*
Cheeseburger* with Relishes

Buttered Zucchini

Tossed Green Salad with Blue Cheese
   Dressing

Praline Peach Rice Pudding
Chilled Bing Cherries

Bread:
White	Whole-Wheat	Rye
Butter	Margarine	Jelly
Coffee	Decaf.	Tea
Milk	Skim Milk	Buttermilk
Cream	Half & Half	Sugar
Salt	Pepper	Lemon

Snacks:

Name _____
Room _____
Diet _____
Date _____

Vegetarian Diet Breakfast

Orange Juice
Prune Juice
Banana
Raisins

Shredded Wheat
Oatmeal

French Toast with Syrup and Margarine
Pancakes with Syrup and Margarine
Bran Muffin

Scrambled Egg
Poached Egg

Toast:
White	Whole-Wheat	Rye	
Butter	Margarine	Jelly	Honey
Coffee	Decaf.	Tea	Herbal Tea
Milk	Low-Fat Milk	Nonfat Milk	
Cream	Half & Half	Cocoa	Lemon

Snacks:

Name _____
Room _____
Diet _____
Date _____

Vegetarian Diet Lunch

Fruit Juice
Soup (Vegetarian) with Saltines
Carrot Sticks

Vegetarian Chef's Salad with Cheeses and
   Vegetables
Peanut Butter and Jelly Sandwich on
   Whole-Wheat Bread
Egg Salad Sandwich on Whole-Wheat
   Bread

Buttered Asparagus

Fresh Fruit
Flavored Yogurt
Cookies

Bread:
White	Whole-Wheat	Rye	
Butter	Margarine	Jelly	Honey
Coffee	Decaf.	Tea	Herbal Tea
Milk	Low-Fat Milk	Nonfat Milk	
Cream	Half & Half	Cocoa	Lemon

Snacks:

Name _____
Room _____
Diet _____
Date _____

Vegetarian Diet Dinner

Fruit Juice
Tossed Green Salad* with Dressing
Walnuts

Cottage Cheese Fruit Plate
Omelet
Cheese Sandwich on Whole-Wheat Bread

Buttered Zucchini

Fresh Fruit
Flavored Yogurt
Ice Cream

Bread:
White	Whole-Wheat	Rye	
Butter	Margarine	Jelly	Honey
Coffee	Decaf.	Tea	Herbal Tea
Milk	Low-Fat Milk	Nonfat Milk	
Cream	Half & Half	Cocoa	Lemon

Snacks:

Index